Vascular Surgery

Third Edition

George Geroulakos • Bauer Sumpio
(Editors)

Vascular Surgery

Cases, Questions, and Commentaries

Third Edition

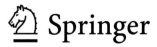 Springer

Editors

George Geroulakos, MD, FRCS, FRCSE, DIC, PhD
President, Section of Vascular Medicine
Royal Society of Medicine
London, UK
and
Consultant Vascular Surgeon
Charing Cross Hospital
London, UK
and
Senior Lecturer
Imperial College
London, UK

Bauer Sumpio, MD, PhD, FACS
Professor of Surgery and Radiology
Yale University, New Haven, CT, USA
and
Chief, Vascular Surgery Service
Yale-New Haven Hospital
New Haven, CT, USA
and
Director, Heart and Vascular Center of
Excellence, Yale Medical Center
New Haven, CT, USA
and
Director, Vascular Surgery Residency
and Fellowship Training Program
Yale Medical Center,
New Haven, CT, USA

ISBN 978-1-84996-355-8 3rd edition   e-ISBN 978-1-84996-356-5 3rd edition
ISBN 978-1-85233-963-0 2nd edition   e-ISBN 978-1-84628-211-9 2nd edition
ISBN 978-1-85233-533-5 1st edition
DOI 10.1007/978-1-84996-356-5
Springer London Dordrecht Heidelberg New York

British Library Cataloguing in Publication Data
A catalogue record for this book is available from the British Library

Library of Congress Control Number: 2010930072

© Springer-Verlag London Limited 2011
First published 2003
Second edition 2006
Third Edition 2011

Cover design: eStudioCalamar, Figueres/Berlin

Printed on acid-free paper

Springer is part of Springer Science+Business Media (www.springer.com)

Union Européenne des Médecins Spécialistes

SECTION AND BOARD
OF VASCULAR SURGERY

President of the Section of Vascular Surgery: F. Benedetti-Valentini
Secretary / Treasurer of the Section and Board of Vascular Surgery:
M. Cairols

President of the Board of Vascular Surgery: K. Balzer
Vice President of the Board of Vascular Surgery:
A. Nevelsteen

Barcelona, March 2006

Vascular Surgery is a discipline that deals with one of the true plagues of the 20th century. Moreover, atherothrombosis will continue to be the main cause of death in the near future.

New developments in the investigation, and endoluminal treatment of vascular disease have recently attracted significant publicity from the mass media and patient groups, and have significantly changed the management of the vascular patient.

The provision of a high quality vascular service is closely linked with the need to give residents an appropriate training and to further introduce Vascular Surgery as an outstanding specialty.

The book, "Vascular Surgery; Cases, Questions and Commentaries," by Mr. Geroulakos, Prof Hero van Urk and Dr. R W Hobson II, will indeed contribute to a better understanding of Vascular Surgery as a specialty that deals with the pathology of arteries, veins and lymphatics. The experience and the teaching capabilities of the authors are unquestionable.

This book, being so comprehensive, enhances the idea of considering Vascular Surgery as an independent entity from other specialties. Before achieving adequate competence to deal with the variety of cases shown in the book, the need for an appropriate training is obvious. Besides, the present text will help candidates to better prepare for the EBSQ-Vasc examination. The book utilises a time proven concept for teaching by questions and answers based on real problems, an essential part of CME. The book proposes learning following the Socratic method, by exercising our mind rather than reading told facts. On the other hand, it may improve our clinical practice and care of our vascular patients, as it incites Continuous Professional Development as a step forward in CME.

The European Board of Vascular Surgery congratulates the authors for their initiative and gladly endorses the book.

Marc Cairols
Secretary General
UEMS Section and Board of Vascular Surgery

Foreword to the First Edition

This book is rather unique among textbooks in vascular surgery. Most cover the surgical management of vascular diseases, in whole or in part, in standard textbook fashion, with the text organized to cover the topics methodically in a didactic manner, and supported by tables, illustrations and references. Others have special purposes, such as atlases on technique or algorithm based books on decision-making. All have their place, but if the educational goals are training of the young surgeon, self-assessment and continuing medical education for the practitioner or preparation for oral examination, this book fills a special need, and fills it very well by breaking away from the didactic approach.

It has long been recognized by educators that retention of knowledge, i.e. true learning, are much better achieved using the Socratic method of questions and answers, as opposed to simply reading or being told facts. In this book this approach is developed and presented in a very effective manner. In each "chapter," one is presented with a case report representing a real life scenario. The case reports-scenarios in this book together cover most of vascular surgery experience. Following the case report, one is presented with questions and answers based on various aspects of the case, forcing the reader to commit to an answer. Whether the answer is right or wrong is not critical, in fact getting a wrong answer may be more beneficial in terms of correcting knowledge and retaining information. The commentary and conclusions that follow analyze the choice of answers, correct and incorrect, and discuss them in concise, authoritative detail, many of which are truly "pearls of information." The conclusion then summarizes the current state of knowledge on the clinical issues under consideration. Numerous references are included. Together, these components constitute one of the most effective vehicles for self-education in vascular surgery today. Importantly, all aspects of management are covered: diagnostic evaluation and appropriate treatment, whether it is non-operative or interventional, endovascular or open surgery.

To accomplish their goals the editors have gathered together a large number of experienced contributors, many well-known for their special areas of interest within vascular surgery, reflected in the contributions they make to this book. As such, the book should be useful to future and practicing vascular surgeons all over the world. It is full of statements covering most of the current state of knowledge in vascular surgery, and it does so in an entertaining and effective manner.

Robert B. Rutherford

Preface to the First Edition

This book is a unique collection of real life case histories written by experts that highlight the diversity of problems that may be encountered in vascular surgery. Each case scenario is interrupted by several questions that aim to engage the reader in the management of the patient and to give him the opportunity to test his knowledge. The comments reflect to as much as possible the principles of evidence based medicine and provide the answers to the questions.

Several chapters are authored by individuals that contributed to the development of innovations in the management and prevention of vascular disease and are of interest for both the vascular trainee and the experienced vascular specialist.

The goal of this book is to help vascular trainees review for Board and other examinations as well as to provide vascular surgeons who wish to expand or refresh their knowledge with an update and interactive source of information relevant to case scenarios that could be encountered in their practice.

The European Boards in Vascular Surgery is a relatively new examination. Although the American Boards in Vascular Surgery were established many years earlier, there are no "dedicated" guides to cover the needs of these examinations. We hope that our book will provide a helpful hand that does not come from the standard text books, but directly from daily practice and therefore contains a high content of "how to do it" and "why we do it." The references show the close relation between daily practice and "evidence based" practice, and we hope the two are not too different.

We would like to thank all the authors who have contributed generously their knowledge and time to this project.

George Geroulakos
Hero van Urk
Keith D. Calligaro
Robert W. Hobson II

Preface to the Second Edition

The author's principal objective of the first edition was the presentation of the principles of vascular and endovascular surgery through interactive real life clinical scenarios. The success of the first edition has been gratifying. We have received many suggestions for additions and changes from vascular trainees, specialists and teachers at various institutions in Europe, USA and other parts of the world. These comments have been well received and have been important in improving and expanding the second edition. We wish to acknowledge our appreciation and gratitude to our authors and publishers.

London   George Geroulakos
Rotterdam   Hero van Urk
New Jersey   Robert W. Hobson II

Preface to the Third Edition

The third edition updated most chapters that were focusing on the endovascular management of arterial and venous disease providing the reader with practical and updated, well referenced information on the full spectrum of options for the management of vascular disease. We are pleased to report the translation of the second edition of our book to Portuguese. We wish to express our thanks to our authors and publishers for their contribution to this project.

London   George Geroulakos
Yale, New Haven   Bauer Sumpio

Contents

Contributors

Cherrie Z. Abraham, MD, FRCS
Jewish General Hospital,
Montreal QC, Canada

Fahad S. Alasfar, MD
Department of Surgery,
Temple University Hospital,
Philadelphia PA, USA

Anders Albäck, MD
Department of Vascular Surgery,
Helsinki University Central Hospital,
Helsinki, Finland

Nasser Alkhamees, MD
Department of Cardiac Surgery,
McGill University,
Montreal QC, Canada

**Christopher T. Andrews, MB, ChB,
FRCS**
Department of Orthopaedic Surgery,
Royal Victoria Hospital,
Belfast, UK

Zachary M. Arthurs, MD
Department of Vascular Surgery,
The Cleveland Clinic Foundation,
Cleveland OH, USA

Enrico Ascher, MD, FACS
The Vascular Institute of New York,
Brooklyn NY, USA

Dwayne Badgett, MD
Department of Surgery,
Temple University Hospital,
Philadelphia PA, USA

Frederico M.V. Bastos Gonçalves, MD
Vascular Surgery Department,
Santa Marta Hospital, CHLC,
Lisbon, Portugal and Erasmus University
Medical Center, Rotterdam,
The Netherlands

Jeroen J. Bax, MD, PhD
Department of Cardiology,
Leiden University Medical Center,
Leiden, The Netherlands

Hernan A. Bazan, MD
Ochsner Clinic Foundation,
Department of Surgery,
Section of Vascular /Endovascular Surgery,
New Orleans, LA, USA

Jean-Pierre Becquemin, MD
Department of Vascular and Endocrine
Surgery, Henri-Mondor Hospital,
Créteil, France

**David Bergqvist, MD, PhD, FRCS,
FEBVS**
Department of Surgery,
Uppsala University Hospital,
Uppsala, Sweden

Ramon Berguer, MD, PhD
Cadiovascular Center,
The University of Michigan,
Ann Arbor MI, USA

Paul H.B. Blair, MD, FRCS
Vascular Surgery Unit,
Royal Victoria Hospital,
Belfast, UK

Francesco Boccardo, MD
Professorial Unit of Medical Oncology,
University and National Cancer
Research Institute,
Genoa, Italy

Marcus Brooks, MA, MD, FRCS
Department of Vascular Surgery,
University Hospitals Bristol NHS
Foundation Trust, Bristol, UK

Marc A. Cairols, MD, PhD, FRCS
Department of Vascular Surgery,
University of Barcelona,
Spain

Keith D. Calligaro, MD
Section of Vascular Surgery and
Endovascular Therapy,
Vascular Surgery Fellowship,
Pennsylvania Hospital, Clinical Professor
of Surgery, University of Pennsylvania
School of Medicine, 700 Spruce
St - Suite 101,
Philadelphia, PA 19106

Corradino Campisi, MD, PhD
Department of General Surgery,
University Hospital, San Martino,
Genoa, Italy

Joseph M. Caruso, MD
Division of Vascular Surgery,
Department of Surgery,
New Jersey Medical School,
University of Medicine
and Dentistry of New Jersey,
Newark NJ, USA

Jeannie K. Chang, MD
Section of Vascular Surgery,
University of Pennsylvania Health System,
Pennsylvania Hospital,
Philadelphia PA,
USA

Constantina Chrysochou, MRCP
Department of Renal Medicine,
Salford Royal Hospital and
University of Manchester,
Manchester, UK

**Anthony J. Comerota, MD,
FACS, FACC**
Department of Surgery,
Temple University Hospital,
Philadelphia PA, USA

Torbjørn Dahl, MD, PhD
Department of Surgery,
St. Olavs Hospital,
University Hospital of Trondheim,
Trondheim, Norway

Guðmundur Daníelsson, MD, PhD
Department of Vascular Surgery,
The National University Hospital
of Iceland, Fossvogi, 108 Reykjavík,
Iceland

Daniel Danzer, MD
Department of Vascular and Endocrine
Surgery, Henri-Mondor Hospital,
Créteil, France

**Stella S. Daskalopoulou, MD, MSc,
DIC, PhD**
Department of Medicine,
McGill University, Montreal QC,
Canada

Luca di Marzo, MD
Department of Surgery P Valdoni,
Sapienza University of Rome,
Rome, Italy

Shiva Dindyal, BSc, MB, BS, MRCS
Department of General Surgery,
The Royal London Hospital,
London, UK

Matthew J. Dougherty, MD
Section of Vascular Surgery,
University of Pennsylvania Health System,
Pennsylvania Hospital,
Philadelphia PA, USA

Jonothan J. Earnshaw, DM, FRCS
Department of Surgery,
Gloucestershire Royal Hospital,
Gloucester, UK

Bo Eklöf, MD, PhD
John A. Burns School of Medicine,
University of Hawaii,
Honolulu HI, USA
University of Lund,
Sweden

Jonathan L. Eliason, MD
Section of Vascular Surgery,
Department of Surgery,
University of Michigan Cardiovascular
Centre, University of Michigan Medical
School, Ann Arbor MI,
USA

George Geroulakos, MD, FRCS, FRCSE, DIC, PhD
Imperial College of Science Technology
and Medicine, Charing Cross Hospital,
and Ealing Hospital,
London, UK

Christopher P. Gibbons, MA, DPhil, MCh, FRCS
Department of Vascular Surgery,
Morriston Hospital,
Swansea, UK

Peter Gloviczki, MD
Division of Vascular and Endovascular
Surgery, Gonda Vascular Center,
Mayo Clinic,
Rochester MN, USA

J. Michael Henderson, MD
Division of Surgery,
Cleveland Clinic Foundation,
Cleveland OH, USA

Joke M. Hendriks, MD
Department of Vascular Surgery,
Erasmus University Medical Center,
Rotterdam, The Netherlands

Ariane L. Herrick, MD, FRCP
University of Manchester,
Manchester Academic Health Science
Centre, Salford Royal NHS Foundation
Trust, Salford M6, 8HD, UK

Anil P. Hingorani, MD
The Vascular Institute of New York,
Brooklyn NY, USA

Larry H. Hollier, MD
Louisiana State University Health
Sciences Center, School of Medicine,
New Orleans LA, USA

Jeffrey Indes, MD
Department of Vascular Surgery,
Yale University School of Medicine,
New Haven CT, USA

Reda Jamjoom, MD, MEd, FRCSC
McGill University, Montreal QC,
Canada

Jørgen J. Jørgensen, MD, PhD
Department of Vascular Surgery,
Oslo University Hospital, Aker,
Oslo, Norway

Milla Kallio, MD
Department of Vascular Surgery,
Helsinki University Central Hospital,
Helsinki, Finland

Philip A. Kalra, MD, FRCP
Department of Renal Medicine,
Salford Royal Hospital and
University of Manchester,
Manchester, UK

Steven S. Kang, MD
Department of Surgery,
Florida International University School
of Medicine,
Miami FL, USA

Vikram S. Kashyap, MD, FACS
Department of Vascular Surgery,
The Cleveland Clinic Foundation,
Cleveland OH, USA

Duk-Kyung Kim, MD, PhD
Division of Cardiology,
Department of Medicine, Samsung
Medical Center, Sungkyunkwan
University School of Medicine,
Seoul, Korea

Young-Wook Kim, MD, PhD
Division of Vascular Surgery,
Department of Surgery,
Samsung Medical Center,
Sungkyunkwan University School
of Medicine,
Seoul, Korea

Fabien Koskas, MD, PhD
Service of Vascular Surgery, Groupe
Hospitalier Pitié-Salpétrière,
Paris, France

Andries J. Kroese, MD, PhD
Department of Vascular Surgery,
Oslo University Hospital,
Aker, Oslo, Norway

**Constantinos Kyriakides, MB, ChB,
MD, FRCS**
Department of General Surgery,
The Royal London Hospital,
London, UK

James Laredo, MD, PhD, FACS
Department of Vascular Surgery,
Georgetown University School
of Medicine,
Washington DC, USA

Jon Largiadèr, MD
University Hospital of Zürich,
Zürich, Switzerland

**Christopher R. Lattimer, MB, BS,
FRCS, FdIT, MS**
Department of Vascular Surgery,
Ealing Hospital NHS Trust,
Middlesex, UK

Miltos K. Lazarides, MD, EBSQvasc
Department of Vascular Surgery,
Demokritos University Hospital,
Alexandroupolis, Greece

Byung-Boong Lee, MD, PhD, FACS
Department of Vascular Surgery,
Georgetown University School of Medicine,
Washington DC, USA

Mauri J.A. Lepäntalo, MD, PhD
Department of Vascular Surgery,
Helsinki University Central Hospital,
Helsinki, Finland

Michel Makaroun, MD
Division of Vascular Surgery,
University of Pittsburgh Medical Center,
Pittsburgh PA, USA

Dimitri P. Mikhailidis, BSc, MSc, MD, FCP, FFPM, FRCP
Department of Clinical Biochemistry
(Vascular Disease Prevention Clinics)
Royal Free Hospital campus,
University College London Medical
School, University College London,
London, UK

Wesley S. Moore, MD
Division of Vascular Surgery, UCLA,
Los Angeles CA, USA

Nicholas J. Morrissey, MD
Columbia University,
New York NY, USA

Hans O. Myhre, MD, PhD
Department of Surgery,
St. Olavs Hospital,
University Hospital of Trondheim,
Trondheim, Norway

Bernard H. Nachbur, MD
University of Berne,
Berne, Switzerland

Adrian K. Neill, MRCS
Department of Vascular Surgery,
Royal Victoria Hospital,
Belfast, UK

Andre Nevelsteen†, MD, PhD, FRCS
Department of Vascular Surgery,
University Hospital Gasthuisberg,
Leuven, Belgium

Cassius Iyad N. Ochoa Chaar, MD, MS
General Surgery Department,
Yale New Haven Hospital,
New Haven CT, USA

William P. Paaske, MD, FRCS, FRCSEd, FACS
Department of Cardiothoracic
and Vascular Surgery,

Aarhus University Hospital,
Aarhus, Denmark

Frank T. Padberg Jr, MD
Division of Vascular Surgery,
Department of Surgery,
New Jersey Medical School,
University of Medicine and
Dentistry of New Jersey,
Newark NJ, USA

Olivier Page, MD
Section of Vascular Surgery and
Vascular Intervention,
University of Poitiers Medical School,
Poitiers, France

Theodossios Perdikides, MD
Vascular and Thoracic Surgery
Department, Hellenic Air Force Hospital,
Athens, Greece

Tomas Pfeiffer, MD
Klinik für Gefäßchirurgie und
Nierentransplantation,
Universitätsklinikum Düsseldorf
Heinrich-Heine-Universität,
Düsseldorf, Germany

Don Poldermans, MD, PhD, FESC
Department of Vascular Surgery,
Erasmus MC, Rotterdam,
The Netherlands

Seshadri Raju, MBBS, MS
Department of Surgery,
University of Mississippi Medical
Center, Flowood MS,
USA

Daniel J. Reddy, MD
Department of Surgery,
Wayne State University,
Detroit MI, USA

Jonathan S. Refson, MBBS, MS, FRCS
Department of Vascular Surgery,
Princess Alexandra Hospital,
Harlow, UK

Lutz Reiher, MD
Klinik für Gefäßchirurgie und
Nierentransplantation,
Universitätsklinikum Düsseldorf
Heinrich-Heine-Universität,
Düsseldorf, Germany

Jean-Baptiste Ricco, MD, PhD
Section of Vascular Surgery and
Vascular Intervention,
University of Poitiers Medical School,
Poitiers, France

Norman M. Rich
Department of Surgery,
F Edward Hébert School of Medicine,
Uniformed Services University
of the Health Sciences,
Bethesda, MD, USA

Ellen V. Rouwet, MD
Department of Vascular Surgery,
Erasmus University Medical Center,
Rotterdam, The Netherlands

Richard J. Sanders
Department of Surgery, University
of Colorado Health Science Center,
Aurora CO, USA

Wilhelm Sandmann, MD
Department of Vascular Surgery and
Kidney Transplantation,
University Clinic of Düsseldorf,
Düsseldorf, Germany

Susanna Shin, MD
Division of Vascular Surgery,
University of Pittsburgh Medical Center,
Pittsburgh PA, USA

William L. Smead, MD
Department of Surgery,
The Ohio State University,
Columbus OH, USA

James C. Stanley, MD
Section of Vascular Surgery,
Department of Surgery,
University of Michigan Cardiovascular
Centre, University of Michigan
Medical School, Ann Arbor MI,
USA

Jean Starr, MD, FACS
Division of Vascular Diseases and Surgery,
The Ohio State University,
Columbus OH, USA

Lars E. Staxrud, MD
Department of Vascular Surgery,
Oslo University Hospital, Aker,
Oslo, Norway

Bauer E. Sumpio, MD, PhD, FACS
Department of Vascular Surgery, Yale
University School of Medicine,
New Haven, CT, USA

Magdiel Trinidad-Hernandez, MD
Division of Vascular and Surgery,
Gonda Vascular Center, Mayo Clinic,
Rochester MN, USA

Vasilios D. Tzilalis, MD
Department of Vascular Surgery,
General Military Hospital,
Athens, Greece

Patrick Vaccaro, MD, FACS
Division of Vascular Diseases and
Surgery, The Ohio State University,
Columbus OH, USA

Marc R.H.M. van Sambeek, MD
Department of Vascular Surgery,
Erasmus University Medical Center,
Rotterdam, The Netherlands

Hero van Urk, MD
Department of Vascular Surgery,
Erasmus University Medical Center,
Rotterdam, The Netherlands

Hence J.M. Verhagen, MD, PhD
Department of Vascular Surgery,
Erasmus University Medical Center,
Rotterdam, The Netherlands

Mark-Paul F.M. Vrancken Peeters, MD
Department of Vascular Surgery,
Erasmus University Medical Center,
Rotterdam, The Netherlands

Mitchell R. Weaver, MD
Henry Ford Medical Group,
Henry Ford Hospital,
Detroit MI, USA

Jeffrey S. Weiss, MD
Department of Vascular Surgery,
Yale University School of Medicine,
New Haven CT, USA

Barbara Theresia Weis-Müller, MD
Department of Vascular Surgery
and Kidney Transplantation,
University Clinic of Düsseldorf,
Düsseldorf, Germany

Jarlis Wesche, MD, PhD
Department of Surgery,
Akershus University Hospital,
University of Oslo,
Lørenskog, Norway

Geoffrey H. White, MD
Endovascular Research Unit,
Department of Surgery,
University of Sydney,
Sydney, Australia

John H.N. Wolfe, MS, FRCS
Regional Vascular Unit,
St. Mary's Hospital,
London, UK

Yolanda Y.L. Yang, MD, PhD
Department of General Surgery,
Cleveland Clinic Foundation,
Cleveland OH, USA

Robert W. Zickler, MD
Division of Vascular Surgery,
Department of Surgery,
New Jersey Medical School,
University of Medicine and Dentistry of
New Jersey, Newark NJ, USA

Kenneth R. Ziegler, MD
Department of Vascular Surgery,
Yale University School of Medicine,
New Haven CT, USA

Part I

Arterial Aneurysms

Preoperative Cardiac Risk Assessment and Management of Elderly Men with an Abdominal Aortic Aneurysm

Don Poldermans and Jeroen J. Bax

A 72-year-old male presented with an abdominal aortic aneurysm. He had a history of chest pain complaints and underwent percutaneous transluminal coronary angioplasty (PTCA) 6 years ago. After the PTCA procedure he had no chest pain symptoms until 2 years ago. The chest pain complaints are stable and he was able to perform moderate exercise, such as a round of golf, in 4.5 h. Physical examination showed a friendly man, with blood pressure 160/70 mmHg and pulse 92 bpm. Examination of the chest revealed no abnormalities of the heart. Palpation of the abdomen showed an aortic aneurysm with an estimated diameter of 7 cm. The patient was referred to the vascular surgeon. Blood test showed an elevated fasting glucose of 10.0 mmol/l and low-density lipoprotein (LDL) cholesterol of 4.1 mmol/l. Electrocardiography showed a sinus rhythm and pathological Q-waves in leads V1–V3, suggestive of an old anterior infarction.

Question 1

Which of the following statements regarding postoperative outcome in patients undergoing major vascular surgery is correct?

A. Cardiac complications are the major cause of perioperative morbidity and mortality.
B. Perioperative myocardial infarctions are related to fixed coronary artery stenosis in all patients.
C. Perioperative cardiac events are related to a sudden, unpredictable progression of a nonsignificant coronary artery stenosis in all patients.
D. Perioperative cardiac complications are related to both fixed and unstable coronary artery lesions.

This patient experienced angina pectoris in the past. He was successfully treated with a PTCA procedure, but recently angina pectoris reoccurred. Because of the multiple risk factors and the planned high-risk surgery a dobutamine stress echocardiography was performed. Figure 1.1 shows the normal stress protocol, with increasing doses of dobutamine and test

D. Poldermans (✉)
Department of Vascular Surgery, Erasmus MC, Rotterdam, The Netherlands

G. Geroulakos and B. Sumpio (eds.), *Vascular Surgery*,
DOI: 10.1007/978-1-84996-356-5_1, © Springer-Verlag London Limited 2011

endpoints. In Fig. 1.2 the scoring of the left ventricle for wall motion abnormalities is shown. Figure 1.3 is an example of a normal resting echocardiogram, showing respectively, apical views and one short-axis view. In Fig. 1.4, the different stages of the stress test are shown for the apical four-chamber view: rest, low-dose dobutamine, peak dose dobutamine, and recovery. As indicated by arrows, the posterior septum shows an outward movement during peak stress, suggesting dyskinesia, and myocardial ischemia of the posterior septum.

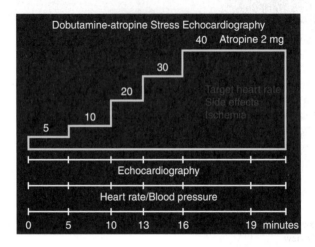

Fig. 1.1 The normal stress protocol, with increasing doses of dobutamine and test endpoints

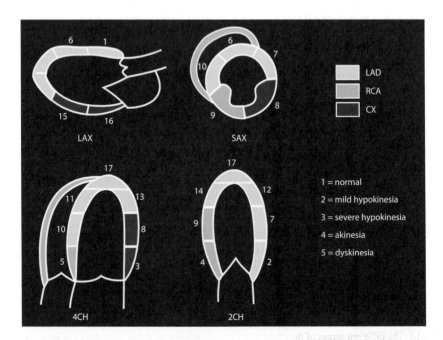

Fig. 1.2 The scoring of the left ventricle for wall motion abnormalities. LAX, long axis; SAX, short axis; 4CH, four.chambers; 2CH, two chambers; LAD, left anterior descending artery; RCA, right coronary artery; LCX, left circumflex artery

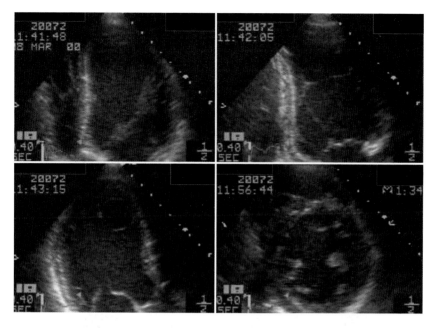

Fig. 1.3 An example of a normal resting echocardiogram, showing respectively, apical views and one short-axis view

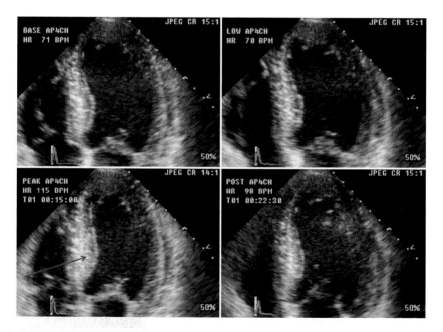

Fig. 1.4 The different stages of the stress test of the apical four-chamber view, rest, low-dose dobutamine, peak dose dobutamine, and recovery. As shown and indicated with arrows, the posterior septum shows an outward movement during peak stress, suggestive of dyskinesia, and also myocardial ischemia of the posterior septum

Question 2

Postoperative outcome in patients undergoing major vascular surgery has been improved in those taking beta-blockers and statins. Medical therapy may reduce the need for additional preoperative testing for coronary artery disease as the incidence of perioperative cardiac mortality is reduced to less than 1%, and may even reduce the indications for preoperative coronary revascularization.

A. Beta-blockers are associated with a reduced perioperative cardiac event rate in patients undergoing vascular surgery, both in retrospective and prospective studies.
B. Statin use is associated with an improved postoperative outcome.
C. Statin use is not associated with an increased incidence of perioperative myopathy.
D. Beta-blockers and statins are independently associated with an improved postoperative outcome.

Question 3

Preoperative beta-blocker therapy is widely used. However, the dose and duration of preoperative therapy is uncertain.

A. Beta-blockers should be started preferably 30 days prior to surgery.
B. Beta-blockers should be initiated several hours before surgery.
C. Heart rate control should be aimed at a heart rate between 90 and 100 bpm.
D. Heart rate control should be aimed at a heart rate between 60 and 70 bpm.

In this patient beta-blockers were started 6 weeks before surgery. Starting dose of bisoprolol was 2.5 mg; the dose was increased to 5.0 mg to obtain a resting heart between 60 and 70 bpm.

Question 4

Perioperative statin therapy has recently been introduced to improve postoperative outcome.

A. Statins improve postoperative outcome by reducing the cholesterol level.
B. Withdrawal of perioperative statin therapy is associated with an increased perioperative cardiac event rate.
C. Perioperative statin use is associated with an increased incidence of myopathy.
D. Perioperative statin use is associated with a reduced perioperative cardiac event rate in vascular surgery patients only.

Statins were prescribed in this patient, Lescol (fluvastatin) XL 80 mg daily, at the same time as beta-blockers were introduced.

Question 5

Preoperative coronary revascularization seems to be an attractive option to improve not only direct postoperative outcome in high-risk patients but also long-term survival after surgery.

A. Preoperative coronary revascularization improves postoperative outcome in all patients with significant coronary artery disease prior to major vascular surgery.

B. Preoperative coronary revascularization in patients with one- or two-vessel disease is not associated with an improved postoperative outcome compared to patients receiving medical therapy.

C. Preoperative coronary revascularization is associated with an improved 2-year outcome compared to medical therapy.

D. Patients with proven coronary artery disease who are treated medically are at increased risk of late coronary revascularization after surgery. After late revascularization, long-term outcome is similar to that with revascularization prior to surgery.

This 72-year-old male had multiple cardiac risk factors: elderly age, angina pectoris, diabetes mellitus, and a previous MI. He underwent a noninvasive stress test, dobutamine stress echocardiography, which showed myocardial ischemia, suggesting left anterior descending artery (LAD) disease. Beta-blockers and statins were prescribed and continued during surgery. Surgery was uneventful; after 2 years angina pectoris complaints increased and a PTCA procedure was successfully performed on the LAD.

1.1
Commentary

Cardiac complications are the major cause of perioperative morbidity and mortality, which may occur in 1–5% of unselected patients undergoing major vascular surgery.[1] **[Q1: A]** This high frequency of cardiac complications is related to the high prevalence of coronary artery disease; 54% of patients undergoing major vascular surgery have advanced or severe coronary artery disease and only 8% of patients have normal coronary arteries.[2] Perioperative cardiac complications are equally caused by prolonged myocardial ischemia or by coronary artery plaque rupture with subsequent thrombus formation and coronary artery occlusion.[1,3] **[Q1: B, C, D]** Prolonged perioperative myocardial ischemia usually occurs from either increased myocardial oxygen demand or reduced supply, or from a combination of the two. There are several perioperative factors that can increase myocardial oxygen demand including tachycardia and hypertension resulting from surgical stress, postoperative pain, interruption of beta-blocker use, or the use sympathomimetic drugs. Decreased oxygen supply, on the other hand, can occur as a result of hypotension, vasospasm, and anemia, hypoxia or coronary artery plaque rupture. Beta-blockers primarily reduce myocardial oxygen demand, while statins may prevent coronary artery plaque rupture. **[Q2: A, B]**

1.2
Beta-Adrenergic Antagonists

Several retrospective and prospective clinical trials have shown that perioperative use of beta-blockers is associated with reduction in the incidence of postoperative myocardial ischemia, nonfatal myocardial infarction and cardiac death.[4-6] [Q2: A] The majority of these studies were small in sample size, and the studies were designed to explore the protective effect of beta-blockers for the reduction of perioperative myocardial ischemia. To overcome the limitations of these studies two randomized clinical trials addressed the issue of perioperative use of beta-blockers for the prevention of cardiac death and myocardial infarction. Mangano et al.[7] studied the effect of atenolol on mortality and cardiovascular morbidity after noncardiac surgery including vascular surgery. The investigators enrolled and randomized 200 patients to atenolol (given intravenously before and immediately after surgery and orally thereafter for the duration of hospitalization) or placebo. No difference was observed in 30-day mortality but mortality was significantly lower at 6 months following discharge (0% vs. 8%, $p<0.001$), over the first year (3% vs. 14%, $p=0.005$), and over 2 years (10% vs. 21%, $p = 0.019$). The apparent lack of a perioperative cardioprotective effect of atenolol in this study was probably related to the small sample size, and the fact that patients at low risk for cardiac complications were studied. In a more recent study, Poldermans et al.[8] clearly demonstrated the cardioprotective effect of perioperative beta-blocker use for the reduction of perioperative cardiac death and myocardial infarction in high-risk patients undergoing major vascular surgery. In total, 112 high-risk vascular patients were selected using a combination of cardiac risk factors and positive results on dobutamine stress echocardiography. Patients were then randomly assigned to standard care or standard care with bisoprolol use. Bisoprolol was started at least 30 days prior to surgery; the dose was adjusted to aim at a resting heart rate of 60–70 bpm. [Q3: A, B, C, D] The results showed that the incidence of the combined endpoint of cardiac death and myocardial infarction within 30 days of surgery was significantly lower in patients using bisoprolol compared to patients in the control group (combined endpoint 3.3% in the bisoprolol group vs. 34% in the control group). Based on the findings of these studies, beta-blocker use has been recommended by the ACC/AHA Guidelines on Perioperative CardiovascularEvaluation for Noncardiac Surgery in high-risk patients with a positive stress test as a level one recommendation.[4]

1.3
3-Hydroxy-3-Methylglutaryl Coenzyme A Reductase Inhibitors (Statins)

Although perioperative use of beta-blockers has been associated with a significant reduction in cardiac mortality and morbidity, still some patients with multiple cardiac risk factors and positive stress test results may remain at considerable risk for perioperative cardiac mortality.[9] For these patients additional cardioprotective medication such as statin use may offer an important addition to preoperative risk reduction strategies. The association between statin use and possible reduction in perioperative cardiac complications may result from the favorable actions of statins on atherosclerosis and from their vascular properties other than those attributed to cholesterol lowering.[10–12] **[Q4: A, B, C]** These so-called pleiotropic effects of statins may attenuate coronary artery plaque inflammation and influence plaque stability in addition to antithrombogenic, antiproliferative and leukocyte-adhesion inhibiting effects.[13–15] All these effects of statins may stabilize unstable coronary artery plaques, thereby reducing myocardial ischemia and subsequent myocardial damage.

There are only a few studies that have evaluated the beneficial effects of perioperative statin use in reducing perioperative cardiac complications.[16–18]

Poldermans et al.,[16] using a case–control study design in 2,816 patients who underwent major vascular surgery, showed that controls more often were statin users than cases, which resulted in a fourfold reduction in all-cause mortality within 30 days after surgery. This finding was consistent in subgroups of patients according to type of vascular surgery, cardiac risk factors and beta-blocker use. **[Q2: D]** Similar to these findings, Durazzo et al.[17] also reported a significantly reduced incidence of cardiovascular events within 6 months of vascular surgery in patients who were randomly assigned to atorvastatin compared with placebo (atorvastatin vs. placebo, 8.3% vs. 26.0%). Finally, the study results of Lindenauer et al.[18] indicated that statin use was associated with 28% relative risk reduction of in-hospital mortality compared to no statin use in 780,591 patients undergoing major noncardiac surgery. **[Q4: D]** The results of these studies are important indications of the possible beneficial effect of perioperative statin use. However, certain limitations such as the retrospective nature of the study of Poldermans et al. and Lindenauer et al., the relatively small sample size (*n* = 100 patients) of the study of Durazzo et al., and the lack of information about the optimal timing and duration of statin therapy warrant future clinical trials to confirm the effectiveness and safety of statin therapy in patients undergoing major noncardiac surgery. Initially, statin use was contraindicated in the perioperative period as it was thought that drug interactions might increase the incidence of myopathy and in combination with analgesics this might even remain asymptomatic. However, a recent study showed no increased incidence of myopathy among statin users.[19] Statin users undergoing vascular surgery at the Erasmus MC were screened for myopathy by measuring creatine kinase (CK) levels at regular intervals and checking for clinical symptoms. In 981 patients no relation was found between statin use and CK levels. Also, no patient experienced myopathy symptoms. Importantly, no deleterious effect of temporary statin interruption was observed. The most recent data are provided by the DECREASE-III study, studying the effect of Leschol XL 80 mg (fluvastatin) in vascular surgery patients compared to placebo, on top of optimal beta-blocker therapy. As shown in almost 500 patients, there was a nearly 50% reduction of the composite end point of myocardial ischemia and myocardial infarction. Importantly, these results were achieved in patients with a slightly elevated LDL-cholesterol level and associated with a reduction of inflammation markers such as interleukin 6 and high-sensitive CRP.[20] **[Q2: C] [Q4: B, C]**

Preoperative cardiac risk evaluation may identify high-risk patients for whom the risk of perioperative cardiac complications without further coronary assessment and subsequent intervention could be too high. For these patients either percutaneous transluminal coronary angioplasty (PTCA) or coronary artery bypass grafting (CABG) may be considered.

1.4
Percutaneous Revascularization

There have been several studies evaluating the clinical utility of PTCA in high-risk patients undergoing major noncardiac surgery including vascular surgery. In the studies of Elmore et al.[21] and Gottlieb et al.,[22] retrospective data were collected of patients who underwent PTCA prior to surgery. These patients were referred for PTCA because of the need to relieve symptomatic angina or to treat myocardial ischemia identified by noninvasive testing. The findings of these studies indicated that the incidence of perioperative cardiac death and myocardial infarction was low, but the investigators in these studies failed to use a comparison group of patients with coronary artery disease not treated with PTCA. The apparent limitations of these studies prompted Posner et al.[23] to conduct their own investigation to compare adverse cardiac outcomes after noncardiac surgery in patients with prior PTCA, patients with non-revascularized coronary artery disease and normal controls. The results showed that patients treated with PTCA within 90 days of noncardiac surgery had a similar incidence of perioperative events to matched patients with coronary artery disease who had not been revascularized. [Q5: A] Those patients who underwent a PTCA procedure 90 days earlier then the day of noncardiac surgery had a lower risk of cardiac events than non-revascularized patients but not as low as normal controls. Furthermore, the effect of revascularization was limited to a reduction in the incidence of angina pectoris and congestive heart failure and there was no reduction in the incidence of death and nonfatal myocardial infarction. Indeed, the recent findings of the Coronary Artery Revascularization Prophylaxis (CARP) trial[24] also showed that coronary revascularization with PTCA or CABG prior to vascular surgery in high-risk cardiac stable patients did not provide short-term survival benefit or better long-term event-free survival rate. [Q5: B, C, D] The findings of the study indicated that patients undergoing coronary revascularization prior to vascular surgery had a 3.1% mortality rate within 30 days of vascular surgery compared to a 3.4% rate for those not having coronary revascularization ($p=0.87$). Additionally, the rate of perioperative nonfatal myocardial infarction as detected by troponin elevation was also similar in coronary revascularization patients and patients not undergoing coronary revascularization (11.6% vs. 14.3%, $p = 0.37$). Furthermore, the results of the trial also indicated that coronary revascularization prior to vascular surgery was associated with delay or cancellation of the required vascular operation. Apart from these findings, it is also important to note that if a PTCA procedure and coronary stent placement are performed less than 6 weeks before major noncardiac surgery, the risk of perioperative coronary thrombosis or major bleeding complications may be substantially increased.[24,25] Two separate small-scale studies reported an increased rate of serious bleeding complications if antithrombotic therapy was continued until the time of surgery, and in patients in whom antiplatelet drugs were interrupted one or two days before surgery an increased rate of fatal events was observed due to stent thrombosis.[25,26] The risk of these complications persisted for 6 weeks after coronary stent placement. Patients who underwent surgery more than 6 weeks after coronary stent placement experienced no adverse cardiac events. These observations indicate that if PTCA with stenting is planned in the weeks or months before noncardiac surgery then a delay of at least 6 weeks should occur before noncardiac surgery to allow for completion of the dual antiplatelet therapy and re-endothelialization of the stent.

1.5
Coronary Artery Bypass Grafting

The results of the largest retrospective study to date indicated that CABG had a protective effect prior to noncardiac surgery.[27] Data for 3368 patients analyzed from the Coronary Artery Surgery Study (CASS) registry showed that patients who underwent CABG before abdominal, vascular, thoracic, or head and neck surgery had a lower incidence of perioperative mortality (3.3% vs. 1.7%) and myocardial infarction (2.7% vs. 0.8%) compared with medically treated patients. The largest reduction in perioperative mortality was observed in patients with a history of advanced angina and in patients with multivessel coronary artery disease. In a more recent study, data analyzed from a random sample of Medicare beneficiaries showed that preoperative coronary revascularization was associated with a reduction in 1-year mortality for patients undergoing aortic surgery but showed no effect on mortality in those undergoing infrainguinal procedures.[28] Hassan et al.,[29] using data from the Bypass Angioplasty Revascularization Investigation, showedthere was no difference in the incidence of cardiac death and myocardial infarction between patients who underwent coronary angioplasty or CABG and subsequent noncardiac surgery (coronary angioplasty group, 1.6% vs. CABG group, 1.6%). **[Q5: A]** As mentioned above under "Percutaneous revascularization," the recent findings of the CARP trial showed that high-risk patients randomized to coronary revascularization prior to vascular surgery had no better perioperative and longterm cardiac complication rates than medically treated patients. Therefore, in the light of these findings a decision to proceed with coronary angioplasty and selective revascularization before high-risk surgery should be made independent of the need for major noncardiac surgery.[4]

References

1. Mangano DT. Perioperative cardiac morbidity. *Anesthesiology*. 1990;72(1):153-184.
2. Hertzer NR, Beven EG, Young JR, et al. Coronary artery disease in peripheral vascular patients. A classification of 1000 coronary angiograms and results of surgical management. *Ann Surg*. 1984;199(2):223-233.
3. Dawood MM, Gutpa DK, Southern J, Walia A, Atkinson JB, Eagle KA. Pathology of fatal perioperative myocardial infarction: implications regarding pathophysiology and prevention. *Int J Cardiol*. 1996;57(1):37-44.
4. Eagle KA, Berger PB, Calkins H, et al. ACC/AHA guideline update for perioperative cardiovascular evaluation for noncardiac surgery – executive summary: a report of the American College of Cardiology/American Heart Association Task Force on Practice Guidelines (Committee to Update the 1996 Guidelines on Perioperative Cardiovascular Evaluation for Noncardiac Surgery). *Circulation*. 2002;105(10):1257-1267.
5. Eagle KA, Rihal CS, Mickel MC, Holmes DR, Foster ED, Gersh BJ. Cardiac risk of noncardiac surgery: influence of coronary disease and type of surgery in 3368 operations. CASS Investigators and University of Michigan Heart Care Program. Coronary Artery Surgery Study. *Circulation*. 1997;96(6):1882-1887.
6. Boersma E, Poldermans D, Bax JJ, et al. Predictors of cardiac events after major vascular surgery: role of clinical characteristics, dobutamine echocardiography, and beta-blocker therapy. *JAMA*. 2001;285(14):1865-1873.

7. Mangano DT, Layug EL, Wallace A, Tateo I. Effect of atenolol on mortality and cardiovascular morbidity after noncardiac surgery. Multicenter Study of Perioperative Ischemia Research Group. *N Engl J Med*. 1996;335(23):1713-1720.
8. Poldermans D, Boersma E, Bax JJ, et al. The effect of bisoprolol on perioperative mortality and myocardial infarction in high-risk patients undergoing vascular surgery. Dutch Echocardiographic Cardiac Risk Evaluation Applying Stress Echocardiography Study Group. *N Engl J Med*. 1999;341(24):1789-1794.
9. Devereaux PJ, Leslie K, Yang H. The effect of perioperative beta-blockers on patients undergoing noncardiac surgery – is the answer in? *Can J Anaesth*. 2004;51(8):749-755.
10. Takemoto M, Liao JK. Pleiotropic effects of 3-hydroxy-3-methylglutaryl coenzyme A reductase inhibitors. *Arterioscler Thromb Vasc Biol*. 2001;21(11):1712-1719.
11. Huhle G, Abletshauser C, Mayer N, Weidinger G, Harenberg J, Heene DL. Reduction of platelet activity markers in type II hypercholesterolemic patients by a HMG-CoA-reductase inhibitor. *Thromb Res*. 1999;95(5):229-234.
12. Hernandez-Perera O, Perez-Sala D, Navarro-Antolin J, et al. Effects of the 3-hydroxy-3-methylglutaryl- CoA reductase inhibitors, atorvastatin and simvastatin, on the expression of endothelin-1 and endothelial nitric oxide synthase in vascular endothelial cells. *J Clin Invest*. 1998;101(12):2711-2719.
13. Stamler JS, Loh E, Roddy MA, Currie KE, Creager MA. Nitric oxide regulates basal systemic and pulmonary vascular resistance in healthy humans. *Circulation*. 1994;89(5):2035-2040.
14. Kurowska EM. Nitric oxide therapies in vascular diseases. *Curr Pharm Des*. 2002;8(3):155-166.
15. van Haelst PL, van Doormaal JJ, May JF, Gans RO, Crijns HJ, Cohen Tervaert JW. Secondary prevention with fluvastatin decreases levels of adhesion molecules, neopterin and C-reactive protein. *Eur J Intern Med*. 2001;12(6):503-509.
16. Poldermans D, Bax JJ, Kertai MD, et al. Statins are associated with a reduced incidence of perioperative mortality in patients undergoing major noncardiac vascular surgery. *Circulation*. 2003;107(14):1848-1851.
17. Durazzo AES, Machado FS, Ikeoka DT, et al. Reduction in cardiovascular events after vascular surgery with atorvastatin: a randomized trial. *J Vasc Surg*. 2004;39(5):967-975.
18. Lindenauer PK, Pekow P, Wang K, Gutierrez B, Benjamin EM. Lipid-lowering therapy and in-hospital mortality following major noncardiac surgery. *JAMA*. 2004;291(17):2092-2099.
19. Schouete O, Kertai MD, Bax JJ, et al. Safety of statin use in high-risk patients undergoing major vascular surgery. *Am J Cardiol*. 2005;95(5):658-660.
20. Schouten O, Boersma E, Hoeks SE, et al. Dutch Echocardiographic Cardiac Risk Evaluation Applying Stress Echocardiography Study Group. Fluvastatin and perioperative events in patients undergoing vascular surgery. *N Engl J Med*. 2009;361:980-989.
21. Elmore JR, Hallett JW Jr, Gibbons RJ, et al. Myocardial revascularization before abdominal aortic aneurysmorrhaphy: effect of coronary angioplasty. *Mayo Clin Proc*. 1993;68(7):637-641.
22. Gottlieb A, Banoub M, Sprung J, Levy PJ, Beven M, Mascha EJ. Perioperative cardiovascular morbidity in patients with coronary artery disease undergoing vascular surgery after percutaneous transluminal coronary angioplasty. *J Cardiothorac Vasc Anesth*. 1998;12(5):501-506.
23. Posner KL, Van Norman GA, Chan V. Adverse cardiac outcomes after noncardiac surgery in patients with prior percutaneous transluminal coronary angioplasty. *Anesth Analg*. 1999;89(3):553-560.
24. McFalls EO, Ward HB, Moritz TE, et al. Coronary-artery revascularization before elective major vascular surgery. *N Engl J Med*. 2004;351:2795-2804.
25. Kaluza GL, Joseph J, Lee JR, Raizner ME, Raizner AE. Catastrophic outcomes of noncardiac surgery soon after coronary stenting. *J Am Coll Cardiol*. 2000;35(5):1288-1294.
26. Wilson SH, Fasseas P, Orford JL, et al. Clinical outcome of patients undergoing non-cardiac surgery in the two months following coronary stenting. *J Am Coll Cardiol*. 2003;42(2):234-240.

27. Eagle KA, Rihal CS, Mickel MC, Holmes DR, Foster ED, Gersh BJ. Cardiac risk of noncardiac surgery: influence of coronary disease and type of surgery in 3368 operations. CASS Investigators and University of Michigan Heart Care Program. Coronary Artery Surgery Study. *Circulation.* 1997;96(6):1882-1887.
28. Fleisher LA, Eagle KA, Shaffer T, Anderson GF. Perioperative- and long-term mortality rates after major vascular surgery: the relationship to preoperative testing in the Medicare population. *Anesth Analg.* 1999;89(4):849-855.
29. Hassan SA, Hlatky MA, Boothroyd DB, et al. Outcomes of noncardiac surgery after coronary bypass surgery or coronary angioplasty in the Bypass Angioplasty Revascularization Investigation (BARI). *Am J Med.* 2001;110(4):260-266.

Abdominal Aortic Aneurysm

2

Daniel Danzer and Jean-Pierre Becquemin

A 59-year-old man presented with an abdominal aortic aneurysm (AAA) discovered on Duplex-scan examination of the abdomen. The AAA was 56-mm large with a slightly conic infra renal neck and an aneurysmal right common iliac artery. The patient was otherwise asymptomatic, with no abdominal or back pain. His medical history was significant for hypertension controlled by bitherapy, non-insulin-dependent diabetes diagnosed 5 years previously, and a smoking history of 30 packs/year. He had neither history of myocardial infarction (MI), angina pectoris nor claudication. He could still play 18 holes of golf and run once a week wi thout difficulties.

His family history revealed that his father died of an aortic aneurysm rupture. He has a 66 year old brother without apparent health problems. On examination, the patient was slightly overweight, no abdominal mass could be palpated. His past surgical history was only relevant for a groin hernia repair in his mid thirties.

A computed tomography (CT) scan was performed (Figs. 2.1 and 2.2). Routine blood tests were normal as well has is electrocardiogram and chest X-ray.

Question 1

The AAA of this patient was found by a systematic screening. In which group(s) of population is Duplex scan screening for AAA justified?

A. Uncomplicated hypertensive patients.
B. Patients with a family history of aneurysmal disease.
C. Patients with a smoking history.
D. Patients with peripheral vascular disease.
E. Obese patients with vascular risk factors
F. All men, starting at the age of 50 years.

D. Danzer (✉)
Department of Vascular and Endocrine Surgery, Henri-Mondor Hospital, Créteil, France

G. Geroulakos and B. Sumpio (eds.), *Vascular Surgery*,
DOI: 10.1007/978-1-84996-356-5_2, © Springer-Verlag London Limited 2011

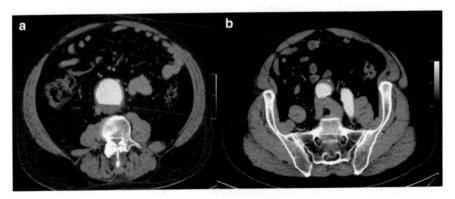

Fig. 2.1 (**a** and **b**): CT scan demonstrating the aortic aneurysm as well as the right common iliac aneurysm

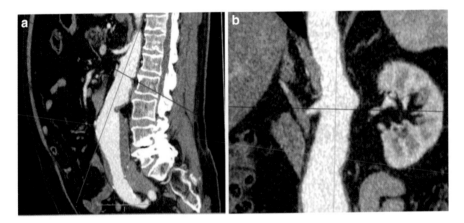

Fig. 2.2 (**a** and **b**): After 3D processing, biplanar reconstruction centered on the renal arteries showing a mild conic shape (**a**) with posterior thrombus (**b**)

Question 2

Without treatment this patient is at risk of rupture. Among the following factors which one(s) have been proved to be associated with an increased risk of rupture?

A. Diameter > 60 mm
B. Association with an hypogastric aneurysm
C. Diabetic patient
D. Lower limb occlusive disease
E. Smoking
F. COPD

Question 3

With the imaging you have been provided with, is (are) there any reason(s) for performing an arteriogram

A. No need, CT-scan is sufficient
B. An angiogram is mandatory to facilitate the planning of the surgical procedure in case of difficult anatomy
C. Angiogram would be needed in case of endovascular treatment
D. Angiography is necessary to rule out any asymptomatic associated visceral arterial stenosis

Question 4

To assess the operative cardiac risk would you need any further test in our patient.

A. None, ECG is sufficient.
B. Cardiac scintigraphy.
C. Cardiac echography.
D. Cardiac echography with Dobutamine test.
E. Coronary angiography.

Question 5

If an operation were being considered, which of the following factors are associated with an increased post-operative mortality?

A. Diameter > 60 mm
B. Association with an hypogastric aneurysm
C. Diabetic patient
D. Renal insufficiency
E. Smoking

Question 6

With the current information you got from the case report, what would you recommend to the patient (a) and which in case of a higher operative risk (b)

A. Duplex scan surveillance every 3 months
B. Aorto bifemoral through a midline incision
C. Aorto bifemoral graft through a left retroperitoneal incision
D. Aorto bi iliac graft through a left retroperitoneal incision
E. Stent-graft

The patient underwent, via a left retroperitoneal approach, an aorto-right and left common iliac bypass with end-to-end anastomosis. The aortic anastomosis was performed just at the level of the renal artery with a supra renal clamping of 10 min. This was justified by the necessity of suturing the prosthesis on the healthiest segment of aorta as possible. Therefore the retroperitoneal route gave a better access to the supra renal aorta. A cell saver was used and no heterogeneous blood had to be transfused.

The patient's postoperative course was uneventful, and he was discharged on the ninth post operative day.

Question 7

During open operation for AAA cell-saver autotransfusion (CSA) can be used. Which of the following is/are correct?

A. It should be used systematically.
B. It should be reserved for when the expected blood loss is significant.
C. It should be substituted in all cases with preoperatively deposited autologous blood transfusion.
D. It presents fewer complications than unwashed cell autotransfusion.
E. It should not be used in case of ruptured aneurysm.

Question 8

Does a genetic predisposition to AAA exist? Describe the pathogenesis of AAA.

Question 9

A duplex scan has been performed to the patient's brother which found a 40 mm abdominal aneurysm.

What recommendation(s) would you give this patient's brother?

A. Serial duplex studies at 3-monthly intervals, and intervention when the diameter reaches 5.5 cm.
B. Serial duplex studies at 6-monthly intervals, and intervention if the diameter reaches or exceeds 5 cm.
C. Serial duplex studies at 12-monthly intervals until the diameter reaches 4.5 cm, then every 6 months until the diameter reaches 5 cm, then every 3 months, and then intervention when the aneurysm reaches 5.5 cm.
D. Schedule the patient for surgery as he is a smoker and therefore his aneurysm will most likely require intervention.

2.1
Commentary

The question of the optimal format for population screening and its cost effectiveness for AAA is still under debate. Many studies have attempted to identify high-risk populations in order to reduce healthcare costs and maximize the yield. Simon et al.[1] have demonstrated a prevalence of AAA of 11% in male patients aged 60–75 years with a systolic blood pressure greater than 175 mmHg. No patient with uncomplicated hypertension had AAA. Claudication was the only cardiovascular complication associated independently with AAA (relative risk 5.8). Baxter et al. found a prevalence of 9% in patients older than 65 years old regardless of cardiovascular risk factors.[2] Furthermore, preliminary results from the Aneurysm Detection and Management (ADAM) study revealed that smoking was the most important risk factor associated with AAA (odds ratio [OR] 5.57), followed by a positive family history (OR 1.95), age, height, coronary artery disease, atherosclerosis, high cholesterol level and hypertension.[3] Similar results were found in the later Multicentre Aneurysm Screening Study (MASS) demonstrating that screening in male patients older than 65 years old would be cost effective.[4] Therefore, most vascular surgeons agree that all men over the age of 65 years and women who did smoke[5] should systematically be offered an abdominal ultrasound, the screening should be done at 55 years if indicated family history.[6] [Q1: B, C, D]

Natural history of aneurysms and risk of rupture are better understood with the results of the UK small aneurysms trial[7] and the ADAM trial. As in former cohort studies of patients who refused early operation[8] or who were considered to be inoperable, risk of rupture increased with size, and intervention seems justified over 5.5 cm, in patients with sufficient life expectancy. Growth is recognized as related to tobacco use but diabetes mellitus and female gender are protective. Controversial opinion regarding other risk factors persist as recent data suggests no influence of hypertension, statin use and ACE on aneurysm growth as published in former studies.[9] Rupture is strongly correlated with persistent tobacco use, female gender, aneurysm size, diminution of FEV1, HTA and presence of transplant. [Q2: A, E, F]

Pre-operative planning is of outmost importance in order to avoid intra-operative unexpected findings, shortening of the surgery and/or evaluate the possibility of endovascular treatment. Nowadays, the CT scanner with 3D reconstruction, the gold standard, and invasive conventional angiography, is only needed for treatment of subsequent visceral significant and symptomatic stenosis. Albeit relatively frequently in patients requiring AAA surgery, visceral arterial stenosis[10–12] should be treated separately if needed and via endovascular means when possible. One stage surgery with visceral reconstruction increases the operative difficulty and consequently the operative risk.[13] Actual data shows better assessment of vessel morphology with CT reconstruction than angiography for EVAR[14] but is also useful in open surgery to evaluate the vessels morphology and planning of surgery in case of any anatomical anomaly (e.g. horseshoe kidney). [Q3: A]

Concerning a pre-operative work-out; routine coronary angiography in vascular patients has shown that 60% of them have severe coronary artery disease.[15] However a large randomized study in patients with stable angina have clearly demonstrated that pre-operative coronary bypass or angioplasty do not improve the post-operative and 5 year survival rate.[16] Beta blockers, statins and antiplatelets have all contributed to the reduction of cardiac events following major vascular surgery. Thus pre-operative investigation can be restricted to patients with poor functional capacity and at least three identified predictive factors of severe coronary artery disease.[17] In the current case diabetes, hypertension and mild renal insufficiency are three of these markers and pre-operative cardiac screening would have been indicated if the patient hadn't shown a good functional capacity.[18] [**Q4: A**] When mandatory cardiac echography with dobutamine probably is the most reliable test.[19] And pre-operative coronary revascularization is only indicated for those patients with acute ST elevation MI, unstable angina, or stable angina with left main coronary artery or three-vessel disease, as well as those patients with two-vessel disease that includes the proximal left anterior descending artery, and either ischemia on non-invasive testing or an ejection fraction of less than 0.50.

Analysis of predictive factor of mortality in patients submitted to open repair of AAA have shown that age, cardiac status, renal insufficiency and pulmonary status were strongly predictive of post operative complications and deaths. Difficult operations are also associated with an increased operative risk mostly related to the increase of blood loss. Unilateral or bilateral hypogastric aneurysm increased the operative risk.[20] [**Q5: B, D**]

In this case surveillance was not recommended due to the aneurysm size and the relatively young age of the patient.

Open surgery via a trans abdominal or retroperitoneal approach is a wise option in case of low operative risk and difficult anatomy as in our case where the infrarenal neck was not suitable for a regular endovascular graft implantation. We choose a retroperitonal approach because of the better exposure of the aorta at the level of the visceral arteries and his obesity. A retroperitoneal approach is an appealing way especially in case of obese patient or the need for preparation of the aorta at the level or upper the renal arteries. Nevertheless the distal right iliac axis remains the Achilles heel's of this approach which would have required a second contra lateral incision for reconstruction of the right external iliac axis if needed. In our case the aneurysm involved only the proximal right common iliac artery and the right iliac anastomosis could be achieved with a slight enlargement of the retroperitoneal route toward the midline.

Femoral anastomosis is not recommended because of the increased infection rate after a groin incision. [**Q6a: D**]

Although a retroperitoneal approach provides a better access to the suprarenal aorta, the former advocated superiority of the retroperitonal route in terms of pain. Bowel and respiratory function was never supported by randomized trials especially in the era of perioperative peridural analgesia. No actual data support the systematic use of trans versus retro peritoneal approach in terms of post operative outcome, therefore the choice should be based on the anatomical features and surgeon preference.

Less invasive with a lower operative mortality (1.5% vs. 4.6% for Open Repair[21]), a shorter in-hospital stay and recovery time, EVAR could have been considered if the patient had a suitable aortic neck, major comorbidities or hostile abdomen. Although the two major early randomized trials (EVAR 1 and DREAM) failed to show sustained benefit of the post-operative mortality at 2 years, no death in the EVAR group was aneurysm related,[22,23] and a former survey showed an incidence of ongoing aneurysm related mortality after EVAR of 1% per year.[24] A large retrospective case match cohort study including more than 40,000 participants did not show inferiority of the long term results of EVAR compared to Open Repair and the rate of secondary procedure in the EVAR group was largely overwhelmed by the rate of wound hernia after OR. Subsequently secondary procedure frequency seems to decrease after the first year following EVAR.[25]

Therefore EVAR is considered by many teams as the first option in case of adequate anatomy. Usual recommendation for endovascular aneurysm treatment requires a proximal neck length under the renal artery of 15 mm, a limited angulation of the aorta (<;60°) or iliac arteries (90°) and healthy landing zones (no or minor dilatation, parietal thrombus or circumferential calcifications).

As already mentioned the infra renal neck seemed inappropriate for conventional graft placement but could have been amenable for a fenestrated or branched graft as in Fig. 2.3 with good midterm results.[26] Branched iliac grafts can treat aneurysmal distal landing zone avoiding the traditional selective hypogastric coiling before endo-graft deployment down to the external iliac artery which has a subsequent risk of ischemic complication in up to 30% in case of bilateral hypogastric sacrifice.[27] [**Q6b: E**]

Over the past 3 decades, with the appreciation of the risk of transfusion related transmission of infectious diseases, a large body of research and instrumentation has emerged on auto transfusion. The current options are:

- Preoperative deposit of autologous blood.
- Intraoperative salvage and washing of red blood cells (cell saver).
- Intraoperative salvage of whole blood without washing.

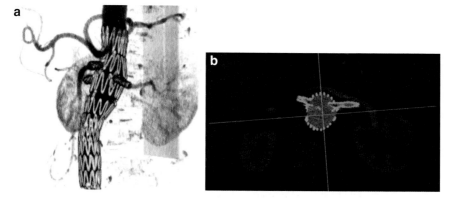

Fig. 2.3 (**a** and **b**): 3D reconstruction of a fenestrated graft with detailed view at the renal arteries level in a patient with a very short infrarenal neck

Although both whole-blood autotransfusion (WBA) and cell saver auto transfusion (CSA) are currently in use, the magnitude of hemostatic and hemolytic disturbances, as well as the clinical side effects, after WBA compared with CSA are still in debate. While Ouriel et al.[28] showed the safety of WBA in 200 patients undergoing AAA repair, others have demonstrated a lower content of hemolytic degradation products and fewer coagulation disturbances after retransfusion of cell-saver blood.[29] Although cell salvage reduce allogenic blood requirement with reduced intensive care and post operative stay no significant impact on the outcome could be demonstrated.[30] Nevertheless its use seems to lower mortality in ruptured aneurysm surgery.[31] Despite its widespread use, several studies have found that CSA is not cost effective and should be limited to patients who have an expected blood loss of at least 1,000 ml, which includes patients with large, complicated aneurysms.[32,33] Finally, transfusion of predonated autologous blood is associated with some of the disadvantages of homologous transfusions, i.e., dilutional hypofibrinoginemia, thrombocytopenia and hypothermia. [**Q7: B, D**]

The causes of AAA are numerous, and may include inflammation, infection with mycotic aneurysm commonly due to Salmonella or Staphyloccous species, nowadays rarely to syphilis infection, aortic dissection, Ehler–Danlos type IV and Marfan syndrome although aneurysm degeneration is rarely seen in Marfan patient without prior dissection. Presence of a common variant of 9p21 is associated with an 31% increased risk for AAA. It is estimated that 15% of patients presenting with an AAA have a first-degree relative with the same condition. Male siblings are at higher risk, but current evidence also supports an autosomal dominant pattern of inheritance.[34]However, more than 90% of all AAAs are associated with atherosclerosis and are classified as either atherosclerotic or degenerative aneurysms. Although aneurysmal and atherosclerotic changes share several common risk factors, atherosclerotic lesions are predominantly intimal with foam cell formation, whereas oxidative stress, immune mediated inflammation leading to matrix degradation and smooth cell apoptosis occurs in the media and adventitial layers in aneurysmal disease.[35]

As ongoing research tends to prove that oxidative stress is the hallmark of aneurysm formation there might be a place in the future for immuno-modulator treatment to cure or prevent arterial aneurysms.[36,37] [**Q8**]

The management and surveillance of small AAAs has been debated for many years. The UK small aneurysm trial has attempted to shade some light on this subject.[38] The participants of this trial concluded that early surgical intervention did not offer any long-term survival advantages for aneurysm under 5.5 cm. Their recommendations, based on the trial methodology, were serial duplex every 6 months for aneurysms of size 4–4.9 cm, and every 3 months for aneurysms of size 5–5.5 cm. In another, larger analysis, the recommendations were yearly duplex for aneurysms measuring 4–4.5 cm on the initial scan.[39] However this study and the later from Thompson et al.[9] did show that only 25% and 50% respectively didn't needed surgery or ruptured during follow up.

Chronic obstructive pulmonary disease (COPD) and continuation of smoking have been associated with aneurysm expansion, but the rate of expansion does not justify intervention on 4-cm aneurysms.[40] Therefore only smoking cessation and careful survey are the only actual recommended treatment for small aneurysms as well as management of frequently associated cardio-vascular co-morbidities. [**Q9: C**]

References

1. Simon G, Nordgren D, Connelly S, Schultz PJ. Screening for abdominal aortic aneurysms in a hypertensive population. *Arch Intern Med*. 1996;156:2084-2088.
2. Baxter BT, Terrin MC, Dalman RL. Medical management of small abdominal aortic aneurysms. *Circulation*. 2008;117:1883-1889.
3. Lederle FA, Aneurysm Detection and Management (ADAM) Veterans Affairs Cooperative study group. Prevalence and association of AAA detected through screening. *Ann Intern Med*. 1997;126:441-449.
4. Multicentre Aneurysm Screening Study Group. Multicentre aneurysm screening study (MASS): cost effectiveness analysis of screening for abdominal aortic aneurysms based on four year results from randomized trial. *BMJ*. 2002;325:1135.
5. Wanhainen A, Lundkvist J, Bergqvist D, Bjorck M. Cost-effectiveness of screening women for abdominal aortic aneurysm. *J Vasc Surg*. 2006;43:908-914.
6. Chaikof EL PhD, Brewster DC, Dalman RL, et al. The care of patients with an abdominal aortic aneurysm: the society for vascular surgery practice guidelines. *JVS*. 2009;50(4Suppl): S2-S49.
7. UKSAT, UK Small Aneurysm Trial participants. Final 12-year follow-up of surgery versus surveillance in the UK Small Aneurysm Trial. *Br J Surg*. 2007;94:702-708.
8. Lederle FA, Johnson GR, Wilson SE, et al. Rupture rate of large abdominal aortic aneurysms in patients refusing or un.t for elective repair. *JAMA*. 2002;287:2968-2972.
9. Thompson R, Cooper JA, Ashton HA, Hafez H. Growth rates of small abdominal aortic aneurysms correlate with clinical events. *BJS*. 2010;97:37-44.
10. Valentine RJ, Martin JD, Myers SI, Rossi MB, Clagett GP. Asymptomatic celiac and SMA stenoses are more prevalent among patients with unsuspected renal artery stenoses. *J Vasc Surg*. 1991;14:195-199.
11. Brewster DC, Retana A, Waltman AC, Darling RC. Angiography in the management of aneurysms of the abdominal aorta. *N Engl J Med*. 1975;292:822-825.
12. Piquet P, Alimi Y, Paulin M, et al. Anévrisme de l'aorte abdominal et insuffisance rénale chronique. In: Kieffer E, ed. *Les Anévrysmes de l'Aorte Abdominal sous-renale*. Paris: Editions AERCV; 1990.
13. Williamson WK, Abou-Zamzam AM Jr, Moneta GL, et al. Prophylactic repair of renal artery stenosis is not justified in patients who require infrarenal aortic reconstruction. *J Vasc Surg*. 1998;28:14-20.
14. Filis KA, Arko FR, Rubin GD, Zarins CK. Three dimensional CT evaluation for endovascular abdominal aortic aneurysm repair. Quantitative assessment of the infrarenal aortic neck. *Acta Chir Belg*. 2003;103:81-86.
15. Hertzer NR, Beven EG, Young JR, et al. Coronary artery disease in peripheral vascular patients. A classification of 1000 coronary angiograms and results of surgical management. *Ann Surg*. 1984;199:223-233.
16. McFalls EO, Ward HB, Moritz TE, et al. Coronary-artery revascularization before elective major vascular surgery. *N Engl J Med*. 2004;351:2795-2804.
17. Kertai MD, Boersma E, Bax JJ, et al. Optimizing long-term cardiac management after major vascular surgery: role of beta-blocker therapy, clinical characteristics, and dobutamine stress echocardiography to optimize long-term cardiac management after major vascular surgery. *Arch Intern Med*. 2003;163:2230-2235.
18. Fleisher LA, Beckman JA, Brown KA, et al. ACC/AHA 2007 Guidelines on perioperative cardiovascular evaluation and care for noncardiac surgery: executive summary. *Circulation*. 2007;116:1971-1996.
19. Kertai MD, Boersma E, Bax JJ, et al. A meta-analysis comparing the prognostic accuracy of six diagnostic tests for predicting perioperative cardiac risk in patients undergoing major vascular surgery. *Heart*. 2003;89:1327-1334.

20. Becquemin JP, Chemla E, Chatellier G, Allaire E, Melliere D, Desgranges P. Peroperative factors influencing the outcome of elective abdominal aorta aneurysm repair. *Eur J Vasc Endovasc Surg*. 2000;20:84-89.
21. Sajid MS, Desai M, Zishan H, Baker DM, Hamilton G. Endovascular aortic aneurysm repair (EVAR) has significantly lower perioperative mortality in comparison to open repair: a systematic review. *Asian J Surg*. 2008;31(3):119-123.
22. Blankensteijn JD, De Jong SECA, Prinssen M, et al. Two-Year Outcomes after Conventional or Endovascular Repair of Abdominal Aortic Aneurysms. *N Engl J Med*. 2005;352: 2398-2405.
23. EVAR trial participants. Comparison of endovascular aneurysm repair with open repair in patients with abdominal aortic aneurysm (EVAR trial 1), 30-day operative mortality results: randomized controlled trial. *Lancet*. 2004;364:843-848.
24. Harris PL, Vallabhaneni SR, Desgranges P, Becquemin JP, van Marrewijk C, Laheij RJ. Incidence and risk factors of late rupture, conversion, and death after endovascular repair of infrarenal aortic aneurysms: the EUROSTAR experience. European Collaborators on Stent/graft techniques for aortic aneurysm repair. *J Vasc Surg*. 2000;32:739-749.
25. Schermerhorn ML, O'Malley AJ, Jhaveri A, Cotterill P, Pomposelli F, Landon BE. Endovascular vs. open repair of abdominal aortic aneurysms in the medicare population. *N Engl J Med*. 2008;358:464-474.
26. Scurr JRH, Brennan JA, Gilling-Smith GL, Harris PL, Vallabhaneni SR, McWilliams RG. Fenestrated endovascular repair for juxtarenal aortic aneurysm. *Br J Surg*. 2008;95:326-332.
27. Verzini F, Parlani G, Romano L, De Rango P, Panuccio G, Cao P. Endovascular treatment of iliac aneurysm: concurrent comparison of side branch endograftversus hypogastric exclusion. *J Vasc Surg*. 2009;49:1154-1161.
28. Ouriel K, Shortell CK, Green RM, DeWeese JA. Intraoperative autotransfusion in aortic surgery. *J Vasc Surg*. 1993;18:16-22.
29. Bartels C, Bechtel JV, Winkler C, Horsch S. Intraoperative autotransfusion in aortic surgery: comparison of whole blood autotransfusion versus cell separation. *J Vasc Surg*. 1996;24:102-108.
30. Tawfick WA, O'Connor M, Hynes N, Sultan S. Implementation of the continuous Auto Transfusion System (C.A.T.S) in open abdominal aneurysm repair: an observational comparative cohort study. *Vasc Endovasc Surg*. 2008;42:32-39.
31. Jarvis NE, Haynes SL, Calderwood R, Mc Collum CN. Does cell salvage influence outcome in ruptured abdominal aortic aneurysm repair? *Br J Surg*. 2008;95(S3):27.
32. Goodnough LT, Monk TG, Sicard G, Satterfield SA, Allen B, Anderson CB. Intraoperative salvage in patients undergoing elective abdominal aortic aneurysm repair: an analysis of cost and benefit. *J Vasc Surg*. 1996;24:213-218.
33. Huber TS, McGorray SP, Carlton LC, et al. Intraoperative autologous transfusion during elective infrarenal aortic reconstruction: a decision analysis model. *J Vasc Surg*. 1997;25: 984-994.
34. Majumder PP, St Jean PL, Ferrell RE, Webster MW, Steed DL. On the inheritance of abdominal aortic aneurysm. *Am J Hum Genet*. 1991;48:164-170.
35. Miller FJ Jr, Sharp WJ, Fang X, Oberley LW, Oberley TD, Weintraub NL. Oxidative stress in human abdominal aortic aneurysms: a potential mediator of aneurysmal remodeling. *Thromb Vasc Biol*. 2002;22:560-565.
36. Satoh K, Nigro P, Matoba T, et al. Cyclophilin A enhances vascular oxidative stress and the development of angiotensin II induced aortic aneurysms. *Nat Med*. 2009;15:649-656.
37. Neal L. Understanding abdominal aortic aneurysm. *N Engl J Med*. 2009;361:11. nejm.org.
38. UK Small Aneurysm Trial participants. Final 12-year follow-up of surgery versus surveillance in the UK Small Aneurysm Trial. *Br J Surg*. 2007;94:702-708.
39. Grimshaw GM, Thompson JM, Hamer JD. A statistical analysis of the growth of small abdominal aneurysms. *Eur J Vasc Surg*. 1994;8:741-746.
40. Macsweeney STR, Ellis M, Worell PC, Greenhalgh RM, Powell JT. Smoking and growth rate of small abdominal aortic aneurysms. *Lancet*. 1994;344:651-652.

Endoluminal Treatment of Infra-renal Abdominal Aortic Aneurysm

3

Frederico M. V. Bastos Gonçalves, Geoffrey H. White, Theodossios Perdikides, and Hence J. M. Verhagen

A 68-year-old male was referred for investigation and management of an asymptomatic abdominal aortic aneurysm (AAA), diagnosed coincidently during an abdominal ultrasound. His prior medical history included smoking and a coronary artery bypass graft 3 years before. The physical examination revealed an expansible pulsatile abdominal mass and all peripheral pulses were present.

Question 1

What is the optimal method of preoperative AAA assessment?

A. Abdominal duplex ultrasound (DUS)
B. Contrast-enhanced high-resolution (64-detector or higher) computer tomography angiography (CTA) of the aorta, iliac and femoral arteries
C. DUS and calibrated digital subtraction angiography (DSA) of the aorta and iliac arteries
D. Abdominal CTA and DSA

A CTA was obtained and visualized using dedicated 3D reconstruction software. This revealed an infra-renal AAA with a maximum diameter of 62 mm. The proximal aneurysm neck (area from the lowermost renal artery to the start of the aneurysm) was 21 mm in diameter and 31 mm in length. Neck angulation was calculated at 25° supra-renal and 65° infra-renal. The distance from the lowest renal artery to the aortic bifurcation was 136 mm and there was a further distance to the orifice of the internal iliac artery of 26 mm on the right side and 31 mm on the left. The right internal iliac was aneurismatic, measuring 44 mm in diameter. Minimum luminal diameters of the external iliac arteries were 5 mm on the right and 9 mm on the left (Figs. 3.1 and 3.2).

F.M.V.B. Gonçalves (✉)
Vascular Surgery Department, Santa Marta Hospital, CHLC, Lisbon, Portugal and
Erasmus University Medical Center, Rotterdam, The Netherlands

G. Geroulakos and B. Sumpio (eds.), *Vascular Surgery*,
DOI: 10.1007/978-1-84996-356-5_3, © Springer-Verlag London Limited 2011

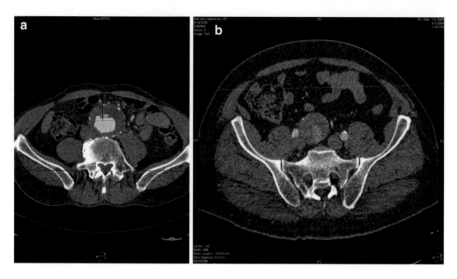

Fig. 3.1 CTA axial slices of maximal AAA and right internal iliac aneurysm diameters

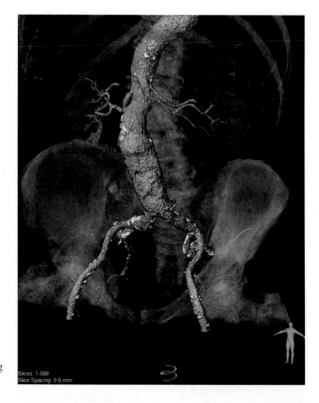

Fig. 3.2 Volume rendering
reconstruction of AAA using
dedicated software

Question 2

What is the approximate annual risk of rupture of an AAA with a maximum diameter of 62 mm?

A. Less than 5%
B. Between 5% and 10%
C. Between 10% and 20%
D. Greater than 20%

Question 3

Regarding intervention in asymptomatic AAA

A. Current evidence supports operative management for aneurysms greater than 55 mm in diameter
B. Rupture risk is higher for women and a lower threshold for intervention in this group has been proposed
C. All diagnosed aneurysms warrant expeditious intervention as they will inevitably grow
D. Surveillance is safe for aneurysms with diameters ranging from 40 to 55 mm
E. Fast growth is not associated to increased risk of rupture in asymptomatic aneurysms under 55 mm in diameter. Close surveillance is the best option

Question 4

In anatomically similar aneurysms, suitable for both open and endovascular repair

A. Open repair is a safer option for high-risk patients
B. The early survival benefit of EVAR applies only to high-risk patients
C. The presence of chronic renal failure is an absolute contra-indication for EVAR
D. Patient preference should be weigh significantly in the decision process
E. Level I evidence has shown that EVAR results in a threefold reduction in 30-day operative mortality compared to open repair in low-risk patients

Question 5

Which anatomical features may limit EVAR?

A. Length and diameter of the aneurysm sac
B. Length and diameter of the aneurysm neck
C. Angulation of the aneurysm neck

D. Tortuosity and luminal diameter of the iliac arteries

E. Associated common iliac aneurysms, provided antegrade flow in at least one internal iliac artery can be preserved

After informed consent, an endovascular procedure was planned. Measurements were performed using center-lumen line reconstruction and a modular bifurcated endovascular graft with a supra-renal open stent and active proximal fixation was selected. Virtual angiography was used to determine the exact C-arm rotation and angulation for optimal deployment, both proximally and distally (Figs. 3.3 and 3.4).

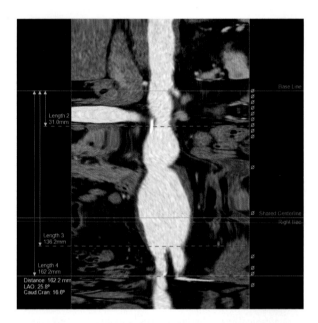

Fig. 3.3 Center-lumen line reconstruction following the right iliac artery, showing measurements

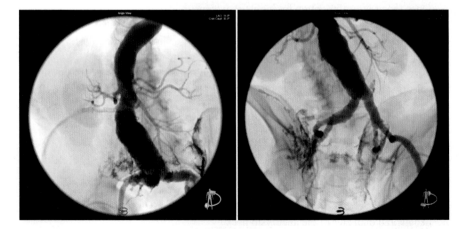

Fig. 3.4 Virtual angiogram with angle selection for optimal visualization of the neck and left iliac bifurcation

Question 6

Endoprosthesis with supra-renal open stent fixation

A. Are associated with a higher rate of migration
B. Are associated with a higher rate of renal complications, particularly embolism and occlusion
C. Are particularly useful in unfavorable aneurysm necks
D. May complicate a conversion procedure

Question 7

In choosing a suitable endoluminal graft, one should

A. Take the graft that resembles your measurements most closely
B. Oversize all diameters by 5%
C. Oversize all diameters by 15–20%
D. Oversize the proximal diameter by 20% and the limb diameters by 30%
E. Undersize all diameters by 10% and balloon-expand them to proper size at the end of the procedure

Question 8

Fenestrated grafts are best applied in

A. Ruptured juxta-renal AAAs
B. Elective juxta-renal or supra-renal AAAs
C. Very angulated aneurysm necks, to avoid migration
D. All cases, being limited only by availability and cost

Question 9

At 2 years, outcomes after EVAR using fenestrated grafts

A. Are equivalent to standard EVAR
B. Are generally worse than those of open repair for juxta-renal or supra-renal AAA
C. Closely relate to the expertise of the operating center
D. Are linked to branch vessel complications, particularly renal artery stenosis or occlusions
E. Are worse than those of standard EVAR, because of a higher percentage of type I and III endoleaks

Question 10

Unilateral common iliac aneurismal involvement

A. Makes EVAR unadvisable
B. May be treated using branched limbs, in order to preserve pelvic blood flow
C. May be treated by internal iliac occlusion and extension of the limb into the external iliac artery
D. Favors the use of aorto-uni-iliac devices and femoro-femoral crossover
E. Should be treated by open repair

The patient was operated under general anesthesia. The abdomen and both groins were prepared into a sterile field, and the common femoral arteries surgically exposed through short oblique incisions. Sheaths were inserted and the patient was given 5,000 U of non-fractioned heparin. Wires were placed under fluoroscopy and the main-body device was advanced via the left side to the level of L1. An angiogram was performed at this level, using the previously determined C-arm angulation. The top-stent was deployed separately in a very controlled fashion and the contra-lateral limb cannulated. The right internal iliac artery distal to the aneurysm was coiled and the limb extended to the external iliac artery, covering the iliac bifurcation. A completion angiogram confirmed the successful exclusion of the aneurysm, without type I or III endoleaks and with maximum proximal seal. A type II endoleak was observed in the late phase of the angiogram, however (Figs. 3.5 and 3.6).

Question 11

The correct intra-operative attitude regarding on-table documentation of a type II endoleak is

A. Do nothing
B. Laparoscopic ligation of the inferior mesenteric artery and lumbar arteries
C. Endovascular coil embolization of the responsible vessels
D. Laparotomy and surgical ligation of responsible vessels
E. Conversion to open repair

Question 12

The correct attitude regarding late follow-up documentation of a type II endoleak without change in aneurysm size is

A. Laparoscopic ligation of the inferior mesenteric artery and lumbar arteries
B. Endovascular coil embolization of the responsible vessels
C. Percutaneous or laparoscopic aortic fenestration
D. Conversion to open repair
E. Close surveillance

Fig. 3.5 Intra-operative completion angiogram showing a type II endoleak (*arrow*)

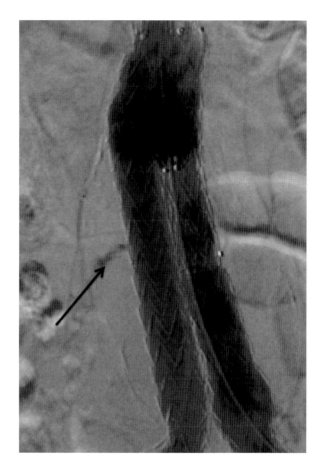

CTA at 3 years showed regression of aneurysm size, despite the presence of a small type II endoleak. No migration or device-related complications were documented. At the appointment, the patient's blood tests revealed deteriorating renal function (Fig. 3.7).

Question 13

Regarding prolonged follow-up in patients with renal insufficiency

A. Non-contrasted CT scans may provide enough information as long as aneurysm size is not increasing
B. Gadolinium-enhanced magnetic resonance angiography (MRA) is the best alternative to CTA and is safe in patients with renal insufficiency
C. DUS is a good alternative for surveillance in expert hands
D. Pain abdominal radiograms provide no additional information when associated with other surveillance methods and should be avoided

Fig. 3.6 CTA volume rendering reconstruction showing successful exclusion of the internal iliac aneurysm by distal coiling and overstenting (*arrow shows coils*)

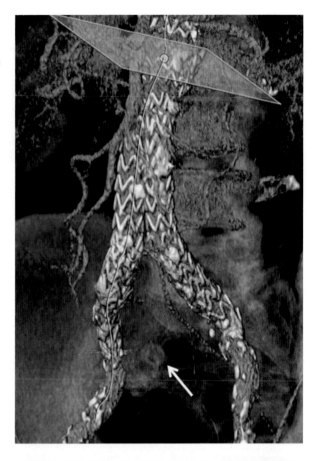

Fig. 3.7 CTA axial slice showing small type II endoleak, associated with a patent inferior mesenteric artery

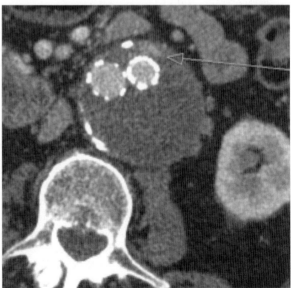

Question 14

According to available data, what is the estimated probability of annual secondary intervention for this patient?

A. <1%
B. 2–4%
C. 5–10%
D. 10–20%
E. >20%

3.1
Commentary

AAAs are typically a disease of elderly white males. In men, occurrence starts in the fifth decade of life, reaching a peak incidence of about 350/100,000 person-years by the age of 80. The prevalence of AAAs measuring at least 3 cm in diameter in men over 65 years old is 7.6%. In women, AAAs tend to occur a few years later in life. The age-adjusted incidence is four to six times greater in men than in women. The risk factors with the largest impact on AAA prevalence are smoking (fivefold), male gender (5.6-fold) and age (1.7-fold each 7 years).[1-3] The course of the disease is usually silent until rupture occurs. This major complication is associated with an overall mortality over 80% and ranks as the 15th cause of death in the United States of America. The aim of elective treatment is essentially to prevent death from rupture.

Although ultrasonography is the method of choice for population screening or follow-up measurements in patients with known aneurysms, ultrasound imaging alone gives insufficient information for preoperative assessment. For open repair, most surgeons recommend preoperative imaging with CTA, which provides accurate information regarding aneurysm size, morphology and relationship with branch vessels, as well as any anatomical variations. Detailed imaging is particularly important when an endovascular treatment is considered. 64-detector (or higher) technology offers great special resolution and submilimetric slices and allows for quick and accurate post-processing.[4,5] Visualization of the entire iliac and common femoral arteries is useful for access planning anticipating difficulties related to stenosis, calcification or tortuosity. Furthermore, optimal projection angles of the C-arm may be obtained using virtual angiography, thus improving deployment accuracy, reducing operative time and minimizing radiation exposure and contrast administration. CTA and post-processing with dedicated software have made conventional calibrated angiography measurements redundant in nearly all cases. **[Q1: B]**

Deciding whether and how to treat a AAA remains a difficult process in which the following variables play a role: risk of rupture, operative risk, anatomical suitability, patient fitness, life expectancy and patient preference (informed consent). Rupture risk will always be an estimate, because of significant interpersonal variability and because no large numbers of patients were ever followed-up without intervention. Using available data from the UK Small Aneurysm Trial and the Veterans Administration Aneurysm Detection and Management (ADAM) Trial, the annual risk of rupture is less than 1% when the maximum diameter is 40–55 mm, although this estimation may be tampered by the fact that many patients received surgery before they reached 55 mm for reasons other than rupture.[6,7] With increasing diameters, the annual rupture rates have been estimated to be the as follows: 50–60 mm, 5–10%; 60–70 mm, 10–20%; 70–80 mm, 20–40%; greater than 80 mm, around 50%.[8] [Q2: C]

The 30-day operative mortality in these two trials ranged from 2.7% to 5.8%, leading to the current concept that aneurysms can be safely observed until they reach 55 mm in diameter. The generally lower operative mortality for EVAR has challenged this view, and two trials are currently under way to compare EVAR and surveillance for small aneurysms.[9,10] Women have been found to have a higher probability of rupture at any given diameter, and a lower threshold of 45 mm for surgery in this group has been proposed.[11] This may be offset partially by the fact that women also have a 1.5-fold higher mortality and mobility both for open repair and for EVAR.[12,13] Faster growth rate has also been associated with a higher likelihood of rupture. Most authors defend treatment of rapidly expanding AAAs (over 5 mm in 6 months or 7 mm in a year) regardless of maximum diameter.[7,11] [Q3: A, B, D]

The benefit gained from EVAR is believed to be greater for higher-risk patients, but those with low-risk should not be denied an endovascular repair. Importantly, patient preference should weigh considerably in candidates for both options, as current evidence demonstrates non-superiority of one over the other. EVAR has demonstrated to result in an important threefold reduction in 30-day mortality, compared to open repair, in patients fit for both procedures. Hospital stays were shorter, recovery was easier and postoperative quality of life was better. At 4 years, though, the early survival advantage of the EVAR groups was lost, mainly due to a higher rate of coronary events. EVAR also required more re-interventions, closer follow-up involving nephrotoxic contrast and radiation exposure and was more expensive.[14,15] However, recent years have witnessed a steady increase in early and late success rates, with decreasing rates of re-interventions, device-related complications and late rupture, for which technological advances and accumulated knowledge are probably responsible.[16,17] While important in demonstrating the efficacy and safety of endovascular repair, the first randomized trials comparing EVAR to open repair are probably already outdated. The presence of renal failure is not an absolute contra-indication for EVAR, as various measures may be used to protect the kidneys and minimize damage, such as intravenous hydration, antioxidant medications or temporary dialysis. The contrast use in straightforward EVAR procedures is 40–100 mL, which is less than the quantity used in most CTA protocols. [Q4: D, E]

Not all aneurysms are suitable for EVAR due to anatomical restrains. Generally, endografts require areas of reasonably healthy vessel wall proximally and distally to be able to seal off blood flow. The most important feature for suitability is the size and morphology of the proximal neck (area between the lowermost renal artery and the beginning of the aneurysm). It should consist of relatively normal aorta over a minimum length of 10 mm, and the diameter should not exceed 32 mm. Neck angulation is another important limitation – infra-renal angulation over 60°–75° or iliac angulation over 90° may result in treatment failure or late complications. Efforts have been undertaken to overcome short or unfavorable sealing zones. Recent devices, more flexible and compliant, have shown to be efficient in aneurysms with severe angulation, though mid and long-term results are still unavailable. Most modern devices offer introducer diameters of 18–22F (main body) and 12–16F (contra-lateral limb and extensions), corresponding roughly to 7 and 5 mm, respectively. Hydrophilic coating of sheaths further improves "pushability" and minimizes injury to access vessels. **[Q5: B, C, D]**

Graft selection should be individualized, as different brand devices show specific advantages over others. Proximal fixation is achieved through radial force, in addition to hooks barbs or anchors in most available devices. An open supra-renal stent with hooks seems to be associated with less downward migration and is advantageous in more complex neck morphology. To date, supra-renal fixation has not been related to embolic or thrombotic complications of the renal arteries. A potential disadvantage supra-renal stents is the added complexity in the unlikely need of a conversion to open repair. Distal fixation usually relies solely on radial force. Bifurcated grafts are preferred, but aorto-uni-iliac (AUI) devices may be used when one of the iliac axis is compromised or the aortic lumen is very narrow. Some prefer these devices for rupture cases. The reasons for this are alleged reduced time until aneurysm exclusion and the need for a smaller off-the-shelf stock. The major disadvantage of AUI devices is the necessary addition of a femoro-femoral cross-over, with concerns over patency, altered hemodynamics and graft infection. **[Q6: C, D]**

Proximal and distal stent-graft diameters should be oversized in 15–20% of the original vessel diameter. Failure to do so will most likely result in failure to achieve adequate proximal or distal seal, thus allowing for continued pressurization of the aneurysm sac (Type I endoleak). More than 20% oversizing may, in turn, cause infolding of the graft fabric, prone to failure in achieving seal. Oversizing has been blamed for continued aortic neck enlargement, which in turn may lead to late treatment failure. While stent radial force at the aneurysm neck seems implicated in neck enlargement, this happens predominantly during the first 6 months and does not usually exceed the diameter of the prothesis.[18,19] **[Q7: C]**

In juxta-renal or supra-renal aneurysms three endovascular options remain. Debranching provides extra-anatomical retrograde revascularization of visceral vessels (with inflow from either the infra-renal aorta or more commonly the iliac arteries) and subsequent coverage of the visceral segment (a so called hybrid procedure). It's a valid alternative with satisfactory mid-term results, but the procedure itself is complex and not without significant operative risk.[20,21] The other two options are fenestrated and branched grafts, offering an all-endovascular solution. Fenestrated grafts have "holes" for the visceral ostia, while branched grafts include ramifications that are intra-operatively extended into visceral branches with covered stents. These grafts are custom-made to match the anatomy of the patient. Time required for manufacturing (around 3 months), high cost and complexity of the procedure have tampered its widespread use, which is limited today to high-risk patients with challenging anatomies. In particular, renal complications seem to be more frequent than observed in the standard devices. In contrast, type I and III endoleak occurrence and aneurysm-related mortality show no significant difference. Despite concerns over the long-term durability of the branch revascularizations, promising short and mid-term results and on-going efforts to reduce cost and availability will likely broaden the use of these devices in the future.[22,23] **[Q8: B] [Q9: C, D]**

Iliac aneurismal involvement is a frequent finding in the diagnostic workup of AAA. Absence of a distal landing zone in the common iliac artery may be overcome by over-stenting the internal iliac artery (occluding it) or by means of a bifurcated iliac branch, with vessel preservation. The first option often requires occlusion of the internal iliac artery by means of coil embolization or using an endovascular plug. This may be avoided if the internal iliac artery is already occluded, stenosed or small and the landing zone in the external iliac artery is long. Internal iliac aneurysms are best treated distal occlusion with coils and overstenting. Infrequently, unilateral occlusion of the internal iliac artery may result in buttock claudication and/or sexual dysfunction, especially if the contra-lateral vessel is occluded and pelvic collateralization is poor. Branched iliac grafts may be used in these selected cases, although they are costly, technically demanding and increase contrast load and radiation exposure. The presence of concomitant iliac aneurysms has been related with a higher risk of distal type I endoleaks.[24] **[Q10: B, C]**

Endoleaks represent the presence of blood flow outside the endograft but within the aneurysm sac after endovascular treatment. They are classified according to their origin (Table 3.1). About one third of patients will present with an endoleak during follow-up, but its significance is related to type and to changes in aneurysm morphology. Type I endoleaks are rare and should be repaired in most instances, as they indicate on-going risk of rupture. This may be achieved by further balloon expansion, placement of a proximal or distal extension or ultimately by conversion. Type II endoleaks are very frequent and their documentation is increasing as image methods become more accurate. Early type II endoleaks tend to disappear spontaneously and additional measures need not be applied when they are present intra-operatively. The true significance of persistent type II endoleaks is still a matter of debate. The pressure transmitted to the aneurysm sac is known to be low and reported ruptures related to these are extremely rare. Unless significant aneurysm growth occurs, most authors defend a conservative approach and closer surveillance. Type III endoleaks are rare and require treatment for the same reason as Type I, usually with additional stent-grafts. Type IV endoleaks were frequent with early devices, but have nearly disappeared with newer generation systems. Endotension may represent undetected endoleaks or fluid accumulation. Although treatment is seldom required, expansion of the

Table 3.1 Endoleak classification

Endoleak type	Origin
Type I a	Proximal graft attachment zone
Type I b	Distal graft attachment zone
Type I c	Iliac occluder failure (in AUI devices)
Type II a	Patent inferior mesenteric artery
Type II b	Patent lumbar, accessory renal or internal iliac arteries
Type III a	Disconnection of components
Type III b	Mid-graft fabric tear
Type IV	Graft fabric porosity
Endotension	Undefined origin

sac may warrant intervention. Anecdotal reports of percutaneous or laparoscopic aneurysm fenestration have been successful. **[Q11: A] [Q12: A]**

EVAR follow-up remains essential for evaluation of long-term aneurysm exclusion and timely detection of complications (Table 3.2). General recommendations include a physical examination and CTA scan within 1 month, then 12 months after operation, and then annually. Gadolinium-enhanced MRA is not an alternative in patients with renal insufficiency, as it may provoke nephrogenic systemic fibrosis, a highly incapacitating and potentially deadly complication. Moreover, prosthetic materials create significant artifacts, especially in endografts using stainless steel stents. Advances in MRA protocols may partially overcome the need for contrast enhancement and diminish artifacts. With strict protocols, CT without contrast may prove to be a valuable alternative for CTA when renal insufficiency is present. Color-flow DUS is emerging as an alternative to CTA for follow-up. Recent evidence shows that it may be comparable to CTA for detection of endoleaks.[25–27] Addition of a four-plane abdominal radiogram to surveillance protocols will allow detection of stent-related complications that would otherwise be missed with DUS. **[Q13: A, C]**

The prognosis of patients with AAA is highly related to the underlying atherosclerotic disease. Cardiovascular complications are responsible for more than two thirds of late deaths after AAA repair. The annual aneurysm rupture risk after EVAR was around 1% with earlier devices, but this figure is estimated to be much lower today and will likely continue to decrease as newer generation grafts become predominant. Also decreasing is the rate of secondary intervention, shown to be around 20% at 4-years in earlier trials.[14–17] Trial and registry data suggests that annual secondary intervention rate today is around 3%.[28,29] Secondary intervention for aneurysm-related complications after open repair was

Table 3.2 EVAR follow-up imaging options

	Advantages	Disadvantages	Limitations
Computed tomography angiography	Accessible Easy to interpret	Nephrotoxic contrast Ionizing radiation exposure	Renal insufficiency
Magnetic resonance angiography (gadolinium enhanced)	No radiation exposure May have higher sensitivity for endoleak detection	Time consuming and expensive Endograft-induced artifacts	Metallic implants Renal insufficiency Claustrophobic patients
Color-flow duplex ultrasound	Cheaper No radiation exposure No contrast needed May be performed at bed-side	Operator and equipment dependent	Adverse body habitus Poor window
Plain abdominal radiogram	Cheap Very low radiation exposure	Limited information Must be used in addition to other methods	None

shown to be 6% at 4 years in the EVAR1 trial (vs 20% for EVAR) but the outcome of these was much worse, as implied by the 3% advantage in aneurysm-related mortality for the endovascular group. Further results from on-going trials and registries are expected to support the trend for less re-intervention and lower aneurysm-related mortality (and hence improved long-term results) for EVAR. **[Q14: B]**

3.2
Case Analysis Quiz

A number of pre and postoperative imaging examples are shown in pictures 8–12. Determine the favorable and unfavorable features shown regarding EVAR adequacy, planning and follow-up (Figs. 3.8–3.12).

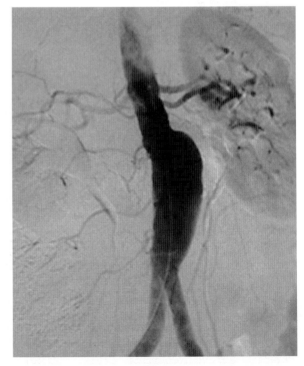

Fig. 3.8 Aortic angiogram showing a very favorable anatomy for endovascular repair: the neck is straight and long, without irregular features of the wall. In addition, the aneurysm sac is straight, and both iliac arteries are non-aneurismal and relatively straight. Notice duplication of the renal arteries, a frequent finding. In long necks, coverage of a polar renal artery is unnecessary and may result in serious morbidity. Efforts should be made to identify the lowest renal artery and cover only below that

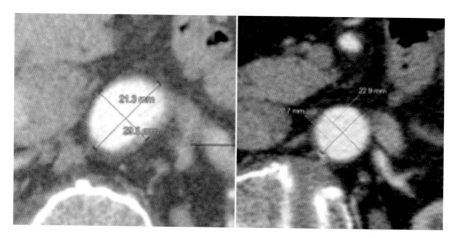

Fig. 3.9 Axial CTA slice of the aneurysm neck. After center-lumen line reconstruction, it is clear that true diameter can differ significantly from that measured in the axial plane, due to vessel tortuosity. Sizing using a workstation is more precise and therefore advisable. Volume-rendering reconstructions are luminograms and thus do not reveal the true diameter of vessels. These should be used for appreciation of the anatomy but for not assessing true aneurysm size

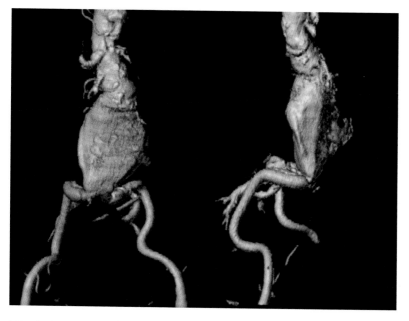

Fig. 3.10 The iliac arteries show severe angulation. This feature is unfavorable for access of the deployment sheaths and is associated with a higher risk of distal type I endoleak. The wide patent lumen and patent IMA are also a risk factor for type II endoleaks, although its significance is not yet fully understood. These two features (iliac angulation and wide patent AAA lumen) will make cannulation of the contra-lateral limb more challenging. An alternative is to canulate in a reversed fashion from the main-body (cross-over technique) or from a brachial access and snare the guide wire

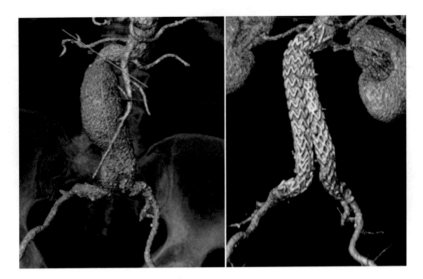

Fig. 3.11 The aneurysm neck is severely angulated and short. These features have been recognized as risk factors for proximal type I endoleak and migration. Newer and more flexible stent-grafts adapt to adverse neck anatomy and seem to reduce this risk. Advances in planning and deployment precision allow treatment for short necks, as the entire possible length of seal is used

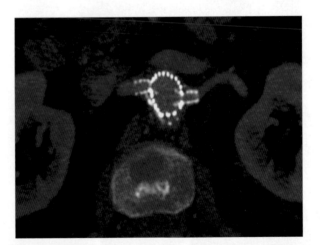

Fig. 3.12 Axial slice of a follow-up CTA – a fenestrated endograft with renal balloon-expandable stents is in situ. In fenestrations, stenting of branch vessels is advised in order to guarantee early patency and preserve flow over time. A small portion (3–4 mm) of the stents should protrude into the luminal side of the aorta, while a minimum of 15 mm should prolong onto the treated artery. Notice the flaring of the intra-aortic segment of the stents, creating a desired "rivet" configuration. This is achieved by partially dilating the stent with an oversized angioplasty balloon and subsequently adjusting the flare with a compliant aortic balloon

References

1. Lederle FA, et al. The aneurysm detection and management study screening program: validation cohort and final results. Aneurysm Detection and Management Veterans Affairs Cooperative Study Investigators. *Arch Intern Med.* 2000;160(10):1425-1430.
2. Ashton HA, Buxton MJ, Day NE, et al. Multicentre Aneurysm Screening Study Group. The Multicentre Aneurysm Screening Study (MASS) into the effect of abdominal aortic aneurysm screening on mortality in men: a randomized controlled trial. *Lancet.* 2002 (Nov 16); 360(9345):1531-1539.
3. Melton LJ 3rd, Bickerstaff LK, Hollier LH, et al. Changing incidence of abdominal aortic aneurysms: a population-based study. *Am J Epidemiol.* 1984;120:379-386.
4. Diehm N, Kickuth R, Gahl B, et al. Intraobserver and interobserver variability of 64-row computed tomography abdominal aortic aneurysm neck measurements. *J Vasc Surg.* 2007 (Feb);45(2):263-268.
5. Higashiura W, Sakaguchi S, Tabayashi N, Taniguchi S, Kichikawa K. Impact of 3-dimensional-computed tomography workstation for precise planning of endovascular aneurysm repair. *Circ J.* 2008 (Dec);72(12):2028-2034.
6. The UK. Small Aneurysm Trial Participants. Mortality results for randomized controlled trial of early elective surgery or ultrasonographic surveillance for small abdominal aortic aneurysms. *Lancet.* 1998;352(9141):1649-1655.
7. Lederle FA, Wilson SE, et al. Immediate repair compared with surveillance of small abdominal aortic aneurysms. *N Engl J Med.* 2002;346(19):1437-1444.
8. Schermerhorn ML, Cronenwett JL. Natural history and decision making for abdominal aortic aneurysms. In: Zelenock GB, ed. *Mastery of Vascular and Endovascular Surgery.* 1st ed. Philadelphia: Lippincott Williams & Wilkins; 2006:71-78.
9. Cao P, CAESAR Trial Collaborators. Comparison of surveillance vs Aortic Endografting for Small Aneurysm Repair (CAESAR) trial: study design and progress. *Eur J Vasc Endovasc Surg.* 2005 (Sept);30(3):245-251.
10. Ouriel K. The PIVOTAL study: a randomized comparison of endovascular repair versus surveillance in patients with smaller abdominal aortic aneurysms. *J Vasc Surg.* 2009 (Jan);49(1):266-269.
11. Brown LC, Powell JT. Risk factors for aneurysm rupture in patients kept under ultrasound surveillance. UK Small Aneurysm Trial Participants. *Ann Surg.* 1999 (Sep);230(3):289-296.
12. Abedi NN, Davenport DL, Xenos E, Sorial E, Minion DJ, Endean ED. Gender and 30-day outcome in patients undergoing endovascular aneurysm repair (EVAR): an analysis using the ACS NSQIP dataset. *J Vasc Surg.* 2009 (Sep);50(3):486-491. 491.e1-4.
13. Egorova N, Giacovelli JK, Gelijns A, et al. Defining high-risk patients for endovascular aneurysm repair. *J Vasc Surg.* 2009 (Dec);50(6):1271-1279. e1.
14. Greenhalgh RM, Brown LL, Kwong GP, Powell JJ, THompson SG. Comparison of endovascular repair with open repair in patients with AAA (EVAR trial 1) 30 day operative mortality results: randomised controlled trial. *Lancet.* 2004;364:843-848.
15. Prinssen M, Verhoeven ELG, Buth J, et al. A randomized trial comparing conventional and endovascular repair of abdominal aortic aneurysms. *N Engl J Med.* 2004;351:1607-1618.
16. Lederle FA, Freischlag JA, Kyriakides TC, et al.; Open Versus Endovascular Repair (OVER) Veterans Affairs Cooperative Study Group. Outcomes following endovascular vs open repair of abdominal aortic aneurysm: a randomized trial. *JAMA.* 2009 (Oct) 14;302(14):1535-1542.
17. Abbruzzese TA, Kwolek CJ, Brewster DC, et al. Outcomes following endovascular abdominal aortic aneurysm repair (EVAR): an anatomic and device-specific analysis. *J Vasc Surg.* 2008 (July);48(1):19-28.

18. van Prehn J, Schlosser FJ, Verhagen HJM, et al. Oversizing of aortic stent grafts for abdominal aneurysm repair: a systematic review of the benefits and risks. *Eur J Vasc Endovasc Surg.* 2009;38(1):42-53.

19. Sampaio SM, Panneton JM, et al. Aortic neck dilation after endovascular abdominal aortic aneurysm repair: should oversizing be blamed? *Ann Vasc Surg.* 2006;20(3):338-345.

20. Black SA, Wolfe JH, Clark M, Hamady M, Cheshire NJ, Jenkins MP. Complex thoracoabdominal aortic aneurysms: endovascular exclusion with visceral revascularization. *J Vasc Surg.* 2006 (Jun);43(6):1081-1089.

21. Biasi L, Ali T, Loosemore T, Morgan R, Loftus I, Thompson M. Hybrid repair of complex thoracoabdominal aortic aneurysms using applied endovascular strategies combined with visceral and renal revascularization. *J Thorac Cardiovasc Surg.* 2009 (Dec);138(6):1331-1338.

22. Greenberg RK, Sternbergh WC, Makaroun M, et al. Fenestrated Investigators. Intermediate results of a United States multicenter trial of fenestrated endograft repair for juxtarenal abdominal aortic aneurysms. *J Vasc Surg.* 2009 (Oct);50(4):730-737. e1.

23. Verhoeven EL, Vourliotakis G, Bos WT, Tielliu IF, Zeebregts CJ, Prins TR, Bracale UM, van den Dungen JJ. Fenestrated stent grafting for short-necked and juxtarenal abdominal aortic aneurysm: an 8-year single-centre experience. *Eur J Vasc Endovasc Surg.* 2010 (Mar 2) [Epub ahead of print].

24. Hobo R, Sybrandy JE, et al. Endovascular repair of abdominal aortic aneurysms with concomitant common iliac artery aneurysm: outcome analysis of the EUROSTAR experience. *J Endovasc Ther.* 2008;15(1):12-22.

25. Chaer RA, et al. Duplex ultrasound as the sole long-term surveillance method post-endovascular aneurysm repair: a safe alternative for stable aneurysms. *J Vasc Surg.* 2009;49(4):845-849.

26. Beeman BR, et al. Duplex ultrasound imaging alone is sufficient for midterm endovascular aneurysm repair surveillance: a cost analysis study and prospective comparison with computed tomography scan. *J Vasc Surg.* 2009;50(5):1019-1024.

27. Badri H, et al. Duplex ultrasound scanning (DUS) versus computed tomography angiography (CTA) in the follow-up after EVAR. *Angiology.* 2010;61(2):131-136.

28. Hobo R, Buth J. Secondary interventions following endovascular abdominal aortic aneurysm repair using current endografts. A EUROSTAR report. *J Vasc Surg.* 2006;43(5):896-902.

29. Nordon I, Karthikesalingam A, Hinchliffe R, Holt P, Loftus I, Thompson M. Secondary interventions following endovascular aneurysm repair (EVAR) and the enduring value of graft surveillance. *Eur J Vasc Endovasc Surg.* 2009 (Nov 23) [Epub ahead of print].

Ruptured Abdominal Aortic Aneurysm

4

Jeffrey S. Weiss and Bauer E. Sumpio

A 70-year-old white male presents to the emergency department with sudden onset of severe back pain. The pain is described as severe and constant without alleviating or aggravating symptoms. He has never had pain like this before. He denies chest pain, shortness of breath, or loss of consciousness. He denies any history of an abdominal aortic aneurysm. His past medical history is significant for hypertension, and chronic obstructive pulmonary disease that requires home oxygen therapy. He had bilateral inguinal herniorrhaphy some years ago, but has never had a laparotomy.

His vital signs yielded a pulse at 90 bpm and a blood pressure of 110/60 mm Hg. He is appropriately conversant and appears older than his stated age. He was without abdominal tenderness or masses and no bruits were heard; however, his belly was slightly obese and the examination was difficult. He has bilaterally palpable lower extremity pulses.

Question 1

What symptoms are considered the classic presenting triad for ruptured abdominal aortic aneurysm (rAAA)?

A. Abdominal/back pain, shortness of breath, and a pulsatile mass.
B. Abdominal/back pain, syncope, and a pulsatile mass.
C. Abdominal/back pain, nausea, and syncope.
D. Abdominal/back pain, chest pain, and hematochezia.

The patient remained stable while the emergency department staff obtained laboratory results and cross-matched blood, and performed an electrocardiogram (ECG).

B.E. Sumpio (✉)
Department of Vascular Surgery, Yale University School of Medicine, New Haven, CT, USA

G. Geroulakos and B. Sumpio (eds.), *Vascular Surgery*,
DOI: 10.1007/978-1-84996-356-5_4, © Springer-Verlag London Limited 2011

Question 2

If this patient is considered to have a ruptured AAA, which of the following factors does not adversely contribute to prognosis?

A. Diabetes
B. Serum creatinine = 1.8 mg/dL
C. Age = 75 years
D. Preoperative blood pressure = 80 mm Hg (systolic)
E. Syncope

The patient's ECG shows normal sinus rhythm, the creatinine was 1.7 mg/dL, and the hematocrit was 32%. He remains hemodynamically stable. Your resident feels he is stable enough for a computed tomography (CT) scan (Fig. 4.1).

Question 3

Which of the following statements is true?

A. Patients with unknown AAA history and symptoms should undergo further diagnostic imaging if they are hemodynamically stable.
B. Symptomatic AAA should undergo emergency repair to prevent possible rupture.
C. Patients with an unknown AAA history must have diagnostic imaging confirmation of an AAA before proceeding to the operating theatre.
D. An ECG demonstrating ischemic changes in a patient with epigastric pain, hypotension and tachycardia is the sine qua non for a myocardial infarction and any operation should be postponed.
E. CT scans are reserved for elective evaluation of AAA and have no place in the workup of a symptomatic AAA.

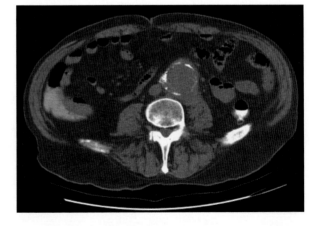

Fig. 4.1 Non-contrast computed tomography (CT) scan of abdomen reveals an aortic aneurysm rupture in a left posterior location with extravasation into the retroperitoneum

Question 4

If an ultrasound (Fig. 4.2) was obtained instead of a CT scan, what statements could be made regarding this study?

A. Ultrasound is more reliable than CT scan for the diagnosis of ruptured AAA.
B. The location of the rupture is typical for most ruptured AAAs.
C. Ultrasound can be performed quickly at the bedside.
D. Ultrasound can be used to provide endograft measurements.
E. Ultrasound is best used in unstable patients to confirm the presence of a known AAA.

After the confirmation of ruptured AAA by radiology, the patient is taken immediately to the operating room.

Question 5

All of the following measures are indicated in the perioperative management of a ruptured AAA, except:

A. Surgical preparation and drape before induction.
B. Preoperative resuscitation to normal blood pressure.
C. Passive cooling of the patient.
D. Heparinization before cross-clamping.
E. Blood recuperation and autotransfusion devices.

The patient is prepared and draped, the anesthetic administered, and operation commenced. The medical student asks if this could be done via an endovascular approach.

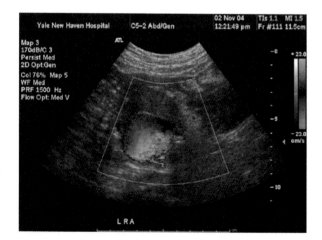

Fig. 4.2 Abdominal ultrasound with duplex color demonstrating rupture of aneurysm at the level of the left renal artery with a fluid collection in the left retroperitoneum

Question 6

Currently, what are the contraindications for endovascular repair of ruptured AAAs?

A. Infrarenal neck diameter >30 mm.
B. Infrarenal neck length <10 mm.
C. Systolic blood pressure <100 mm Hg.
D. Endograft or "endograft team" not available.
E. Thrombus present at infrarenal neck.

The patient was determined to have too large a neck diameter for an endovascular stent, so you decide to proceed with an open repair. After induction, the patient´s blood pressure falls to a systolic of 60 mm Hg. A supraceliac clamp is quickly placed and the aneurysm exposed. The rupture was contained to the retroperitoneum, but is rather large. The supraceliac clamp is moved to an infrarenal position after about 10 min. Anesthesia quickly catches up and his systolic blood pressure rises to 100 mm Hg. The inferior mesenteric artery was not patent and the iliac arteries were without aneurysms, allowing a Dacron tube graft to be placed. The clamp is slowly removed and he remains hemodynamically stable. The bowel appears well perfused and distal pulses are palpable before closure. Postoperatively, the patient recovers in the surgical intensive care unit.

Question 7

The most common complication following repair of ruptured AAAs is?

A. Aortoenteric fistula.
B. Bowel ischemia.
C. Myocardial ischemia.
D. Atheroemboli.
E. Acute renal failure.

He is noted to have a creatinine that rises to 4.7 mg/dL 2 days after operation and his urine output falls to less than 100 mL/day. He is eventually placed on intermittent hemodialysis because of volume overload. Over the next 2 weeks he is weaned off the ventilator, his urine output slowly increases, and his creatinine levels stabilizes at 2.0 mg/dL. He is discharged to a convalescence facility 19 days after operation.

4.1
Commentary

The optimal treatment of rAAA is prevention; unfortunately close to 70% of presenting patients have no prior diagnosis.[1] The overall mortality rates for rAAA are 80–90% with operative mortality around 50%.[2-4] Although more than three-quarters of patients with an rAAA report either abdominal or back pain, they can present with a myriad of symptoms and signs that are both broad and inconsistently present.[5] The triad of hypotension, abdominal pain, and a pulsatile mass **[Q1: B]** are found together in only half of cases.[6] A great deal of effort has been applied to identifying perioperative risk factors for patients who have a decreased survival advantage. Preoperative risk factors include: age <75–76 years, hypotension = 80–95 mm Hg, creatinine = 1.8–1.9 mg/dL, loss of consciousness, ECG ischemia or dysrhythmia, CHF congestive heart failure, hemoglobin <9 g/dL, base deficit >8, and free rupture.[7–10] **[Q2: A]** Intraoperative risk factors include: blood loss >2–3.5 L, duration of surgery >200 min, aortic cross-clamp time >47 min, lack of autotransfusion devices, bifurcated grafts, and technical complications (i.e., left renal vein injury).[11–13] Postoperative risk factors include renal failure, coagulopathy, and cardiac complications. Hardman et al.[10] found that possession of three or more preoperative risk factors correlated with 100% mortality. Currently, no recommendation exists to withhold surgery for patients with any or all of these risk factors; this decision is made on a case-by-case basis, making risk factor analysis useful mostly from the standpoint of guiding patient decisions on surgery and family discussions on prognosis.

Patients who present with symptoms of a rAAA can be divided into two groups based on whether or not they have a known AAA (Fig. 4.3).[14] Unstable patients with known AAAs present the least diagnostic challenge as they belong in the operating room. In contrast, the unstable patient without known AAA can be the hardest to evaluate. If an rAAA is suspected, this patient needs to be assessed expeditiously with an ECG as myocardial infarction can often mimic these symptoms. If cardiogenic shock is clinically apparent, resuscitation should override emergent surgery; however, cardiac ischemia secondary to hypovolemic shock from a rupture needs both rapid resuscitation and emergent surgery as the underlying cause of shock is the rupture and not the heart. Patients without hemodynamic instability allow the examiner the time to proceed with radiological confirmation.[15] **[Q3: A]** Ultrasound is fast and convenient as it allows an examination while resuscitation is taking place at the bedside. The sensitivity is as high as 100% for detecting an AAA, but it is inaccurate on diagnosing rupture (49%).[12,16] This study is ideal on hemodynamically stable patients without known AAA, minimal operative risk factors, and symptoms or signs suggestive of rupture. **[Q4: B, C]** In this case, the mere presence of an AAA would warrant surgery without delay. CT scans are more difficult to obtain and place the patient at some increased risk because of time delay and interruption of resuscitation. They are clearly only indicated for patients who are stable and offer the advantage of being able to diagnosis rupture. The groups of patients most likely to benefit from CT scan are those with significant comorbidities where delay could allow preoperative optimization.[17] The sensitivity and specificity of CT scan for diagnosing rupture is quoted to be as high as 94% and 95%, respectively.[15]

Once the decision to operate has been made, several preoperative measures should be undertaken. A natural instinct is to bolus intravenous (IV) fluid in an attempt to normalize the blood pressure; this should be avoided. Instead, adopting a *permissive hypotensive* strategy will allow the patient's own physiologic response to minimize blood loss.[18] Although there are times when fluids are necessary, this strategy can be effective in preventing accelerated blood loss until the aorta is clamped or occluded. Every effort should be made to keep the patient warm with blankets, raising the operating room temperature, and utilizing warmed IV fluids and blood products.[8] The patient should be prepared and draped before induction as the loss of sympathetic tone with anesthesia may cause a marginally compensated patient to collapse.

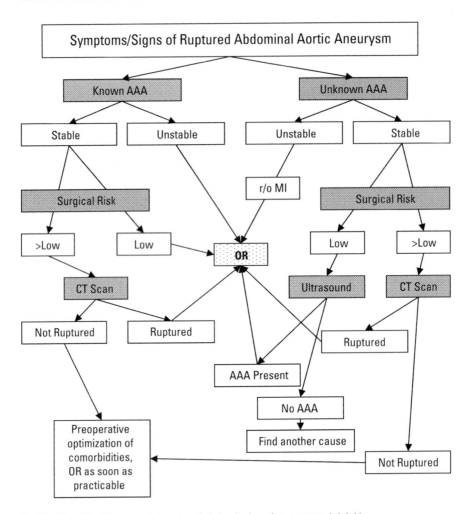

Fig. 4.3 Algorithm for suspected ruptured abdominal aortic aneurysm (rAAA)

A midline laparotomy provides the quickest route of entry and best exposure in most cases. A low threshold to obtain supraceliac control will prevent inadvertent venous injury, especially in cases with large retroperitoneal hematomas. This control is obtained by incising the gastrohepatic ligament and diaphragmatic crura, and then bluntly dissecting the periaortic tissue; a preoperative nasogastric tube can aid in identification of the laterally positioned esophagus. A clamp or manual pressure is applied to the supraceliac aorta. The transverse colon is reflected cephalad and the small bowel eviscerated. The supraceliac control can then be moved to the infrarenal neck after it is carefully dissected out. Systemic heparinization is avoided and heparinized saline (10 units/mL) is used locally down both iliacs before balloon occlusion. The use of intraoperative blood recuperation and autotransfusion devices is crucial in minimizing postoperative mortality by limiting homologous blood transfusions.[13] The use of a tube graft, typically knitted Dacron or PTFE polytetrafluoroethylene, will shorten operative times and restore flow sooner than a bifurcated graft; this may necessitate leaving aneurysmal iliac arteries alone.[14] **[Q5: B, C, D]** After completion of grafting, bowel and lower extremity perfusion are assessed, usually by inspection and Doppler probe. The aneurysm sac is closed around the graft in an attempt to prevent later aortoenteric fistulas. Depending on the size of retroperitoneal hematoma and degree of resuscitation, the abdomen may not close easily. In these cases, it is best to perform a temporary closure with plans to return to the operating room for washout and definitive closure at a later, more stable time.

The dismal mortality following open repair of rAAA and the expansion of endovascular techniques has prompted recent exploration into application of stent grafts for primary therapy. Patient candidacy for an endovascular repair of AAA (EVAR) is the first hurdle when considering this approach. Measurements to determine this are typically done by CT angiography, although the Montefiore group have been successful utilizing digital subtraction angiography in two views.[19] The concern of sending a potentially unstable patient with known or suspected ruptured AAA to the CT scanner was recently addressed by Lloyd et al.[20] from Leicester; they found that 87.5% of patients survived longer than 2 h after admission, with 92% of these patients having systolic blood pressures greater than 80 mm Hg. Ruptured or symptomatic AAAs are found to have larger infrarenal neck diameters and smaller neck lengths.[21] Despite these morphological differences, several reports have found amazingly high feasibility rates for EVAR, ranging from 46% to 80%.[22,23] Dimensional requirements for endografts are constantly shifting as new devices improve the field, but currently an infrarenal neck = 10 mm and a diameter = 30 mm are needed.[24] **[Q6: A, B, D]** The next hurdle is availability of an endograft team and the graft itself. The importance of a knowledgeable and experienced team cannot be overstated as any program without this is destined for failure. A variety of grafts are being utilized, with favor towards a modular aorto-uniiliac device; this set-up decreases the need for large inventories.[23,24] The Montefiore group have developed an aorto-unifemoral graft which they use in conjunction with a crossover femoral-femoral graft.[19] Surprisingly few patients are rejected for EVAR secondary to unfavorable hemodynamics. Supraceliac balloon occlusion via a brachial or femoral route under fluoroscopic guidance can allow proximal aortic control under local anesthesia; a technique being utilized by some for control prior to laparotomy in open cases.[25] Prospective randomized studies are underway to examine the morbidity and mortality rates of EVAR with respect to open repair, but preliminary nonrandomized results are already favoring this approach.[19,24,26]

The most common complication of rAAA repair is renal failure, followed by ileus, sepsis, myocardial infarction, respiratory failure, bleeding, and bowel ischemia.[1,11] **[Q7: E]** Postoperative renal failure has been found by several authors to correlate with mortality.[1,11] Minimizing suprarenal clamp time and use of mannitol before cross-clamping the aorta to initiate brisk diuresis may limit renal damage. The inflammatory mediators and cytokines released from the shock state, visceral hypoperfusion, and massive transfusions associated with open repair can lead to multi-organ system failure; the avoidance of supraceliac clamping and lower blood loss are some of the potential advantages of the EVAR approach. But EVAR has its own unique complications which include endoleaks, graft malfunction, and groin wound issues.

References

1. Noel AA, Gloviczki P, Cherry KJ, et al. Ruptured abdominal aortic aneurysms: the excessive mortality rate of conventional repair. *J Vasc Surg*. 2001;34:41-46.
2. Dardik A, Burleyson GP, Bowman H, Gordon TA, Webb TH, Perler BA. Surgical repair of ruptured abdominal aortic aneurysms in the state of Maryland: factors influencing outcome among 527 recent cases. *J Vasc Surg*. 1998;28:413-421.
3. Heller JA, Weinberg A, Arons R, et al. Two decades of abdominal aortic repair: have we made any progress? *J Vasc Surg*. 2000;32:1091-1100.
4. Bengtsson H, Bergqvist D. Ruptured abdominal aortic aneurysm: a population-based study. *J Vasc Surg*. 1993;18:74-80.
5. Rose J, Civil I, Koelmeyer T, Haydock D, Adams D. Ruptured abdominal aortic aneurysms: clinical presentation in Auckland 1993–1997. *Aust NZ J Surg*. 2001;71:341-344.
6. Wakefield TW, Whitehouse WM, Wu SC, et al. Abdominal aortic aneurysm rupture: statistical analysis of factors affecting outcome of surgical treatment. *Surgery*. 1982;91:586-596.
7. Sasaki S, Yasuda K, Yamauchi H, Shiya N, Sakuma M. Determinants of the postoperative and long-term survival of patients with ruptured abdominal aortic aneurysms. *Surg Today*. 1998;28:30-35.
8. Piper G, Patel N, Chandela S, et al. Short-term predictors and long-term outcome after ruptured abdominal aortic aneurysm repair. *Am Surg*. 2003;63:703-710.
9. Shackelton CR, Schechter MT, Bianco R, Hildebrand HD. Preoperative predictors of mortality risk in ruptured abdominal aortic aneurysm. *J Vasc Surg*. 1987;6:583-589.
10. Hardman DT, Fisher CM, Patel MI, et al. Ruptured abdominal aortic aneurysms: who should be offered surgery? *J Vasc Surg*. 1996;23:123-129.
11. Donaldson MC, Rosenberg JM, Bucknam CA. Factors affecting survival after ruptured abdominal aortic aneurysm. *J Vasc Surg*. 1985;2:564-570.
12. Markovic M, Davidovic L, Maksimovic Z, et al. Ruptured abdominal aortic aneurysm predictors of survival in 229 consecutive surgical patients. *Herz*. 2004;29:123-129.
13. Marty-Ane CH, Alric P, Picot MC, Picard E, Colson P, Mary H. Ruptured abdominal aortic aneurysm: influence of intraoperative management on surgical outcome. *J Vasc Surg*. 1995;22:780-786.
14. Hallett JW, Rasmussen TE. Ruptured abdominal aortic aneurysm. In: Cronenwett JL, Rutherford RB, eds. *Decision Making in Vascular Surgery*. Philadelphia: Saunders; 2001: 104-107.
15. Kvilekval KH, Best IM, Mason RA, Newton GB, Giron F. The value of computed tomography in the management of symptomatic abdominal aortic aneurysms. *J Vasc Surg*. 1990;12: 28-33.
16. Tayal VS, Graf CD, Gibbs MA. Prospective study of accuracy and outcome of emergency ultrasound for abdominal aortic aneurysm over two years. *Acad Emerg Med*. 2003;10: 867-871.
17. Sullivan CA, Rohrer MJ, Cutler BS. Clinical management of the symptomatic but unruptured abdominal aortic aneurysm. *J Vasc Surg*. 1990;11:799-803.
18. Owens TM, Watson WC, Prough DS, Uchida T, Kramer GC. Limiting initial resuscitation of uncontrolled hemorrhage reduces internal bleeding and subsequent volume requirements. *J Trauma*. 1995;39:200-209.
19. Veith FJ, Ohki T, Lipsitz EC, Suggs WD, Cynamon J. Treatment of ruptured abdominal aneurysms with stent grafts: a new gold standard? *Semin Vasc Surg*. 2003;16:171-175.
20. Lloyd GM, Bown MJ, Norwood MG, et al. Feasibility of preoperative computer tomography in patients with ruptured abdominal aortic aneurysm: a time-to-death study in patients without operation. *J Vasc Surg*. 2004;39:788-791.

21. Lee WA, Huber TS, Hirneise CM, Berceli SA, Seeger JM. Eligibility rates of ruptured and symptomatic AAA for endovascular repair. *J Endovasc Ther*. 2002;9:436-442.
22. Reichart M, Geelkerken RH, Huisman AB, van Det RJ, de Smit P, Volker EP. Ruptured abdominal aortic aneurysm: endovascular repair is feasible in 40% of patients. *Eur J Vasc Endovasc Surg*. 2003;26:479-486.
23. Hinchliffe RJ, Braithwaite BD, Hopkinson BR. The endovascular management of ruptured abdominal aortic aneurysms. *Eur J Vasc Endovasc Surg*. 2003;25:191-201.
24. Peppelenbosch N, Yilmaz N, van Marrewijk C, et al. Emergency treatment of acute symptomatic or ruptured abdominal aortic aneurysm. Outcome of a prospective intent-to-treat by EVAR protocol. *Eur J Vasc Endovasc Surg*. 2003;26:303-310.
25. Matsuda H, Tanaka Y, Hino Y, et al. Transbrachial arterial insertion of aortic occlusion balloon catheter in patients with shock from ruptured abdominal aortic aneurysm. *J Vasc Surg*. 2003;38:1293-1296.
26. Lee WA, Huber TS, Hirneise CM, Berceli SA, Seeger JM. Impact of endovascular repair on early outcomes of ruptured abdominal aortic aneurysms. *J Vasc Surg*. 2004;40:211-215.

Thoracoabdominal Aortic Aneurysm

5

Hernan A. Bazan, Nicholas J. Morrissey, and Larry H. Hollier

A 72-year-old white male presented to his primary-care physician with a history of left chest pain for the past month. The pain was dull and constant and radiated to the back, medial to the scapula. He denied a new cough or worsening shortness of breath. He had no recent weight loss, and his appetite was good. He had a history of hypertension, which was currently controlled medically, and a significant 60 pack-a-year smoking history. In addition, he suffered a myocardial infarction (MI) 5 years ago. The patient denied any history of claudication, transient ischaemic attacks or stroke. He had undergone surgery in the past for bilateral inguinal hernias, and underwent cardiac catheterization after his MI.

On physical examination, the patient was thin but did not appear malnourished.

Vital signs were heart rate 72 beats/min, blood pressure 140/80 mmHg, respiratory rate 18/min, and temperature 36.8°C. His head and neck examination was remarkable for bilateral carotid bruits. Cardiac examination revealed a regular rate and rhythm without murmurs. Abdominal examination revealed no bruits and a palpable aortic mass. His femoral and popliteal pulses were normal (2+); Posterior tibial pulses were 1+ bilaterally, and dorsalis pedis signals were detectable only by Doppler. No prominent popliteal pulses were appreciated. Routine blood work was unremarkable, and an electrocardiogram (ECG) revealed changes consistent with an old inferior wall MI and left ventricular (LV) hypertrophy. Chest X-ray (Fig. 5.1) was remarkable for a tortuous aorta, which had calcification within the wall and appeared dilated. There were no pleural effusions, but both hemidiaphragms did demonstrate some flattening, and bony structures were normal. Lung fields were clear of masses or consolidation.

H.A. Bazan (✉)
Ochsner Clinic Foundation, Department of Surgery, Section of Vascular/Endovascular Surgery,
New Orleans, LA 70121, USA
e-mail: hbazan@ochsner.org

G. Geroulakos and B. Sumpio (eds.), *Vascular Surgery*,
DOI: 10.1007/978-1-84996-356-5_5, © Springer-Verlag London Limited 2011

Fig. 5.1 Chest X-ray
demonstrating a tortuous
and dilated descending
thoracic aorta suggestive of
a thoracoabdominal aortic
aneurysm

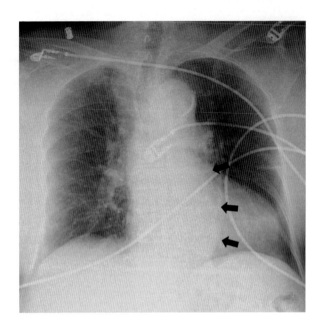

Question 1

Which of the following is the single most likely diagnosis causing this man's pain?

A. Acute MI
B. Acute aortic dissection
C. Thoracic aortic aneurysm
D. Lung cancer
E. Pneumonia

Question 2

Which of the following studies should be performed in this patient in order to plan therapy?

A. Aortography
B. Computed tomography (CT) scan of chest
C. Carotid duplex studies
D. Cardiac stress test
E. Arterial blood gas (ABG) analysis

Although aortography was routinely done before, CT scan of the chest and abdomen was obtained (Fig. 5.2) and deemed sufficient for operative planning. Findings were consistent with a thoracoabdominal aneurysm without concomitant dissection of the aorta. There was

Fig. 5.2 CTA scan
demonstrating aneurysmal
dilatation of the descending
thoracic aorta

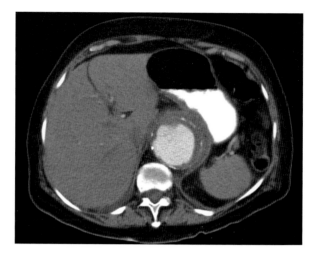

no evidence for acute leak or rupture, and the maximal diameter of the thoracic aorta
was 7.3 cm.

Question 3

In the Crawford classification system for thoracoabdominal aortic aneurysms (TAAAs),
which represents the most extensive TAAA?

A. Type I
B. Type II
C. Type III
D. Type IV

The patient underwent a cardiac stress test, which was normal. Carotid duplex studies
revealed minimal atherosclerotic disease with bilateral stenoses of less than 50%. ABG
analysis showed pH 7.38, pCO2 42 and pO276 on room air.

Question 4

Which of the following management schemes seems most reasonable for this patient?

A. Observation with annual follow-up chest CT
B. Repair of thoracoabdominal aneurysm after bilateral carotid endarterectomies
C. Cardiac catheterization followed by repair of TAAA
D. Elective repair of TAAA

The patient is scheduled for elective repair of his TAAA. He expresses concern about the
possibility of complications from the surgery. You explain to him the most likely complications related to this surgery.

Question 5

Of the following, which is *not* a common complication following TAAA repair?

A. Pulmonary
B. Cardiac
C. Renal
D. Gastrointestinal

The patient seems most concerned about the risk of postoperative paralysis. You explain to him that there are things you can do to decrease his risk of suffering these complications, although nothing can eliminate the risk.

Question 6

Which of the following technical modifications is *not* believed to be beneficial in the prevention of spinal cord dysfunction following TAAA repair?

A. Tumor necrosis factor-α monoclonal antibody
B. Cerebrospinal fluid drainage
C. Reimplantation of key intercostal arteries
D. Epidural cooling

The patient undergoes repair of TAAA and tolerates the procedure well. Postoperatively, the chest tubes are draining 100–150 cm³ blood/h for the first 3 h. In addition, urine output is steady at 500 cm³/h. The patient has transient drops in blood pressure to a systolic blood pressure in the 70s, with central venous pressure dropping to 5 mmHg.

Question 7

(a) Outline the initial work-up and potential correction of the bleeding problem described above in order to prevent a return to the operating room. (b) What fluid resuscitation approach should be taken to stabilize this patient's hemodynamic status?

The patient's temperature is 34.6°C, international normalized ration (INR) is 1.7 and partial thromboplastin time (PTT) is 50 s (control, 34 s). Platelet count is 33,000. After infusion of warm fluids, the use of a warming blanket, and platelet and fresh frozen plasma (FFP) transfusions, the parameters return to normal and the drainage from the chest tubes decreases to about 10–20 cm³/h. On the second postoperative day, the patient is noted to have loss of motor function in his lower extremities.

Question 8

What therapeutic intervention, if carried out in a timely fashion, may restore this patient's neurological function partially or fully?

Following appropriate intervention, the patient's neurological function returns to normal. The patient's recovery is otherwise uneventful, and he is discharged on postoperative day 8 with clean incisions, intact neurological status and adequate analgesia.

Question 9

Following a successful recovery from his surgery, this gentleman's approximate predicted 5-year survival is:

A. 20%
B. 50%
C. 70%
D. 90%

Question 10

Is there a role for endovascular or hybrid repair of this TAAA?

5.1
Commentary

TAAAs are less common than infrarenal abdominal aortic aneurysms. One population-based study suggested an incidence of 5.9 TAAAs per 100,000 person-years.[1] Although TAAAs are more common in males, the male:female ratio of 1.1–2.1:1 is not as weighted as the ratio of abdominal aortic aneurysm (AAA). The aetiology of TAAAs is related to atherosclerotic medial degenerative disease (82%) and aortic dissection (17%) in most cases.[2] About 45% of TAAAs are asymptomatic and detected during work-up of other systems, usually on chest X-ray or cardiac echocardiography examinations. Patients with TAAAs tend to be older than AAA patients and, therefore, may have more severe comorbidities. When present, symptoms are usually chest or back pain related to compression of adjacent structures by the aneurysm or cough from compression/erosion of airways. Fistulization is rare but erosion into the bronchial tree presents with massive haemoptysis, while erosion into the esophagus presents with upper-gastrointestinal bleeding. Presentation with acute, severe pain may reflect leak, acute expansion or dissection of the aneurysm and require urgent evaluation and treatment. The risk factors associated with TAAA are smoking, hypertension, coronary artery disease, chronic obstructive pulmonary disease (COPD), and disease in other vascular beds. Syphilitic aneurysms are a rare cause of TAAA in this era but, when present, usually involve the ascending aorta.

Other causes of vague chest and back pain in a patient such as this include myocardial ischemia, pulmonary neoplasm, acute dissection, pneumonia, and bony metastases. **[Q1: C]**

The clinical and X-ray findings in this particular case argue against these other possibilities. The work-up of patients with TAAA requires assessment of the aneurysm extent, size, and condition of the remaining aorta. Before any studies are carried out, a thorough history and physical examination, including vascular assessment, are needed. **[Q2: B]** With marked improvements in non-invasive imaging in the past decade, computed tomography angiography (CTA) has replaced invasive aortography for defining the extent of TAAA, status of aortic branches, delineation of any associated dissection, and presence of leak. Magnetic resonance imaging (MRI) and magnetic resonance angiography (MRA) have also improved dramatically and offer unique benefits over CT, such as lack of radiation and non-nephrotoxic contrast agents. However, MRA has yet to achieve the resolution of CTA and its use is contraindicated in unstable patients. Transesophageal echocardiography can assess the status of the aortic valve as well as cardiac function. Significant aortic insufficiency is a contraindication to thoracic aortic cross-clamping, unless a shunt or pump is used to bypass the left heart.

The Crawford classification **[Q3: B]** is used to characterise TAAAs.[3] According to this system, aneurysms beginning just distal to the left subclavian artery and involving the aorta up to, but not below, the renals are termed type I. Type II TAAAs are the most extensive – they begin just beyond the left subclavian and continue into the infrarenal aorta. Type III aneurysms involve the distal half of the thoracic aorta, usually originating at the level of T6, and varying extents of the abdominal aorta. Type IV TAAAs refer to those aneurysms involving the entire abdominal aorta, up to the diaphragm and including the visceral segments. This classification scheme has been useful for predicting morbidity and mortality following repair of TAAAs.

In addition to assessment of the aneurysm, the high incidence of comorbidities in this patient population mandates thorough evaluation of cardiac, as well as pulmonary reserve. Preoperative studies should include electrocardiography and cardiac stress testing. Further work-up is dictated by the presence of positive findings. Screening chest X-ray and preoperative ABG provides information regarding the patient's pulmonary status. Formal pulmonary function tests should be reserved for those patients with evidence of significant pulmonary compromise. Since the risk factors for TAAA are the same as those for atherosclerotic disease, a careful history and physical will dictate whether there is a need to work up disease in other vascular beds (carotid, mesenteric, renal, lower extremity). Carotid duplex studies may be done routinely preoperatively and significant carotid stenoses are treated before TAAA repair. The status of the patient's clotting system must be determined and optimized, if necessary. In the absence of indications to carry out other operations first, this patient with a TAAA of >6 cm should undergo elective repair of his aneurysm.

[Q4: D] Observation with follow-up imaging studies is dangerous and puts the patient at risk of death due to aneurysm rupture. The natural history of TAAAs is related to size and growth rate. Understanding the behaviour of these lesions is of crucial importance when determining treatment. Crawford's series of 94 TAAAs followed for 25 years demonstrated 2-year survival of 24%, with about half of deaths due to rupture.[4] This series included dissected as well as non-dissected aneurysms. A more recent series of non-dissected TAAAs revealed rupture rates of 12% at 2 years and 32% at 4 years; for aneurysms greater than 5 cm in diameter, rupture rates increased to 18% at 2 years.[5] Rupture is uncommon in aneurysms measuring less than 5 cm in diameter. Another risk factor for rupture seems to be an increased expansion rate, with aneurysms growing more than 5 mm in 6 months at higher risk than those growing more slowly. Survival in non-operated patients was 52% at 2 years and 17% at 5 years. Patients who underwent repair of TAAA had a 5-year survival of 50%. Another series revealed 61% 5-year survival following TAAA repair. Survival decreased to 50% for patients with dissecting TAAA.[6]

Operative repair is usually through a left thoracotomy with a paramedian abdominal extension, depending on the distal extent of the aneurysm. A retroperitoneal approach to the abdominal segment is used. The distal extent of the aneurysm determines which inter-costal space will be used for a thoracotomy. The incision is made in the fourth or fifth intercostal space for type I or high type II TAAAs, while an incision in the seventh, eighth or ninth intercostal spaces is appropriate for types III or IV.[7] Careful identification and re-implantation of visceral vessels is important, as is re-attachment of intercostal arteries when feasible. Successful repair of TAAA results from careful yet quick technique, as well as maintenance of optimal physiology by the anaesthesia and surgical teams. Distal aortic perfusion is accomplished either with left heart bypass and selective visceral perfusion or an axillary-femoral artery bypass before thoracotomy. Distal aortic perfusion manoeuvres are important for the prevention of major systemic morbidity following TAAA repair.

Patients undergoing TAAA repair frequently are older and have significant cardiac, pul-monary and other vascular comorbidities. These factors, combined with the magnitude of the operation and extent of aortic replacement, can lead to significant rates of mortality and serious morbidity. **[Q5: D]** *Pulmonary* complications remain the most common and result from a combination of preoperative tobacco use, chronic obstructive pulmonary disease (COPD), and the effect of the thoracoabdominal incision on postoperative pulmonary mechanics. Reperfusion injury may also lead to pulmonary microvascular injury and sub-sequent pulmonary dysfunction.[8] *Cardiac* complications remain the next most common, in spite of preoperative cardiac optimisation. Avoidance of hypotension, close monitoring perioperatively with pulmonary artery catheters, and minimisation of strain on the left ven-tricle can help decrease postoperative cardiac dysfunction. Using the bypass circuit to con-trol ventricular afterload can reduce the risk of cardiac complications.[9] *Renal* insufficiency preoperatively increases the risk of postoperative renal failure and mortality. Minimising ischaemic time, selective renal perfusion during cross-clamping, distal aortic perfusion techniques, and avoidance of hypovolaemia are important in preventing renal failure.[10]

Perhaps the most devastating complication following TAAA repair is *paraplegia*. Despite years of research and development of protective strategies, paraplegia rates following TAAA repair remain between 5% and 30%, with an average of 13%.[6] Risk factors for postoperative paraplegia include extent of aneurysm (and therefore most common in Type II TAAAs), cross-clamp time, postoperative hypotension, previous abdominal aortic reconstruction, and oversewing of intercostal arteries. Cross-clamp times of less than 30 min are generally safe, while those in the range of 30–60 min are associated with increasing risk; cross-clamp times of more than 60 min carry the highest risk for neurological complications. Minimizing cross-clamp time and avoiding hypotension will decrease the risk of paraplegia. Sequential reperfusion of intercostal vessels by moving the cross clamp caudally as segments are reim-planted is useful to re-establish flow to these vessels quickly. In addition, avoiding pro-longed mesenteric ischemia, which may worsen reperfusion injury to the lungs, heart and possibly spinal cord through release of cytotoxic cytokines, is beneficial.

Numerous adjuncts have been studied for their ability to prevent paraplegia. **[Q6: A]** The use of *cerebrospinal fluid (CSF) drainage* to keep CSF pressure at less than 10 mmHg has been shown to decrease the incidence of postoperative paraplegia, when combined with distal aortic perfusion and/or moderate hypothermia.[11] *Reimplantation of intercostal vessels*, particularly in the important segment of T8–T12, is most likely beneficial in preventing postoperative paraplegia, provided this manoeuvre does not excessively prolong clamp time.[12] *Epidural cooling* by continuous infusion of cool saline via catheter has been reported to decrease the incidence of paraplegia following TAAA repair in a high-volume centre.[13] *Preoperative angiographic localisation of the artery of Adamkiewicz* followed by successful *reimplantation* of this vessel during surgery has resulted in no neurological sequelae in another Centre's series.[14] Patients who did not have preoperative localisation, or in whom reimplantation was unsuccessful, had a 50% paraplegia rate. These results have not been reproduced, and angiographic localisation has not gained widespread acceptance. General anesthetic agents can also help to prevent paraplegia, with propofol being the most protective. When left heart bypass is performed using pump techniques, moderate hypothermia can be used to protect the spinal cord. Other pharmacological adjuncts that may be beneficial include steroids and mannitol. Free-radical scavengers and inhibitors of excitatory neurotransmitter pathways have shown benefit experimentally but have not been proven clinically.[15] At present, the best strategy for preventing spinal cord complications appears to involve a combination of physiological optimization of the patient perioperatively, avoidance of intra-operative hypotension, intraoperative use of spinal drainage and some form of distal aortic perfusion, reimplantation of patent intercostal vessels, and minimisation of cross-clamp time. Other protective adjuncts are used based on surgeon preference and experience.

Repair of a TAAA represents a major physiological insult. Excellent anesthesia care and post-operative critical care monitoring are essential components of a successful operation. Postoperatively, large volumes of urine output must be replaced on a 1:1 basis in order to avoid hypovolaemia. Use of warmed, balanced electrolyte solutions is preferred. **[Q7]** Coagulopathy in the postoperative period is usually related to incomplete replacement of clotting factors and hypothermia. In addition, supracoeliac aortic clamping has been shown to result in a state of fibrinolysis that may exacerbate bleeding.[17] The aneurysm itself can be responsible for chronic coagulation factor consumption and a subsequent increased tendency to perioperative coagulopathy.[18] Ongoing bleeding after TAAA repair may require reoperation, and results in an increase in major morbidity and mortality. It is important to ensure that any increased prothrombin and partial thromboplastin times are corrected with plasma transfusions. Platelets should be replaced if thrombocytopenia occurs in the face of ongoing bleeding. Since hypothermia is often used intraoperatively as a spinal cord protective measure, it may persist as a problem postoperatively. Aggressive correction with warm fluids, blood products and warming blankets is needed to restore normothermia and proper function of coagulation as well as other enzymatic systems. Reoperation is reserved for ongoing significant bleeding following correction of coagulopathy and hypothermia. Reoperation for bleeding results in mortality rates of 25% or greater in these patients.[19]

Some patients, as in the case we present here, will awake neurologically intact only to develop paraplegia hours to days later. **[Q8]** This phenomenon of delayed-onset paraplegia may represent reperfusion injury to areas of the spinal cord at risk from intraoperative hypoperfusion. Avoidance of postoperative hypoperfusion may decrease the incidence of this complication. The epidural catheter is left in place for 3 days postoperatively. In cases of delayed-onset paraplegia, maintenance of CSF pressure below 10 mmHg may permit restoration of function. There are anecdotal reports of reversal of delayed-onset paraplegia by placement of an epidural catheter after onset of paralysis and removal of CSF to decrease pressure to below 10 mmHg.[16] Lowering the CSF pressure may increase cord perfusion pressure enough to rescue the threatened regions of neuronal tissue. Lowering the CSF pressure to below 5 mmHg may cause intracerebral haemorrhage, therefore the pressure must be monitored closely and maintained in the safe range. **[Q9: B]** Patients undergoing successful TAAA repair have a 5-year survival of 50–61%[5, 6] [also please refer to discussion following **Q4**].

[Q10] Since the patient presented did not have any significant contraindications to an open thoracoabdominal repair, endovascular repair of his TAAA would not have been appropriate at this time. However, various institutional studies have demonstrated the feasibility and safety of endovascular repair of TAAAs for patients at significant risk for open repair.[20] Pre-operative planning with high-resolution, thin-cut CTA is mandatory. Fenestrated endografts may be used for treatment of juxta-renal aortic aneurysms or more extensive type IV and other TAAAs. Fenestrations are circular openings in the aortic graft fabric that are circumferentially reinforced with a nitinol ring, which is ultimately matted with a balloon-expandable stent graft into the target visceral vessel. Branched endografts are aortic endografts with side branches pre-sewn to the graft fabric; these in combination with fenestrations, help treat even the most complex TAAAs. A recent French series of 33 patients undergoing treatment of TAAAs with fenestrated and branched endografts for a variety of TAAAs types (type I [3%], II [21%], III [37%], IV [13%]) demonstrated an in-hospital mortality of 9%.[21] Type II and III endoleaks were present in 15% of patients and transient spinal cord ischemia occurred in 12% of patients, though permanent paraplegia remained in only 3%. A review of six single-institution series encompassing 496 patients with TAAAs, demonstrated a 30-day mortality of fewer than 9%, spinal cord ischemia of 2.7–20%, and remarkably high branch patency rates (96–100%). As potential loss of visceral branch vessels is a feared complication of fenestrated and branched endografts repair, mid- and long-term results with larger patient populations will be important to determine whether material fatigue and fracture, migration, and/or component separation occur. Aside from fenestrated or branched endograft repair, early follow-up demonstrated no renal of visceral branch vessel occlusion; all 109 vessels were patent in this high-volume centre single centre study.

Recently, Lachat et al. have introduced a novel hybrid open and endovascular approach that may be particularly useful for the treatment of Type IV TAAAs.[22] This technique involves placement of a self-expanding stent graft (Viabahn grafts, Gore and Associates, Flagstaff, Az) thru a retrograde Seldinger technique into the origin of the renal or visceral vessel. Using this Viabahn Open Rebranching TEChnique (VORTEC) technique, the distal end of the self-expanding stent graft is deployed in the visceral or renal vessel and partially projects outside the vessel. The proximal end of the graft is then anastomosed to the debranching graft, which may originate from a common iliac artery; the proximal stump of the visceral vessel is ligated to avoid retrograde perfusion of the aneurysm and endoleak after subsequent endovascular aneurysm repair. VORTEC may be particularly useful in re-do operations, where entire dissection of the visceral vessel is not necessary. This novel hybrid technique remains a single institution experience and more broad experience is necessary to establish reproducibility and safety.

References

1. Bickerstaff LK, Pairolero PC, Hollier LH, et al. Thoracic aortic aneurysms: a population based study. *Surgery*. 1982;92:1103-1108.
2. Panneton JM, Hollier LH. Nondissecting thoracoabdominal aortic aneurysms: part I. *Ann Vasc Surg*. 1995;9:503.
3. Crawford ES, Crawford JL, Safi HJ, et al. Thoracoabdominal aortic aneurysms: preoperative and intraoperative factors determining immediate and long term results of operations in 605 patients. *J Vasc Surg*. 1986;3:389-404.
4. Crawford ES, DeNatale RW. Thoracoabdominal aortic aneurysm: observations regarding the natural course of the disease. *J Vasc Surg*. 1986;3:578-582.
5. Cambria RA, Gloviczki P, Stanson AW, et al. Outcome and expansion rate of 57 thoracoabdominal aortic aneurysms managed nonoperatively. *Am J Surg*. 1995;170:213-217.
6. Panneton JM, Hollier LH. Dissecting descending thoracic and thoracoabdominal aortic aneurysms: Part II. *Ann Vasc Surg*. 1995;9:596-605.
7. Hollier LH. Technical modifications in the repair of thoracoabdominal aortic aneurysms. In: Greenlagh RM, ed. *Vascular Surgical Techniques*. London: W.B. Saunders; 1989:144-151.
8. Paterson IS, Klausner JM, Goldman G, et al. Pulmonary edema after aneurysm surgery is modified by mannitol. *Ann Surg*. 1989;210:796-801.
9. Hug HR, Taber RE. Bypass flow requirements during thoracic aneurysmectomy with particular attention to the prevention of left heart failure. *J Thorac Cardiovasc Surg*. 1969;57:203-213.
10. Kazui T, Komatsu S, Yokoyama H. Surgical treatment of aneurysms of the thoracic aorta with the aid of partial cardiopulmonary bypass: an analysis of 95 patients. *Ann Thorac Surg*. 1987;43:622-627.
11. Safi HJ, Miller CC 3rd, Huynh TT, et al. Distal aortic perfusion and cerebrospinal fluid drainage for thoracoabdominal and descending thoracic aortic repair: ten years of organ protection. *Ann Surg*. 2003;238:372-380.
12. Safi HJ, Estrera AL, Azizzadeh A, Coogan S, Miller CC 3rd. Progress and future challenges in thoracoabdominal aortic aneurysm management. *World J Surg*. 2008;32:355-360.
13. Black JH, Davison JK, Cambria RP. Regional hypothermia with epidural cooling for prevention of spinal cord ischemic complications after thoracoabdominal aortic surgery. *Semin Thorac Cardiovasc Surg*. 2003;15:345-352.
14. Webb TH, Williams GM. Thoracoabdominal aneurysm repair. *Cardiovasc Surg*. 1999;7:573-585.
15. Wisselink W, Money SR, Crockett DE, et al. Ischemia-reperfusion of the spinal cord: protective effect of the hydroxyl radical scavenger dimethylthiourea. *J Vasc Surg*. 1994;20:444-450.
16. Hollier LH, Money SR, Naslund TC, et al. Risk of spinal cord dysfunction in patients undergoing thoracoabdominal aortic replacement. *Am J Surg*. 1992;164:210-214.
17. Gertler JP, Cambria RP, Brewster DC, et al. Coagulation changes during thoracoabdominal aneurysm repair. *J Vasc Surg*. 1996;24:936-945.
18. Fisher DF, Yawn DH, Crawford ES. Preoperative disseminated intravascular coagulation caused by abdominal aortic aneurysm. *J Vasc Surg*. 1986;4:184-186.

19. Svensson LG, Crawford ES, Hess KR, Coselli JS, Safi HJ. Experience with 1509 patients undergoing thoracoabdominal aortic operations. *J Vasc Surg*. 1993;17:357-370.
20. D'Elia P, Tyrrell M, Sobocinski J, Azzaoui R, Koussa M, Haulon S. Endovascular thoracoabdominal aortic aneurysm repair: a literature review of early and mid-term results. *J Cardiovasc Surg*. 2009;50:439-445.
21. Haulon S, D'Elia P, O'Brien N, et al. Endovascular repair of thoracoabdominal aortic aneurysms. *Eur J Vasc Endovasc Surg*. 2009;50(4):475-481.
22. Donas KP, Lachat M, Rancic Z, et al. Early and midterm outcome of a novel technique to simplify the hybrid procedures in the treatment of thoracoabdominal and pararenal aortic aneurysms. *J Vasc Surg*. 2009;50:1280-1284.

Endovascular Management of Thoracic Aneurysm

6

Reda Jamjoom, Nasser Alkhamees, and Cherrie Z. Abraham

A 75-year-old male has been referred to your service after a contrast–enhanced spiral computed tomography (CT) performed for investigation of chronic cough revealed an incidental finding of a 7.3 cm thoracic aortic aneurysm (TAA).

Past medical history includes moderate chronic obstructive pulmonary disease (COPD), hypertension, insulin-dependent diabetes and a history of coronary artery catheterization and stenting 5 years ago. The patient denies current angina symptoms. On examination, vital signs are stable, cardio-respiratory examination is within normal limits, and arterial examination reveals no carotid bruits, normal heart sounds without murmurs, no palpable abdominal masses and all upper and lower limb distal pulses are palpable. His routine blood work is within normal range.

Question 1

What is your next investigation?

A. Ankle brachial index (ABI)
B. Contrast-enhanced computed tomography angiography (CTA) of chest, abdomen and pelvis with 3D reconstruction
C. Duplex ultrasound of the abdomen
D. Cardiac stress test

CTA was obtained (Fig. 6.1). It demonstrates a 7.3 cm saccular thoracic aortic aneurysm, beginning 3 cm distal to the subclavian artery. External iliac artery diameters are 8 mm on the right and 9 mm on the left. Due to the patient's age and medical comorbidities, endovascular repair was the sole treatment option offered to the patient, who subsequently consented to the procedure.

R. Jamjoom (✉)
McGill University, Montreal, QC, Canada

G. Geroulakos and B. Sumpio (eds.), *Vascular Surgery*,
DOI: 10.1007/978-1-84996-356-5_6, © Springer-Verlag London Limited 2011

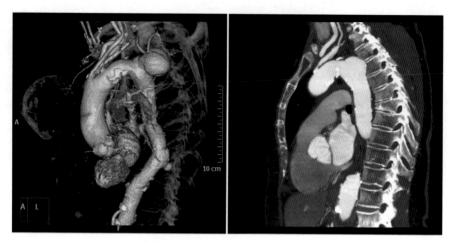

Fig. 6.1 CTA of chest demonstrating 7.3 cm TAA in size

Question 2

What are the contraindications for standard TEVAR?

A. Diseased (<7mm) external iliac artery
B. No landing zone distal to the subclavian (<2cm)
C. Concurrent abdominal aortic aneurysm
D. Circumferential thrombus in proximal and distal landing zones

Question 3

How would you position the patient in the operating room?

A. Supine with bilateral arm extension (90°)
B. Supine with left arm tucked in and right arm extended
C. Supine with both arms tucked in
D. Supine with right arm tucked in and left arm extended

Right common femoral artery exposure is performed and arterial access is gained for positioning of the extra-stiff 260–300 cm guide wire.

Question 4

Optimal distal position of the tip of the stiff wire is:

A. Distal to subclavian
B. In the left ventricle

C. Above the aortic valve

D. Proximal to subclavian

In the left groin you place a percutaneous 5Fr sheath and place the pigtail catheter in the ascending aorta.

Question 5

What are possible intra-operative complications of TEVAR?

Question 6

What are the options to induce hypotension during graft deployment to ensure accurate placement?

A. Rapid ventricular pacing

B. Administration of Adenosine

C. Administration of nitrates

D. Partial right atrial inflow balloon occlusion

Question 7

List possible methods to prevent spinal cord ischemia during and after TEVAR?

Question 8

What are the most important parameters to observe in the early postoperative period?

A. Neurological exam

B. Renal function

C. Compartment syndrome

D. Cardiac enzymes

Question 9

How would you follow up your patient postoperatively?

A. Chest X-ray and renal function at 6 weeks and every 3 month

B. CTA and renal function at 3, 6 and 12 months, then every 12 month

C. CTA and renal function every 6 month

D. Abdominal ultrasound and chest X-ray every 6 month

A 76-year old male, otherwise healthy, is sent to your clinic after an incidental finding of TAA during investigation of a possible pulmonary embolus. Subsequent CTA is ordered and is shown in Fig. 6.2

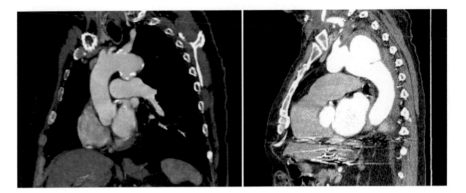

Fig. 6.2 CTA of chest demonstrating TAA 6.2 cm in size, starting just proximal to the subclavian artery. The distance between the left common carotid and left subclavian is 1.5 cm and between the left subclavian and innominate is 2.5 cm

Question 10

What is your endovascular option of treatment?

A. Direct antegrade bypass to the left common carotid artery and the subclavian artery from the ascending thoracic aorta and TEVAR
B. Right to left carotid-carotid bypass and left carotid subclavian bypass and TEVAR
C. Carotid subclavian bypass and TEVAR
D. Transposition of the subclavian to the carotid artery and TEVAR

Question 11

What is another important investigation you need to do before proceeding with your bypass?

A. MRI brain
B. ABI
C. Carotid Duplex ultrasound
D. Abdominal ultrasound

You have obtained a Carotid Duplex ultrasound that shows no significant stenosis.

Question 12

In which circumstances is left carotid subclavian bypass strongly recommended before covering the left subclavian artery?

A. Dominant left vertebral artery
B. History of CABG using LIMA
C. Covering more than 20 cm of thoracic aorta
D. Left carotid stenosis > 80%

You perform a carotid–carotid bypass and carotid–subclavian bypass with ligation of the proximal left carotid and endovascular occlusion of the subclavian artery proximal to the left vertebral artery. Two weeks later you book your patient for TEVAR under general anesthesia. Pre-deployment angiogram is demonstrated in Fig. 6.3.

Question 13

What are the advantages of staged procedures?
   You were successful with the procedure and your completion intraoperative angiogram is shown in Fig. 6.4. Patient is discharged 2 days postoperatively and booked for a follow-up CTA in 3 months.

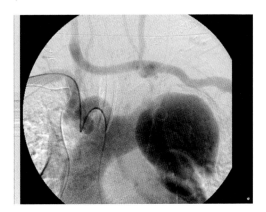

Fig. 6.3 Intraoperative angiography, demonstrating the TAA and right carotid to left carotid and subclavian bypass

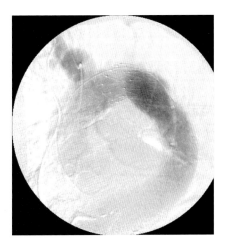

Fig. 6.4 Intraoperative completion angiography

6.1
Commentary

Parodi and associates reported the first successful endovascular aneurysm repair of an abdominal aortic aneurysm in 1991.[1] Dake et al. followed in 1994 with the first report of EVAR for a thoracic aortic aneurysm (TEVAR).[2]

TEVAR and open surgical repair (OSR) share similar indications for treatment of TAA. These indications include: TAA ≥ 6 cm, symptomatic thoracic aneurysm regardless of size, and TAA growth rate >3 mm/year.[3,4] However, whereas OSR is appropriate only for relatively physiologically fit patients, TEVAR has the advantage of being able to treat less fit patients who might otherwise be turned down for open repair. Most surgeons treating this pathology favour TEVAR as their first option given the fact that the chest cavity does not need to be opened thus avoiding the common pulmonary complications that are associated with OSR. Perhaps the most important advantage of TEVAR is that the thoracic aorta does not need to be cross-clamped. This can obviously lead to deleterious consequences in any patient with cardiac insufficiency or valvular abnormalities. Relative contraindications for standard TEVAR include inadequate proximal and distal landing zone (<2 cm in length), significant tortuosity, extensive aortic arch thrombus, and extensive calcification at the proximal and distal fixation sites.[5,6] Patient selection should be based on CTA findings, clinical presentation, and past medical history. **[Q2: A, B, D]**

Compared to OSR, TEVAR has demonstrated a reduction in 30-day mortality from 11.7% to 2.1%, decreased length of hospital stay, and a lower risk of stroke, end organ failure, spinal cord ischemia, and cardiopulmonary complications. However, TEVAR does result in a higher number of re-interventions compared to OSR, although the majority of these are minimally invasive in nature. There is no difference between TEVAR and OSR of the thoracic aorta in terms of late mortality.[7]

Preoperative cardiac investigation is indicated for patients who display active ischemic heart symptoms and signs but is not necessary in the majority of patients as balloon aortic occlusion is limited to a few seconds during the procedure. CTA is the preferred imaging modality as it demonstrates the most useful information for both planning and sizing of the endograft procedure. **[Q1: B] [Q9: B]**

In general TAA occurs in patients with advanced age who commonly have a diseased, angulated and tortuous aortic arch. For this reason, proximal fixation of the thoracic stent graft is often the greatest challenge to success. Two centimeters of normal healthy cylindrical aorta (neck) is the absolute minimum for optimal results, with a 20–30% oversizing recommended for the endoprosthesis.[3]

Positioning may vary depending on surgeon preference. The authors generally prefer the supine patient's left arm tucked in and the right arm extended. If the case is performed under C-arm fluoroscopy, and lateral views are necessary in order to identify the celiac artery for accurate distal graft placement, then positioning both arms extended is recommended to improve the lateral image. Femoral cutdown is performed on the intended side of delivery of the endoprosthesis. The authors prefer accessing the vessel through concentric double pursestring 5–0 prolene sutures of the femoral artery instead of formal arteriotomy. Contralateral percutaneous access is obtained in standard fashion. After obtaining appropriate sheath access to both femoral arteries, standard endovascular technique is used to gain access to the ascending aorta with an extra stiff double curved lunderquist wire (Cook Medical, Inc., Indiana, USA) and the distal wire tip is placed above the aortic valve. A pigtail catheter is placed via the contralateral access just proximal to the subclavian artery. The device is delivered on the stiff wire to the desired location. Digital subtraction angiography (DSA) is preformed under breath holding/apnea state. If absolute accurate positioning is required in reference to the supra-aortic vessels, induced hypotension is recommended using rapid ventricular pacing technique during deployment of the device. This is very well tolerated in the majority of cases but may be contraindicated in patients with significant cardiac insufficiency. The pigtail is retrieved with wire support. In general, we recommend compliant balloon molding of the proximal stent only in the event of obvious type I endoleak and certainly in the presence of induced hypotension to reduce the chance of migration. [Q3: B] [Q4: C]

Permissive hypotension is a technique that permits accurate device deployment, as well as avoiding migration during balloon molding. It can be accomplished by permissive "low grade" hypotension during the deployment and molding balloon phase with the help of nitrates.[8] Acute short acting hypotension can be achieved by the use of adenosine, which usually results in resumption of normotension within seconds of hypotension but can often be unpredictable.[9,10] The authors prefer rapid ventricular pacing which is safe, reliable, and short acting with resumption of normotension usually occurring only a few seconds after turning off the pacing device.[11–13] [Q6: A, B, D]

TEVAR devices generally require a large-profile delivery system ranging in size 22-27 French (Fr). This clearly necessitates the presence of large, femoral-iliac arteries and represents a significant contributor to the risks of access vessel injury. Access vessel injury is the most significant cause of serious morbidity and mortality. The most common site of rupture is the proximal external iliac artery. Iliac accessibility can often be tested with careful use of endovascular dilators, which should clarify the issue of whether the operator should attempt transfemoral introduction or proceed to an iliac conduit.[14] As an alternative to conduit placement, the authors prefer directly accessing the common iliac vessel through double concentric 4–0 prolene sutures. Other intra-operative complications include aortic rupture, dissection, aortic branch vessel occlusions, and lower extremity embolism. During deployment, the utmost care should be exercised to avoid an unnecessary windsock effect that may, in some cases, lead to instability or even migration or displacement of the proximal end of the device. This undesirable consequence may be avoided by continuous fluoroscopic visualization during deployment, permissive hypotension techniques described, and the use of devices with modifications designed to counter this effect such as the newest generation Cook TX2 thoracic device. Severely angulated aortic arches can often lead to non-apposition of the inferior aortic wall with the fabric of the proximal covered stent leading to the characteristic "Birds Beak" appearance on angiography with possible consequential type I endoleak. This issue appears to be resolved with a technological modification of the Cook TX2 thoracic graft with Cook's most recent generation TX2 Pro-Form graft.

Post-implantation syndrome can sometimes occur with transient elevation of body temperature and C-reactive protein with mild leukocytosis. This phenomenon is often observed in cases of large segment coverage and the use of multiple devices and/or extensions.[2,15]

Stroke has been identified as a common complication of TEVAR, with an incidence ranging from 0% to 8%. Risk factors for stroke include history of preoperative stroke, CT grade IV atheroma (5 mm) in the aortic arch, proximal descending aorta coverage, and long segment coverage.[16] **[Q5]**

TEVAR is also associated with a 3–6% incidence of spinal cord ischemia. Risk factors for spinal cord ischemia include prior abdominal aortic repair, length of thoracic aortic coverage, hypogastric artery interruption, subclavian artery coverage, emergent repair, intra-operative hemorrhage and sustained hypotension.[17–20]

Coverage of the thoracic aorta may be categorized as in Fig. 6.5 below.

A-coverage from the origin of the left subclavian artery to the T6 vertebral level, B-coverage from T6 to the diaphragm and C-coverage of the entire descending thoracic aorta from the left subclavian artery to the diaphragm.[20,21] This can often be helpful in conveying spinal cord ischemia risk to patients and their families. Category C obviously has the highest risk of paraplegia (5–10%).

With respect to post-procedural care, all patients should be transferred to a monitored setting postoperatively. Multiple parameters should be monitored closely. Most importantly, blood pressure should be controlled (MAP>80 mmHg), avoiding high blood pressure (SBP>160) to minimize the chance of stent migration as well as hypertensive medical complications such as stroke. Urine output should be recorded, and regular neurological assessment should be carried out to assess for stroke and spinal cord ischemia. Patients with cerebrospinal fluid (CSF) drains should have continuous CSF pressure monitoring and CSF should be drained according to a standardized protocol.[22,23] **[Q7] [Q8: A, B, C, D]**

Case number 2 describes a situation in which there is inadequate length of healthy aorta distal to the left carotid artery for an adequate seal. A hybrid procedure consisting of extra-anatomic bypass (right to left carotid-carotid bypass with or without a left carotid-subclavian bypass) and TEVAR was chosen as the treatment option.[24] Recently, technological innovation has demonstrated the possibility of circumventing debranching

Extent A
(L. subclavian a. to T6)

Extent B
(T6 to diaphragm)

Extent C
(L. subclavian a. to diaphragm)

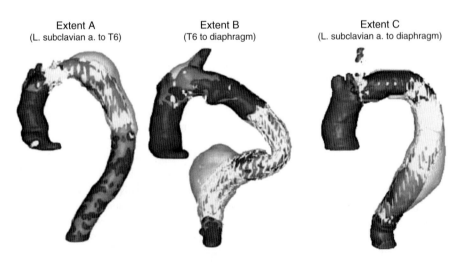

Fig. 6.5 Extent of aortic coverage during TEVAR

procedures with fenestrated/scalloped and branched arch grafts. However, further cases and published case series are necessary before these procedures become ready for prime time. **[Q10: A, B]**

If extra-anatomic bypass is being considered for aortic arch debranching, carotid duplex ultrasound is mandatory to assess for occlusive disease as well as vertebral artery flow dynamics. Carotid endarterectomy may need to be performed in conjunction with the bypass. **[Q11: C]**

In some instances, it is acceptable to cover the origin of the subclavian artery with the thoracic aortic stent graft without subclavian revascularization, however carotid-subclavian bypass should be considered in patients who have radiological evidence of a dominant left vertebral artery and in patients who demonstrated the following: aberrant origin of the left vertebral artery, history of CABG using the left internal mammary artery, history of AAA repair, occluded or diseased hypogastric arteries, patent left axillary-femoral bypass graft, functional left arm arteriovenous fistula, and in any patients who require long segment coverage with TEVAR (B, C extent).[16,25] **[Q12: A. B, C]**

The authors prefer staging the extra-anatomic debranching procedures when possible. Advantages to this method include minimizing operative time, and identifying the etiology of potential neurological complications after each procedure. **[Q13]**

References

1. Parodi JC, Palmaz JC, Barone HD. Transfemoral intraluminal graft implantation for abdominal aortic aneurysms. *Ann Vasc Surg.* (Nov) 1991;5(6):491-499.
2. Dake MD, Miller DC, Semba CP, Mitchell RS, Walker PJ, Liddell RP. Transluminal placement of endovascular stent-grafts for the treatment of descending thoracic aortic aneurysms. *N Engl J Med.* (Dec 29) 1994;331(26):1729-1734.
3. Katzen BT, Dake MD, MacLean AA, Wang DS. Endovascular repair of abdominal and thoracic aortic aneurysms. *Circulation.* (Sept 13) 2005;112(11):1663-1675.
4. Cambria RP, Crawford RS, Cho JS, et al. A multicenter clinical trial of endovascular stent graft repair of acute catastrophes of the descending thoracic aorta. *J Vasc Surg.* (Dec) 2009;50(6):1255-1264. e1251-1254.
5. Jones LE. Endovascular stent grafting of thoracic aortic aneurysms: technological advancements provide an alternative to traditional surgical repair. *J Cardiovasc Nurs.* (Nov–Dec) 2005;20(6):376-384.
6. Patel HJ, Williams DM, Upchurch GR Jr, et al. A comparison of open and endovascular descending thoracic aortic repair in patients older than 75 years of age. *Ann Thorac Surg.* (May) 2008;85((5):1597-1603. discussion 1603-1594.
7. Ueda T, Fleischmann D, Rubin GD, Dake MD, Sze DY. Imaging of the thoracic aorta before and after stent-graft repair of aneurysms and dissections. *Semin Thorac Cardiovasc Surg.* (Winter) 2008;20(4):348-357.
8. Bernard EO, Schmid ER, Lachat ML, Germann RC. Nitroglycerin to control blood pressure during endovascular stent-grafting of descending thoracic aortic aneurysms. *J Vasc Surg.* (Apr) 2000;31(4):790-793.
9. Dorros G, Cohn JM. Adenosine-induced transient cardiac asystole enhances precise deployment of stent-grafts in the thoracic or abdominal aorta. *J Endovasc Surg.* (Aug) 1996;3(3):270-272.

10. Kahn RA, Moskowitz DM, Marin ML, et al. Safety and efficacy of high-dose adenosine-induced asystole during endovascular AAA repair. *J Endovasc Ther.* (Aug) 2000;7(4):292-296.

11. Pornratanarangsi S, Webster MW, Alison P, Nand P. Rapid ventricular pacing to lower blood pressure during endograft deployment in the thoracic aorta. *Ann Thorac Surg.* (May) 2006;81(5):e21-23.

12. David F, Sanchez A, Yanez L, et al. Cardiac pacing in balloon aortic valvuloplasty. *Int J Cardiol.* (Apr 4) 2007;116(3):327-330.

13. Webb JG, Pasupati S, Achtem L, Thompson CR. Rapid pacing to facilitate transcatheter prosthetic heart valve implantation. *Catheter Cardiovasc Interv.* (Aug) 2006;68(2):199-204.

14. Criado FJ. Iliac arterial conduits for endovascular access: technical considerations. *J Endovasc Ther.* (Jun) 2007;14(3):347-351.

15. Criado FJ, Barnatan MF, Rizk Y, Clark NS, Wang CF. Technical strategies to expand stent-graft applicability in the aortic arch and proximal descending thoracic aorta. *J Endovasc Ther.* 2002;9(Suppl 2):II32-38.

16. Gutsche JT, Szeto W, Cheung AT. Endovascular stenting of thoracic aortic aneurysm. *Anesthesiol Clin.* (Sept) 2008;26(3):481-499.

17. Buth J, Harris PL, Hobo R, et al. Neurologic complications associated with endovascular repair of thoracic aortic pathology: incidence and risk factors. A study from the European Collaborators on Stent/Graft Techniques for Aortic Aneurysm Repair (EUROSTAR) registry. *J Vasc Surg.* (Dec) 2007;46(6):1103-1110. discussion 1110-1101.

18. Chiesa R, Melissano G, Marrocco-Trischitta MM, Civilini E, Setacci F. Spinal cord ischemia after elective stent-graft repair of the thoracic aorta. *J Vasc Surg.* (Jul) 2005;42(1):11-17.

19. Kawaharada N, Morishita K, Kurimoto Y, et al. Spinal cord ischemia after elective endovascular stent-graft repair of the thoracic aorta. *Eur J Cardiothorac Surg.* (Jun) 2007;31(6): 998-1003. discussion 1003.

20. Gutsche JT, Cheung AT, McGarvey ML, et al. Risk factors for perioperative stroke after thoracic endovascular aortic repair. *Ann Thorac Surg.* (Oct) 2007;84(4)):1195-1200. discussion 1200.

21. Feezor RJ, Martin TD, Hess PJ Jr, et al. Extent of aortic coverage and incidence of spinal cord ischemia after thoracic endovascular aneurysm repair. *Ann Thorac Surg.* (Dec) 2008;86(6): 1809-1814. discussion 1814.

22. Estrera AL, Miller CC 3rd, Chen EP, et al. Descending thoracic aortic aneurysm repair: 12-year experience using distal aortic perfusion and cerebrospinal fluid drainage. *Ann Thorac Surg.* (Oct) 2005;80(4):1290-1296. discussion 1296.

23. Hnath JC, Mehta M, Taggert JB, et al. Strategies to improve spinal cord ischemia in endovascular thoracic aortic repair: outcomes of a prospective cerebrospinal fluid drainage protocol. *J Vasc Surg.* (Oct) 2008;48(4):836-840.

24. Cina CS, Safar HA, Lagana A, Arena G, Clase CM. Subclavian carotid transposition and bypass grafting: consecutive cohort study and systematic review. *J Vasc Surg.* (Mar) 2002;35(3):422-429.

25. Feezor RJ, Lee WA. Management of the left subclavian artery during TEVAR. *Semin Vasc Surg.* (Sept) 2009;22(3):159-164.

Aortic Dissection

7

Barbara Theresia Weis-Müller and Wilhelm Sandmann

7.1
Dissection: Stanford A

A 68-year-old woman spontaneously and suddenly developed severe retrosternal pain during her holiday in Turkey. Without knowing the diagnosis, she flew home 2 days later. Computed tomography (CT) scans taken immediately after arrival revealed a dissection of the ascending aorta, the aortic bow and the descending aorta.

Question 1

How would you classify the aortic dissection?

A. Stanford A dissection.
B. Stanford B dissection.
C. de Bakey I dissection.
D. de Bakey II dissection.
E. de Bakey III dissection

On the same day, she underwent an emergency operation. The dissected ascending aorta with the entry of dissection was incised in a cardiopulmonary bypass and replaced by a graft using the in-graft technique. The aortic valve was patent and remained in situ. For reconstruction of the aortic root, the sandwich technique was used. Two Teflon strips were placed externally and into the true lumen to reattach the dissected membrane to the aortic wall. The aortic graft was then sutured into the reconstructed aortic root.

B.T. Weis-Müller (✉)
Department of Vascular Surgery and Kidney Transplantation, University Clinic of Düsseldorf, Düsseldorf, Germany

G. Geroulakos and B. Sumpio (eds.), *Vascular Surgery*,
DOI: 10.1007/978-1-84996-356-5_7, © Springer-Verlag London Limited 2011

Question 2

Which of the following statements are wrong?

A. Stanford A dissections should be treated medically.
B. Stanford A dissections should undergo operation immediately.
C. Stanford B dissections without ischemic complications should be treated medically.
D. Stanford B dissections require operative intervention immediately.
E. Stanford A dissections require an aortic stent graft immediately.

The postoperative course was uneventful at the beginning. However, 3 days later, renal function deteriorated and the patient required haemofiltration. Moreover, the patient developed severe hypertension and had to be treated with three different antihypertensive drugs. Contrast CT scans revealed that the right kidney was without function due to an old hydronephrosis, while the left renal artery was probably dissected. Furthermore, the patient developed left leg ischemia and was transferred to our centre. We explored the abdomen via the transperitoneal approach. The pulsation of the left iliac artery was weak due to aortic and left iliac dissection. Infrarenal aorto-iliac membrane resection was performed to restore the blood flow to the extremities. Then the left renal artery was explored; the renal artery dissection was found to extend towards the hilus of the kidney.

Revascularisation was achieved with a saphenous vein interposition graft placed between the left iliac artery and the distal left renal artery (Fig. 7.1).

Question 3

Which of the following statements are correct?

A. Complications of Stanford A dissection are aortic valve insufficiency and perforation into the pericardium.
B. Stroke is a typical complication of Stanford B dissection.
C. Paraplegia is a typical complication of aortic dissection.
D. Most patients with Stanford B dissections die of aortic perforation.
E. Typical complications of aortic dissection are organ and lower-extremity ischaemia.

The postoperative course was uneventful. The patient recovered promptly from the operative intervention, while renal function and blood pressure improved substantially. Urine production and laboratory findings became normal, and only one antihypertensive drug (a beta-blocker) was necessary to maintain normal blood pressure. The postoperative angiography showed a patent iliac-renal interposition graft and normal perfusion of the left kidney (Fig. 7.1). CT scans taken 2 years later displayed a hypertrophic, well-functioning left kidney, while the right kidney was small and hydronephrotic (Fig. 7.2).

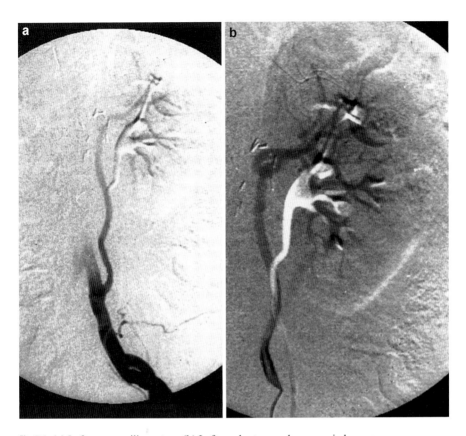

Fig. 7.1 (**a**) Left common iliac artery. (**b**) Left renal artery saphenous vein bypass

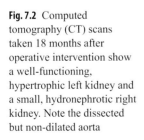

Fig. 7.2 Computed tomography (CT) scans taken 18 months after operative intervention show a well-functioning, hypertrophic left kidney and a small, hydronephrotic right kidney. Note the dissected but non-dilated aorta

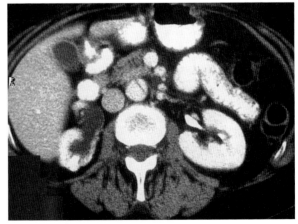

7.2
Dissection: Stanford B

A 54-year-old woman was admitted to another hospital with the provisional diagnosis of a myocardial infarction (MI). She experienced a sudden chest pain. Some hours later, she developed paraesthesia in both legs, which improved spontaneously. Subsequently, she felt abdominal discomfort and developed diarrhoea and vomiting. The patient had been normotensive throughout her life, but now she required five different antihypertensive drugs to stabilise blood pressure. Some laboratory data were abnormal, including leucocytes, transaminases, lactic dehydrogenase and lactate. Duplex sonography and transoesophageal echocardiography revealed an aortic dissection of the thoracic and abdominal aorta beginning distal to the left subclavian artery; blood flow into the visceral arteries and the right renal artery was reduced. Contrast CT scans confirmed Stanford B aortic dissection.

Question 4

What diagnostic methods are involved in acute aortic dissection?

A. Computed tomography.
B. Magnet resonance imaging.
C. Angiography.
D. Transoesophageal echocardiography.

The patient was first treated medically with parenteral therapy and antihypertensive drugs (including beta-blockers). Under this management, clinical outcome and laboratory findings improved, but 3 weeks later the patient deteriorated again and developed severe right upper abdominal pain.

She was referred to our hospital for operation. CT scans displayed the aortic dissection and a dissected superior mesenteric artery. The true aortic lumen was very small and partially thrombosed (Fig. 7.3). Abdominal exploration via the transperitoneal approach revealed borderline ischaemia of all intra-abdominal organs due to aortic dissection. The dissection had affected the coeliac trunk, the superior mesenteric artery and the right renal artery. The right upper abdominal pain was caused by an ischaemic cholecystitis. The gallbladder had to be removed. The para-aortic tissue displayed severe inflammation; therefore no fenestration and membrane resection could be carried out. Instead, intestinal and renal blood flow was restored by a 12-mm Dacron graft, which was placed end to side into the left iliac artery and end to end to the coeliac trunk. The superior mesenteric artery was implanted directly into the Dacron graft, while the right renal artery was attached by means of a saphenous vein interposition graft (Fig. 7.4).

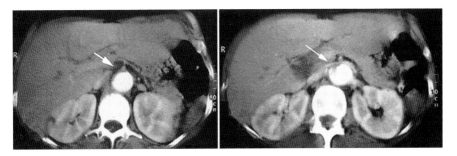

Fig. 7.3 Aortic dissection, with a small, partially thrombosed "true" aortic lumen and dissected superior mesenteric artery

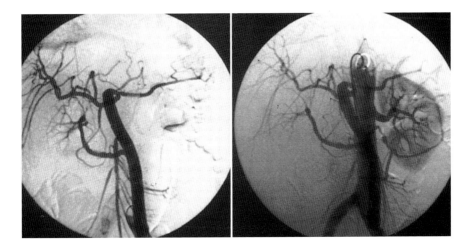

Fig. 7.4 Extra-anatomical reconstruction with a Dacron graft, which was placed end to side between the left common iliac artery and end to end to the coeliac trunk. The superior mesenteric artery was implanted directly into the graft, while the right renal artery was implanted via the interposition of a saphenous vein. The left renal artery originates from the aorta

Question 5

What techniques are used to restore blood flow to the visceral organs and extremities following ischaemia from aortic dissection? Which of the following statements are wrong?

A. Aortic stent graft.
B. Percutaneous transluminal angioplasty (PTA) of organ and limb arteries and stenting.
C. Aortic fenestration and membrane resection.
D. Cardiopulmonary bypass.
E. Extra-anatomic revascularisation, e.g. axillo-femoral bypass.

The complication of postoperative retroperitoneal bleeding from the reconstructed right renal artery had to be managed by relaparotomy and single vascular stitches, and clinical recovery was delayed. The patient required 4 months of rehabilitation until she had regained her previous health status. At this point, digestion and renal function had recovered, laboratory findings became normal, and hypertension had to be treated with only one drug (beta-blocker). Postoperative angiographies showed good perfusion of all visceral and renal arteries via the Dacron graft (Fig. 7.4).

7.3
Commentary

The life-threatening aortic dissection starts with an intimal tear (entry) in the ascending aorta (Stanford A, de Bakey I or II) or distally to the left subclavian artery (Stanford B, de Bakey III). De Bakey II dissection affects the ascending aorta only, while de Bakey I and III dissections also involve the descending aorta.[1, 2] **[Q1: A, C]** Most patients with acute aortic dissection present with severe chest pain, which might be misinterpreted as acute MI.[3,4]

Echocardiography, particularly by the transoesophageal approach, is a reliable and rapid method for diagnosis of aortic dissection and differentiation into Stanford A or B type.[5] Nevertheless, the evaluation of organ arteries and their blood flow by ultrasound may be difficult in acute dissection. In our opinion, contrast thoracic and abdominal CT scans, especially using the spiral technique, are appropriate diagnostic methods for determining the extension of dissection and the relation of its dissecting membrane to major branches of the aorta. The perfusion of abdominal organs, and often of their arteries, can be seen easily. In the case of organ malperfusion, angiography may be helpful to determine whether the ischaemia is caused by the dissecting membrane of the aorta or whether the dissection extends into the organ arteries.[6] Magnetic resonance imaging (MRI) or magnetic resonance angiography (MRA) are effective alternatives in the diagnosis of patients with dissection and renal failure.[7] **[Q4: A–D]**

Without treatment, the prognosis of acute aortic dissection is very poor. In 1958, Hirst et al. reviewed 505 cases of aortic dissection and found that 21% of patients died within 24 h of onset and only 20% survived the first month.[3] Causes of death in patients with Stanford A dissection include intrapericardial and free intrapleural rupture, acute aortic valve insufficiency, and, to a minor extent, cerebral and coronary malperfusion. In patients with type B dissections, free rupture of the aorta is less frequent. Dissection of the descending aorta may lead, in about 30% of cases, to obstruction of visceral, renal and extremity arteries, resulting in visceral ischaemia, renal insufficiency and acute limb ischaemia, which may be lethal without prompt and adequate therapy.[8–10] **[Q3: A, C, E]**

To improve the natural course of the disease, in 1955 de Bakey et al. started to treat acute aortic dissections surgically. Within only a few years, they had developed the current principles of operative intervention in acute Stanford A dissection with replacement of the ascending aorta by a graft in cardiopulmonary arrest. Their results were outstanding, with an overall mortality of 21%.[1,11]

However, the surgical experiences of other workgroups were not so successful. Therefore, Wheat et al. developed a new medical treatment with ganglionic blockers, sodium nitroprusside or beta-blockers to influence the hydrodynamic forces of the bloodstream based on the theory that blood pressure and the steepness of the pulse wave are propagating the dissecting haematoma.[12] In 1979, a meta-analysis of 219 patients with acute aortic dissection from six centres revealed that Stanford A patients treated medically had a mortality of 74%, whereas 70% of patients survived after surgical therapy. On the other hand, in patients with acute type B dissection, drug therapy alone had a survival rate of 80%, whereas 50% died after operative intervention.[13] Therefore in most centres, current therapy for acute dissection type Stanford A is surgical,[14–17] and for uncomplicated Stanford B dissection it is medical.[18–22] **[Q2: A, D, E]**

An acute dissection, involving the ascending aorta, should be considered a surgical emergency. The aim of operative intervention is to prevent or treat dilation or rupture of the aortic root, and to maintain aortic valve function. The following reconstructive approach is recommended: in patients in whom the root is not involved by dissection, a tubular graft is anastomosed to the sinotubular ridge. In the presence of commissural detachment, the valve is resuspended before supra-commissural graft insertion. If the aortic valve is affected by congenital or acquired abnormalities, then it is generally replaced.[15]

Patients with acute uncomplicated Stanford B dissection should be treated medically. Careful monitoring is obligatory, while antihypertensive drugs, such as beta-blockers,[23] and analgesics are administered. The aim of treatment is to stabilise the dissected aortic wall within 2 weeks and to prevent further extension of dissection or perforation. Careful clinical and laboratory examinations are necessary to detect symptoms of organ or extremity malperfusion in time. Limb, renal and visceral ischaemia can be observed frequently, but paraplegia due to malperfusion of intercostal arteries is rare.[6, 8–10]

If peripheral vascular complications occur, several therapeutic strategies are possible. Newer publications describe endovascular procedures, for example emergency aortic stenting to close the "entry" and the false aortic lumen.[24–27] Ultrasound-guided endovascular catheter aortic membrane fenestration was performed to restore the blood flow to the aortic branches. Dilation and stenting of dissected organ or iliac arteries were performed to resolve stenosis and restore blood flow.[28–30] These new therapeutic methods need to be evaluated in long-term follow-up.

Aortic surgery in the acute stage of aortic dissection is a dangerous procedure. The dissected aortic wall is extremely friable and does not hold sutures well. Therefore we, and many other centres, try to leave the aorta itself untouched and to restore organ or extremity blood flow by extra-anatomical bypass procedures. Extra-anatomical revascularisation also becomes necessary if the aortic branches themselves are dissected.[6, 8, 15] Normally, we use one common iliac artery as the donor vessel for extra-anatomical bypass grafting, but the distal lumbar aorta might also be suitable. If only one aortic branch requires revascularisation, then the iliac-visceral bypass is performed with the saphenous vein (Fig. 7.1). If two or more branches are affected, then a Dacron graft is used and the visceral arteries can be implanted into the graft directly or via interposition of the saphenous vein (Fig. 7.4). Blood flow to the legs can be restored with a femoral-femoral crossover bypass or with an axillo-(bi)-femoral graft. If several organ arteries are occluded by the aortic dissecting membrane, and the visceral arteries are undissected, then abdominal aortic fenestration and membrane resection combined with thrombectomy of the organ arteries can also be performed.[31-34] We prefer the latter to treat paraplegia caused by acute aortic dissection. [Q5: D]

Our only indication for total aortic replacement in the acute stage of dissection is aortic penetration or perforation.

References

1. De Bakey ME, Henly WS, Cooley DA, et al. Surgical management of dissecting aneurysm of the aorta. *J Thorac Cardiovasc Surg*. 1965;49:130.
2. Daily PO, Trueblood HW, Stinson EB, Wuerflein RD, Shumway NE. Management of acute aortic dissections. *Ann Thorac Surg*. 1970;10:237-47.
3. Hirst AE, Johns VJ, Kime SW. Dissecting aneurysm of the aorta: a review of 505 cases. *Medicine*. 1958;37:217.
4. De Bakey ME, McCollum CH, Crawford ES, et al. Dissection and dissecting aneurysms of the aorta: twenty year follow up of five hundred twenty seven patients treated surgically. *Surgery*. 1982;92:1118-34.
5. Nienaber CA, von Kodolitsch Y, Nicolas V, et al. The diagnosis of thoracic aortic dissection by non-invasive imaging procedures. *N Engl J Med*. 1993;328:1-9.
6. Müller BT, Grabitz K, Fürst G, Sandmann W. Die akute Aortendissektion: Diagnostik und Therapie von ischämischen Komplikationen. *Chirurg*. 2000;71:209.
7. Nienaber CA, von Kodolitsch Y. Bildgebende Diagnostik der Aortenerkrankungen. *Radiologie*. 1997;37:402.
8. Cambria RP, Brewster DC, Gertler J, et al. Vascular complications associated with spontaneous aortic dissection. *J Vasc Surg*. 1988;7:199-209.
9. Da Gama AD. The surgical management of aortic dissection: from university to diversity, a continuous challenge. *J Cardiovasc Surg*. 1991;32:141.
10. Fann JI, Sarris GE, Mitchell RS, et al. Treatment of patients with aortic dissection presenting with peripheral vascular complications. *Ann Surg*. 1990;212:705-713.
11. De Bakey ME, Cooley DA, Creech O. Surgical considerations of dissecting aneurysm of the aorta. *Ann Surg*. 1955;142:586.
12. Wheat MW, Palmer RF, Bartley TD, Seelmann RC. Treatment of dissecting aneurysm of the aorta without surgery. *J Thorac Cardiovasc Surg*. 1965;49:364.
13. Wheat MW, Wheat MD Jr. Acute dissecting aneurysms of the aorta: diagnosis and treatment. *Am Heart J*. 1979;99:373.
14. Borst HG, Laas J, Frank G, Haverich A. Surgical decision making in acute aortic dissection type A. *Thorac Cardiovasc Surg*. 1987;35:134.
15. Borst HG, Heinemann MK, Stone CD. Indications for surgery. In: *Surgical Treatment of Aortic Dissection*. New York: Churchill Livingstone; 1996:103.
16. Heinemann M, Borst HG. Kardiovaskuläre Erkrankungen des Marfan Syndroms. *Dt ärztebl*. 1996;93B:934.
17. Vecht RJ, Bestermann EMM, Bromley LL, Eastcott HHG. Acute dissection of the aorta: long term review and management. *Lancet*. 1980;i:109.
18. Bavaria JE, Brinster DR, Gorman RC, et al. Advances in the treatment of acute type A dissection: an integrated approach. *Ann Thorac Surg*. 2002;74:S1848.
19. Vecht RJ, Bestermann EMM, Bromley LL, Eastcott HHG. Acute aortic dissection: historical perspective and current management. *Am Heart J*. 1981;102:1087.

20. Fradet G, Jamieson WR, Janusz MT, et al. Aortic dissection: a six year experience with 17 patients. *Am J Surg*. 1988;155:697-700.
21. Glower DD, Speier RH, White WD. Management and long-term outcome of aortic dissection. *Ann J Surg*. 1990;214:31.
22. Hashimoto A, Kimata S, Hosada S. Acute aortic dissection: a comparison between the result of medical and surgical treatments. *Jpn Circ J*. 1991;55:821.
23. Shores J, Berger KR, Murphy EA, Pyeritz R. Progression of aortic dilatation and the benefit of long-term beta-adrenergic blockade in Marfan's syndrome. *N Engl J Med*. 1994;330:1335.
24. Nienaber CA, Fattori R, Lund G, et al. Nonsurgical reconstruction of thoracic aortic dissection by stent-graft replacement. *N Engl J Med*. 1999;340:1539-1545.
25. Dake MD, Kato N, Mitchell RS, et al. Endovascular stent-graft replacement for treatment of acute aortic dissection. *N Engl J Med*. 1999;340:1546.
26. Leurs LJ, Bell R, Drieck Y, et al. Endovascular treatment of thoracic aortic diseases: combined experience from EUROSTAR and United Kingdom thoracic Endograft registries. *J Vasc Surg*. 2004;40:670-680.
27. Hansen CJ, Bui H, Donayre CE. Complications of endovascular repair of high-risk and emergent descending thoracic aortic aneurysms and dissections. *J Vasc Surg*. 2004;40:228-234.
28. Chavan A, Hausmann D, Dresler C, et al. Intravasal ultrasound guided percutaneous fenestration of the intimal flap in the dissected aorta. *Circulation*. 1997;96:2124-2127.
29. Farber A, Gmelin E, Heinemann M. Transfemorale Fensterung und Stentimplantation bei aorto-ili-akaler Dissektion. *Vasa*. 1995;24:389.
30. Slonim SM, Nyman U, Semba CP, Miller DC, Mitchell RS, Dake MD. Aortic dissection: percutaneous management of ischemic complications with endovascular stents and balloon fenestration. *J Vasc Surg*. 1996;23:241-251.
31. Gurin D, Bulmer JW, Derby R. Dissecting aneurysm of the aorta: diagnosis of operative relief of acute arterial obstruction due to this cause. *NY State J Med*. 1935;35:1200.
32. Elefteriades JA, Hammond GL, Gusberg RJ, Kopf GS, Baldwin JC. Fenestration revisited. A safe and effective procedure of descending aortic dissection. *Arch Surg*. 1990;125:786-790.
33. Harms J, Hess U, Cavallaro A, Naundorf M, Maurer PC. The abdominal aortic fenestration procedure in acute thoraco-abdominal aortic dissection with aortic branch artery ischemia. *J Cardiovasc Surg (Torino)*. 1998;39:273-280.
34. Webb TH, Williams GM. Abdominal aortic tailoring for renal, visceral and lower extremity mal-perfusion resulting from acute aortic dissection. *J Vasc Surg*. 1997;26:474.

Popliteal Artery Aneurysms

8

Susanna Shin and Michel Makaroun

A 62-year-old male patient presented to the emergency department with a cool right foot. On examination, his femoral pulse is intact and a pulsatile mass is appreciated in the popliteal fossa. His right foot is cool but motor and sensory function are intact. No pedal pulses are palpable and faint Doppler signals are audible.

Question 1

The presence of a popliteal artery aneurysm increases a patient's risk for:

A. Contralateral popliteal artery aneurysm
B. Infra-renal abdominal aortic aneurysm
C. Other peripheral artery aneurysms
D. All of the above

Question 2

Which of the following is the initial diagnostic test of choice for popliteal artery aneurysm?

A. Magnetic resonance imaging
B. Contrast arteriography
C. Duplex ultrasonography
D. Computed tomography angiography

Duplex ultrasonography demonstrates giant bilateral popliteal artery aneurysms and a 4.5 cm infra-renal abdominal aortic aneurysm. A computed tomography (CT) angiogram is obtained to further evaluate the aortic aneurysm and both lower extremities are included (Fig. 8.1). The right (symptomatic) popliteal artery aneurysm is resected through a posterior approach with the ipsilateral greater saphenous vein used as an interposition graft. After his recovery from this repair, the same approach is used to repair the contralateral aneurysm.

S. Shin (✉)
Division of Vascular Surgery, University of Pittsburgh Medical Center, Pittsburgh, PA, USA

G. Geroulakos and B. Sumpio (eds.), *Vascular Surgery*,
DOI: 10.1007/978-1-84996-356-5_8, © Springer-Verlag London Limited 2011

Fig. 8.1 Computed tomography angiogram demonstrating bilateral giant popliteal artery aneurysms

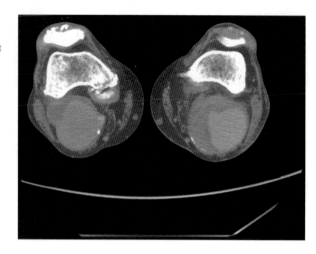

Question 3

Popliteal aneurysms can present with

A. Distal embolization
B. Acute thrombosis
C. Swelling from venous compression
D. Asymptomatic

Question 4

Emergent repair of popliteal artery aneurysms results in similar graft patency and limb preservation when compared to elective repair.

A. True
B. False

An 82-year-old female patient is referred for evaluation of a right blue second toe. She complains of a painful toe that has been blue for quite some time. On examination, her femoral pulse is intact with a prominent popliteal pulse on the right with thready pedal pulses bilaterally. A duplex ultrasound demonstrates a 2.0 cm popliteal artery aneurysm with 3–4 cm of normal artery proximal and distal to the aneurysm. The left popliteal artery is normal in size without thrombus. A CT angiogram is obtained and confirms a partially thrombosed 2.0 cm popliteal artery aneurysm (Fig. 8.2). The patient has a history of CAD, CHF with a left ventricular ejection fraction of 25%. The right lower extremity angiogram shows the runoff (Fig. 8.3).

Fig. 8.2 Computed tomography angiogram demonstrat-
ing a 2.0 cm right popliteal
artery aneurysm that is
partially thrombosed

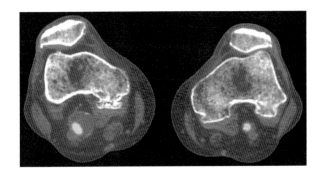

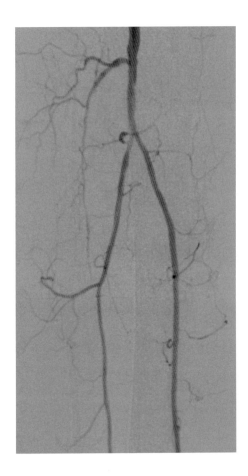

Fig. 8.3 Diagnostic angiogram demonstrating three-vessel distal runoff

Question 5

Which of the following are acceptable options in the treatment of a popliteal artery aneurysm?

A. Thrombolytics followed by ligation and bypass of an acutely thrombosed aneurysm
B. Resection and interposition vein graft of an aneurysm causing local compressive symptoms
C. Endovascular stent graft of an aneurysm in a 78-year-old COPD patient with severe CAD
D. Thrombectomy alone of an acutely thrombosed aneurysm

This patient is at high risk for operative repair of the popliteal artery aneurysm and endovascular exclusion would offer her better peri-operative morbidity and mortality. The anatomy of her aneurysm is acceptable for endovascular repair with adequate landing zones proximal and distal to the aneurysm with three-vessel runoff. A 6 mm (diameter) by 10 cm (long) stent graft is placed in the popliteal artery to exclude the aneurysm. Completion angiogram demonstrates preserved runoff and no kinking of the stent graft with the knee bent (Fig. 8.4).

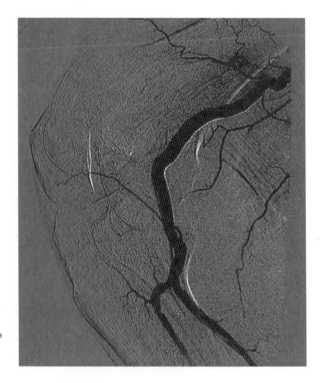

Fig. 8.4 Completion angiogram demonstrating no kinking with the knee bent and preserved runoff

8.1
Popliteal Artery Aneurysm

Popliteal artery aneurysms are the most common peripheral artery aneurysm. The popliteal artery is considered aneurysmal at a diameter of 1.5 cm and complications usually occur once the aneurysm grows to 2 cm or greater. Atherosclerosis is the primary underlying pathology in the formation of most popliteal artery aneurysms and they affect a predictable population, occurring most often in men in their 60s and 70s.[1–4] The presence of a popliteal artery aneurysm increases the risk for other aneurysms; 36–54% are bilateral and 25–54% occur synchronously with infrarenal abdominal aortic aneurysms.[1–6] **[Q1: D]** Diagnosis of a popliteal artery aneurysm is suspected with the detection of a prominent pulse or pulsatile mass in the popliteal fossa on physical exam. This is confirmed with duplex ultrasonography which can differentiate the aneurysmal segment from other masses in the popliteal fossa and demonstrate mural thrombus. **[Q2: C]** Angiography can be an important adjunctive exam to determine distal run-off in preparation for surgical repair. Although a significant percentage of these aneurysms are diagnosed incidentally, the majority (58–71%) of popliteal artery aneurysms are symptomatic at the time of diagnosis.[1,3,5,7] Most common presentations are distal embolization or acute thrombosis, followed by compressive symptoms.[6] Compression of adjacent structures of the popliteal fossa can cause venous obstruction (deep venous thrombosis) and pain (compression of adjacent nerves). Rupture can occur rarely, in less than 5% of the presentations.[1,6] **[Q3: A, B, C, D]** Distal embolization can cause minor or major tissue loss but more importantly, it destroys distal run-off, decreasing patency of operative repair.

Indications for repair include size of 2 cm and greater, the presence of significant mural thrombus, compression of adjacent structures causing pain and/or venous obstruction and symptoms of embolization. Elective repair in asymptomatic patients results in excellent graft patency and limb preservation. Conversely, repair in symptomatic patients has decreased graft patency and limb salvage rates, particularly in emergent repair for acute thrombosis and rarely rupture.[1,2,7,8] **[Q4: B]** Therefore, popliteal aneurysms are better repaired in the asymptomatic state once they reach 2 cm, or when associated with significant thrombus. Options for repair include open bypass with ligation using a medial approach, open aneurysmorrhaphy via a posterior approach or endovascular stent grafting. Open repair is the gold standard in the treatment of popliteal artery aneurysm. The medial approach is most often utilized as it offers the best exposure of the distal superficial femoral artery, the trifurcation and the greater saphenous vein. The posterior approach is sometimes preferred in cases with limited extent of the disease especially when ligation of all branches of the aneurysm is necessary to relieve compressive symptoms. Endovascular repair of a popliteal artery aneurysm is a minimally invasive approach that has gained acceptance recently with the addition of kink resistant stent grafts. It is a good alternative to open repair in patients with suitable anatomy especially poor operative candidates. A good runoff and suitable landing zones are important determinants of success. Small studies have shown excellent results with endovascular repair with similar patency at intermediate follow-up and faster/shorter recovery.[8] Contraindications to endovascular stent grafting for popliteal artery aneurysms include compressive symptoms and single-vessel run-off. An acutely thrombosed popliteal artery aneurysm often presents as an acutely ischemic limb and requires emergent therapy. Systemic anti-coagulation should be initiated immediately and directed thrombolytics improve distal run-off in preparation for surgical repair. [**Q5: A, B, C**]

References

1. Lichtenfels E, Frankini AD, Bonamigo TP, et al. Popliteal artery aneurysm surgery: the role of emergency setting. *Vasc Endovasc Surg.* 2008;42(2):159-164.
2. Ravn H, Wanhainen A, Bjorck M. Surgical technique and long-term results after popliteal artery aneurysm repair: results from 717 legs. *J Vasc Surg.* 2007;46(2):236-243.
3. Martelli E, Ippoliti A, Ventoruzzo G, et al. Popliteal artery aneurysms. Factors associated with thromboembolism and graft failure. *Int Angiol.* 2004;23(1):54-65.
4. Huang Y, Gloviczki P, Noel AA, et al. Early complications and long-term outcome after open surgical treatment of popliteal artery aneurysms: is exclusion with saphenous vein bypass still the gold standard? *J Vasc Surg.* 2007;45(4):706-713. discussion 713-115.
5. Ascher E, Markevich N, Schutzer RW, et al. Small popliteal artery aneurysms: are they clinically significant? *J Vasc Surg.* 2003;37(4):755-760.
6. Ravn H, Bergqvist D, Bjorck M. Nationwide study of the outcome of popliteal artery aneurysms treated surgically. *Br J Surg.* 2007;94(8):970-977.
7. Pulli R, Dorigo W, Troisi N, et al. Surgical management of popliteal artery aneurysms: which factors affect outcomes? *J Vasc Surg.* 2006;43(3):481-487.
8. Antonello M, Frigatti P, Battocchio P, et al. Open repair versus endovascular treatment for asymptomatic popliteal artery aneurysm: results of a prospective randomized study. *J Vasc Surg.* 2005;42(2):185-193.

Renal Artery Aneurysm

9

Lutz Reiher, Tomas Pfeiffer, and Wilhelm Sandmann

A 45-year-old woman presented with a 10-year history of arterial hypertension. After initially successful conservative therapy with two antihypertensive drugs, arterial blood pressure was not controlled well during the last months. To exclude a renovascular origin of hypertension, an angiography was performed, which showed fibrodysplastic disease of the right renal artery with several stenotic segments and aneurysms (Fig. 9.1).

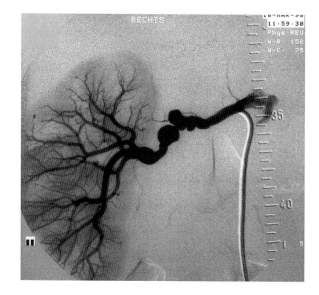

Fig. 9.1 Selective intra-arterial renal artery angiography revealed renal artery aneurysm (RAA) combined with renal artery stenosis (RAS) due to fibromuscular dysplasia.

L. Reiher (✉)
Klinik für Gefäßchirurgie und Nierentransplantation, Universitätsklinikum Düsseldorf, Heinrich-Heine-Universität, Düsseldorf, Germany

G. Geroulakos and B. Sumpio (eds.), *Vascular Surgery*,
DOI: 10.1007/978-1-84996-356-5_9, © Springer-Verlag London Limited 2011

Question 1

Which of the following statements regarding renal artery aneurysm (RAA) is correct?

A. It has a marked female preponderance.
B. It is usually diagnosed during examination for flank pain.
C. It may cause arterial hypertension.
D. It typically leads to proteinuria by compression of the renal vein.
E. It can cause haematuria in rare cases.

Question 2

Which statements about the aetiology of the RAA are true?

A. The most frequent underlying diseases of RAA are aortic coarctation with con-comitant disease of the renal artery and renal artery dissection.
B. Fibromuscular dysplasia of the renal artery may present with renal artery stenosis (RAS), RAA or both.
C. Arteriosclerosis is a frequent cause of RAA.
D. Some RAA present with inflammation of the arterial wall.
E. The incidence of RAAs is increased in Ehlers–Danlos syndrome and Marfan´s syndrome.

Question 3

Which risks of the spontaneous course of the RAA should you explain to your patient?

A. The RAA may rupture and lead to a life-threatening bleeding.
B. The risk of rupture decreases during pregnancy and childbirth.
C. Hypertension in RAA may be caused by concomitant stenosis of the renal artery or its branches.
D. In cases of RAA and hypertension the angiography of the renal artery always shows an additional RAS.
E. The RAA may be a source of embolisation leading to a loss of renal function.

Question 4

Which of the following statements regarding the indication of renal artery repair (RAR) for RAA is correct?

A. There is an indication for RAR only in cases of symptoms other than hypertension.
B. There is no reason to perform RAR in women of childbearing age if there is no arterial hypertension.
C. There is a good indication for RAR if a concomitant RAS is found.
D. There is a good indication for RAR only if the RAA is larger than 5.5 cm.
E. There is an indication for RAR in patients presenting with RAA and hypertension even if an additional RAS is not detectable.

Fig. 9.2 Postoperative angiography demonstrates a patent aortorenal venous graft.

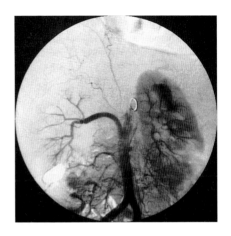

For RAR, a midline abdominal incision was performed for direct access to the infrarenal aorta, where an end-to-side anastomosis was performed with a segment of the patient's greater saphenous vein. After Kocher's manoeuvre, the distal renal artery was transected and anastomosed to the saphenous vein, which had been placed on the renal hilus dorsal to the inferior vena cava. Good results were shown by postoperative angiography (Fig. 9.2). At re-examination 3 years after the operation, the patient had a normal blood pressure without antihypertensive medication.

Question 5

Which of the following statements regarding the management of RAA is correct?

A. Replacement of the diseased renal artery by prosthetic graft is the RAR of first choice.

B. Protection of the kidney against ischaemic injury is performed only during ex situ reconstruction of the renal artery.

C. RAA exclusion and aortorenal vein graft interposition, or RAA resection and end-to-end anastomosis or aneurysmorrhaphy, are valuable methods for RAR.

D. Ex situ repair of the renal artery may be needed in cases presenting with lesions of the distal branch arteries.

E. Tailoring of RAA often leads to recurrent aneurysmatic dilation of the renal artery.

9.1
Commentary

RAAs do not usually cause symptoms, and generally they are diagnosed accidentally during work-up for hypertension, as in our patient. In rare cases, flank pain has been described as the initial symptom, which may be due either to the size of the RAA or to a renal artery dissection. Rupture of the aneurysm into the urinary tract will lead to haematuria. [Q1: A, C, E] The underlying disease is most frequently dysplasia of the arterial wall followed by arteriosclerosis. In our case, fibromuscular dysplasia was found to be the aetiology of the RAA. Rare causes of RAA may be atypical aortic coarctation with concomitant disease of the renal arteries, inflammation of the arterial wall, dissection or trauma, or disorders of the elastic and collagen fibres (i.e. Ehlers–Danlos syndrome or Marfan´s syndrome). [Q2: B, C, D, E]

RAA is found about twice as often in the right renal artery as in the left. Selective angiography often reveals concomitant RAS of mainstem and segmental arteries, and seg-mental arteries may also be aneurysmal. Concomitant renal artery dissection is rare.

Rupture of RAA, development or deterioration of arterial hypertension, and loss of renal function by thrombosis or embolisation, are impending spontaneous consequences of RAA.

As with all arterial aneurysms, rupture is a possible complication of RAA. While Tham et al.[1] experienced no rupture of RAA in 69 patients who had been treated conservatively during a mean observation time of 4.3 years, Henriksson et al.[2] observed RAA rupture in four cases (10.2%), and at the time of rupture only a nephrectomy could be performed. There are several case reports about RAA rupture in pregnancy and childbirth,[3-5] and one author found the probability of RAA rupture during pregnancy to be as high as 80%.[6]

As high arterial blood pressure is in itself a risk factor for rupture of arterial aneurysms of any localisation, one can argue that hypertension per se is an indication to remove an RAA. Hypertension was found in 90% of all patients with ruptured RAA.[7]

The larger the diameter of the RAA, the more likely the danger of rupture seems to be, which can be explained by Laplace's law. However, RAAs of any diameter can rupture. In one patient cohort,[8] the smallest (1 cm) and the largest (16.5 cm) RAAs ruptured.

About 80% of patients with RAA have arterial hypertension.[9, 10] If RAA is accompa-nied by RAS on the same or the contralateral side, as in our patient, then it is reasonable to remove both, with the intention to improve hypertension and eliminate the risk of rupture. However, an ipsilateral stenosis may be missed by angiography due to overprojection of the aneurysm. Furthermore, aneurysmal disease includes not only dilation of vessels but also elongation, which might cause kinking with a relevant stenosis.[11] [Q3: A, C, E]

There is an absolute indication to remove RAAs in all patients with arterial hyperten-sion with and without concomitant RAS and in women of childbearing age. [Q2: C] RAAs with a diameter greater than 2 cm should be removed, even if there is no hypertension. There are good long-term results for autologous RAR; therefore, there is a relative indica-tion for operation in younger patients without hypertension and concomitant RAS with RAA of diameter of 1 cm or more. [Q4: C, E]

The most promising method of RAR is by autogenous reconstruction. Methods of RAR are replacement of the renal artery by the greater saphenous vein, resection of dis-eased sections and reanastomosis. The autoplastic reconstruction by tailoring (synonym: aneurysmorrhaphy) is another appropriate technique. Although the aneurysmatic wall is only resected partially, recurrent RAAs have not been observed. The in situ reconstruc-tion is less traumatic, but ex situ repair of the renal artery may be necessary in cases in which not only the distal mainstem artery but also the segmental arteries are involved. [Q5: C, D]

If arterial repair is restricted to renal arteries only, and if concomitant repair of the aorta is not necessary, then a postoperative mortality less than 1% can be expected. Postoperative morbidity is due to temporary kidney insufficiency, graft thrombosis, bleeding, thrombosis and pancreatitis. Affected kidneys can be preserved in more than 85% of cases. The number of patients who benefit from surgical therapy in terms of improvement of arterial hypertension varies considerably between authors, ranging from 5% to 50% and from 25% to 62%, respectively.[12]

References

1. Tham G, Ekelund L, Herrlin K, Lindstedt EL, Olin T, Bergentz SE. Renal artery aneurysms. Natural history and prognosis. *Ann Surg*. 1983;197:348-352.
2. Henriksson C, Lukes P, Nilson AE, Pettersson S. Angiographically discovered, non-operated renal artery aneurysms. *Scand J Urol Nephrol*. 1984;18:59-62.
3. Rijbroek A, Dijk HA, Roex AJM. Rupture of renal artery aneurysm during pregnancy. *Eur J Vasc Surg*. 1994;8:375-376.
4. Smith JA, Macleish DG. Postpartum rupture of a renal artery aneurysm to a solitary kidney. *Aust N Z J Surg*. 1985;55:299-300.
5. Whiteley MS, Katoch R, Kennedy RH, Bidgood KA, Baird RN. Ruptured renal artery aneurysm in the first trimester of pregnancy. *Eur J Vasc Surg*. 1994;8:238-239.
6. Love WK, Robinette MA, Vernon CP. Renal artery aneurysm rupture in pregnancy. *J Urol*. 1981;126:809-811.
7. Abud O, Chelile GE, Sole-Balcells F. Aneurysm and arteriovenous malformation. In: Novick AC, Scoble J, Hamilton G, eds. *Renal Vascular Disease*. London: Saunders; 1996:35-46.
8. Hupp T, Allenberg JR, Post K, Roeren T, Meier M, Clorius JH. Renal artery aneurysm: surgical indications and results. *Eur J Vasc Surg*. 1992;6:477-486.
9. Martin RSD, Meacham PW, Ditesheim JA, Mulherin JL Jr, Edwards WH. Renal artery aneurysm: selective treatment for hypertension and prevention of rupture. *J Vasc Surg*. 1989;9:26-34.
10. Brekke IB, Sodal G, Jakobsen A, et al. Fibro-muscular renal artery disease treated by extracorporeal vascular reconstruction and renal autotransplantation: short- and long-term results. *Eur J Vasc Surg*. 1992;6:471-476.
11. Poutasse EF. Renal artery aneurysms. *J Urol*. 1975;113:443-449.
12. Pfeiffer T, Reiher L, Grabitz K, et al. Reconstruction for renal artery aneurysm: operative techniques and long-term results. *J Vasc Surg*. 2003;37:293-300.

Anastomotic Aneurysms

10

Jonothan J. Earnshaw

A 70-year-old woman presented with bilateral pulsatile groin masses (Fig. 10.1). Six years ago, she had an elective aorto-bifemoral graft for a 6-cm abdominal aortic aneurysm involving both iliac arteries, from which she made a full recovery. She first found the larger, right-sided mass 4 months ago, and she had noted gradual enlargement since then. She had no symptoms of claudication or leg ischemia. Her past medical history included a myocardial infarction (MI) 18 months ago, but without limitation to her exercise tolerance. On examination, she appeared well. There was a well-healed midline laparotomy scar from the previous operation. Abdominal examination was unremarkable, and there were no bruits on auscultation. Two well-defined expansile masses were palpable in the middle third of the femoral scars, measuring approximately 2 cm on the left and 4 cm on the right. The masses were not tender. There was no evidence of compromise to the distal circulation, and all pulses were palpable. Duplex imaging identified anastomotic false aneurysms in both groins, measuring 1.8 cm on the left and 3.5 cm on the right.

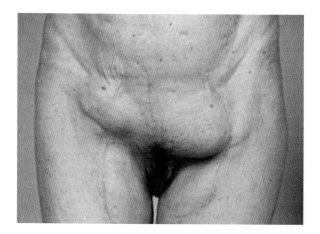

Fig. 10.1 Female patient with bilateral anastomotic aneurysms from an aortobifemoral graft

J.J. Earnshaw
Department of Surgery, Gloucestershire Royal Hospital, Gloucester, UK

G. Geroulakos and B. Sumpio (eds.), *Vascular Surgery*,
DOI: 10.1007/978-1-84996-356-5_10, © Springer-Verlag London Limited 2011

Question 1

Which of the following statements regarding the etiology of anastomotic false aneurysms are correct?

A. Anastomotic false aneurysms occur in 3–5% of anastomoses to the femoral artery in the groin
B. Forty per cent are found in the groin
C. Primary degeneration of the arterial wall is an etiological factor
D. Continued smoking is an etiological factor
E. At reoperation, approximately one-third will be found to be infected with pathogenic bacteria

Question 2

The patient wished to know the risks of leaving the aneurysm alone. Rank the potential complications of anastomotic aneurysms in order of frequency.

A. Rupture
B. Embolization
C. Pressure symptoms
D. Pain
E. Secondary hemorrhage

Question 3

Which of the following non-operative treatments are also available?

A. Embolization
B. Ultrasound-guided compression
C. Thrombin injection
D. Intravascular stent graft

The larger of the two aneurysms was repaired surgically. The previous surgical incision was reopened and extended. A large false aneurysm was confirmed; the graft appeared to have become detached from the artery. There were no signs of infection. The aneurysm was replaced by straight 8-mm gelatin-coated woven Dacron interposition graft (soaked in rifampicin solution 10 mg/mL) taken end to end from the old graft and sutured end to side over the common femoral bifurcation. The thrombus and old graft were sent for microbiology. The patient made a good postoperative recovery. All bacterial cultures were negative, so perioperative antibiotic prophylaxis was stopped after 48 h.

Question 4

Rank the following surgical procedures in order of value for the management of anastomotic aneurysm in the groin (least useful first):

A. Resuture or local repair
B. Ligation and bypass
C. Prosthetic patch
D. Vein patch
E. Interposition graft

This patient at 2-year follow-up had no evidence of recurrence of the anastomotic aneurysm in her right groin. A follow-up ultrasound scan of her left groin revealed that the left anastomotic aneurysm remained 2 cm in maximum diameter.

Question 5

Which of the following statements are false.

A. Surgery cures 50% of all anastomotic aneurysms.
B. Surgery cures 90% of all anastomotic aneurysms.
C. Surgery cures 50% of all recurrent anastomotic aneurysms.
D. Surgery cures 90% of all recurrent anastomotic aneurysms.
E. Long-term follow-up of retroperitoneal anastomotic aneurysms is not necessary.

10.1
Commentary

The incidence of anastomotic aneurysms is increasing, due primarily to the increased frequency of prosthetic vascular reconstructions involving groin anastomosis. The overall incidence following vascular anastomoses is about 2%, but this increases to 3–8% when the anastomosis involves the femoral artery.[1-4] Although they are most common after prosthetic bypass, anastomotic aneurysms occasionally occur after vein bypass, semi-closed endarterectomy, and open endarterectomy with a vein patch. Anastomotic aneurysms can occur anywhere, but they frequently develop near to a joint. About 80% occur at the groin,[1] presumably due to movement-related strains. **[Q1: A, C, D, E]**

The etiology is summarized in Fig. 10.2; there are three primary factors and a number of secondary factors. One of the first documented causes was suture failure, when braided silk was employed for vascular anastomoses.[5] Since monofilament sutures have been used, suture failure has become a less common factor, although occasionally reported disasters highlight the importance of careful suture handling to avoid cracking of the polypropylene.[6]

Primary factors

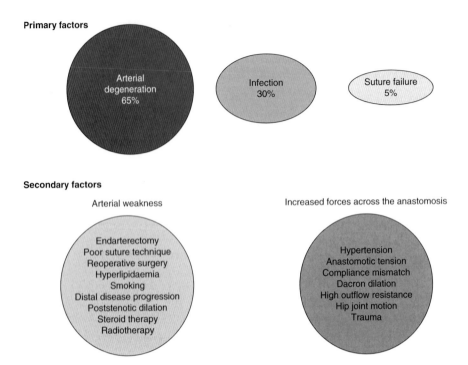

Secondary factors

Fig. 10.2 Etiology of anastomotic aneurysms

Arterial degeneration is the most common primary factor. The disease process that mandated the bypass continues after its insertion.[1,7,8] Histologically, a chronic inflammatory response can be identified at an anastomosis.[9] Secondary factors are numerous and compound the process of arterial degeneration.[10] Poor technique, failing to suture all layers of the artery, use of Dacron, and the need for endarterectomy all weaken the arterial graft complex.[1] Hypertension and high outflow resistance may theoretically increase strains at the anastomosis, together with physical disruption from both hip motion and poststenotic dilation as the graft passes under the inguinal ligament.[9] These and other factors can cause compliance mismatch, which may also be a factor.[8] Anastomotic aneurysms can be caused by local infection. Infection with high-virulence bacteria, such as *Staphylococcus aureus*, usually presents early with clinical graft infection. Late anastomotic rupture is often caused by low-virulence organisms, such as *Staphylococcus epidermidis*. Up to 30% of anastomotic aneurysms can be shown to harbor pathogenic bacteria at reoperation.[7] This has implications for surgical repair (see below). **[Q2: D, C, B, A, E]**

10.2
Indications for Intervention

Treatment of anastomotic aneurysms is aimed at controlling symptoms or preventing the onset of complications. Symptoms of pain are associated with the enlarging mass or pressure on adjacent structures, such as the femoral nerve. Complications may be local or distal. The enlarging aneurysm may occlude the underlying vessel, causing distal ischaemia. Emboli associated with flow disruption may be propagated distally. Aneurysm rupture represents the greatest worry but is relatively rare. Complications are related to aneurysm size. Therefore, conservative management may be undertaken if the aneurysm is small and easily accessible, and demonstrates no evidence of progressive enlargement or symptoms. Aneurysms less than 2 cm in diameter can be observed safely.[1] Above this size, the incidence of complications rises and intervention should be considered. However, the medical state of the patient may necessitate selected aneurysms larger than 2 cm being managed conservatively by watchful waiting.

False aneurysms caused iatrogenically following direct arterial puncture must be differentiated from anastomotic aneurysms because their treatment differs substantially. False aneurysms following sterile arterial puncture may be treated by arterial compression under duplex imaging.[11] More recently, injection of thrombin into these false aneurysms has been shown to be safe and effective, even in anticoagulated patients.[12] This technique is not suitable for anastomotic aneurysms. Other radiological techniques may be used selectively for false aneurysms in inaccessible positions, such as the renal or subclavian arteries, where coil embolization may be used to occlude the feeding vessel.[13] Again, this is rarely suitable for anastomotic aneurysms. Occasionally, endovascular treatment with a covered stent can be employed across an anastomotic aneurysm to produce aneurysm sac thrombosis[14, 15] and to maintain normal distal flow. This technique is particularly valuable for intra-abdominal aortoiliac anastomotic aneurysms, where reoperation carries substantial risk. It is important that endovascular techniques are not used in situations where there is any risk that the false aneurysm is due to infection. The most common site for anastomotic aneurysm is the groin, where non-operative techniques have not been found to be effective. The groin is also easily accessible for surgery, so direct operation is the usual intervention in this situation. [Q3: A, B, C, D] [Q4: A, C, D, E, B]

10.3
Treatment for Anastomotic Aneurysms

Surgical repair should be undertaken in fit patients with large or symptomatic anastomotic aneurysms. Local repair is usually possible in non-infected aneurysms, although graft replacement may be necessary. If infection is the cause of the aneurysm, then more extensive repairs with ligation and remote bypass or replacement of the entire initial graft may be needed.[16]

Anastomotic aneurysms usually occur in arteriopathic patients. Careful preoperative planning is needed to make the patient as fit as possible. General anesthesia is needed to allow adequate exposure, and the surgery is carried out under antibiotic and heparin cover. Once vascular control above and below the aneurysm has been obtained with minimal dissection, the aneurysm should be opened, along with the entire abnormal artery. Occlusion balloon catheters are often helpful in obtaining vascular control in this situation. The false aneurysm is usually resected and the ends of the graft and artery freshened for reanastomosis. Interposition grafting is likely to be needed to ensure that the new anastomosis is created without tension. Autologous saphenous vein is the graft of choice, although often polytetrafluoroethylene (PTFE) or Dacron may be better for size matching. **[Q5: A, C, E]** Retroperitoneal anastomotic aneurysms present more of a challenge. Proximal aortic anastomotic aneurysms may require supracoeliac clamping or balloon occlusion catheters.[17] Aneurysms associated with the distal portion of an aortoiliac graft may present late and catastrophically, illustrating the potential importance of monitoring these grafts for a prolonged period.[18] As previously stated, and endovascular approach is used increasingly in this situation.

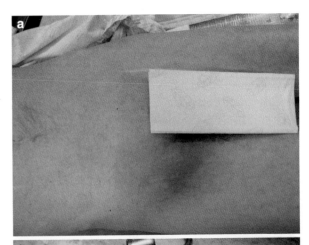

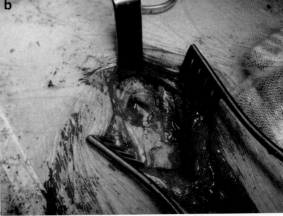

Fig. 10.3 (a) This man presented with sudden pain in the right groin. A false aneurysm of a previous axillobifemoral graft was diagnosed on ultrasound imaging. Note the inflammatory nature of the lump suggesting infection. (b) At operation the hood of the graft had separated completely from the artery. There was no sign of sepsis, and all bacterial cultures were negative

10.4
Infection in Anastomotic Aneurysms

Some 80% of anastomotic aneurysms occur in the groin, and they have the highest incidence of infection as their primary cause; approximately 30% contain pathogenic bacteria. A high level of clinical suspicion of infection must be maintained, and Gram staining of all clots and removed graft should be carried out as a matter of routine. Perioperative antibiotics should be continued until results are available (Fig. 10.3).

The diagnosis of infection is usually obvious if the graft is surrounded by pus. If the graft is frankly infected, it should be excised completely with an extra-anastomotic bypass to restore the distal circulation with prolonged, high-dose antibiotic cover. An obturator bypass may be used for an infected femoral false aneurysm, or a femoral crossover with saphenous vein. Aortic stump oversewing and axillobifemoral grafting can treat the (fortunately rare) infected aortic anastomotic aneurysm. Morbidity and mortality rates are high. Grafts with a more indolent level of infection that becomes apparent only after microbiological investigation may be treated less radically. It is safest to assume that all femoral anastomotic aneurysms are contaminated. If prosthetic material is needed for repair, then measures used to reduce the chance of reinfection include the use of a rifampicin-soaked, gelatin-coated Dacron graft and gentamicin beads laid in close proximity. The reinfection rate after such procedures is 10%.[19]

10.5
Outcome

Outcome depends on the initial site of the aneurysm and any confounding factors.[20] As the most common site for anastomotic aneurysms, the femoral artery has one of the highest rates of successful outcome. About 90% of surgical procedures are successful, and those that recur still have a 90% success rate from a second or subsequent operation. In comparison, anastomotic aneurysms that are intra-abdominal have a high complication rate when repaired surgically. A small anastomotic aneurysm in a superficial position can be monitored by ultrasound or by repeated examination by a clinician or the motivated patient. The success rate of operation at these sites is good.[21] Retroperitoneal aneurysms require long-term ultrasound follow-up. [Q6: F, T, F, T, F] If possible, minimally invasive techniques should be used for repair to avoid the high morbidity and mortality associated with surgery (providing infection is not present). In patients fit for surgery, excision and graft interposition has excellent long-term results.

References

1. Szilagyi DE, Smith RF, Elliott JP, Hageman JH, Dall'Olmo CA. Anastomotic aneurysms after vascular reconstruction: problems of incidence, etiology and treatment. *Surgery*. 1975;78: 800-816.
2. Waibel P. False aneurysm after reconstruction for peripheral arterial occlusive disease. Observations over 15–25 years. *Vasa*. 1994;23:43-51.
3. Stone PA, AbuRhama AF, Flaherty SK, Bates MC. Femoral pseudoaneurysms. *Vasc Endovasc Surg*. 2006;40:109-117.
4. Corriere MA, Guzman RJ. True and false aneurysms of the femoral artery. *Semin Vasc Surg*. 2005;18:216-223.
5. Moore WS, Hall AD. Late suture failure in the pathogenesis of anastomotic false aneurysms. *Ann Surg*. 1970;172:1064-1068.
6. Berridge DC, Earnshaw JJ, Makin GS, Hopkinson BR. A ten-year review of false aneurysms in Nottingham. *Ann R Coll Surg Engl*. 1988;70:253-256.
7. Wandschneider W, Bull O, Deneck H. Anastomotic aneurysms: an unsolvable problem. *Eur J Vasc Endovasc Surg*. 1988;2:115-119.
8. Gayliss H. Pathogenesis of anastomotic aneurysms. *Surgery*. 1981;90:509-515.
9. Sladen JG, Gerein AN, Miyagishima RT. Late rupture of prosthetic aortic grafts. *Am J Surg*. 1987;15:453-458.
10. De Monti M, Ghilardi G, Sgroi G, Longhi F, Scorza R. Anastomotic pseudoaneurysm, true para-anastomotic aneurysm and recurrent aneurysm following surgery for abdominal aortic aneurysm. Is a unifying theory possible? *Minerva Cardioangiol*. 1995;43:367-373.
11. Hajarizadeh H, LaRosa CR, Cardullo P, Rohrer MJ, Cutler BS. Ultrasound guided compression of iatrogenic femoral psuedoaneurysm: failure, recurrence and long term results. *J Vasc Surg*. 1995;22:425-430.
12. Kang SS, Labropoulos N, Mansour MA, et al. Expanded indications for ultrasound-guided thrombin injection of pseudoaneurysms. *J Vasc Surg*. 2000;31:289-298.
13. Uflacker R. Transcatheter embolisation of arterial aneurysms. *Br J Radiol*. 1986;59:317-324.
14. Manns RA, Duffield RG. Intravascular stenting across a false aneurysm of the popliteal artery. *Clin Radiol*. 1997;52:151-153.
15. Brittenden J, Gillespie I, McBride K, McInnes G, Bradbury AW. Endovascular repair of aortic pseudoaneurysms. *Eur J Vasc Endovasc Surg*. 2000;19:82-84.
16. Clarke AM, Poskitt KR, Baird RN, Horrocks M. Anastomotic aneurysms of the femoral artery: aetiology and treatment. *Br J Surg*. 1989;76:1014-1016.
17. Ernst CB. The surgical correction of arteriosclerotic femoral aneurysm and anastomotic aneurysm. In: Greenhalgh RM, Mannick JA, eds. *The Cause and Management of Aneurysms*. London: W.B. Saunders; 1990:245-256.
18. Treiman GS, Weaver FA, Cossman DV, et al. Anastomotic false aneurysms of the abdominal aorta and the iliac arteries. *J Vasc Surg*. 1988;8:268-273.
19. Earnshaw JJ. Anastomotic/false aneurysms. In: Horrocks M, ed. *Arterial Aneurysms: Diagnosis and Management*. Bath: Butterworth Heinemann; 1995:209-221.
20. Ylonen K, Biancari F, Leo E, et al. Predictors of development of anastomotic femoral pseudoaneurysms after aortobifemoral reconstruction for abdominal aortic aneurysm. *Am J Surg*. 2004;187:83-87.
21. Woodburn K. False aneurysms. In: Earnshaw JJ, Parvin S, eds. *Rare Vascular Disorders*. Tfm Publishing, Ltd.; 2005:283–292.

False Aneurysm in the Groin Following Coronary Angioplasty

11

A 70-year-old female with a history of hypertension developed chest pain and came to the Emergency Room. Her electrocardiogram showed ST segment elevation. The patient was administered aspirin, clopidogrel, and intravenous heparin. Within 60 min, she underwent coronary angiography, which showed a critical stenosis of the left anterior descending artery. The lesion was treated with angioplasty and stent placement. The right femoral artery sheath was left in place overnight, and heparin was continued. The following morning after stopping heparin, the sheath was removed and a FemoStop device was placed over the groin for 4 h. Heparin was then restarted.

The next day, the patient was without any chest pain, but she did have mild discomfort in the right groin. There was a large hematoma in the right groin. The overlying skin had ecchymosis. The femoral pulse was prominent, and popliteal and pedal pulses were normal. A systolic bruit was heard over the femoral artery.

Question 1

What test should be obtained at this time?

A. Computed tomography scan with intravenous contrast
B. Duplex ultrasound
C. Magnetic resonance angiogram
D. Contrast arteriogram

A false aneurysm was suspected and confirmed by duplex ultrasound examination. It was arising from the common femoral artery (CFA). The flow cavity measured 3 cm in diameter (Fig. 11.1).

S.S. Kang
Department of Surgery, Florida International University School of Medicine, Miami, FL, USA

G. Geroulakos and B. Sumpio (eds.), *Vascular Surgery*,
DOI: 10.1007/978-1-84996-356-5_11, © Springer-Verlag London Limited 2011

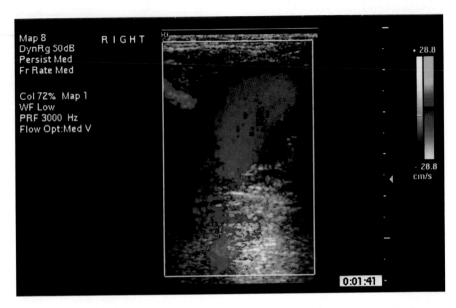

Fig. 11.1 Duplex ultrasound demonstrates a false aneurysm arising from the common femoral artery

Question 2

The incidence of postcatheterization false aneurysms in the groin is higher under which of the following situations?

A. Puncture of the CFA instead of the superficial femoral artery (SFA)
B. Use of larger sheaths
C. Use of postprocedural anticoagulation
D. Patients with hypertension
E. Manual compression versus mechanical compression with a FemoStop after catheter removal

Question 3

Which of the following statements about postcatheterization false aneurysms is/are true?

A. Urgent surgical repair is indicated
B. This aneurysm is likely to undergo spontaneous thrombosis if observed
C. Spontaneous thrombosis is less common in patients who are anticoagulated
D. They may cause deep venous thrombosis

Heparin was discontinued and ultrasound-guided compression repair (UGCR) was attempted.

Question 4

Which are disadvantages of UGCR?

A. Thrombosis of the underlying artery is a frequent complication
B. Most patients find it painful
C. It is less successful in patients who are anticoagulated
D. Approximately 30% of successfully thrombosed false aneurysms recur

Due to patient discomfort, intravenous morphine and midazolam were administered. After 60 min of compression, the false aneurysm still had flow. Vascular surgery was consulted for ultrasound-guided thrombin injection.

Question 5

Which of the following statements regarding ultrasound-guided thrombin injection is/are true?

A. It requires direct injection of thrombin into the neck of the false aneurysm
B. It involves simultaneous compression of the false aneurysm
C. It is less painful but less effective than UGCR
D. It works well in anticoagulated patients
E. It is appropriate only for femoral false aneurysms

Bovine thrombin solution (1,000 units/mL) was loaded into a small syringe and a 22-gauge spinal needle was attached. Under ultrasound guidance, the needle was placed into the center of the false aneurysm (Fig. 11.2) and 0.3 mL thrombin was injected slowly. Within 15 s, the false aneurysm was thrombosed completely (Fig. 11.3). The procedure was tolerated well. Flow in the underlying artery was preserved and pedal pulses were intact. As the patient was otherwise stable, she was discharged soon afterwards.

Question 6

What are the reported complications of thrombin injection?

A. Anaphylaxis
B. Intra-arterial thrombosis
C. Prolonged urticaria
D. Mad cow disease

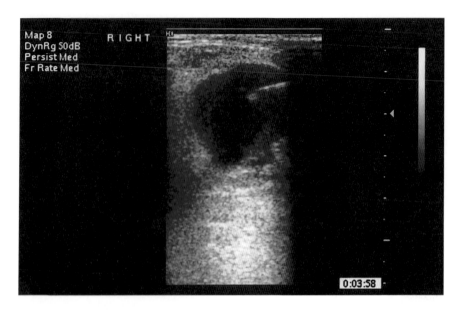

Fig. 11.2 The tip of the needle is visible within the false aneurysm cavity

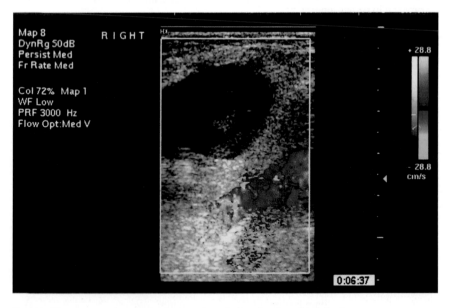

Fig. 11.3 The aneurysm is completely thrombosed 15 s after thrombin injection

11.1
Commentary

A false aneurysm after catheterization is suspected when there is a hematoma, especially an enlarging one, at the puncture site hours or days after the procedure. There is often significant ecchymosis of the overlying skin. There may be a bruit, but a continuous bruit is usually associated with an arteriovenous fistula. There may be pain or neuralgia, and the site is often tender. A pulsatile mass is usually palpable, but a simple hematoma overlying the artery may give the same impression. Only a minority of false aneurysms are diagnosed unequivocally by physical examination. The diagnosis of a femoral false aneurysm has become very easy with duplex ultrasound. [Q1: B]

The incidence of postcatheterization femoral false aneurysms varies from less than 0.5% to more than 5%.[1] Some of the factors that increase the likelihood of false aneurysm formation include larger sheaths, longer procedure times, multiple catheter exchanges, and peri- and postprocedure anticoagulation. Puncture of the superficial femoral or deep femoral artery instead of the CFA is found to be associated with higher rates of false aneurysm formation. Direct manual compression after catheter removal is better than compression devices, such as the FemoStop or C-clamp. Patient characteristics that may increase the likelihood of false aneurysm formation include atherosclerosis of the punctured artery, obesity and hypertension. [Q2: B, C, D]

The potential complications of untreated false aneurysms are well known. Rupture is the most dramatic and life-threatening complication. Compression of surrounding tissues can cause pain, neuropathy, venous thrombosis, and necrosis of the overlying skin. Thrombosis of, or embolisation into, the femoral artery may occur. Infection of these false aneurysms is less common. Because of these potential outcomes, early surgical repair had been advocated in the past. However, in the 1990s, several series showed that the majority of small false aneurysms will develop spontaneous thrombosis.[2-4] It is less likely to occur for larger false aneurysms or in patients who are on anticoagulants. [Q3: C, D] Thrombosis may occur within days, or it may take weeks. Once thrombosis occurs, the false aneurysm is then a simple hematoma that gets resorbed slowly over time. The defect in the artery heals uneventfully in most cases.

In 1991, Fellmeth et al.[5] described the method of UGCR of postcatheterization femoral false aneurysms and arteriovenous fistulas. The ultrasound transducer is used to apply downward pressure on the neck of the false aneurysm to arrest flow. Pressure is maintained until the blood in the aneurysm becomes thrombosed. After the introduction of UGCR, numerous reports were published verifying the efficacy and overall safety of this procedure.[6-9] The typical success rate was between 60% and 90%. There were only a few published complications, including thrombosis of the underlying artery or the femoral vein from the compression, rupture during compression, rupture after successful compression, skin necrosis caused by prolonged pressure on the skin, and vasovagal reactions. Therefore, UGCR was shown to be a good alternative to surgical repair or observation, and most centers made it the initial treatment method.

There are several disadvantages to the procedure. It is time-consuming, requiring an average of 30–60 min of compression. In most hands, the results are significantly poorer for patients on anticoagulants.[10] The recurrence rate is about 4–11%, but it is as high as 20% for anticoagulated patients.[6] About 10% of patients cannot be treated with UGCR because they have false aneurysms that are not compressible or cannot be compressed without also collapsing the underlying artery, which would increase the chance of arterial thrombosis. For most patients, the compression is painful, and intravenous sedation or analgesia is often necessary. Some patients have required epidural or general anesthesia to allow compression. Applying compression is also very uncomfortable for the operator. [Q4: B, C]

Various endovascular treatments have been described for false aneurysms that have failed compression. They usually require catheterization of the feeding artery or false aneurysm from a remote access site. Embolisation coils can be used to occlude the neck or to fill the cavity of the false aneurysm.[11,12] Stent grafts can be placed in the femoral artery to exclude the false aneurysm, but late occlusion of the grafts is not uncommon.[13] They certainly should not be the initial method of treatment. However, for false aneurysms arising from other, less easily accessible arteries, these techniques may have a role.

Because of the shortcomings of UGCR, we developed a new method of treating false aneurysms with ultrasound-guided thrombin injection.[14,15] Thrombin causes the cleavage of fibrinogen into fibrin, which then polymerises into a solid. It is the final product of the coagulation cascade, and this reaction occurs naturally whenever blood clots. Thrombin has been used topically for many years to control surface bleeding in the operating room. Our technique is as follows: The ultrasound transducer is centered over the false aneurysm. Thrombin at a concentration of 1,000 U/mL is placed into a small syringe, and a 22G spinal needle is attached. The needle is inserted at an angle into the false aneurysm along the same plane as the transducer, and the tip is positioned near the center of the false aneurysm. About 0.5 mL thrombin solution is injected slowly into the false aneurysm. Within seconds, thrombosis of the false aneurysm is seen. The procedure is not painful, and patients do not require any analgesia or sedation. We allow patients to get out of bed immediately after treatment, and outpatients are sent home soon after the procedure.

So far, we have had great success with this procedure. We have treated 165 false aneurysms. Most (149) developed after groin puncture. There were also false aneurysms in six brachial, three subclavian, two radial, two tibial, one distal SFA, and one superficial temporal arteries, and in one arm arteriovenous fistula. Forty-seven patients were anticoagulated at the time of thrombin injection. It was initially successful in 161 of 165 patients. The other four (all femoral) had partial thrombosis. One of these had complete thrombosis 3 days later when brought back for repeat injection. Three had surgical repair. There were early recurrences in twelve patients who had initial successful thrombin injection. Seven were reinjected successfully at the time the recurrence was diagnosed. One had spontaneous thrombosis several days after recurrence was identified. Four had surgical repair. Overall, only 7 of 165 required surgical repair. There were three complications. A brachial artery false aneurysm had injection of thrombin directly into its neck, which caused thrombosis of the brachial artery. A femoral false aneurysm had a relatively large volume of thrombin injected and developed a thombus in the posterior tibial artery. Both of these thromboses resolved after intravenous heparin. A femoral false aneurysm with a short neck that was about 10 mm wide had partial thrombosis of the aneurysm. Further injection was not able to thrombose the remaining cavity but instead caused a tail of thrombus to form in the SFA. The patient underwent surgical thrombectomy and repair of the aneurysm. **[Q5: D]**

Our results show that intra-arterial thrombosis after thrombin injection is uncommon. The high concentration of thrombin results in almost immediate conversion of the solution into a solid (thrombus) when it mixes with relatively stagnant blood. Since the neck of the false aneurysm is usually much narrower than the aneurysm cavity, the thrombus cannot enter the artery. As long as the volume of the thrombin injected does not approach or exceed the volume of the false aneurysm, which may result in forcing some of the solution out of the cavity, then the risk of native artery thrombosis should be small. It is likely to be higher when the neck is very wide. Other complications that have been reported include single cases of anaphylaxis[16] and prolonged urticaria.[17] **[Q6: A, B, C]** Repeated exposure to bovine thrombin can also lead to development of antibodies to bovine factor V, which may cross-react with autogenous factor V, causing hemorrhagic complications.[18] Recently available recombinant human thrombin should be similarly effective in treating false aneurysms with fewer immunologic complications.[19]

Many others have also had good results with this procedure. In the largest series, the success rate is around 96% and the complication rate less than 2% (Table 11.1). Given its simplicity, efficacy, and safety, ultrasound-guided thrombin injection should be considered the initial treatment of choice for postcatheterization false aneurysms.

Table 11.1 Results of ultrasound-guided thrombin injection

	Cases	Successes (%)	Complications
Current	165	158 (96)	3
Khoury[20]	131	126 (96)	3
Paulson[21]	114	110 (96)	4
Maleux[22]	101	99 (98)	0
Mohler[23]	91	89 (98)	1
La Perna[24]	70	66 (94)	0
Total	672	648 (96)	11 (1.6)

References

1. Skillman JJ, Kim D, Baim DS. Vascular complications of percutaneous femoral cardiac interventions. Incidence and operative repair. *Arch Surg.* 1988;123:1207-1212.
2. Kent KC, McArdle CR, Kennedy B, Baim DS, Anninos E, Skillman JJ. A prospective study of the clinical outcome of femoral pseudoaneurysms and arteriovenous fistulas induced by arterial puncture. *J Vasc Surg.* 1993;17:125-131.
3. Kresowik TF, Khoury MD, Miller BV, et al. A prospective study of the incidence and natural history of femoral vascular complications after percutaneous transluminal coronary angioplasty. *J Vasc Surg.* 1991;13:328-333.

4. Toursarkissian B, Allen BT, Petrinec D, et al. Spontaneous closure of selected iatrogenic pseudoaneurysms and arteriovenous fistulae. *J Vasc Surg*. 1997;25:803-808.
5. Fellmeth BD, Roberts AC, Bookstein JJ, et al. Postangiographic femoral artery injuries: non-surgical repair with US-guided compression. *Radiology*. 1991;178:671-675.
6. Cox GS, Young JR, Gray BR, Grubb MW, Hertzer NR. Ultrasound-guided compression repair of postcatheterization pseudoaneurysms: results of treatment in one hundred cases. *J Vasc Surg*. 1994;19:683-686.
7. Hajarizadeh H, LaRosa CR, Cardullo P, Rohrer MJ, Cutler BS. Ultrasound-guided compression of iatrogenic femoral pseudoaneurysm failure, recurrence, and long-term results. *J Vasc Surg*. 1995;22:425-430.
8. Hertz SM, Brener BJ. Ultrasound-guided pseudoaneurysm compression: efficacy after coronary stenting and angioplasty. *J Vasc Surg*. 1997;26:913-916.
9. Hood DB, Mattos MA, Douglas MG, et al. Determinants of success of color-flow duplex-guided compression repair of femoral pseudoaneurysms. *Surgery*. 1996;120:585-588.
10. Hodgett DA, Kang SS, Baker WH. Ultrasound-guided compression repair of catheter-related femoral artery pseudoaneurysms is impaired by anticoagulation. *Vasc Surg*. 1997;31:639-644.
11. Jain SP, Roubin GS, Iyer SS, Saddekni S, Yadav JS. Closure of an iatrogenic femoral artery pseudoaneurysm by transcutaneous coil embolization. *Catheter Cardiovasc Diagn*. 1996;39:317-319.
12. Pan M, Medina A, Suarez DL, et al. Obliteration of femoral pseudoaneurysm complicating coronary intervention by direct puncture and permanent or removable coil insertion. *Am J Cardiol*. 1997;80:786-788.
13. Thalhammer C, Kirchherr AS, Uhlich F, Walgand J, Gross CM. Postcatheterization pseudoaneurysms and arteriovenous fistulas: repair with percutaneous implantation of endovascular covered stents. *Radiology*. 2000;214:127-131.
14. Kang SS, Labropoulos N, Mansour MA, Baker WH. Percutaneous ultrasound guided thrombin injection: a new method for treating postcatheterization femoral pseudoaneurysms. *J Vasc Surg*. 1998;27:1032-1038.
15. Kang SS, Labropoulos N, Mansour MA, et al. Expanded indications for ultrasound-guided thrombin injection of pseudoaneurysms. *J Vasc Surg*. 2000;31:289-298.
16. Pope M, Johnston KW. Anaphylaxis after thrombin injection of a femoral pseudoaneurysm: recommendations for prevention. *J Vasc Surg*. 2000;32:190-191.
17. Sheldon PJ, Oglevie SB, Kaplan LA. Prolonged generalized urticarial reaction after percutaneous thrombin injection for treatment of a femoral artery pseudoaneurysm. *J Vasc Interv Radiol*. 2000;11:759-761.
18. Ofusu FA, Crean S, Reynolds MW. A safety review of topical bovine thrombin-induced generation of antibodies to bovine proteins. *Clin Ther*. 2009;31:679-691.
19. Chapman WC, Singla N, Genyk Y, et al. A phase 3, randomized, double-blind comparative study of the efficacy and safety of topical recombinant human thrombin and bovine thrombin in surgical hemostasis. *J Am Coll Surg*. 2007;205:256-265.
20. Khoury M, Rebecca A, Greene K, et al. Duplex scanning-guided thrombin injection for the treatment of iatrogenic pseudoaneurysms. *J Vasc Surg*. 2002;35:517-521.
21. Paulson EK, Nelson RC, Mayes CE, Sheafor DH, Sketch MH Jr, Kliewer MA. Sonographically guided thrombin injection of iatrogenic femoral pseudoaneurysms: further experience of a single institution. *AJR Am J Roentgenol*. 2001;177:309-316.
22. Maleux G, Hendrickx S, Vaninbroukx J, et al. Percutaneous injection of human thrombin to treat iatrogenic femoral pseudoaneurysms: short- and midterm ultrasound follow-up. *Eur Radiol*. 2003;13:209-212.
23. Mohler ER 3rd, Mitchell ME, Carpenter JP, et al. Therapeutic thrombin injection of pseudoaneurysms: a multicenter experience. *Vasc Med*. 2001;6:241-244.
24. La Perna L, Olin JW, Goines D, Childs MB, Ouriel K. Ultrasound-guided thrombin injection for the treatment of postcatheterization pseudoaneurysms. *Circulation*. 2000;102:2391-2395.

Acute Thrombosis

12

Zachary M. Arthurs and Vikram S. Kashyap

A 72-year-old female presents with a 2-week history of abdominal/back pain and lower extremity fatigue. She was evaluated by her physician and diagnosed with lumbosacral neuritis. Initial treatment involved lumbar corticosteroid injections. Secondary to sudden onset lower extremity weakness she presented to the emergency department. Her past history included diabetes, hyperlipidemia, and obesity. In the past month, she had undergone heart catheterization which was significant for multi-vessel coronary artery disease. She denied any prior surgeries.

On examination, her pulse is 75 bpm, and blood pressure is 175/60. Heart sounds reveal a regular rhythm. The abdomen is soft and nontender. She has absent pulses and diminished strength in both lower extremities. Both feet are insensate. There are venous Doppler signals in the feet, but no arterial signals. Creatinine on arrival was 0.9 mg/dL, and white blood cell count was 23,000. Pre-operative CTA demonstrates infrarenal aortic occlusion with bilateral renal infarcts.

Question 1

Native arterial or graft thrombosis can be differentiated from embolic occlusion by the following:

A. The presence of palpable pulses in the contralateral extremity
B. A history of cardiac arrhythmias
C. The location of the occlusion
D. The degree of profound ischemia in the affected extremity
E. All of the above

Z.M. Arthurs (✉)
Department of Vascular Surgery, The Cleveland Clinic Foundation, Cleveland, OH, USA

G. Geroulakos and B. Sumpio (eds.), *Vascular Surgery*,
DOI: 10.1007/978-1-84996-356-5_12, © Springer-Verlag London Limited 2011

Question 2

What is the SVS/ISCVS category of limb ischemia in this patient?

A. Category I
B. Category II a
C. Category II b
D. Category III

Question 3

What sign differentiates SVS/ISCVS Category IIa from IIb ischemia?

A. Pulselessness
B. Sensory loss
C. Motor loss
D. Loss of venous doppler signals

Question 4

In acute embolism, the sequence of events is:

A. Pulselessness, pain, pallor, paresthesia, paralysis
B. Paralysis, pain, paresthesia, pulselessness, pallor
C. Pulselessness, pain, pallor, paralysis, paresthesia

The patient is taken to the endovascular suite, and based on the preoperative CTA, the left groin is accessed utilizing ultrasound guidance. An angiogram is performed from the sheath that reveals an occluded left iliac system with an isolated common femoral artery. A glide wire is traversed through the iliac system into the aorta. After confirmation of position, an aortogram is performed (Fig. 12.1).

Question 5

Treatment options for this patient include which of the following:

A. Aortobifemoral bypass
B. Operative thrombo-embolectomy
C. Extra-anatomic bypass
D. Mechanical thrombectomy, thrombolysis and endovascular intervention
E. Intravenous thrombolysis
F. Anticoagulation with heparin and coumadin

Fig. 12.1 Aortography via a left femoral approach documents infrarenal aortic and bilateral iliac occlusions

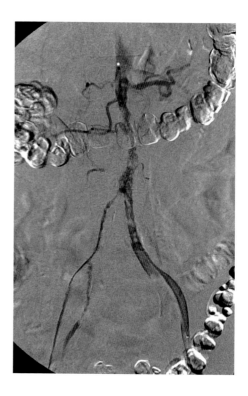

Question 6

After thrombolysis, long-term outcome is predicated on:

A. Unmasking a "culprit lesion" that is treated via either endovascular or surgical means
B. The dose of thrombolytic agent used
C. The duration of thrombolysis
D. The arterial outflow
E. Assuring all acute thrombus is lysed

This patient underwent lysis from the left groin with a 20 cm infusion catheter. Thrombolysis (TPA, tissue plasminogen activator, dose = 1 mg/h) was performed through a multi-side hole infusion catheter, and the following day, there was significant resolution of thrombus in the aorta/left common iliac system (Fig. 12.2). A combination of a hydrophilic wire and catheter was used to cross occlusion in the right common iliac system and gain access to the native femoral system (Fig. 12.3). A second infusion catheter was placed through this occlusion, and thrombolytic therapy was continued. After another 24 h of therapy, the patient was returned to the endovascular suite. While there was significant improvement, there was still residual thrombus at the origin of the right hypogastric artery and right external iliac artery (Fig. 12.4). Thrombolytic therapy was continued another 24 h at 0.5 mg/h TPA.

Fig. 12.2 After 24 h of thrombolysis, there was significant clot resolution throughout the aorta and common iliac segment. The left hypogastric artery is occluded

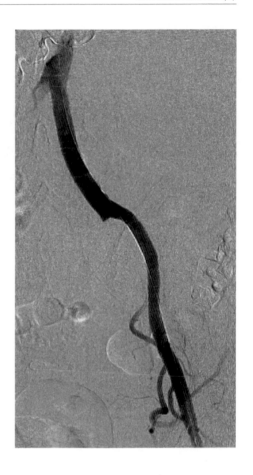

Fig. 12.3 From the left groin, the right common iliac thrombus has been crossed, and angiography confirms a patent external iliac and femoral system. A second 10-cm infusion catheter was positioned across this region

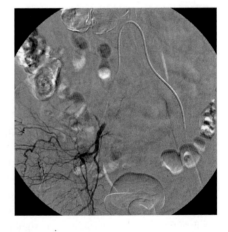

Fig. 12.4 After 48 h of thrombolysis, the right common iliac system was cleared of thrombus; however, there was still residual thrombus in the external iliac and hypogastric arteries. Thrombolysis was continued in attempt to clear the residual thrombus

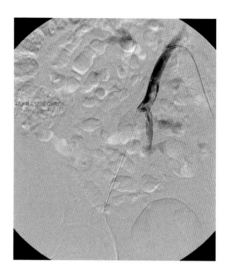

Question 7

During thrombolytic therapy for peripheral arterial occlusion, the most frequent complication is:

A. Pulmonary failure
B. Myocardial infarction
C. Intracranial hemorrhage
D. Vascular access bleeding

After 72 h of thrombolysis, there was still residual thrombus at the right hypogastric artery and external iliac artery origins (Fig. 12.5). Because of concerns over pelvic ischemia and residual thrombus in the left hypogastric artery, efforts were made to preserve the right hypogastric artery. The right hypogastric artery occlusion lesion was traversed from the left groin; the right groin was accessed and a second wire was positioned across the right external iliac artery (Fig. 12.6). From this position, opposing self-expanding stents were placed at the origins of both the external and internal iliac arteries restoring perfusion to the right lower extremity without embolization (Figs. 12.7 and 12.8).

The patient had palpable pedal pulses at completion of the procedure. In the postoperative period, a transesophageal echocardiogram documented cardiac thrombus as the source of aortoiliac embolization. She was discharged on anticoagulation.

12.1
Commentary

The etiology of acute limb ischemia can be classified into two groups. Thrombotic events occur in the setting of native arterial disease or bypass graft stenoses. In contrast, embolic phenomena usually occur in normal vessels and tend to lodge at arterial bifurcations.[1]

Fig. 12.5 After 72 h of thrombolysis, the residual clot remained at the origins of the external iliac artery and hypogastric artery

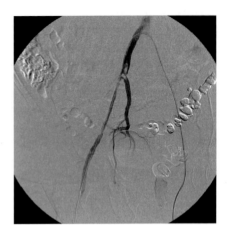

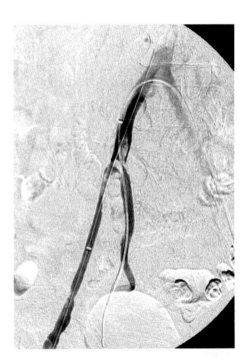

Fig. 12.6 Access was obtained from the right groin, and a wire was positioned retrograde across the external iliac thrombus. From the left groin, the right hypogastric artery was selected

Thrombotic occlusions are thought to represent progression of atherosclerotic disease and occur at sites along the arterial tree and most notably the superficial femoral artery at the adductor canal. In comparison, autologous grafts fail at sites of intimal hyperplasia, or fibrotic valves. Due to preexisting collaterals, native arterial thrombosis seldom presents with the profound ischemia seen with embolic ischemia. The presence of palpable pulses on the contralateral limb and a history of cardiac arrhythmia assist in differentiating acute embolus as opposed to thrombotic occlusions.[1]

Fig. 12.7 Two self-expanding stents were deployed in an "opposing fashion" in order to maintain patency of both the external iliac and hypogastric arteries. The right hypogastric artery was treated because of concerns for pelvic ischemia and possible residual left hypogastric thrombus

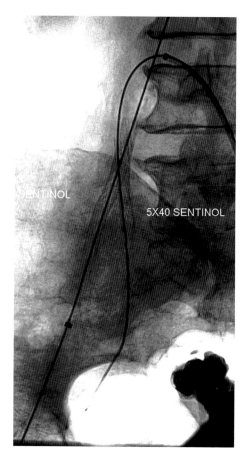

[Q1: E] All of the factors listed can help in differentiating embolic versus thrombotic occlusions. Often, a definitive diagnosis cannot be made preoperatively. However, identifying an embolic source for acute limb ischemia is helpful both for the acute and long-term management of the patient.

Clinical classification and diagnosis of acute occlusion of the lower extremity is based on the symptoms of the patient. The severity of symptoms is associated with the extent of the occlusion and the presence of pre-existing vessels. Patients with thrombotic occlusions from underlying disease of the SFA at the adductor canal may only experience worsening claudication while embolic events are usually associated with rapid onset and severe ischemia because of the lack of preexisting collateral flow. Limb ischemia has been classified into three categories by an SVS/ISCVS ad hoc committee, based on severity of ischemia.[2] Category I limbs are viable, not immediately threatened and have no motor or sensory loss. There are clearly audible arterial Doppler signals in the foot. Category II includes threatened limbs where salvage may be possible with timely intervention. Importantly, this category is divided into two subgroups, a and b which distinguish the time interval necessary for treatment. Group IIa require prompt treatment whereas Group IIb need immediate therapy to prevent amputation. In Group

Fig. 12.8 Completion imaging documents rapid flow through the aortoiliac system without any residual thrombus. Bilateral lower extremity runoff documented good runoff without embolization

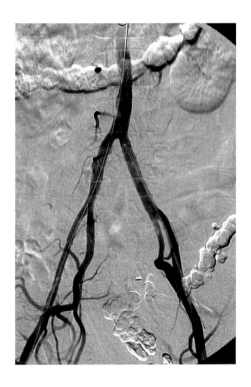

II, audible venous Doppler signals are present, but there is no arterial signal in the foot. Group IIa patients have minimal sensory loss and have no motor loss. However, patients with Group IIb ischemia, have muscle weakness, and sensory loss encompasses more than the toes. Category III is characterized by irreversible ischemia with profound and permanent neuromuscular damage where amputation may be the only recourse.

[Q2: C] This patient has Category IIb limb ischemia characterized by lack of distal arterial signals in the foot, sensory loss, and motor weakness. [Q3: C] Motor loss separates Category IIa from IIb ischemia and determines the urgency on which to proceed to revascularization.

The sequence of clinical events in patients with lower extremity ischemia is often predictable. [Q4: A] Most patients with acute ischemia, especially from of an embolic nature, will have pulselessness followed by pain and pallor. Paresthesia indicates sensory nerve ischemia and occurs usually from 1 to 3 h after the onset of acute ischemia. Paralysis indicates motor nerve damage that is often irreversible. In the setting of acute ischemia without collateral flow, paralysis occurs approximately 6 h after the onset of ischemia.[3] Any motor dysfunction should be seen as a worrisome sign and should prompt urgent intervention. Poikilothermia indicates that the foot or limb has approximated ambient temperature. In these irreversible cases (Category III), amputation may be the only option and often has to be done quickly to avoid systemic complications.

Both the diagnosis and localization of acute arterial occlusion is based upon the findings on physical exam and imaging studies. A "waterhammer" pulse signifies outflow obstruction, as observed with a common femoral embolus. By contrast, calcified vessels are common with thrombosis from underlying atherosclerotic disease. Multiple options are available for localization of the occlusion. Noninvasive testing with segmental pressures, pulse volume recording and measurement of the ankle brachial indices can provide a baseline study for comparison after treatment. Both vertical and horizontal pressure gradients of 30 mmHg or more in the lower extremity can accurately identify the site of occlusion. Duplex ultrasonography can also be utilized to examine the femoral and popliteal vessels and localize area of occlusion. Other causes such as thrombosed popliteal aneurysm can be easily diagnosed in this manner. MRA and CTA are emerging as noninvasive techniques for arteriographic imaging and localization of thrombosis. However, angiography remains the gold standard for localization of arterial occlusion. As importantly, angiography allows percutaneous access to the site of thrombosis and an array of treatment options for restoring blood flow to the limb.

Treatment for limb ischemia has evolved over the past two decades with advances in both pharmacologic therapy and endovascular options. **[Q5: B, C, D]** In patients with acute limb ischemia secondary to iliac occlusion, operative thrombectomy of the occluded iliac system may be feasible. In the setting of profound ischemia and a diseased iliac artery precluding successful thrombectomy, extra-anatomic bypass can be performed to provide expeditious blood flow into the ischemic limb. In these cases, either femoral-femoral bypass or axillo-femoral bypass can be contemplated depending on the inflow source. Aortofemoral bypass is a very durable option for patients with chronic occlusion and chronic ischemia of the limb. However, in patients with acute ischemia ill-prepared for major surgery, proceeding with direct reconstruction with the aorta as the inflow is sometimes hazardous. Multiple endovascular devices are available in the setting of acute thrombosis. Percutaneous mechanical thrombectomy with thrombolysis either via the power-pulse technique or via a standard infusion often quickly resolves the acute ischemia. Continued thrombolytic infusion is required for complete resolution of thrombus. Often, a "culprit" lesion will be unmasked by dissolving all of the acute thrombus, allowing percutaneous treatment of the offending lesion. Systemic thrombolytic therapy has been used to treat peripheral arterial occlusions, but results have been disappointing owing to a significant incidence of bleeding complications. Currently, systemic therapy is usually used for venous thromboembolic states. Regional intravascular infusion of the lytic agent avoids some of the systemic complications and is largely used for peripheral arterial thromboses and graft occlusions. Because a systemic lytic state may occur with prolonged regional intravascular thrombolytic therapy, patient selection is critical. Absolute contraindications include active internal bleeding, recent surgery or trauma to the area to be perfused, recent cerebrovascular accident, or documented left heart thrombus.[3] Relative contraindications include recent surgery, gastrointestinal bleeding or trauma, severe hypertension, mitral valve disease, endocarditis, hemostatic defects, or pregnancy.

[Q6: A, D, E] Several multicenter trials have examined groups of patients treated with surgical therapy or thrombolysis. The Rochester trial randomized patients to surgery or thrombolysis and demonstrated a lower mortality in the thrombolysis group.[4] Following successful thrombolysis, unmasked "culprit lesions" were treated with angioplasty or surgery of a lesser magnitude, thereby reducing the severity of the intervention and overall morbidity. The finding of a lesion that precipitated the thrombosis is critical to avoiding re-thrombosis. The STILE trial (Surgery versus Thrombolysis for Ischemia of the Lower

Extremity) compared optimal surgical therapy to intraarterial catheter-directed thrombolysis for native arterial or bypass graft occlusions.[5,6] Stratification by duration of ischemic symptoms revealed that patients with ischemia of less than 14 days duration had lower amputation rates with thrombolysis and shorter hospital stays, while patients with ischemia for longer than 14 days who were treated surgically had less ongoing or recurrent ischemia and trends toward lower morbidity. At 6 months, amputation-free survival was improved in patients with acute ischemia treated with thrombolysis, but patients with chronic ischemia had lower amputation rates when treated surgically. Fifty-five percent of patients treated with thrombolysis had a reduction in magnitude of their surgical procedure. Of note, no difference was seen between the use of rt-PA and urokinase.[5]

A multicenter, randomized, prospective trial comparing thrombolysis to surgery for acute lower extremity ischemia of less than 14 days duration has been performed. The Thrombolysis or Peripheral Arterial Surgery trial (TOPAS) randomized 757 patients to surgery or thrombolytic therapy.[7] The most effective dose for recombinant urokinase was determined to be 4,000 U/min with complete thrombolysis in 71% (mean duration of therapy 24 ± 0.8 h) of patients. After successful thrombolytic therapy, either surgical or endovascular intervention was performed on the lesion responsible for the occlusion if found. When compared to the surgical arm, the 1-year limb salvage rates and mortality were not statistically different. However, although no statistical differences between the two groups were seen with respect to amputation-free survival, thrombolysis was associated with a reduction in the number and magnitude of open surgical interventions over a 1-year follow up period.

Perhaps, unlike thrombolysis in coronary or venous systems, dissolution of the larger peripheral arterial thrombi requires direct infusion of thrombolytic agent into the clot. The thrombosed artery or bypass graft must be accessed with a wire, followed by placement of an infusion system into the thrombus. There are multiple dosing regimens for urokinase (UK), t-PA and other thrombolytic agents. A plethora of strategies for thrombolysis have been used and are described in a consensus document.[8] In this comprehensive review, 33 recommendations were made by a panel of experienced hematologists, radiologists, and vascular surgeons from North America and Europe. Of note, over 40 dosage schemes were reviewed and described for thrombolytic infusion. This included strategies of continuous versus stepwise infusion, bolusing or lacing the clot, and intraoperative thrombolysis. The most popular strategies included using UK 4,000 u/min for 4 h, and then decreasing to 2,000 u/min for a maximum of 48 h, t-PA at a dose of 1 mg/h and lacing the clot to increase thrombolytic efficiency. Our preferred current technique is to use low-dose t-PA (0.5–1.0 mg/h) after initial percutaneous mechanical thrombectomy. Low-dose heparin (300–400 u/h) is infused via the arterial sheath side arm to prevent pericatheter thrombosis, but full anticoagulation is avoided.

Following successful thrombolysis, any unmasked lesion can be addressed with balloon angioplasty and stenting or with an open surgical procedure. Even when a surgical procedure is necessary, it can usually be performed electively, in a well-prepared patient and is often of a lesser magnitude than what would have been required without thrombolysis. Thrombolytic therapy is an effective option for selected patients with acute thrombotic occlusion.

[Q7: D] Both pulmonary failure and myocardial infarction are more common with surgical revascularization and relatively infrequent complications in patients treated with thrombolytic therapy. Bleeding complications are the most frequent complications associated with thrombolytic therapy, and these are typically related to access bleeding that requires transfusion. The access-related bleeding rates ranged from 7% to 12.5% in the Rochester, STILE, and TOPAS trials compared to intracranial hemorrhage rates ranging from 0.5% to 2.5%. STILE found low fibrinogen levels to be associated with bleeding complications, while TOPAS found therapeutic heparin to increase the risk of complications. It is important to note that these trials limited therapy to 24–48 h for fear of bleeding complications. Bleeding, unexplained drop in hemoglobin, neurological changes, or fibrinogen levels falling below 100 mg/dL usually require cessation of thrombolytic therapy. The patient in this case represents an aggressive approach to extensive clot burden throughout the aortoiliac segment. In this example, therapy was extended to 72 h, longer than our usual arterial thrombolytic case, in order to fully dissolve all of the thrombus.

References

1. Blaisdell FW, Steele M, Allen RE. Management of acute lower extremity arterial ischemia due to embolism and thrombosis. *Surgery*. 1978;84:822-834.
2. Rutherford RB, Baker JD, Ernst C, et al. Recommended standards for reports dealing with lower extremity ischemia: Revised version. *J Vasc Surg*. 1997;26:517-538.
3. Kashyap VS, Quinones-Baldrich WJ. Principles of thrombolytic therapy. In: Rutherford RB, ed. *Vascular Surgery*. 5th ed. Philadelphia, PA: W.B. Saunders; 2000:457-475.
4. Ouriel K, Shortell CK, DeWeese JA, et al. A comparison of thrombolytic therapy with operative revascularization in the initial treatment of acute peripheral arterial ischemia. *J Vasc Surg*. 1994;19:1021-1030.
5. The STILE Investigators. Results of a prospective randomized trial evaluating surgery versus thrombolysis for ischemia of the lower extremity, The STILE Trial. *Ann Surg*. 1994;220:251-268.
6. Weaver F, Camerato A, Papanicolau G, et al. Surgical revascularization versus thrombolysis for non-embolic lower extremity native artery occlusions: results of a prospective randomized trial. The STILE Investigators. *J Vasc Surg*. 1996;24:513-523.
7. Ouriel K, Veith FJ, Sasahara AA. A comparison of recombinant urokinase with vascular surgery as initial treatment for acute arterial occlusion of the legs. *N Engl J Med*. 1998;338:1105-1111.
8. Working Party on Thrombolysis in the Management of Limb Ischemia. Thrombolysis in the management of lower limb peripheral arterial occlusion – a consensus document. *J Vasc Interv Radiol*. 2003 (Sept);14(9 Pt 2):S337-S349.

Part II

Acute Ischemia

Arterial Embolism

13

Andre Nevelsteen[†]

A 65-year-old man presented with acute severe pain in his right leg. Medical history revealed non-insulin-dependent diabetes mellitus for 3 years and a myocardial infarction (MI) some 5 years ago. The pain in the right leg developed suddenly over 6 hours without associated trauma and became worse over time. On admission, the right leg looked pale distally from the level of the knee. There was loss of light touch sensation on examination of the foot. The patient had difficulties in wiggling the toes. Plantarflexion and dorsiflexion of the toes were still possible. Palpation of the calf showed soft but tender muscles. Clinical examination of the abdomen showed no abnormalities. There was no pulsating mass. Irregular but bounding pulsations were felt in the right femoral artery. Popliteal artery and tibial artery pulsations were absent. Normal pulsations were felt in the left popliteal and posterior tibial artery.

Question 1

What is the aetiology of arterial embolism?

A. The aetiology of arterial embolism is most frequently unknown.
B. The most frequent cause of arterial embolism is cardiac valve destruction by rheumatic heart disease or endocarditis.
C. The most frequent cause of arterial embolism is atrial fibrillation in association with atherosclerotic heart disease.
D. Deep venous thrombosis might represent a rare cause of arterial embolism.
E. Arterial embolism is most frequently seen in the presence of increased blood viscosity.

With the diagnosis of acute arterial ischaemia in mind, a full dose of intravenous heparin was administered immediately.

A. Nevelsteen
Department of Vascular Surgery, University Hospital Gasthuisberg, Leuven, Belgium

G. Geroulakos and B. Sumpio (eds.), *Vascular Surgery*,
DOI: 10.1007/978-1-84996-356-5_13, © Springer-Verlag London Limited 2011

Question 2

What is the place of heparin in the treatment of arterial embolism?

A. Heparin can dissolve an arterial embolus, avoiding the need for subsequent operation.

B. Heparin will avoid subsequent arterial thrombosis, which can complicate treatment of arterial embolism.

C. Heparin will avoid subsequent arterial thrombosis, which can complicate treatment of arterial embolism. In addition, heparin will prevent recurrent emboli.

D. The use of heparin is contraindicated since it may lead to fragmentation of an arterial embolism and induce microembolisation in the peripheral arteries.

A chest film X-ray showed no abnormalities. Electrocardiogram (ECG) revealed atrial fibrillation and signs of an old MI. Laboratory studies were normal. Duplex examination showed a thrombotic occlusion of the right femoral bifurcation and the superficial femoral artery. A weak flow sign was present in the popliteal artery. The tibial arteries were not visualised.

Question 3

The preferred treatment of arterial embolism is:

A. Local excision of the vessel and reconstruction with interposition graft.

B. Continued heparinisation and wait and see.

C. Simple Fogarty catheter embolectomy with peroperative angiographic control.

D. Simple Fogarty catheter embolectomy, but percutaneous aspiration thromboembolectomy might be a good alternative in selected cases.

After placement of a central venous catheter, the patient was taken to the operating theatre and the right femoral bifurcation was exposed under local anaesthesia. A transverse arteriotomy confirmed complete thrombotic occlusion of the femoral bifurcation. There was good inflow. Thrombi were removed from the femoral bifurcation, and pulsatile backflow was obtained from the profunda femoris artery.

Multiple thrombi were removed from the superficial femoral artery and the popliteal artery after several passages of Fogarty embolectomy catheters numbers 3 and 4. Intraoperative angiography showed good patency of the superficial, popliteal and peroneal arteries. The anterior tibial artery was completely occluded. The posterior tibial was patent in its first portion but occluded distally. A small catheter was inserted into the popliteal artery, and 350,000 units of urokinase were infused as a dripping infusion over 30 min. Repeated angiography showed further clearance of the posterior tibial artery to the level of the ankle joint. The anterior tibial artery was still occluded. It was decided to accept the situation. The arteries were flushed with a diluted heparinised saline solution, and the transverse arteriotomy was closed with the aid of a Dacron patch. Sodium bicarbonate was administered intravenously before reperfusion.

Question 4

Reperfusion syndrome after arterial embolectomy:

A. Will never be seen after peripheral but only after aortic embolism.
B. Cannot be prevented medically.
C. Will be prevented by early ambulation.
D. Is induced by metabolic acidosis and myoglobinuria.

Postoperatively, the foot was well vascularised and the patient was able to wiggle his toes almost normally. Pulsations were felt in the posterior tibial artery. Intravenous heparin was continued. Brisk diuresis was maintained with mannitol and alkalisation of the urine. Repeated laboratory studies showed no evidence of acidosis or hyperkalaemia.

Question 5

Fasciotomy:

A. Has become obsolete and swelling of the limb should be treated by elevation and bed rest.
B. Is best routinely performed in any patient, treated for arterial embolism of the lower limbs.
C. The indication to fasciotomy needs to be based on objective parameters such as the presence of reperfusion syndrome and postoperative compartmental pressure measurements.
D. In daily practice, the indication for fasciotomy is most frequently based on individual preference and clinical feeling.

Six hours postoperatively, the patient developed significant limb swelling with augmentation of pain, venous hypertension and sensory impairment of the foot. A perifibular fasciotomy to decompress all four compartments was performed under general anaesthesia. Afterwards, the swelling subsided and the fasciotomy wound was closed in a delayed primary fashion after 1 week.

Question 6

With the pre- and peroperative diagnosis in mind:

A. The patient should be placed under antiplatelet therapy postoperatively in order to prevent another episode of embolism.
B. Heparin and oral anticoagulants remain the treatment of choice during the postoperative period.
C. Subsequent investigation with regard to the source of the embolus is not necessary, because this will not change the medical treatment.
D. Postoperative investigation with regard to the source of embolism can be limited to cardiac examinations such as echocardiography and Holter monitoring.

Abdominal ultrasound performed postoperatively showed atheromatosis of the abdominal aorta but no aneurysmal dilatation. Transthoracic and transoesophageal echocardiography revealed no ventricular aneurysm or intracardiac thrombi. Holter monitoring for 24 h confirmed atrial fibrillation. Pathological examination of the retrieved emboli was compatible with ordinary thrombotic material. Cultures were negative. The problem of atrial fibrillation was handled medically. Oral anticoagulation was initiated, and the patient was discharged after 10 days. Six months later, there were no repeat episodes of acute ischaemia.

13.1
Commentary

Acute ischaemia due to arterial embolism represents a limb-threatening event. Although the carotid or intracranial vessels may be involved in a minority of the cases, the upper or lower extremities are involved in 70–80% in most series of arterial embolisation.[1] The lower extremity is involved five times as frequently as the upper extremity, and the sites of embolic occlusion are most often related to major arterial bifurcations. The common femoral bifurcation is the most frequent site of embolic occlusion, usually noted in 30–50% of all cases.[2] In total, the femoral and popliteal arteries are involved more than twice as often as the aorta.

The heart is by far the predominant source of arterial emboli, seen in 80–90% of cases.[3] Atrial fibrillation is present in approximately 70% of patients. Previously, it was most frequently the reflection of rheumatic heart disease. Since the incidence of rheumatic heart disease has declined steadily over the last 50 years, atrial fibrillation is now associated most frequently with atherosclerotic heart disease.

MI is the second common cause of peripheral embolisation. Left ventricular mural thrombus occurs in 30% of acute transmural infarcts. Clinically evident embolism is seen in only 5% of these patients.[4] One should be aware, however, that silent MI may be present in up to 10% of patients with peripheral emboli, and that embolisation may be the presenting symptom of an acute infarction. Apart from the acute period, MI may also cause emboli after longer intervals. This is usually due to areas of hypokinesis or ventricular aneurysm formation. Although most emboli occur within 6 weeks of MI, much longer intervals may be noted.

Other cardiac diseases are associated less frequently with peripheral emboli. Thromboemboli can, however, arise from prosthetic cardiac valves or from vegetations on the mitral or aortic valve leaflets. Endocarditis should certainly be ruled out. Finally, intracardiac tumours, such as atrial myxoma, may also give rise to clinically evident embolic events.

Non-cardiac sources of peripheral emboli are noted less frequently. Major emboli may arise from aneurysms of the aorta or less frequently from the femoropopliteal vessels.[5] With upper-extremity emboli, one should be aware of unsuspected thoracic outlet syndrome and aneurysmal deformation of the subclavian artery. Paradoxical emboli might be seen with deep venous thrombosis in association with a patent foramen ovale. Primary or secondary lung tumours might invade the pulmonary veins, causing tumour emboli. Finally, apart from rare causes such as foreign body embolisation, it should be recognised that the source of embolisation will remain inapparent in some 10% of patients.[2] **[Q1: C, D]**

The diagnosis of acute ischaemia caused by arterial embolism is usually straight-forward. The most typical signs are characterised by the "five Ps": pulselessness, pain, pallor, paraesthesia and paralysis. The level of occlusion is determined by the presence or absence of palpable pulses. Once the diagnosis of acute arterial ischaemia has been made, 5,000 units of heparin are administered intravenously. This is not meant as effective treatment but it prevents the propagation and fragmentation of the thrombus. Concomitant venous thrombosis, which can occur with prolonged severe arterial ischaemia, might also be avoided. Heparin administration allows time for diagnosis, evaluation and, if necessary, treatment of cardiac disturbances. **[Q2: B]**

Fogarty catheter embolectomy remains the treatment of choice in most patients with peripheral embolisation.[6] The procedure is usually carried out under local anaesthesia and is effective in cases of major emboli. All retrieved emboli should be sent for pathological and microbiological examination. The operative result should be checked by intraoperative fluoroscopy or angioscopy. Remaining thrombi in the distal vessels can be approached directly or by intraoperative thrombolysis.[7] Thrombolytic therapy or percutaneous aspiration thromboembolectomy (Fig. 13.1) may be used as alternatives to Fogarty catheter embolectomy in selected cases with no motor dysfunction or profound sensory loss.[8, 9] **[Q3: C, D]**

All patients undergoing revascularisation of an acutely ischaemic limb are at risk of ischaemia reperfusion syndrome. This was first emphasised by Haimovici,[10] described under its most grave form as the myonephropathic-metabolic syndrome. This reperfusion syndrome is the consequence of muscular hypoxia and the associated metabolic changes. A prolonged period of ischaemia results in accumulation of potassium, lactic acid, myoglobin and other cellular enzymes, leading to a significant fall in blood pH due to anaerobic metabolism, paralysis of the sodium potassium cellular pump and rhabdomyolysis.[11] Acute washout of these products may lead to hyperkalaemia and metabolic acidosis, resulting in myocardial depression or dysrhythmias. Myoglobin and other products of skeletal muscle breakdown can precipitate within the kidney and result in acute renal failure. Myoglobinuria is the first sign. **[Q4: D]** These problems should be anticipated with bicarbonate and/or calcium intravenously just before reperfusion. Induction of forced diuresis with mannitol and alkalisation of the urine might avoid acute renal failure. In addition, mannitol also acts as a scavenger of oxygen-derived free radicals, which are an important intermediary in ischaemia reperfusion injury.[12, 13] It is clear, therefore, that the patient should be monitored carefully postoperatively with regard to electrolyte changes, development of metabolic acidosis and urinary output.

Another problem following revascularisation of an acute ischaemic limb might be significant limb swelling. This may result in secondary muscle or nerve injury, venous compression, further oedema and compartment syndrome, leading to arterial compression and secondary ischaemia. To avoid this, the surgeon might prefer to perform a fasciotomy in conjunction with the embolectomy procedure.[14] Alternatively, the extremity can be assessed immediately and at regular intervals postoperatively for evolving compartment syndrome. As described in different textbooks, there are several ways of performing an adequate fasciotomy. The most important point here is that all four compartments should be decompressed.

Although concomitant fasciotomy can be preferable in some cases of prolonged acute ischaemia, the more conservative approach might avoid unnecessary fasciotomy and

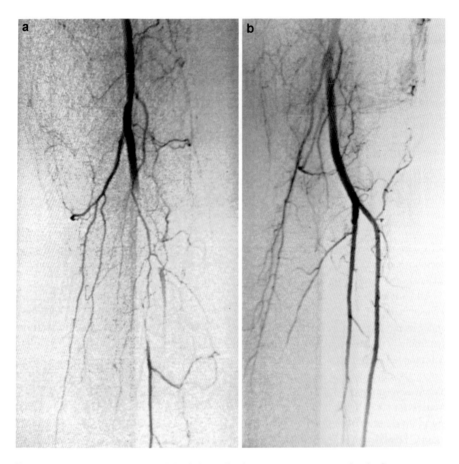

Fig. 13.1 (**a**) Embolic occlusion of the left popliteal artery; treatment consisted of percutaneous aspiration thromboembolectomy. (**b**) Normal patency of the popliteal, anterior tibial and peroneal arteries

unaesthetic scars. Since a Fogarty catheter embolectomy can easily be carried out under local anaesthesia, this wait-and-see approach eliminates the need for systematic general anaesthesia, particularly for patients in a poor general condition.[15]

Despite the fact that the value of postoperative compartmental pressure measurements has been documented by several teams,[16, 17] the decision regarding subsequent fasciotomy is most frequently based upon individual preferences and prior clinical experience. [**Q5: D**]

Every effort should be made in the postoperative period to minimise the incidence of recurrent emboli. The patient should be treated with heparin or oral anticoagulants until the source of the embolus has been taken care of. [**Q6: B**] If extensive investigation fails to show any correctable source, then long-term anti-coagulation is indicated, except in the case of major contraindications.

References

1. Panetta T, Thompson JE, Talkinton CM, Garrett WV, Smith BL. Arterial embolectomy: a 34-year experience with 400 cases. *Surg Clin North Am.* 1986;66:339.
2. Thompson JE, Sigler L, Raut PS, Austin DJ, Patman RD. Arterial embolectomy: a 20-year experience. *Surgery.* 1970;67:212-220.
3. Mills JL, Porter JM. Basic data related to clinical decision making in acute limb ischemia. *Ann Vasc Surg.* 1991;5:96.
4. Keating EC, Gross SA, Schlamowitz RA. Mural thrombi in myocardial infarctions. *Am J Med.* 1983;74:989.
5. Reber PU, Patel AG, Stauffer E, Muller MF, Do DD, Kniemeyer HW. Mural aortic thrombi: an important cause of peripheral embolization. *Vasc Surg.* 1999;30:1084-1089.
6. Abbott WM, Maloney RD, McCabe CC, Lee CE, Wirthlin LS. Arterial embolism: a 44 year perspective. *Am J Surg.* 1982;143:460-464.
7. Beard JD, Nyamekye I, Earnshaw JJ, Scott DJ, Thompson JF. Intraoperative streptokinase: a useful adjunct to balloon-catheter embolectomy. *Br J Surg.* 1993;80:21-24.
8. Heymans S, Vanderschueren S, Verhaeghe R, et al. Outcome and one year follow-up of intra-arterial staphylokinase in 191 patients with peripheral arterial occlusion. *Thromb Haemost.* 2000;83:666-671.
9. Sniderman KW, Kalman PG, Quigley MJ. Percutaneous aspiration embolectomy. *J Cardiovasc Surg (Torino).* 1993;34:255.
10. Haimovici H. Muscular, renal and metabolic complications of acute arterial occlusions: myonephropathic-metabolic syndrome. *Surgery.* 1979;85:461.
11. Fischer RD, Fogarty TJ, Morrow AG. Clinical and biochemical observations of the effect of transient femoral artery occlusion in man. *Surgery.* 1970;68:323.
12. Rubin BB, Walker PM. Pathophysiology of acute skeletal muscle injury: adenine nucleotide metabolism in ischemic reperfused muscle. *Semin Vasc Surg.* 1992;5:11.
13. Pattwell D, McArdle A, Griffiths RD, Jackson MJ. Measurement of free radical production by in vivo microdialysis during ischemia/reperfusion injury to skeletal muscle. *Free Radic Biol Med.* 2001;30:979-985.
14. Padberg FT, Hobson RWII. Fasciotomy in acute limb ischemia. *Semin Vasc Surg.* 1992;5:52.
15. Rush DS, Frame SB, Bell RM, Berg EE, Kerstein MD, Haynes JL. Does open fasciotomy contribute to morbidity and mortality after acute lower extremity ischemia and revascularization? *J Vasc Surg.* 1989;10:343-350.
16. Whitesides TE, Heckman MM. Acute compartment syndrome: update on diagnosis and treatment. *J Am Acad Orthop Surg.* 1996;4:209-218.
17. Janzing HMJ. *The acute compartment syndrome, a complication of fractures and soft tissue injuries of the extremities. A clinical study about diagnosis and treatment of the compartment syndrome.* Doctoral thesis. Leuven University; 1999.

Blast Injury to the Lower Limb

14

Paul H.B. Blair, Adrian K. Neil, and Christopher T. Andrews

A 40-year-old male was admitted to the emergency room approximately 1.5 h after sustaining a blast injury to both lower limbs. He had been resuscitated at his local accident and emergency department prior to transfer. On arrival, his pulse was 120 bpm and his blood pressure 80/40 mm Hg.

Examination revealed that the patient had sustained significant blast injuries to both lower limbs with no obvious torso injuries. The left leg had sustained neurovascular damage above and below the knee with concomitant bone and soft tissue injury; there was no tissue perfusion below the knee. On the right side there was a large wound in the thigh extending anteriorly to the knee joint with profuse bleeding; bony fragments could be seen in the wound and the right foot was pale with no palpable pulses and slight reduction in sensation.

Question 1

The priorities for the care of this patient include:

A. Secure an airway, commence oxygen therapy and obtain adequate intravenous (IV) access.
B. Complete a full survey of the patient before transferring for further management.
C. Wait for blood result before deciding on transfer out of the emergency room.
D. Transfer the patient to theatre for definitive management during primary resuscitation.
E. Discuss treatment options with relatives.

Question 2

Which of the following are "hard" signs of vascular injury?

A. Limb pain.
B. Absence of pulses.
C. Pallor or cyanosis.
D. Cool to the touch.
E. Bruit or thrill.

P.H.B. Blair (✉)
Vascular Surgery Unit, Royal Victoria Hospital, Belfast, UK

G. Geroulakos and B. Sumpio (eds.), *Vascular Surgery*,
DOI: 10.1007/978-1-84996-356-5_14, © Springer-Verlag London Limited 2011

Question 3

Which of the following statements relating to angiography are true?

A. Angiography should be performed in all patients to target surgery.
B. Angiography may be a useful tool in trauma patients with no hard signs of vascular injury.
C. Angiography is reserved for stable patients.
D. Angiography should only be performed in a radiology department.
E. The patient's pre-morbid condition should not influence the decision to perform angiography.

Question 4

For how long will the lower limb tolerate ischemia?

A. 20–30 min
B. 90–120 min
C. 6–8 h
D. 16–20 h
E. 24–36 h

The patient was resuscitated as per advanced trauma life support (ATLS) protocol. Supplementary oxygen was administered in addition to obtaining additional IV access. Pressure dressings were applied to the open wounds and further assessment revealed an injury to the patient's right hand; no other significant injuries were present. The patient was transferred to the operating theatre.

Question 5

What are the primary aims of surgery in such a case?

A. To control life-threatening haemorrhage.
B. To prevent end-organ ischaemia.
C. To restore vascular continuity.
D. To preserve limb function.
E. To detect occult injuries.

Question 6

What factors will influence the decision to perform an amputation?

A. Patient's age
B. Mechanism of injury

C. Time to treatment
D. Degree of contamination
E. All of the above

Question 7

Which of the following statements about complex vein repair are true?

A. Complex vein repair should never be undertaken in the trauma patient.
B. Complex vein repair should only be performed in the absence of major arterial injury.
C. Complex vein repair should be used to improve venous return in unstable patients.
D. Complex vein repair may prevent long-term limb dysfunction.
E. Intraluminal venous shunting is an acceptable intraoperative temporising measure.

In the operating theatre, under general anaesthesia, the patient was placed in the supine position. The lower abdomen and both legs were prepared and draped widely and IV broad spectrum antibiotics were administered. Closer examination revealed that the left leg had sustained extensive injuries. The foot and distal calf were cold, pale and mottled. There was a compound injury to the left femur and tibia with complete disruption of the superficial femoral artery, superficial femoral vein and extensive injury to the sciatic nerve. It was decided that primary amputation of the left limb was required. On examination of the right leg there was complete disruption of the distal superficial/popliteal artery, a ragged laceration of the popliteal vein and significant bruising to branches of the sciatic nerve. There was a shrapnel injury to the right hand involving the thumb and middle finger.

Immediate surgical steps were as follows: (a) a proximal thigh tourniquet was placed on the left leg to arrest haemorrhage prior to formal amputation. The laceration to the right lower leg was then extended distally to facilitate exposure of the neurovascular structures. Control of the superficial femoral and below-knee popliteal artery was obtained and a careful distal embolectomy performed. A Javid shunt was then placed between the right superficial femoral artery and right below-knee popliteal vessel (Fig. 14.1). Significant bleeding from a large defect in the popliteal vein occurred following shunt insertion; this was repaired using a lateral suture. The long saphenous vein was harvested from the left leg, prior to performing above-knee amputation. While the left above-knee amputation was being performed, the orthopaedic surgeons carefully assessed the right lower limb and placed a temporary fixation device traversing the right knee joint (Fig. 14.2). Having obtained bony stability, with an external fixator device, the temporary intraluminal shunt was removed and a definitive bypass performed using reversed left long saphenous vein graft. Formal fasciotomy was performed of the right lower leg using a standard lateral and medial approach; distal pulses were confirmed in the right foot. Further debridement of necrotic muscle was performed and the wound on the medial aspect was partially closed; the anterolateral wounds were debrided and irrigated, as were the fasciotomy sites, with sterile dressings being applied to both.

Fig. 14.1 Extended wound, medial aspect of right leg with a temporary intraluminal shunt between superficial femoral and below-knee popliteal arteries

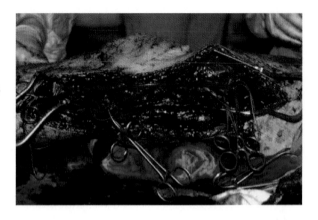

Fig. 14.2 A multidisciplinary approach. Bony stabilization of right leg (after temporary intraluminal shunt placement) by the orthopaedic surgeons, simultaneous with left above-knee amputation by the vascular surgeons

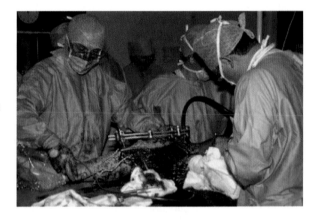

Question 8

In the absence of obvious haemorrhage, when is it appropriate to reinspect the wounds in the postoperative period?

A. 1–2 h
B. 4–6 h
C. 12–16 h
D. 24–48 h
E. 5+ days

Postoperatively the patient was transferred to the intensive care unit where the right limb was elevated to reduce swelling. The right foot was left exposed to allow access for pedal pulses. Broad spectrum IV antibiotics were continued in addition to standard prophylaxis for deep vein thrombosis, and urine was checked for myoglobinuria. The patient was returned to the operating theatre within 48 h for wound inspection and change of dressing. Eventually skin coverage of the right limb was obtained using a combination of split skin grafting and healing by delayed primary intention. Over the next few months the patient required complex orthopaedic surgery including the use of an Ilizarov frame device (Fig. 14.3). He was fitted with an above-knee prosthesis for his left leg and is now fully independent (Fig. 14.4).

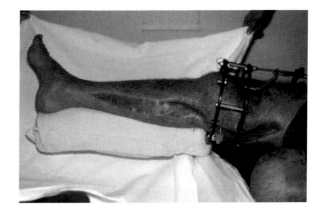

Fig. 14.3 Recovery. Healed traumatic and fasciotomy wounds after skin grafting; Ilizarov frame still in place

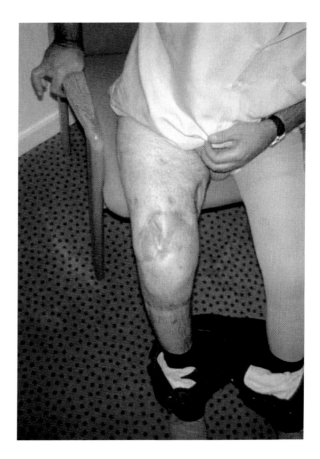

Fig. 14.4 Rehabilitation. An excellent result for limb salvage (right leg) and learning to function with a prosthesis (left)

14.1
Commentary

Lower limb injuries, due to penetrating trauma, can be devastating and occasionally may distract the clinician from less obvious but potentially life-threatening injuries to the head, neck and torso. It is important that some form of resuscitation protocol is followed such as the ATLS system to detect less obvious injuries. Time is of the essence when managing vascular injuries. While delays rarely occur in patients with obvious haemorrhage, it is the prompt instigation of life-saving measures and ongoing diagnosis in parallel with transfer to the operating theatre for definitive care that reduces morbidity and mortality. [Q1: A, D]

The clinical manifestations of vascular injury have traditionally been divided into "hard" and "soft" signs (Table 14.1). [Q2: B, E]

In general, preoperative arteriography may be used in the following situations: (1) to confirm the site and extent of vascular injury in stable patients whose clinical signs and symptoms are equivocal; and (2) to exclude vascular injury in patients with no hard signs, but who are considered to be at risk because of the proximity of the injury. The majority of patients with penetrating extremity trauma and the presence of a single hard sign should be transferred directly to the operating theatre. Possible exceptions to this rule include stable patients with multiple levels of injury, extensive bone or soft tissue injury, blast or shotgun injuries, potential injuries to the subclavian or axillary arteries and the pre-existence of peripheral vascular disease. Some centres report excellent results with emergency room angiography[1] while recent advances in endovascular technique facilitate high-quality imaging in the operating theatre. [Q3: B, C]

Inadequate tissue perfusion due to major vessel disruption is aggravated by hypovolemic shock and associated bone and soft tissue injury. The resulting fall in tissue pO_2 increases capillary membrane permeability, with increased exudation of fluid into the interstitial space. Compromised muscle fibres swell within the fascial compartments, causing further resistance to blood flow, and swelling becomes traumatic when arterial repair and restoration of flow brings about reperfusion injury. The degree of reperfusion injury depends on the duration of ischaemia, and is mediated by the generation of free radicals, activation of neutrophils, and production of arachidonic acid metabolites. Eventually, the microvascular bed of the extremity may undergo widespread thrombosis.[2] It is generally accepted that a warm ischaemia time of more than 6–8 h makes limb survival unlikely. [Q4: C] To achieve optimal results from emergency vascular repair, and to avoid complications

Table 14.1 Signs of vascular injury. Updated

Hard signs	Soft signs
Absent pulse	Haematoma (small)
Bruit or thrill	History of haemorrhage at scene
Haematoma (large or expanding)	Peripheral nerve deficit
Distal ischaemia	

such as compartment syndrome or contracture due to prolonged warm ischaemia and reperfusion injury, surgical exploration should be undertaken expeditiously.

A patient with complex lower limb injuries should be placed in a supine position on an operating table suitable for on-table angiography, if required, when clinical stability has been reached. Some form of warming device should be employed to maintain adequate body temperature. In lower limb trauma, both limbs should be prepared from umbilicus to toes; donor saphenous vein harvesting may be required from the contralateral limb, particularly if ipsilateral venous injury is suspected. Careful attention should be given to correct hypothermia, blood loss, electrolyte imbalance and coagulopathy.

The principal aims of emergency vascular surgery are to control life-threatening haemorrhage and prevent end-organ ischaemia. [Q5: A, B] An assistant should control haemorrhage using a pressure dressing until the patient is prepared and draped appropriately. Haemorrhage control can be difficult if the proximal vessels are not immediately apparent, and the use of a cephalad incision through virgin territory may be a reasonable alternative to obtain rapid proximal control. Care should be taken when making additional incisions, particularly if it seems likely that plastic surgery will be required at a later date. When access to the proximal or distal vessel is difficult, temporary control can be gained by careful cannulation and inflation of an embolectomy catheter. It is important that the surgeon cooperates fully with the anaesthetist during surgery as it may be necessary to pack the wound for a few minutes to facilitate IV fluid resuscitation before proximal vascular control can be obtained. Complex lengthy operations should be avoided in unstable patients and damage limitation surgery should be considered in patients with significant metabolic acidosis, coagulopathy and/or hypothermia.

The use of a temporary intraluminal vascular shunt should be considered in the majority of limb vascular injuries and is particularly important in complex cases with associated bone and soft tissue injury.

Temporary shunts for arterial and venous injuries have been employed in Belfast since the late 1970s.[2] A considerable body of evidence continues to support the use of these intravascular shunts in the management of both penetrating and blunt major vascular trauma.[3-6] Before securing the shunt between the proximal and distal arteries, a careful embolectomy should be performed to remove any thrombus in the distal vessel. If a venous injury is encountered, then an additional shunt can be employed to facilitate venous return. In the absence of coagulopathy or ongoing haemorrhage we use IV heparin routinely. Recent evidence has shown clearly that delayed renewal of venous flow in combined arterial and venous injury compounds ischaemia-reperfusion injury and causes remote lung injury.[7] The advantages of shunting artery and vein are the early restoration of blood flow and venous return, respectively, thus avoiding the complications of prolonged ischaemia and ischaemia-reperfusion injury while ensuring that an optimal vascular repair can be performed.

In patients with concomitant fractures, accurate internal or external fixation of the fracture can be performed with the shunt secured carefully with sloops before definitive vascular repair is performed. This avoids the dilemma of unnecessary haste for both the orthopaedic and vascular surgeons, ensures that a vein graft will be of optimal length, and eliminates the risk of graft disruption during fracture manipulation. Autologous vein is our preferred bypass conduit in the majority of cases because of its durability and suitability in a potentially contaminated wound. Satisfactory results, however, have been reported using synthetic grafts and in critically ill, unstable patients this may be a preferable option.[8]

The acute management of high energy limb trauma can be challenging and significant morbidity and mortality can occur following failed attempts at limb salvage. A number of scoring systems have been devised in an attempt to assist the clinician's decision to either amputate or perform a limb-salvage procedure.[9-13] In each of the systems, a score is assigned based on a range of differing criteria including patient age, "mechanism of injury", time to treatment, degree of shock, warm ischaemia time and the presence of local injuries to the following structures: major artery, major vein, bone, muscle, nerve, skin, and degree of contamination. [Q6: E] All of these scoring systems demonstrate a much higher degree of specificity than sensitivity and are more useful in highlighting the patients who should be considered for a limb-salvage procedure, than identifying those who should proceed straight to primary amputation. Indeed a number of studies have challenged their use at all.[14,15]

It is the authors' opinion that scoring systems can help the surgeon perform a detailed assessment of a complex limb injury. However, the decision to perform a primary amputation must be judged individually in each case. Extensive nerve injuries have a particularly poor prognosis and it is important that such injuries, where possible, are documented before taking the patient to the operating theatre. The patient's life should never be put at risk in a futile attempt to save a severely compromised limb. Where possible, additional specialties such as orthopaedics and plastic surgery should be involved in the decision to perform a primary limb amputation, particularly in a case of upper limb trauma.

Venous injuries can be difficult to manage. Prior to World War II, the traditional treatment for lower extremity venous injuries was ligation. This custom was challenged by Debakey and Simeone[16] in 1946 with an analysis of WWII battle injuries. Since then a number of clinical and laboratory investigations have confirmed that ligation of major veins in conjunction with repair of a traumatically injured arterial system leads to significantly poorer clinical outcomes, such as decreased function or even limb loss.[17,18] Where possible vein repair should be attempted, particularly in the presence of significant lower limb arterial injury, in an attempt to reduce venous hypertension and associated morbidity. While there are few data regarding the long-term outcome of venous repairs, it is the authors' impression that maintaining venous patency, in the initial few days after injury, can significantly help reduce acute post-injury swelling. If the superficial femoral vein requires ligation, it is important to maintain patency of the ipsilateral long saphenous and profunda femoris veins. Complex vein repair should never be attempted in unstable patients who have sustained major blood loss and have significant problems with hypothermia and coagulopathy. In more stable patients, however, temporary intraluminal venous shunting can facilitate the construction of larger calibre panel grafts obtained from the contralateral long saphenous vein. [Q7: D, E]

Postoperative management of patients with complex limb injuries is critically important. The majority of these patients have been transferred immediately to the operating theatre and it is important that a thorough search for occult injuries is performed on admission to the intensive care unit. These patients are at risk of developing multiple organ dysfunction syndrome as a result of their large transfusion requirements and likely reperfusion injury sustained.[19,20] It is important that the vascular surgeon communicates clearly with the staff in the intensive care unit regarding the presence or absence of distal pulses, to ensure that vascular repair remains patent. Young trauma patients with normal blood pressure and temperature should have a palpable distal pulse. If there is any doubt regarding the integrity of the vascular repair, the dressings should be removed and a careful assessment performed by a vascular surgeon using handheld Doppler and/or portable ultrasound device.

Wounds should be reinspected 24–48 h after initial surgery and at that stage definitive plastic surgery may be required to obtain soft tissue and skin cover. **[Q8: D]** Some centres advocate a selective policy with regard to fasciotomy based on compartmental pressures, while many continue to advocate a more liberal policy based on clinical grounds. Prolonged ischaemia time, combined arteriovenous injuries, complex injuries including bone and soft tissue destruction and crush injuries remain absolute indications for fasciotomy. The avoidance of compartment syndrome and restoration of limb function far outweigh the low morbidity associated with liberal use of fasciotomy. These patients are at significant risk of wound and other nosocomial infections and prolonged antibiotic use may be required.

The management of patients with complex injuries can be difficult; however, timely surgery and the involvement of a multidisciplinary team can produce rewarding results. One possible criticism of the above care could be failure to use the great toe, from the amputated left lower limb, to replace the patient's right thumb.

References

1. Itani KM, Burch JM, Spjut-Patrinely V, Richardson R, Martin RR, Mattox KL. Emergency center arteriography. *J Trauma*. 1992;32(3):302-306. discussion 306-37.
2. Barros D'Sa AA. How do we manage acute limb ischaemia due to trauma? In: Greenhalgh RM, Jamieson CW, Nicolaides AN, eds. *Limb Salvage and Amputation for Vascular Disease*. London: WB Saunders; 1998.
3. D'Sa AA. A decade of missile-induced vascular trauma. *Ann R Coll Surg Engl*. 1982;64(1): 37-44.
4. Elliot J, Templeton J, Barros D'Sa AA. Combined bony and vascular trauma: a new approach to treatment. *J Bone Joint Surg Am*. 1984;66B:281.
5. Barros D'Sa AA. The rationale for arterial and venous shunting in the management of limb vascular injuries. *Eur J Vasc Surg*. 1989;3(6):471-474.
6. Barros D'Sa AA, Moorehead RJ. Combined arterial and venous intraluminal shunting in major trauma of the lower limb. *Eur J Vasc Surg*. 1989;3(6):577-581.
7. Harkin DW, D'Sa AA, Yassin MM, et al. Reperfusion injury is greater with delayed restoration of venous outflow in concurrent arterial and venous limb injury. *Br J Surg*. 2000;87(6): 734-741.
8. Lovric Z, Lehner V, Kosic-Lovric L, Wertheimer B. Reconstruction of major arteries of lower extremities after war injuries. Long-term follow up. *J Cardiovasc Surg (Torino)*. 1996;37(3): 223-227.
9. Howe HR Jr, Poole GV Jr, Hansen KJ, et al. Salvage of lower extremities following combined orthopedic and vascular trauma. A predictive salvage index. *Am Surg*. 1987;53(4):205-208.
10. Johansen K, Daines M, Howey T, Helfet D, Hansen ST Jr. Objective criteria accurately predict amputation following lower extremity trauma. *J Trauma*. 1990;30(5):568-572. discussion 572-573.

11. Helfet DL, Howey T, Sanders R, Johansen K. Limb salvage versus amputation. Preliminary results of the Mangled Extremity Severity Score. *Clin Orthop Relat Res*. 1990;256:80-86.
12. Russell WL, Sailors DM, Whittle TB, Fisher DF Jr, Burns RP. Limb salvage versus traumatic amputation. A decision based on a seven-part predictive index. *Ann Surg*. 1991;213(5): 473-480. discussion 480-481.
13. McNamara MG, Heckman JD, Corley FG. Severe open fractures of the lower extremity: a retrospective evaluation of the Mangled Extremity Severity Score (MESS). *J Orthop Trauma*. 1994;8(2):81-87.
14. Bonanni F, Rhodes M, Lucke JF. The futility of predictive scoring of mangled lower extremities. *J Trauma*. 1993;34(1):99-104.
15. Durham RM, Mistry BM, Mazuski JE, Shapiro M, Jacobs D. Outcome and utility of scoring systems in the management of the mangled extremity. *Am J Surg*. 1996;172(5):569-573. discussion 573-574.
16. Debakey ME, Simeone FA. Battle injuries of arteries in World War II: analysis of 2471 cases. *Ann Surg*. 1946;123:534-579.
17. Nanobashvili J, Kopadze T, Tvaladze M, Buachidze T, Nazvlishvili G. War injuries of major extremity arteries. *World J Surg*. 2003;27(2):134-139.
18. Kuralay E, Demirkilic U, Ozal E, et al. A quantitative approach to lower extremity vein repair. *J Vasc Surg*. 2002;36(6):1213-1218.
19. Defraigne JO, Pincemail J. Local and systemic consequences of severe ischemia and reperfusion of the skeletal muscle. Physiopathology and prevention. *Acta Chir Belg*. 1998;98(4):176-186.
20. Foex BA. Systemic responses to trauma. *Br Med Bull*. 1999;55(4):726-743.

Endovascular Management of Aortic Transection in a Multiinjured Patient

15

Shiva Dindyal and Constantinos Kyriakides

A 19-year-old female was admitted to casualty following a road traffic collision. A witness of the incident reported that she was driving her car at approximately 70 km/h in wet conditions and the car skidded off the road when she turned a sharp bend. She collided with a tree and there were no other passengers involved. She was found in her severely damaged car, drowsy and restrained by her seat belt and the dashboard. The car windscreen had a "bulls-eye" on the driver's side and she had a laceration to her forehead, which was profoundly bleeding. She complained of difficulty in breathing and pain in her chest, abdomen and obviously deformed right leg. The paramedics attended the scene with the fire-service who helped extricate her form the wreckage then carefully immobilized her cervical spine.

She was immediately transported by helicopter to the nearest emergency department. There she was treated by the duty surgical trauma team.

Question 1

Which of the following interventions should be performed by the paramedics as their initial management?

A. Reduction, splinting and immobilization of her right femur fracture
B. Intravenous cannulation and bolus fluid administration
C. High flow oxygen administration
D. Administration of analgesia

Primary examination in casualty revealed a patent airway as she was talking but she was short of breath. Her trachea was deviated to the right side, the left chest was hyper-resonant and devoid of breath sounds. Hemodynamically her heart rate was raised (109 beats/min) and blood pressure (120/75 mmHg) was within normal limits. Her abdomen was tender in the left hypochondrium and right femur had an open mid-shaft fracture. Routine trauma blood investigations were requested. Neurologically she was drowsy and becoming increasingly confused.

S. Dindyal (✉)
Department of General Surgery, The Royal London Hospital, London, UK

G. Geroulakos and B. Sumpio (eds.), *Vascular Surgery*,
DOI: 10.1007/978-1-84996-356-5_15, © Springer-Verlag London Limited 2011

Question 2

Which is the most appropriate initial investigation required?

A. Computerized tomography of her head and neck
B. Plain radiographs of the pelvis and right femur
C. Computerized tomography of her abdomen and pelvis
D. Plain portable chest radiograph

Her heart rate further increased (120 beats/min) and blood pressure reduced (110/65 mmHg). She was visibly more confused and breathing was more labored, whilst her abdomen had also become distended. Hemodynamically she was a transient responder to a bolus intravenous fluid replacement.

Question 3

Which is the most appropriate immediate intervention required?

A. Chest drain insertion
B. Emergency laparotomy and damage control surgery
C. Reduction, splinting and immobilization of her right femur fracture
D. Diagnostic peritoneal lavage

Chest imaging revealed a widened mediastinum and left tension pneumothorax. Immediate left chest needle decompression revealed a "whoosh of air" and the trachea centralized (Fig. 15.1). Consequently a left chest drain was inserted. The patient was becoming more confused and combative with a reducing Glasgow Coma Scale (GCS 7), so was intubated and sedated. Initial blood results revealed a low hemoglobin, however her hemodynamics

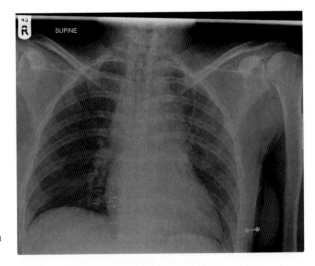

Fig. 15.1 Chest radiograph showing a widened mediastinum and left tension pneumothorax

had returned to values within normal ranges with a continuous fluid infusion and whole blood transfusion. A plain pelvic radiograph and clinical examination were normal.

Question 4

Which investigation or treatment should be performed next?

A. Plain radiographs of the right femur then reduction, splinting and immobilization of her right femur fracture
B. Computerized tomography of head, neck, chest, abdomen and pelvis
C. Emergency laparotomy and damage control surgery
D. Diagnostic angiography

Imaging revealed that she had suffered from polytraumatic injuries. She had bilateral cerebral contusions, left clavicle and cervical vertebra (Fig. 15.2) fractures, multiple rib fractures including the left first rib with a left hemo-pneumothorax and bilateral lung contusions. Her thoracic aorta was disrupted and a pseudoaneurysm of the proximal descending vessel had formed (Figs. 15.3 and 15.4). Her abdominal imaging revealed a liver laceration, large splenic hematoma and free abdominal fluid suggestive of bleeding. Her pelvis was normal but she had an open, displaced fracture of her right femoral shaft.

Clinically she was becoming increasing more difficult to ventilate, and was deteriorating hemodynamically. Her left chest drain continued to swing and bubble however blood was also still draining. Her abdomen had become more distended. She was in hypovolemic shock and was no longer responding to intravenous fluid and blood administration. Her right thigh wound was becoming more tense and swollen.

An arterial blood gas revealed that she was suffering a metabolic acidosis, with a raised lactate, and her hemoglobin level had further dropped. She was taken immediately to the operating room.

She underwent an emergency laparotomy, splenectomy and packing of her liver. Her right femoral shaft fracture was debrided, irrigated, reduced then immobilized with a splint. An intracranial bolt was inserted for pressure measurements. The duty vascular surgeon was called to assess her transected thoracic aorta, he scrutinized the Computerized Tomographic chest imaging.

Question 5

Using Fig. 15.5 below, which is the correct list order of the commonest anatomical sites of traumatic aortic disruption starting with the most frequent to the least common in descending order?

A. 1, 2, 3, 4
B. 4, 2, 3, 1
C. 3, 1, 2, 4
D. 3, 1, 4, 2
E. 1, 4, 2, 3

Fig. 15.2 MRI showing a cervical vertebral fracture

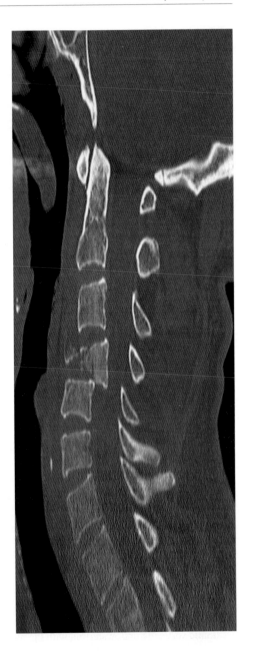

Fig. 15.3 CT scan reconstruction showing a disrupted thoracic aorta with a pseudoaneurysm of the proximal descending vessel

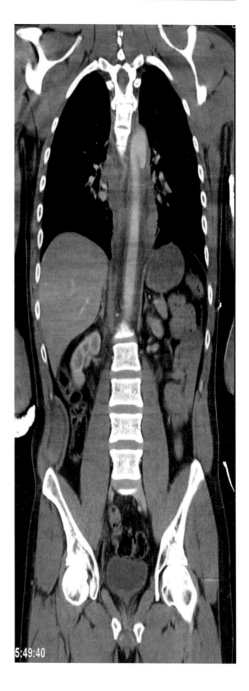

Fig. 15.4 CT scan cross-
sectional slice showing a
disrupted thoracic aorta with
a pseudoaneurysm of the
proximal descending vessel

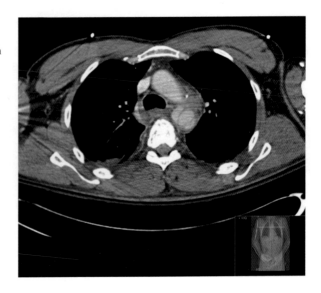

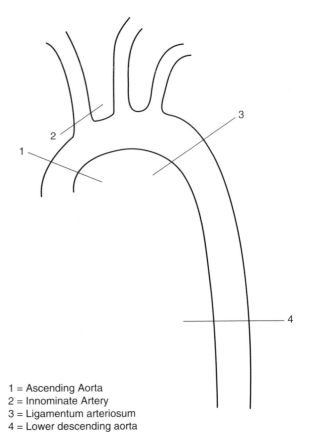

1 = Ascending Aorta
2 = Innominate Artery
Fig. 15.5 Anatomical sites of   3 = Ligamentum arteriosum
traumatic aortic disruption   4 = Lower descending aorta

Question 6

Which of the following is a favorable feature for thoracic endovascular aortic stent graft access?

A. Tortuous iliac arteries
B. Iliac diameter<7 mm
C. Suitable anatomy for conduit formation
D. Patent femoral arteries
E. Calcified iliac arteries

Question 7

Which of the following is a favorable feature for thoracic endovascular aortic stent deployment?

A. Bovine aortic arch
B. Aortic diameter<18 mm
C. Transection is proximal to left subclavian artery
D. Patent vertebral arteries
E. Acute angulated aortic arch

Answer=Q7: A&D

It was felt that her thoracic aorta was anatomically suitable for endovascular stent repair. There was an appropriate stent available in the hospital to use for the procedure. Her condition was much better and her hemodynamics had returned to within normal limits with the use of inotropic support. The vascular surgeons requested that her systolic blood pressure be kept at approximately 100 mmHg.

She underwent successful endovascular stent repair of her transected thoracic aorta (Figs. 15.6 and 15.7) and was transferred to the intensive care unit. After a prolonged hospital stay she returned home and finally achieved independent living. On discharge she was entered onto a thoracic endovascular aortic stent surveillance program.

Question 8

Which of the following are potential complications of thoracic aortic endovascular stent repair?

A. Stroke
B. Aortic rupture
C. Paraplegia
D. Aortic thrombosis
E. Graft infolding
F. Graft collapse

Fig. 15.6 Angiographic
imaging of successful
endovascular stent repair of
a transected thoracic aorta

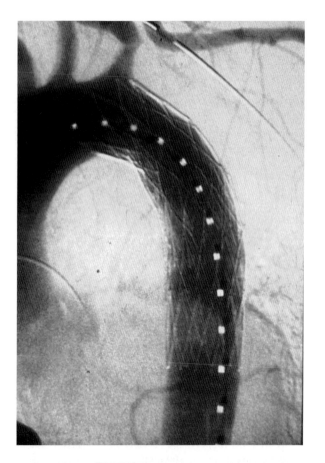

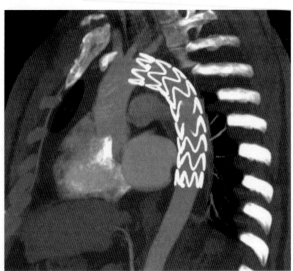

Fig. 15.7 CT reconstruction
of successful endovascular
stent repair of her transected
thoracic aorta

Question 9

What imaging modality is usually employed for thoracic aortic stent surveillance?

A. Thoracic computerized tomography
B. Chest radiography only
C. Diagnostic subtraction angiography
D. Intravascular ultrasound
E. Echocardiography

15.1
Commentary

Road traffic accidents are a common cause of trauma and resultant death for young persons. The injuries sustained are termed polytraumatic, as they occur to a number of anatomical and physiological systems. Deceleration injuries cause blunt trauma and the collision itself can result in penetrating injuries depending what impact is made with. In the case of the young female that we have presented, she collided with a stationary object. She was subjected to a sudden deceleration causing shear forces to her body and on impact she did not suffer from penetrating injuries, however did suffer crush injuries due to the vehicle's compressive forces against the tree.

She suffered head, neck, thoracic (lung and great vessel), abdominal (hepatic and splenic) and long bone (femoral shaft) injuries. All of these in separation are life threatening, however the mortality is significantly greater if they occur simultaneously, as with this case.

When presented with such a patient suffering from polytraumatic injuries pre-hospital or in an emergency department, a clear and systematic approach to treating injuries in order of most life-threatening first should be adopted. A commonly used approach is the Advanced Trauma Life Support taught by the American College of Surgeons.[1] Initially a primary survey is conducted where the common "ABCDE" approach is adopted after cervical spine immobilization, as airway injuries (A) have a higher mortality than breathing (B), than circulatory (C), than disability/neurologically (D) and then environmental/everything (E) else is treated last.

The correct answer to **Question 1** is **C (Q1 = C)**. Administration of high flow oxygen is beneficial to airway and breathing injuries and thus survival compared to the other options available. Answers A and B, address the circulatory system so would follow from airway control. Administration of analgesia is humane, however should not take priority over life-threatening injuries and interventions.

Once the primary survey has been conducted and problems encountered addressed as best as possible for the circumstance, transfer to an appropriate facility is necessary for definitive care. Continuous reassessment of the primary survey is compulsory to detect any evolving injuries and deterioration, especially on arrival at the appropriate facility. Our lady's arrival to an emergency department at a trauma hospital in our case revealed a number of possible injuries which included airway compromise, abdominal and long bone trauma with an evolving head injury. These problems should be addressed immediately to save her life, this approach is termed "damage control." It is advised that a multidisciplinary team approach to trauma should be adopted as there may be a number of synchronous pathologies of which many expert opinions would be beneficial to the patient's survival.

Next, primary radiology is performed. This consists of plain chest and pelvic radiographs with or without cervical spine lateral view, if indicated. The appropriate answer to **Question 2** is **D** (**Q2=D**). Computerized tomography and long bone radiographs can be performed after the primary radiology.

The patient began to deteriorate and hemodynamically started to display signs of hypovolaemic shock. Her heart rate rose and inversely her blood pressure dropped. She also showed signs of cerebral malperfusion by becoming more confused, combative and drowsy. A reduction of consciousness (Glasgow coma scale of <8) should be treated by intubating the patient because the airway may be at risk of obstruction, thus our patient was eventually sedated and intubated.

It is important to note that this patient is young. Young victims and children often initially present with normal hemodynamics as they can compensate for blood loss due to an abundance of physiological reserve, compared to the elderly who usually also possess more comorbidities. However, they may show subtle signs of deterioration and then unexpectedly "crash" their hemodynamics. We know that she suffered from hypovolaemic shock as she was a transient responder to fluid administration, so she was volume depleted. The cause for this patient's hypovolaemic shock could be due to poor oxygen delivery from her lung injuries and tension pneumothorax, her evolving peritoneal bleeding, hemorrhage from her long bone fracture, which can be profuse, or head injury. Bleeding was further confirmed by clinical and investigative reassessment which showed a falling hemoglobin level and profound metabolic acidosis.

The most appropriate injury to address first was her tension pneumothorax with needle decompression then the insertion of a chest drain, so the answer to **Question 3** is **A** (**Q3=A**). Addressing the circulatory injuries to the abdomen and long bones causing bleeding should follow.

Question 4 deals with appropriate diagnostic investigations in a stable patient in hypovolaemic shock responsive to fluid administration when the cause of bleeding is uncertain. Computerized tomography is often readily available in larger centers, but not to all. It offers a rapid cross-sectional multi-cavity imaging which can positively guide definitive management. It must be stressed that unstable patients should receive immediate treatment and not be investigated. Many patients have died due to inappropriate diagnostic imaging when "damage control" operative surgery is indicated. In this lady's case, she was stable and there was a diagnostic uncertainty of the source of her bleeding. She had chest pathology displayed by her tension pneumothorax and widened mediastinum and hemothorax, as well as a tender, distending abdomen. She was also suffering from a head injury and neck injury, so answer **B** is correct (**Q4=B**).

The computerized tomographical imaging demonstrated a number of her injuries in the thorax, abdomen, and head as well as a several bone fractures. She then went for operative treatment of her abdominal (liver and spleen) injuries and femoral shaft fracture.

Whilst "damage control" surgery was undertaken, the duty vascular surgeon and interventional radiologist evaluated the thoracic aortic transection image reconstructions with particular interests to the vessels measurements and anatomical parameters. Some advocate that computerized tomographical angiography with contrast is best, however, if there is a true vascular traumatic transection, then contrast in a hematoma will obscure images.

An aortic transection is a laceration of all three layers of the vessel wall, not to be confused with aortic dissections, which are rarely, associated with trauma and usually longitudinal vessel wall tears. It is usually associated with rapid deceleration and crush injuries from blunt trauma caused from high speed road traffic collisions or falls from heights. Less frequently penetrating trauma such as stab wounds or gunshot injuries can cause transections. The majority of victims die immediately at the scene (80–90%) from exsanguination. Due to the rarity of sufferers actually reaching hospital, most centers have little experience in treating these injuries. These factors in conjunction with subtle and vague clinical signs,[2–5] thus reliant on imaging for diagnosis make the prognosis poor with a consequently high mortality. The concomitant non-aortic injuries can be numerous as with the case presented. Involvement with multiple rib fractures (78%), liver lacerations (61%), head injuries (42%), first rib fracture (42%), splenic lacerations (36%), heart lacerations (34%), sternal fractures (28%) and cervical spinal fractures (26%) are not uncommon.[3,6]

Traditionally, conventional surgical repair of the traumatic transected thoracic aorta has been the gold standard,[3,7] but carries a significant mortality and paraplegia rate ranging from 15% to 30% in contemporary studies.[3,8,9] Endovascular treatment of the thoracic aortic was first described in 1991[10] and has become favorable over conventional open surgical techniques for treating traumatic transections in the polytraumatised patients due to a much lesser mortality and morbidity rate.[3,11] Physiologically these patients are particularly vulnerable and a quick non-invasive procedure would be preferential. There are no randomized control trials of open vs. endovascular repair for traumatic aortic transections. There is an overwhelming abundance of mostly small case series[3,12–30] and meta-analysis[31–34] of these series all generally concluding that endovascular techniques have a reduced mortality and morbidity compared to the alternatives. Endovascular aortic transection repair can be conducted more quickly under local anesthesia in a supine position unlike open surgery which always requires general anesthetic, specific dual cuff intubating and lateral positioning in these polytraumatized subjects often with synchronous lung and cervical spine injuries. Conventional surgery often requires aortic cross-clamping, significant blood loss and use of cardiopulmonary bypass which increase spinal ischemia and thus paraplegia rates[3,16] as well as renal ischemia times and ischemic reperfusion syndromes. Open surgical series have higher stroke and paraplegia rates and consequently have greater mortality and morbidity association. The post-operative pain, recovery,[15] intensive care[13] and monitoring required is significantly greater for open surgical repair.

The consensus is that it will be very unlikely that a randomized control trial will be performed to definitively prove this superior benefit because from overwhelming current endovascular practice and preference, with such good results, a trial would be unethical.[35] In a number of these abundant case series, endovascular repair has been performed on sicker patients with higher severity score compared to conventional surgery series, because these patients were deemed unfit for open repair. A suitable study would also require large numbers of patients to provide adequate statistical power which would be difficult with a prolonged study period due to the rare and acute nature of this traumatic disease.

The third management option which is discussed less by endovascular surgeons is the conservative medical treatment favored by physicians and intensivists. Accurate blood pressure control with short-acting beta-blockade such as esmolol or labetalol, to achieve a systolic blood pressure of approximately 100 mmHg and a relative bradycardia, has been shown to be beneficial to polytraumatised patients with aortic transections, mediastinal hematoma and thus pseudoaneurysm formation (aortic rupture contained by adventitia or peri-aortic tissue). Similarly to patients with thoracic aneurysm rupture or acute dissections, medical management can be used as a stop gap whilst other injuries are addressed and definitive management is planned. The rationale is that aortic wall stress and tension are decreased thus markedly reducing the risk of aortic rupture because wall tension is directly proportional to increases in pressure and inversely proportional to pulse rate.[5] Treatment can be delayed for days, weeks, infrequently months and on a few occasions in the literature years.[3,5,17,23,27,36-38]

Question 5 is concerned with sites of thoracic traumatic transection and the correct answer is **C (Q5=C)**. The commonest site of injury is the aortic isthmus (93%) which is the portion of the proximal descending aorta between the left subclavian artery origin and ligamentum arteriosum.[3,31,39] Fixation and tethering by the ligamentum arteriosum is believed to be accountable for the high frequency of injury in this position. The remaining 7% of injuries exist in the ascending aorta and arch. The order injury frequency is first the ascending aorta, then avulsion of the innominate artery followed by the lower descending aorta.[40] These frequencies are correct for patients presenting to hospital, as mentioned earlier, the majority of patients with the injuries die instantly on scene and post-mortem investigations have showed a higher proportion who die suffer ascending aortic injuries. The percentages listed above have been defined by the American Association for the Surgery of Trauma (AAST), who performed the first prospective multicenter observational study of traumatic transections in 274 patients.[41]

There are a number of factors that determine suitability for thoracic endovascular aortic stent repair (TEVAR). These factors are highlighted in **Question 6**, where the correct answers for access are **D (Q6=C&D)**.

Access for stent device delivery is very important. Current devices require delivery access of at least 20–26 Fr, and thus a minimal iliac diameter of 7.6–9.1 mm. Patent, straight, non-tortuous and non-calcified iliac and femoral arteries are favorable for endovascular delivery of the large stent devices. Despite endovascular techniques being considerably less invasive than conventional open techniques, the older, first generation devices large and cumbersome, so always required femoral artery dissection and arterotomy. Thoracic stent devices are bigger than those used for abdominal aortic repair because the thoracic aorta is bigger and further away from the groin. As time progresses and investment in technology continues delivery systems have become more slim-line and percutaneous stent insertion is more frequently available. Imaging should include views of the iliac arteries to assess size, tortosity and composition, particularly for aneurysms, plaques and calcification. These features make access very difficult and can be a contraindication to this type of treatment due to poorer compliance. An alternative, which is underused in our opinion is endoconduit formation, however this makes the overall procedure more invasive. The common iliacs, upper limb and great vessels can be used as a suitable conduit, if the anatomy is suitable and disease is minimum, to deliver the stent device.

Factors that are favorable for accurate and successful thoracic endovascular aortic stent repair (TEVAR) and deployment are highlighted in **Question 7**, where the correct answers for access are **A and D (Q6=A&D)**.

Aortic size is very important. These groups of trauma patients are young and consequently have a tighter aortic curvature with smaller aortic and iliac diameters than patients suffering from other thoracic pathologies such as aneurysms, acute and chronic dissections.[3,15,37,42] Device sizes are getting smaller with much innovative research but there is still a minimal size that can be treated, so this treatment cannot be offered to all. The smallest currently available aortic stent is 21 mm in diameter, however, smaller stents with diameters of 16–18 mm are in production. Additionally of relevance to our patient is that the thoracic aorta of females is significantly smaller than males, so size and stent availability is particularly relevant to our young female patient in this case.

Stent availability has also been touched-upon. To offer an emergency thoracic endovascular service, one needs to have a wide range of stents and variety of different sizes on consignment. For optimal fixation, stent grafts are commonly oversized by 10–15% compared with the landing zone aortic diameter[3] to enhance conformability and adherence within a vessel. However in trauma, there is the potential for stent undersizing due to the patient's hypovolemia causing a relatively smaller aortic caliber and sympathetic overdrive causing vasoconstriction.[3,43] There are a number of different manufacturers who have devices with particular advantages and disadvantages. To possess an inventory of equipment to suit all is costly, requires storage and needs regular cataloging and replacing.

Thoracic stents exist for treating aortic aneurysms and also for treating dissections.[15,39] These two pathologies are distinctly different and thus require different devices to treat endovascularly. Traumatic thoracic transections are rare and thus there are few dedicated stents developed for these situations, such as the newly released conformable GORE TAG™ stent. One has to, by using best judgment and in-depth knowledge of available stent technology, rapidly assess what is best for the patient. For this reason a vascular specialist with endovascular training should plan these cases.

Despite the significantly smaller mortality and morbidity of endovascular stent repair over conventional surgery, TEVAR still is not without complications and should not be underestimated. Poor preparation and planning of measurements and sizings could lead to inadequate stent positioning. An inappropriately positioned stent can lead to stroke, paraplegia, graft infolding, graft collapse, aortic thrombosis and aortic rupture to name a few. Thus the answer to **Question 8** is *all* of the available options **(Q8=A&B&C&D&E&F)**.

The use of imaging for aortic vessel measurements and to locate the precise anatomical position of the transection is vital. For successful stent deployment and fixation, one requires an appropriate proximal and distal stent landing zone. With the most common site of transection being adjacent to the ligamentum arteriosum, as previously mentioned, the distal landing zone is usually sufficient and not a problem. However, proximal landing zones require particular attention due to the left subclavian artery and other great vessels. A proximal landing zone distance of approximately 20 mm minimum is recommended, however with increased experience, boundaries are expanding and smaller distances are being attempted with correspondingly good results. In some cases when the site of injury is close to the left subclavian artery, partial or total vessel coverage may be required. Conveniently, the arterial tree of this young group of effected patients contains little disease so normally the vertebral circulation to the posterior Circle of Willis is suitable for cerebral collateralization and thus perfusion. However, this may not be the case for an older patient suffering transection. If left subclavian coverage is required then simultaneous carotid-left subclavian vessel bypass may be indicated to prevent posterior circulatory stroke, spinal cord ischemia or subclavian steal syndrome.[44] Peri-operatively, the physiological consequences of left subclavian artery coverage and thus occlusion can be tested by temporary balloon insufflation within the arterial osteum. Some centers routinely bypass all patients for elective thoracic aneurysm and dissection procedures prophylactically during the same operation simultaneously or in a staged alternative sitting.[3,12,17,25,37] Their evidence for this hybrid technique is mostly extrapolated from the EUROSTAR (European Collaborators on Stent Graft Techniques for Thoracic Aortic Aneurysm and Dissection Repair) database and the UK Thoracic Aortic Data Registry,[35,45] which suggests a small complication rate (paraplegia and stroke rate in particular) for bypassing patients. Not all believe and practice this technique. Transections proximal to the left subclavian artery pose a challenge to primary endovascular treatments in the polytraumatised patient who requires a short operation and rapid vigorous re-warming and intensive resuscitation, but hybrid techniques can be conducted such as carotid-carotid arterial bypass.[3]

The "Bovine Aorta" which is present in 20% of the population, may cause particular difficulty. In this variant of aortic structure, the left subclavian artery originates from the innominate artery, thus there is usually an increased stent proximal landing zone length, but any coverage of the innominate origin requires a bypass.

The last anatomical consideration is to the aortic curvature. The lesser and greater aortic curves are exerted to different hemodynamic forces as are the proximal, middle and distal stent fabrics. Also consideration should be paid to the size discrepancy between ascending and descending aorta. The more curved aortic arch may not be ideal for the available devices in stock for these trauma patients and may compromise the final outcome. The high pressures of blood jetted to a stent during deployment can make accurate millimeter positioning more difficult, so a systolic blood pressure of 100 mmHg is recommended and during actual stent deployment, some administer adenosine to temporarily cease cardiac activity and others use rapid cardiac pacing. With such delirious consequences to malpositioning, such as stent collapse, proximal of distal migration, great vessel coverage and stroke, proximal dissection formation, incomplete stent opening, poor seals and endoleaks, these procedures require adequate intraoperative imaging, kit availability and staff with endovascular familiarity and thus expertise. To achieve all of this many vascular surgeons now advocate centralization of such endovascular services.[46-49]

All patients with an abdominal aortic endovascular stent enter a local hospital surveillance program. Similar for all thoracic stented patients, they should undergo lifelong surveillance. The intention of long-term surveillance imaging is to detect endoleaks, occlusions, stent migration, fracture and collapse early and thus evoke early surgical repair.[50] In answer to the final **Question 9**, the most usual imaging technique employed for thoracic stent surveillance is **A (Q9 = A)**. Thoracic Computerized tomography, is the most common modality, however post-stent surveillance is a popular research area and rapid advances include intravascular ultrasound, contrast ultrasound, virtual angiography as well as magnetic resonance imaging will possibly become common place in the future.

This is a controversial area as subjecting a young patient to this technique is attractive, but the long-term implications of lifelong yearly radiation exposure are unknown. Magnetic resonance imaging is particularly appealing in this younger group of patients because they require lifelong surveillance, for a longer duration, compared to stented aneurysm and dissection patients, thus the lack of radiation of this modality is highly attractive. Similarly the longevity of this new technology is undetermined. These young patients are still growing and corresponding have developing aortic diameters. Does growth have an effect on stent stability and durability? Do stents degrade or migrate with time? The answers to these questions are awaited, but will not be available to us until long-term surveillance results from large series are available. Thus surveillance is necessary for this still relatively new technique. Lastly many series have found compliance with surveillance is poor in this young group of patients suffering traumatic transections, making data collection more difficult.[3,16]

This patient required a prolonged hospital stay due to her numerous multiple injuries and also for physical and psycho-social rehabilitation. For these reasons, this young group of patients need a multidisciplinary team input for their multiinjuries to provide a successful outcome.

Acknowledgments   We would like to thank Dr. Nicos Fotiadis (Consultant Interventional Radiologist at Barts and The London NHS Trust) who provided the images for this chapter.

References

1. American College of Surgeons. *Advanced Trauma and Life Support Course for Physicians.* 7th ed. Chicago: Committee on Trauma, American College of Surgeons; 2004.
2. Park SM, Kim DH, Kwak YT, Sohn IS. Triple aortic root injury. *Ann Thorac Surg.* 2009 (Feb);87(2):621-623.
3. Bent CL, Matson MB, Sobeh M, et al. Endovascular management of acute blunt traumatic thoracic aortic injury: a single center experience. *J Vasc Surg.* 2007 (Nov);46:920-927.
4. Parmley LF, Mattingly TW, Manion TW, et al. Nonpenetrating traumatic injury of the aorta. *Circulation.* 1958;12:1086-1101.
5. Fabian TC. Advances in the management of blunt thoracic aortic injury: parmley to the present. *Surgeon.* (Apr) 2009;75:4. Health Module.
6. Williams JS, et al. Aortic injury in vehicular trauma. *ATS.* 1994;57:726-730.
7. Creasy JD, Chiles C, Routh WD, Dyer RB. Overview of traumatic injury of the thoracic aorta. *Radiographics.* 1997;17:27-45.
8. Attar S, Cardarelli MG, Downing SW, et al. Traumatic aortic rupture: recent outcome with regard to neurologic deficit. *Ann Thorac Surg.* 1999;67:959-964.
9. von Oppell UO, Dunne TT, De Groot MK, Zilla P. Traumatic aortic rupture: 20-year meta-analysis of mortality and risk of paraplegia. *Ann Thorac Surg.* 1994;58:585-593.
10. Volodos NL, Karpovich IP, Troyan VI, et al. Clinical experience of the use of self-fixing synthetic prosthetics of the thoracic and the abdominal aorta and iliac arteries through the femoral artery and intraoperative endoprosthesis for aorta reconstruction. *Vasa Suppl.* 1991;33:93-95.
11. Stone DH, Brewster DC, Kwolek CJ, et al. Stent-graft versus open surgical repair of the thoracic aorta: mid-term results. *J Vasc Surg.* 2006;44:1188-1197.

12. Canaud L, Hireche K, Berthet JP, Branchereau P, Marty-Ane C, Alric P. Endovascular repair of aortic arch lesions in high risk patients or after previous aortic surgery: midterm results. *J Thorac Cardiovasc Surg.* 2009 (Nov 16) [Epub ahead of print].

13. Asmat A, Tan L, Caleb MG, Lee CN, Robless PA. Endovascular management of traumatic thoracic aortic transection. *Asian Cardiovasc Thorac Ann.* 2009 (Oct);17(5):458-461.

14. Ryan M, Valazquez O, Martinez E, Patel S, Parodi J, Karmacharya J. Thoracic aortic transection treated by thoracic endovascular aortic repair: predictors of survival. *Vasc Endovascular Surg.* 2010 (Feb);44(2):95-100.

15. Caddell KA, Song HK, Landry GJ, et al. Favorable early outcomes for patients with extended indications for thoracic endografting. *Heart Surg Forum.* 2009 (Aug);12(4):E187-193.

16. Neschis DG, Moainie S, Flinn WR, Scalea TM, Bartlett ST, Griffith BP. Endograft repair of traumatic aortic injury – a technique in evolution: a single institution's experience. *Ann Surg.* 2009 (Sept);250(3):377-382.

17. Botta L, Russo V, Saini C, et al. Endovascular treatment for acute traumatic transection of the descending aorta: focus on operative timing and left subclavian artery management. *J Thorac Cardiovasc Surg.* 2008 (Dec);136(6):1558-1563.

18. Wellons ED, Milner R, Solis M, Levitt A, Rosenthal D. Stent-graft repair of traumatic thoracic aortic disruptions. *J Vasc Surg.* 2004;40:1095-1100.

19. Orford VP, Atkinson NR, Thomson K, et al. Blunt traumatic aortic transection: the endovascular experience. *Ann Thorac Surg.* 2003;75:106-112.

20. Demetriades D, et al. Operative repair or endovascular stent graft in blunt traumatic thoracic aortic injuries: results of an American Association for the Surgery of Traumatic Multicenter Study. *J Trauma.* 2008 (Mar);64(3):561-570. discussion 570-571.

21. Mohan IV, Hitos K, White GH, et al. Improved outcomes with endovascular stent grafts for thoracic aorta transections. *Eur J Vasc Endovasc Surg.* 2008;36:152-157.

22. McCarthy MJ. Is endovascular repair now the first line treatment for traumatic transection of the thoracic aorta? *Eur J Vasc Endovasc Surg.* 2008;36:158-159.

23. Clough RE, Taylor PR. Endovascular repair of aortic transection can be a durable treatment option. *Eur J Vasc Endovasc Surg.* 2009;37:120.

24. Alsac JM, Boura B, Desgranges P, Fabiani JN, Becquemin JP, Leseche G. Immediate endovascular repair for acute traumatic injuries of the thoracic aorta: a multicenter analysis of 28 cases. *J Vasc Surg.* 2008 (Dec);48:1369-1374.

25. Botta L, Russo V, Savini C, et al. Endovascular treatment for acute traumatic transection of the descending aorta: focus on operative timing and left subclavian artery management. *J Thorac Cardiovasc Surg.* 2008 (Dec);136(6):1558-1563.

26. Yamane BH, Tefera G, Hoch JR, Turnipseed WD, Acher CW. Blunt thoracic aortic injury: open or stent graft repair? *Surgery.* 2008 (Oct);144(4):575-580. discussion 580–582. Epub 2008 Aug 29.

27. Go MR, Barbato JE, Dillavou ED, et al. Thoracic endovascular aortic repair for traumatic aortic transection. *J Vasc Surg.* 2007 (Nov);46:928-933.

28. Riesenman PJ, Farber MA, Rich PB, et al. Outcomes of surgical and endovascular treatment of acute traumatic thoracic aortic injury. *J Vasc Surg.* 2007 (Nov);46:934-940.

29. Agostinelli A, Saccani S, Borello B, Franceco N, Larini P, Gherli T. Immediate endovascular treatment of blunt aortic injury: our therapeutic strategy. *J Thorac Cardiovasc Surg.* 2006 (May);131(5):1053-1057.

30. Ott MC, Stewart TC, Lawlor DK, Gray DK, Forbes TL. Management of blunt thoracic aortic injuries: endovascular stents versus open repair. *J Traum.* 2004 (Mar);56(3):565-570.

31. Xenos ES, Abedi NN, Davenport DL, et al. Meta-analysis of endovascular vs open repair for traumatic descending thoracic aortic rupture. *J Vasc Surg.* 2008 (Nov);48(5):1343-1351.

32. Takagi H, Kawai N, Umemoto T. A meta-analysis of comparative studies of endovascular versus open repair for blunt thoracic aortic injury. *J Thorac Cardiovasc Surg.* 2008 (June);135(6):1392-1394.
33. Walsh SR, Tang TY, Sadat U, et al. Endovascular stenting versus open surgery for thoracic aortic disease: systematic review and meta-analysis of perioperative results. *J Vasc Surg.* 2008 (May);47:1094-1098.
34. Tang GL, Tehrani HY, Usman A, et al. Reduced mortaility, paraplegia, and stroke with stent graft repair of blunt aortic transections: a modern meta-analysis. *J Vasc Surg.* 2008 (March);47:671-675.
35. McDonnell CO, Haider SN, Colgan MP, Shanik GD, Moore DJ, Madhavan P. Endovascular management of thoracic aortic pathology. *Surgeon.* 2009 (Feb);7(1):24-30.
36. Bruno VD, Batchelor TJ. Late aortic injury: a rare complication of a posterior rib fracture. *Ann Thorac Surg.* 2009 (Jan);87(1):301-303.
37. Hughes GC, Daneshmand MA, Swaminathan M, et al. "Real world" thoracic endografting: results with the Gore TAG device 2 years after US FDA approval. *Ann Thorac Surg.* 2008 (Nov);86(5):1530-1537. discussion 1537–1538.
38. Tai N, Renfrew I, Kyriakides C. Chronic pseudoaneurysm of the thoracic aorta due to trauma: 30-year delay in presentation and treatment. *Injury Extra.* 2005;36:475-478.
39. Akins CW, Buckley MJ, Dagget W, McIlduff JB, Austen WG. Acute traumatic aortic disruption of the thoracic aorta: a 10-year experience. *Ann Thorac Cardiovasc Surg.* 1981;31: 305-309.
40. Stene JK, Grande CM, Bernhard WN, et al. Perioperative anesthetic management of the trauma patient: thoracoabdominal and orthopaedic injuries. In: Stene JK, Grande CM, eds. *Trauma Anesthesia.* Baltimore: Williams & Wilkins; 1991:218.
41. Shapiro MJ, Yanofsky SD, Trapp J, et al. Cardiovascular evaluation in blunt thoracic trauma using transesophageal echocardiography (TEE). *J Trauma.* 1991;31:835-840.
42. Roche-Nagle G, de Perrot M, Waddell TK, Oropoulos G, Rubin BB. Neoadjuvant aortic endografting. *Ann Vasc Surg.* 2009 (Nov–Dec);23(6):787. El–5. Epub 2009 Sept 12.
43. Hoornweg LL, Dinkelman MK, Goslings JC, et al. Endovascular management of traumatic ruptures of the thoracic aorta: a retrospective multicenter analysis of 28 cases in the Netherlands. *J Vasc Surg.* 2006;43:1096-1102.
44. Riesenman PJ, Farber MA, Mendes RR, Marston WA, Fulton JJ, Keagy BA. Coverage of the left subclavian artery during thoracic endovascular aortic repair. *J Vasc Surg.* 2007;45:90-94.
45. Leurs LJ et al. Endovascular treatment of thoracic aortic diseases: combined experience from the EUROSTAR and United Kingdom Thoracic Endograft registries. *J Vasc Surg.* 2004;40:86-89.
46. Holt PJ, Karthikesalingam A, Poloniecki JD, Hinchliffe RJ, Loftus IM, Thompson MM. Propensity scored analysis of outcomes after ruptured abdominal aortic aneurysm. *Br J Surg.* 2010 (Feb 12) [Epub ahead of print].
47. Holt PJ, Poloniecki JD, Khalid U, Hinchliffe RJ, Loftus IM, Thompson MM. Effect of endovascular aneurysm repair on the volume-outcome relationship in aneurysm repair. *Circ Cardiovasc Qual Outcome.* 2009 (Nov);2(6):624-632. Epub 2009 Sept 22.
48. Holt PJ, Poloniecki JD, Hinchliffe RJ, Loftus IM, Thompson MM. Model for the reconfiguration of specialized vascular services. *Br J Surg.* 2008 (Dec);95(12):1469-1474.
49. Holt PJ, Poloniecki JD, Thompson MM. How to improve surgical outcomes. *BMJ.* 2008 (Apr 26);336(7650):900-901. Epub 2008 Apr 21.
50. Kotelis D, Lopez-Benitez R, Tengg-Kobligk H, Geisbusch P, Bockler D. Endovascular repair of stent graft collapse by stent-protected angioplasty using a femoral-brachial guidewire. *J Vasc Surg.* 2008 (Dec);48(6):1609-1612.

Part III

Management of Chronic Ischemia
of the Lower Extremities

Cardiovascular Risk Factors and Peripheral Arterial Disease

16

Stella S. Daskalopoulou and Dimitri P. Mikhailidis

A 62-year-old man with intermittent claudication was referred for vascular risk factor modification. He had no history of myocardial infarction (MI) or stroke. He was smoking 20 cigarettes/day. His family history was negative for premature vascular events. He was not taking any medication. He was advised to start aspirin 75 mg/day, but he stopped taking these tablets because of "stomach discomfort". The patient's total cholesterol was 228 mg/dL (5.9 mmol/L). His blood pressure required treatment with amlodipine and a thiazide diuretic. The patient eventually stopped smoking after referral to the smoking cessation clinic in our hospital.

Question 1

Which of the following investigations would you order?

A. Fasting serum glucose.
B. Urine glucose to make a diagnosis of diabetes mellitus.
C. Fasting serum triglycerides.
D. Fasting serum high-density lipoprotein cholesterol (HDL-C).
E. Thyroid function tests.

A. Requesting a fasting serum glucose level is an essential test in all patients with vascular disease. In this case the fasting glucose was 87 mg/dL (4.8 mmol/L); this is satisfactory.

Interpretation of fasting glucose values:

There are three categories in which a patient can be placed relative to fasting serum glucose levels:

- *Normal:* fasting glucose <110 mg/dL (<6.0 mmol/L).
- *Impaired fasting glucose (IFG):* fasting glucose 110–125 mg/dL (6.0–6.9 mmol/L).
- *Diabetes mellitus:* fasting glucose ≥126 mg/dL (≥7.0 mmol/L). IFG is associated with an increased risk of vascular events and conversion to diabetes mellitus. Furthermore, a glucose level in the IFG range can be one of the features of the metabolic syndrome (also known as insulin resistance or Reaven's syndrome)[1] (Table 16.1).

S.S. Daskalopoulou (✉)
Department of Medicine, McGill University, Montreal, QC, Canada

G. Geroulakos and B. Sumpio (eds.), *Vascular Surgery*,
DOI: 10.1007/978-1-84996-356-5_16, © Springer-Verlag London Limited 2011

Table 16.1 Features of metabolic syndrome*

1. Abdominal obesity (waist circumference):
   Men ≥ 102 cm (≥40 in.)
   Women ≥ 88 cm (≥36 in.)
2. Triglycerides
   ≥150 mg/dL (≥1.7 mmol/L)
3. High-density lipoprotein cholesterol (HDL-C):
   Men <40 mg/dL (<1.0 mmol/L)
   Women <50 mg/dL (<1.3 mmol/L)
4. Blood pressure: ≥130/≥85 mmHg
5. Fasting glucose: ≥110 mg/dL (≥6.1 mmol/L)

*According to the National Cholesterol Education Program (NCEP) Adult Treatment Panel (ATP) III guidelines,[1] any three or more of these five features are diagnostic of the metabolic syndrome. Other factors that may coexist in these patients include a family history of type 2 diabetes, South Asian ethnicity, decreased physical activity, smoking, elevated serum urate levels and evidence of fatty liver (abnormal levels of aminotransferases, ALT/AST). A new consensus definition of metabolic syndrome has been proposed in 2009.[2] The new definition interpret waist circumference by ethnicity and the glucose value is 100 mg/dL (5.6 mmol/L).

B. This patient's urine was tested when he was first seen in outpatients. The renal threshold for glucose is a serum level of about 180–200 mg/dL (10–11 mmol/L). Therefore, testing urine for glucose will not detect IFG or early/mild diabetes. Clinicians must not rely on a urine glucose test to exclude IFG or early diabetes. In view of the serum glucose value (see **A**, above), it is not surprising that the urine glucose test was negative. However, testing the urine was an opportunity to exclude proteinuria, another indicator of vascular risk.

C. The fasting triglyceride level in this patient was 141 mg/dL (1.6 mmol/L) – this is satisfactory.

Interpretation of fasting triglyceride values:

There has been considerable confusion regarding the importance of triglycerides. There are several reasons for this, including:

- *Interactions with other lipid variables:* serum triglyceride and HDL-C levels are inversely related. HDL-C is a "protective" lipoprotein.
- *Interactions with potential risk factors:* elevated serum triglyceride levels are associated with impaired fibrinolysis and possibly elevated plasma levels of fibrinogen. Both type 2 diabetes and metabolic syndrome are associated with raised serum triglyceride levels.
- There is evidence (post-hoc analysis) from the Scandinavian Simvastatin Survival Study (4S) that IFG and diabetic patients benefit from treatment with simvastatin.[3] More recently, a trial in type 2 diabetic patients without established vascular disease showed a beneficial effect of atorvastatin 10 mg/day (vs. placebo) in reducing the risk of first cardiovascular events, including stroke.[4] Both diabetes and metabolic syndrome are common in patients with peripheral arterial disease (PAD).[5] Furthermore, both diabetes and PAD are considered as coronary heart disease (CHD) equivalent and need to be treated aggressively.[1]

- *Triglyceride levels vary considerably within any individual:* this variability includes the fact that fasting triglycerides may be considerably lower than non-fasting levels in some patients. There is evidence that postprandial triglyceride levels also predict vascular risk, but this measurement is not easily standardised. Therefore, assessment of triglyceride status is best represented by a fasting sample (12- to 14-h overnight fast; water only allowed). Fasting serum triglyceride levels may be independent vascular risk factors.[6] Hypertriglyceridaemia is often associated with secondary causes that aggravate the patient's tendency to this type of dyslipidaemia (Table 16.2). These causes need to be addressed.

Fasting triglyceride levels are defined in the NCEP ATP III guidelines[1]:

- *Borderline high:* 150–199 mg/dL (1.7–2.2 mmol/L).
- *Moderately elevated:* 200–499 mg/dL (2.3–5.6 mmol/L).
- *Severe hypertriglyceridaemia:* ≥500 mg/dL (≥5.6 mmol/L).
  According to these guidelines,[1] the treatment priority for cases with severe hypertriglyceridaemia shifts from LDL-C to the triglyceride levels. This is because of the increased risk of acute pancreatitis associated with severe hypertriglyceridaemia.[1] For milder hypertriglyceridaemia, the priority for treatment remains the LDL-C level.[1]

D. The fasting HDL-C level in this patient was 46 mg/dL (1.2 mmol/L) – this is satisfactory.

Interpretation of fasting HDL-C values:

A raised HDL-C level is a protective factor, whatever the levels of other lipid variables.[1,7, 8] The recent NCEP ATP III guidelines[1] recommend that HDL-C levels should ideally be ≥ 40 mg/dL (≥1.0 mmol/L).[1,7,8] A low HDL-C level is also predictive of the risk of stroke.[9,10] The importance of HDL-C in reducing the risk of vascular events is supported by the findings of a secondary prevention trial (VA-HIT).[10]

E. The thyroid function tests were normal.

It is useful to routinely assess thyroid function in dyslipidaemic patients. This is because hypothyroidism is not uncommon and it is associated with dyslipidaemia (see Table 16.2). There is also some evidence showing that hypothyroid patients are more likely to have "muscle-related" side effects if they are given a statin. Hypothyroidism can also be difficult to spot unless the clinical features are obvious. Replacement with thyroxine is usually associated with a beneficial change in the lipid profile and body weight.

Table 16.2 Secondary causes of hypertriglyceridaemia/hypercholesterolaemia

Excessive alcohol intake
Diabetes mellitus
Hypothyroidism
Some types of liver disease
Some types of renal disease
Obesity/diet
Drugs: beta-blockers, thiazides, oestrogens, anabolic steroids, corticosteroids, tamoxifen, protease inhibitors, retinoids, ciclosporin

Table 16.3 CHD equivalents according to the NCEP ATP III guidelines[1]

Peripheral arterial disease

Abdominal aortic aneurysm

Symptomatic carotid artery disease

Diabetes mellitus

Multiple risk factors conferring a calculated risk for a vascular event ≥ 20% over the next 10 years

Question 2

What drug would you use to treat this patient's dyslipidaemia? What are your target levels?

The main target for lipid-lowering treatment is the LDL-C level. Since PAD is considered a coronary heart disease (CHD) equivalent[1] (Table 16.3), the LDL-C target is 100 mg/dL (2.6 mmol/L) in the USA[1] and 96 mg/dL (2.5 mmol/L) in Europe.[11] The NCEP ATP III guidelines were revised in 2004 to include an optional LDL-C target of 70 mg/dL (1.8 mmol/L) for very high-risk patients.[12] As explained above, the HDL-C and triglyceride levels are secondary targets. A full fasting lipid profile should be obtained before making any decision regarding treatment. In the case presented above, the fasting values were: total cholesterol=228 mg/dL (5.9 mmol/L), HDL-C=46 mg/dL (1.2 mmol/L), LDL-C=155 mg/dL (4.0 mmol/L) and triglycerides=141 mg/dL (1.6 mmol/L). The drug of choice is a statin to achieve the LDL-C target. Statins also improve HDL-C and triglyceride levels, although these latter effects may be relatively small.

There is also evidence that treatment with statins decreases morbidity and mortality and improves symptoms in patients with PAD.[5,13] Furthermore, there is convincing evidence that statins reduce the risk of stroke.[13–15] Several studies have also shown that aggressive lipid lowering is associated with a reduced progression of atherosclerotic carotid artery disease.[14,15] Patients with PAD are likely to have some degree of carotid artery disease. PAD is also a strong predictor of the risk of stroke.

Question 3

What modifiable risk factors would you like to address in a high-risk patient, as in this case?

Smoking

Smoking cessation is of paramount importance. The vast majority of PAD patients are, or have been, smokers. Furthermore, smoking is associated with adverse effects on several variables that predict vascular events. For example, smoking can lower serum HDL-C levels, raise serum triglyceride levels, increase insulin resistance and elevate plasma fibrinogen concentrations.[16] Smoking may even predict the progression of PAD and graft occlusion after infrainguinal bypass surgery.[17] There is evidence that the vascular risk is greater in smokers than in non-smokers, despite the use of statins.[18] In PAD, quitting may improve claudication and reduce the risk of vascular events. There is a need to establish smoking cessation clinics to deliver specialist care. All clinicians should try to motivate patients to quit by spending a few minutes explaining why smoking is harmful to them.

Antiplatelet Agents

This patient could not tolerate aspirin. It is estimated that this problem arises in 10–15% of patients who are prescribed aspirin. There are several alternatives:

- "Cover" aspirin with a proton pump inhibitor (e.g. omeprazole).
- Eradicate *Helicobacter pylori* infection, if present.
- Use clopidogrel: the effectiveness of clopidogrel is based on the findings of major trials (e.g. CAPRIE, CREDO and CURE), but there is no study specifically designed to assess the effectiveness of this drug in PAD.[19] However, patients with PAD had significantly fewer events on clopidogrel than on aspirin in the CAPRIE trial. Unfortunately, this conclusion is limited by the fact that PAD subgroup analysis was not included in the trial protocol.[20]

Due to his intolerance of aspirin, this patient was prescribed clopidogrel 75 mg/day. He tolerated this antiplatelet agent without any problems.

Potential limitations associated with the use of aspirin and/or clopidogrel have inspired clinical investigation into several promising new antiplatelet agents as potential additions or alternatives to standard therapy. The candidates include prasugrel, which has a mechanism similar to that of clopidogrel but with superior pharmacokinetics; ticagrelor, a non-thienopyridine that binds reversibly to the platelet P2Y(12) receptor; cangrelor, an intravenously administered analogue of ticagrelor; and various thrombin receptor antagonists. Current evidence derives from research in cardiovascular disease. Future studies will establish the role of these new therapeutic options in the treatment of PAD.[21]

Blood Pressure (BP)

Strict control of blood pressure (BP) in high risk patients is essential (<140/90 mmHg, ideally around 120/80 mmHg).[20] In order to achieve this objective, there may be a need to use several antihypertensive drugs. Some general recommendations are appropriate:

- Several experts suggest that angiotensin-converting enzyme (ACE) inhibitors and angiotensin II receptor blockers (ARB) should be avoided or used with caution in PAD because these patients may have renal artery stenosis. If an ACE inhibitor or ARB is used, the plasma creatinine concentration should be monitored soon after starting treatment (initiate treatment at the lowest dose).
- There is some debate as to whether beta-blockers adversely affect lower limb circulation in patients with PAD. It would appear reasonable, however, to use a beta-blocker in post-MI patients with PAD.
- Some BP drugs exert beneficial or adverse effects on lipid levels, haemostatic factors and perhaps more importantly, the long-term risk of developing diabetes.

Glucose Status

This topic was discussed above. It is also important to note that if the patient is diabetic, the blood pressure targets become stricter, especially if proteinuria is present (<130/80 mmHg).

Lipids

This topic has been discussed above.

Emerging Risk Factors

These factors[1,5] include:

- *Lipoprotein (a) (Lp(a)):* there is evidence that Lp(a) is a marker of vascular risk, especially in patients with a raised serum LDL-C. Raised Lp(a) levels may also predict the risk of restenosis after surgery for PAD.[17] Serum Lp(a) levels are difficult to lower, but the risk associated with this abnormality may decrease if the LDL-C level is markedly reduced. Correcting hypothyroidism is associated with a fall in serum Lp(a) levels. Similarly, postmenopausal hormone therapy (HT) may reduce serum Lp(a) concentrations. There are, as yet, no intervention trials to show that lowering serum Lp(a) levels (e.g. by using high doses of nicotinic acid) is associated with fewer vascular events.
- *Homocysteine:* raised plasma levels of homocysteine are thought to predict vascular risk possibly by acting synergistically with established risk factors. The link between homocysteine and PAD appears to be stronger than with CHD.[5] However, there is no evidence from intervention trials to show that lowering plasma homocysteine levels (e.g. by folic acid, vitamin B12 or B6 supplements) is associated with a reduced risk of vascular events.
- *Haemostatic and fibrinolytic factors:* plasma fibrinogen concentration may be a predictor of vascular risk. The levels of this coagulation factor also predict the progression of PAD and possibly the risk of restenosis following bypass surgery.[17] Plasma fibrinogen levels can be lowered by some fibrates used to treat dyslipidaemia. However, as with other emerging risk factors, no trial-based evidence is available to show that lowering fibrinogen levels is associated with a decreased risk of vascular events. There is less evidence linking fibrinolytic factors with vascular risk.
- *Markers of inflammation (e.g. high-sensitivity C-reactive protein, CRP):* serum CRP levels predict the risk of a vascular event even when there is no vascular disease present or when lipid levels are "normal". We do not know whether CRP just reflects the inflammatory component of atherosclerosis or whether it is actually involved in its pathogenesis. Statins and fibrates lower serum levels of CRP.[20] Recent evidence suggests that we should also consider CRP levels (in the high sensitivity range) as a target for treatment.[22]

Question 4

Is it relevant to monitor renal function in this patient?

Yes, because about 33% of PAD patients have atherosclerotic renal artery stenosis.[5] It is therefore important to consider this diagnosis, especially if renal function tests are abnormal. There is evidence that renal and vascular disease progress in parallel.[23] Increased plasma creatinine levels are associated with a higher risk of vascular events, even if these values are in the upper end of the reference range. There is evidence that statins exert a renoprotective action in patients with CHD or PAD.[24,25] Impaired renal function may contribute to hyperuricaemia and hyperhomocysteinaemia.[26] These variables may predict increased vascular risk.

References

1. Expert panel on detection evaluation, and treatment of high blood cholesterol in adults. Executive summary of the third report of the National Cholesterol Education Program (NCEP) expert panel on detection, evaluation, and treatment of high blood cholesterol in adults (Adult Treatment Panel III). *JAMA,* 2001;285:2486-2497.
2. Alberti KG, Eckel RH, Grundy SM, Zimmet PZ, Cleeman JI, Donato KA, Fruchart JC, James WP, Loria CM, Smith SC Jr. International Diabetes Federation Task Force on Epidemiology and Prevention. Hational Heart, Lung, and Blood Institute. American Heart Association; World Heart Federation. International Atherosclerosis Society; International Association for the Study of Obesity. Harmonizing the metabolic syndrome: a joint interim statement of the International Diabetes Federation Task Force on Epidemiology and Prevention. National Heart, Lung, and Blood Institute. American Heart Association. World Heart Federation. International Atherosclerosis Society. and International Association for the Study of Obesity. *Circulation.* 2009;120:1640-1645.
3. Haffner SM, Alexander CM, Cook TJ, et al. Reduced coronary events in simvastatin-treated patients with coronary heart disease and diabetes or impaired fasting glucose levels. Subgroup analyses in the Scandinavian Simvastatin Survival Study. *Arch Intern Med.* 1999;159: 2661-2667.
4. Colhoun HM, Betteridge DJ, Durrington PN, et al. CARDS investigators. Primary prevention of cardiovascular disease with atorvastatin in type 2 diabetes in the Collaborative Atorvastatin Diabetes Study (CARDS): multicentre randomised placebo-controlled trial. *Lancet.* 2004;364:685-696.
5. Daskalopoulou SS, Daskalopoulos ME, Liapis CD, Mikhailidis DP. Peripheral arterial disease: a missed opportunity to administer statins so as to reduce cardiac morbidity and mortality. *Curr Med Chem.* 2005;12:443-452.
6. Hokanson JE, Austin MA. Plasma triglyceride level is a risk factor for cardiovascular disease independent of high density lipoprotein cholesterol level: a meta-analysis of the population-based prospective studies. *J Cardiovasc Risk.* 1996;3:213-219.
7. Wood D, Durrington P, Poulter N, McInnes G, Rees A, Wray R, on behalf of the Societies. Joint British recommendations on prevention of coronary heart disease in clinical practice. *Heart.* 1998;80(Suppl 2):S1-S29.
8. Sacks FM, for the Expert Group on HDL Cholesterol. The role of high-density lipoprotein (HDL) cholesterol in the prevention and treatment of coronary heart disease: Expert Group Recommendations. *Am J Cardiol.* 2003;90:139-143.

9. Rizos E, Mikhailidis DP. Are high density lipoprotein (HDL) and triglyceride levels relevant in strokeprevention? *Cardiovasc Res.* 2001;52:199-207.
10. Rubins HB, Robins SJ, Collins D, et al. Gemfibrozil for the secondary prevention of coronary heart disease in men with low levels of high-density lipoprotein cholesterol. *N Engl J Med.* 1999;341:410-417.
11. De Backer G, Ambrosioni E, Borch-Johnsen K, et al. Third Joint Task Force of European and Other Societies on Cardiovascular Disease Prevention in Clinical Practice. European guidelines on cardiovascular disease prevention in clinical practice. *Eur Heart J.* 2003;24:1601-1610.
12. Grundy SM, Cleeman JI, Merz CN, et al. Implications of recent clinical trials for the National Cholesterol Education Program Adult Treatment Panel III guidelines. *Circulation.* 2004;110:227-239.
13. Heart Protection Study Collaborative Group. MRC/BHF Heart Protection Study of cholesterol lowering with simvastatin in 20, 536 high-risk individuals: a randomised placebo-controlled trial. *Lancet.* 2002;360:7-22.
14. Cheng KS, Mikhailidis DP, Hamilton G, Seifalian AM. A review of the carotid and femoral intimamedia thickness as an indicator of the presence of peripheral vascular disease and cardiovascular risk factors. *Cardiovasc Res.* 2002;54:528-538.
15. Rantanen K, Tatlisumak T. Secondary prevention of ischemic stroke. *Curr Drug Targets.* 2004;5:457-472.
16. Tsiara S, Elisaf M, Mikhailidis DP. Influence of smoking on predictors of vascular disease. *Angiology.* 2003;54:507-530.
17. Cheshire NJW, Wolfe JHN, Barradas MA, Chambler AW, Mikhailidis DP. Smoking and plasma fibrinogen, lipoprotein (a) and serotonin are markers for postoperative infrainguinal graft stenosis. *Eur J Vasc Endovasc Surg.* 1996;11:479-486.
18. Milionis HJ, Rizos E, Mikhailidis DP. Smoking diminishes the beneficial effect of statins: observations from the landmark trials. *Angiology.* 2001;52:575-587.
19. Robless P, Mikhailidis DP, Stansby G. Systematic review of antiplatelet therapy for the prevention of myocardial infarction, stroke or vascular death in patients with peripheral vascular disease. *Br J Surg.* 2001;88:787-800.
20. Chobanian AV, Bakris GL, Black HR, et al. National Heart, Lung, and Blood Institute Joint National Committee on Prevention, Detection, Evaluation, and Treatment of High Blood Pressure. National High Blood Pressure Education Program Coordinating Committee. The Seventh Report of the Joint National Committee on Prevention, Detection, Evaluation, and Treatment of High Blood Pressure: the JNC 7 report. *JAMA.* 2003;289:2560-2572.
21. Angiolillo DJ, Bhatt DL, Gurbel PA, Jennings LK. Advances in antiplatelet therapy: agents in clinical development. *Am J Cardiol.* 2009;103(3 Suppl):40A-51A.
22. Ridker PM, Danielson E, Fonseca FA, et al. Rosuvastatin to prevent vascular events in men and women with elevated C-reactive protein. *N Engl J Med.* 2008;359:2195-2207.
23. Rahman M, Brown CD, Coresh J, et al. Antihypertensive and Lipid-Lowering Treatment to Prevent Heart Attack Trial Collaborative Research Group. The prevalence of reduced glomerular filtration rate in older hypertensive patients and its association with cardiovascular disease: a report from the Antihypertensive and Lipid-Lowering Treatment to Prevent Heart Attack Trial. Arch Intern Med. 2003;164:969-976.
24. Athyros VG, Mikhailidis DP, Papageorgiou AA, et al. The effect of statins versus untreated dyslipidaemia on renal function in patients with coronary heart disease. A subgroup analysis of the Greek atorvastatin and coronary heart disease evaluation (GREACE) study. *J Clin Pathol.* 2004;57:728-734.
25. Youssef F, Gupta P, Seifalian AM, Myint F, Mikhailidis DP, Hamilton G. The effect of short-term treatment with simvastatin on renal function in patients with peripheral arterial disease. *Angiology.* 2004;55:53-62.
26. Daskalopoulou SS, Athyros VG, Elisaf M, Mikhailidis DP. Uric acid levels and vascular disease. *Curr Med Res Opin.* 2004;20:951-954.

Lower Limb Claudication Due to Iliac Artery Occlusive Disease

17

Marcus Brooks and Fabien Koskas

A 63-year-old man presents with a history of worsening pain in his left buttock, thigh and calf on walking. During the preceding 3 months, following the introduction of a beta-blocker for newly diagnosed hypertension, the distance he could walk at a "normal" pace had reduced from 200 to 100 m. The pain ceased almost immediately after stopping walking and appeared again after the same interval. A systemic enquiry revealed recently diagnosed hypertension and life-long history of heavy smoking. He had never experienced cerebro-vascular or cardiac symptoms.

Clinical examination revealed sinus rhythm, full upper limb pulses, a diminished left femoral pulse and absent left popliteal and pedal pulses. The right leg pulses were normal. Both feet appeared well perfused. No bruits were audible in the abdomen or groins. The abdominal aorta was not aneurismal. Ankle pressure brachial indices were 0.74 on the left and 0.93 on the right at rest. On treadmill walking for 100 m the left ankle pressure fell to 0.49.

Question 1

Which of the following would be part of your initial management of this patient?

A. A prescription for nicotine replacement therapy.
B. A prescription for warfarin.
C. A prescription for aspirin.
D. A prescription for a statin.
E. Stopping the beta-blocker.

The clinical findings were sufficient to make the diagnosis of peripheral arterial disease (PAD). The patient was advised as to the risk of smoking and referred to the local smoking cessation clinic. Best medical therapy was instituted for PAD. It was decided not to investigate further at this stage but to review in three months. After three months the patient had successfully managed to stop smoking and was taking the medication prescribed. His left leg claudication,

M. Brooks (✉)
Department of Vascular Surgery,
University Hospitals Bristol NHS Foundation Trust, Bristol, UK

G. Geroulakos and B. Sumpio (eds.), *Vascular Surgery*,
DOI: 10.1007/978-1-84996-356-5_17, © Springer-Verlag London Limited 2011

however, had not deteriorated. He was also now complaining of erectile dysfunction. As the patient was shortly to be retiring and was an enthusiastic hunter he was very keen for any intervention that might improve his walking distance and impotence.

Question 2

How would you proceed with your management at this second clinic visit?

A. No further intervention.
B. A prescription for Cilostazol (Pletal™, Otsuka Pharmaceuticals Co.)
C. Obtain arterial imaging to define the pattern of arterial disease.
D. Enrolment of the patient in a supervised exercise programme.

Question 3

Which of the following is *not* an appropriate first line imaging modality?

A. Duplex ultrasound.
B. Contrast-enhanced CT scan (CTA).
C. Contrast-enhanced magnetic resonance angiography (MRA).
D. Intra-arterial digital subtraction contrast angiogram (IADSA).

The patient underwent an arterial duplex scan. This scan showed a significant stenosis at the left internal iliac artery origin and a short but tight stenosis of the proximal left external iliac artery. The contra-lateral iliac system was found to be free from significant disease, as were the femoral and popliteal arteries in both legs. The crural arteries were not formally assessed using duplex. This pattern of disease was confirmed on subsequent angiographic images (Fig. 17.1).

Question 4

Into which of the following TransAtlantic Inter-Society Consensus (TASC) categories would you put both the internal and external iliac artery lesions?

A. TASC A
B. TASC B
C. TASC C
D. TASC D
E. TASC E

Question 5

Which of the following would you consider as possible interventions?

A. Aorto-bifemoral bypass graft.
B. Left aorto-uni-iliac bypass graft.
C. Right femoral to left femoral cross-over graft.

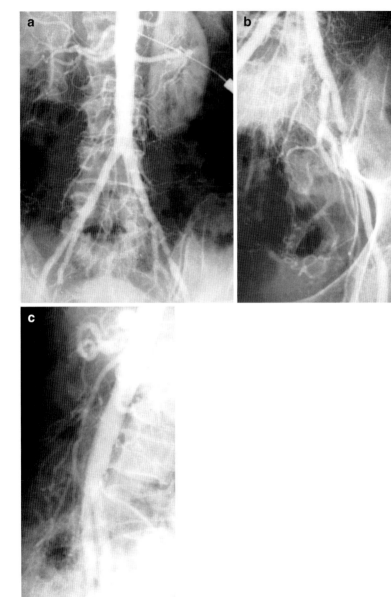

Fig. 17.1 Images from the digital subtraction angiogram showing (**a**) the renal arteries, infrarenal aorta and iliac bifurcation, (**b**) internal iliac and proximal external iliac stenoses, and (**c**) an oblique projection of the left iliac system

D. Percutaneous transluminal angioplasty via a right common femoral puncture.

E. Percutaneous transluminal angioplasty via a left common femoral puncture.

A percutaneous transluminal angioplasty was performed from the left groin under local anaesthesia. First a 4F sheath and pigtail catheter were used to obtain a diagnostic angiogram, as seen in Fig 17.2. The angiogram was performed to visualize the left iliac disease, but also

Fig. 17.2 Angiogram performed for investigation of
the patient's erectile dysfunction and worsening of
left thigh and calf intermittent claudication

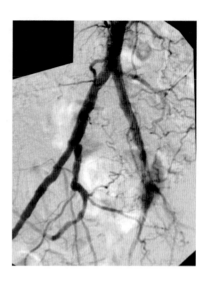

the crural arteries which had not been imaged with duplex. The diagnostic angiogram confirmed the duplex findings and revealed normal runoff arteries below the knee. The sheath
was therefore changed to 6F and systemic heparin given. A SOS OMNI® catheter was used
to direct a guide wire across the bifurcation. The guide wire was then steered first into the
internal iliac and then the external iliac arteries with balloon angioplasties performed.

Question 6

What size of balloon is likely to be needed to dilate the internal and external iliac arteries
in this man?

A. 2 mm
B. 4 mm
C. 7 mm
D. 10 mm
E. 12 mm

A completion diagnostic angiogram confirmed a good result. The right femoral sheath was
removed with manual pressure over the puncture site. The left leg pulses were restored by
the procedure.

Question 7

Which of the following statements describe the optimal follow-up for this patient?

A. Low-dose subcutaneous low-molecular-weight heparin (LMWH) for 3 months.
B. Enrolment of the patient in a supervised exercise programme.

C. Serial duplex scanning to detect recurrent stenosis before symptoms occur.
D. No follow-up.

The patient had post angioplasty ABPI in the left leg of 0.97. His symptoms completely resolved. He was therefore not referred for supervised exercise. Eleven years later he returned complaining of the return of his left leg claudication and a recent onset of erectile dysfunction. In that time period he had re-commenced smoking, but less than he had done previously. He had also undergone a coronary artery bypass graft for unstable angina. Two years following the bypass his angina had recurred. He continued to hunt but by now walking was difficult due to occasional angina attacks, breathlessness up hills and more recently pain in the left thigh and calf. On examination his left femoral pulse was weak, the distal pulses were absent in the left leg and a soft bruit was heard over the right femoral artery.

Question 8

What is the likely aetiology of this man's erectile dysfunction?

A. Advancing age.
B. Side effect of his cardiac medication.
C. Arterial insufficiency.
D. Endocrine failure.

In view of the history of peripheral arterial disease with an internal iliac artery stenosis arterial insufficiency was considered the most likely cause for impotence; this is the most common cause of impotence in this age group. Another angiogram was requested, the angiogram shows that the left internal iliac artery has re-stenosed and the external iliac artery has progressed to an occlusion. The common femoral artery reforms from collaterals and the distal run-off (neither shown) was preserved.

Question 9

Into which of the following The TransAtlantic Inter-Society Consensus (TASC) categories would you put the new occlusion of the external iliac artery?

A. TASC A
B. TASC B
C. TASC C
D. TASC D
E. TASC E

The patient insisted on being relieved from his symptoms "no matter what the risks". Discussion with his cardiologist revealed that the most recent coronary angiogram showed that two of three vein grafts had occluded and that his left ventricle function was poor (28% ejection fraction).

Question 10

Which of the following is your preferred intervention?

A. Aorto-bifemoral bypass graft with revascularisation of both internal iliac arteries.
B. Left aorto-uni-iliac bypass graft with revascularisation of the left internal iliac.
C. Right femoral to left femoral cross-over graft.
D. Percutaneous transluminal angioplasty.
E. No intervention.

The majority of iliac lesions, even occlusions, can now be treated with endovascular therapies. Such an approach was certainly sensible in this man who's cardiac history would put him at significant risk from open aortic surgery. A cross-over graft would relieve his claudication but would be unlikely to improve symptoms of impotence.

Question 11

When performing angioplasty in the iliac arteries which of the following are indications for stent insertion?

A. Never.
B. If there is a significant residual stenosis following angioplasty.
C. When crossing an occlusion.
D. Always.
E. When treating a calcified plaque.

A percutaneous approach was attempted successfully. A diagnostic angiogram was first performed from the right side as in the first procedure. The left common femoral artery was then punctured under ultrasound guidance and a 6F sheath inserted. A hydrophilic guidewire was successfully passed across the external iliac occlusion. This lesion was primarily stented prior to angioplasty of the internal iliac artery stenosis, Fig. 17.3.

Following this procedure all left leg pulses were present with an ABPI of 1.0. Both the symptoms of impotence and claudication resolved.

17.1
Commentary

The majority of patients with peripheral arterial disease smoke.[1] Cessation of smoking slows the rate of progression of peripheral arterial disease and reduces the risk of cardiac

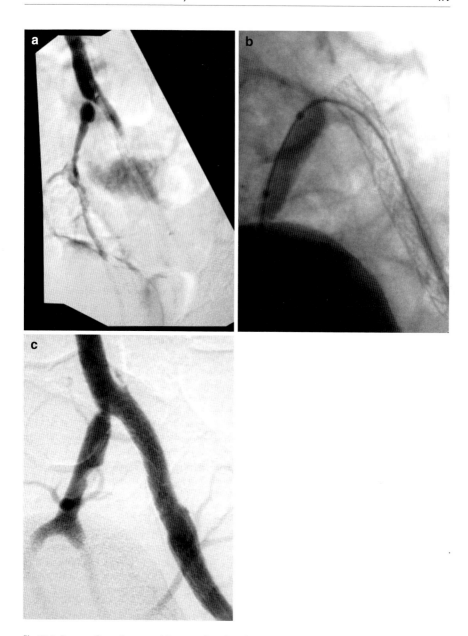

Fig. 17.3 Images from the second intervention showing a retrograde passage of a hydrophilic guide wire across the occluded external iliac artery, b the technical result from angioplasty with stent placement in the external iliac artery and the guide wire now directed into the internal iliac artery and c the completion angiogram

morbidity and mortality.[2] The prescription of nicotine replacement therapy is of benefit in patients who find it difficult to quit.[3] The benefit of exercise for relieving the symptoms of intermittent claudication has long been recognised.[4] The type and frequency of exercise to yield maximum benefit has been examined in a systematic review and Cochrane Collaboration Overview; advice alone is of little benefit but supervised exercise programmes (achieving maximal walking distance for at least 30 min three times a week) can achieve a 150% increase in walking distance or 6-min increase in walking time.[5,6] A systematic review failed to show any association between beta-blockers and worsening claudication.[7] If the beta blocker is stopped another antihypertensive agent, such as a calcium channel blocker or ACE inhibitor, should be substituted for control of hypertension, as treating hypertension reduces the stroke risk by 38%, cardiovascular risk by 14% and peripheral vascular events by 14%.[8] A systematic review by the Anti-platelet Trialists Collaboration has proven the benefit of 75–1,500 mg aspirin daily in achieving a 25% reduction in the risk of death, stroke or myocardial infarction.[9] A post-hoc subgroup analysis of patients with peripheral vascular disease in the CAPRIE trial showed additional benefit for clopidogrel.[10] The additional benefit is small (196 patients on clopidogrel to prevent one death) and not justified except for the 20% of patients who are aspirin intolerant. There is no evidence of benefit from warfarin.[11] It is also important to start the patient on statin therapy as this intervention has been shown to achieve an equivalent reduction in morbidity and mortality to aspirin.[12,13] **[Q1: A, C, D and (E)]**

The patient returns having modified his risk factors and is no better. His claudication is affecting his quality of life. The options for management are persistence with unsupervised exercise, a supervised exercise programme, drug therapy or intervention (angioplasty or bypass). Cilostazol is the only drug shown to be effective at relieving the symptoms of intermittent claudication in a small randomised trial.[14,15] However, it is expensive and the effect is shortlived. Intervention can only be considered once the anatomy of the underlying stenosis is known. As the presenting symptom is intermittent claudication and the patient has a weak left femoral pulse with normal right leg pulses we suspect a single level left iliac stenosis. It was decided to image the lesion. **[Q2: C, (B)]**

The optimal imaging of aortoiliac lesions is dependent on the facilities available. It is preferable to first obtain non-invasive images to allow the approach to a lesion to be planned, ensure the appropriate equipment is available and obtain the appropriate patient consent. Duplex scanning has become a useful tool for non invasive evaluation of aortoiliac occlusive disease.[16] However, duplex in the aortoiliac segment is highly dependent on patient's body habitus and experience of the operator. A helical multi-detector row (32 or 64 detectors) CT scanner can provide highquality cross-sectional images of the aorta, iliac arteries and even arteries down to the feet. CT scans have the advantage to the surgeon of familiarity and show calcified vessel walls. The disadvantages of CTA are the risk of contrast-induced nephropathy, patient exposure to ionising radiation and the time it takes to reformat the images.[17,18] Contrast-enhanced magnetic resonance angiography (MRA) can also image the aortoiliac segment, Fig. 17.4. It is the investigation of choice in patients at risk of contrast-induced renal impairment. In a comparison of CTA and MRA in imaging the aorta and iliac segments, sensitivity and specificity for the detection of lesions were equivalent. CTA took longer to reformat and report; a greater proportion of patients expressed a preference for CTA.[19] MRA is contraindicated in patients with pacemakers and ferromagnetic intracranial aneurysm clips. Intra-arterial digital subtraction angiography now has a limited

Fig. 17.4 Magnetic resonance angiogram (MRA) of another patient demonstrating occlusion of the right external iliac artery

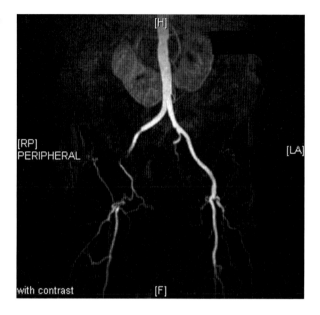

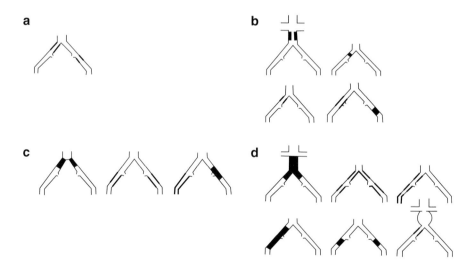

Fig. 17.5 TASC II classification of aorto-iliac lesions

diagnostic role in the aortoiliac segment. Angiography is invasive and is only performed if artefacts from previous implants (i.e. stainless steel stents) degrade threedimensional imaging, if direct pressure measurements across a stenosis are required or, as in this patient, as the first stage of an invasive procedure following non-invasive imaging. **[Q3: D]**

The left internal iliac origin and mid-third external iliac artery lesions are TransAtlantic Inter-Society Consensus (TASC) type A lesions, Fig. 17.5.[20] **[Q4: A]**

The TASC consensus on the management of type A aorto iliac lesions (Recommendation 32) was for endovascular intervention, Table 17.1. Surgical options, endarterectomy or bypass, are reserved for longer stenoses (5–10 cm) or occlusions.[20] The reported primary technical success of angioplasty of type A lesions is 98–99% with 60–80% patency at 5 years.[21] The 5-year patency of open procedures is slightly better, 90% for aorto-bifemoral bypass, but the patient is exposed to the risks of death (2–3 %), erectile dysfunction and graft infection.[22] It is a matter of personal preference whether a left or right percutaneous approach is used for the angioplasty as the lesion is mid-way between the aortic bifurcation and inguinal ligament. The internal iliac artery may be easier to approach from the contra-lateral side. **[Q5: D or E]**

In this case a contra-lateral approach was employed. The size of balloon used for angioplasty depends on the size of the native vessel. 2 and 4 mm balloons are used in the crural arteries, below the knee, and a 15 mm balloon is likely to rupture even a common iliac artery. In this patient a 7 mm balloon was used. **[Q6: C]**

The optimal management of patients following angioplasty has not been evaluated in randomised control trials. The risks to the artery are thrombosis, myointimal hyperplasia and disease progression. All patients should already be on an antiplatelet agent. Patients are formally heparinised during the procedure and for this short stenosis this is probably adequate. There is no evidence that postprocedure low-molecular-weight heparin, or for that matter any pharmacological agent (e.g. ticlopidine), is of benefit. Routine graft surveillance has been shown to improve the secondary patency of infra-inguinal vein bypass

Table 17.1 TASC II recommendations for management of aorto-iliac lesions

Type of lesion	Treatment recommendations
TASC A	Percutaneous angioplasty, with stenting reserved for residual stenosis following treatment.
TASC B	Percutaneous angioplasty, with stenting reserved for residual stenosis or intervention for occlusion.
TASC C	Percutaneous angioplasty, with or without stenting. Surgery occasionally first choice in young 'fit' patient with bilateral disease; alternative unilateral angioplasty then either an ilio-femoral or femoral-femoral cross-over offers a less invasive alternative approach.
TASC D	Open surgical reconstruction (aorto-(bi)femoral bypass or axillo-(bi) femoral bypass) may be indicated, especially an aorto-bi-femoral graft in a patient with aortic aneurysm or occlusion. Increasingly, however, TASC D lesions are managed with combined approach, as for TASC C, with even long CIA and/or EIA occlusions successfully re-canalised.
TASC C/D	CFA disease generally responds poorly to angioplasty and requires surgical endarterectomy, again combined with a proximal angioplasty or surgical inflow procedure.

AAA abdominal aortic aneurysm, *CFA* common femoral artery, *CIA* common iliac artery, *EIA* external iliac artery, *IIA* internal iliac artery (hypogastric artery)
[a]Modified from [31]

grafts.[23] Surveillance has not been evaluated following iliac angioplasty. The MIMIC Trial has shown that the benefit of angioplasty plus supervised exercise are additive for patients who have stopped smoking with iliac artery occlusive disease and mild to moderate intermittent claudication.[24] As myointimal hyperplasia and disease progression both occur, it appears prudent, if not mandatory, to follow up patients. This can be done using clinical examination, arterial duplex or ankle brachial pressure index (ABPI) measurement. Clinical follow-up is cost-effective and in addition is a good way of enforcing a tight control of risk factors. **[Q7: B]**

Erectile dysfunction in this setting is probably due to arterial insufficiency resulting from progression of bilateral iliac occlusive disease. The association of erectile dysfunction with aortoiliac occlusive disease was first described in 1814 by Robert Graham.[25] However, it was Rene Leriche in 1940 who operated on a 29-year-old truck driver "who for two years had been suffering from claudicatio intermittens with severe cramps in the leg musculature already after a few hundred meters of walking, and cramp pains also at night. The last weeks before the operation he complained of not being able to complete an intercourse, as both erection and ejaculation was disturbed".[26] **[Q8: C]**

This patient has suffered disease progression in the intervening years. He has developed a very tight stenosis of the left internal iliac artery, a stenosis or the right internal iliac artery origin, and complete occlusion of the left external iliac. The left external iliac artery occlusion is classified as a TASC type C lesion.[20] **[Q9: C]**

The consensus in 1990, when the TASC guidelines were drawn up, was that definitive recommendations on how to treat such lesions must await more convincing evidence. This situation has not changed. The risks of open aortoiliac bypass surgery and endarterectomy have already been discussed. Remote iliac endarterectomy using Moll ring strippers avoids an abdominal approach and pelvic dissection, has good published technical success rates (88–92%), and 3-year patency just below that of open endarterectomy (60%).[27,28] A potential development for the future is laparoscopic aortoiliac surgery.[29] In this patient a femoral-femoral cross-over graft is not advisable because contralateral lesions may impair the graft inflow and because this procedure would not address the internal iliac stenoses. Had the cardiac antecedents not been present, direct bilateral surgical antegrade revascularization of the lower limbs and one or both internal iliac arteries would have been an excellent solution. However, in the context of unreconstructable coronary artery disease and poor left ventricular function, such a solution is too invasive and carries too great a risk of cardiac death. On the other hand, surgical abstention, although not without justification, seems exaggerated because quality of life is often as important as its length among middle-aged and aged patients. **[Q10: D]**

Stenting is generally reserved for the primary treatment of occlusions to reduce the risk of distal embolisation. Stents are also used in management of lesions with a high risk of primary failure; eccentric calcified plaque, residual stenosis greater than 50% or greater than 10 mmHg pressure gradient or if there is local dissection.[30] Stenting adds considerably to the cost of the procedure. In this patient, stents were placed into both the external and internal iliac arteries, because of the occlusion and a residual stenosis after angioplasty respectively. **[Q11: B, C and possibly E]**

References

1. Kannel WB, The SD, Study F. Cigarettes and the development of intermittent claudication. *Geriatrics.* 1973;28:61-68.
2. Mathieson FR, Larsen EE, Wulff M. Some factors influencing the spontaneous course of arterial vascular insufficiency. *Acta Chir Scand.* 1970;136:303-308.
3. Joseph AM, Norman SM, Ferry LH, et al. The safety of trans-dermal nicotine as an aid to smoking cessation in patients with cardiac disease. *N Eng J Med.* 1996;335:1793-1798.
4. Housley E. Treating claudication in five words. *BMJ.* 1988;296(6635):1483-1484.
5. Gardener AW, Poehlman ET. Exercise rehabilitation programs for the treatment of claudication pain. *JAMA.* 1995;274:975-980.
6. Leng GC, Fowler B, Ernst E. Exercise for intermittent claudication. The Cochrane Database of Systematic Reviews 2000, Issue 2.
7. Radark K, Deck C. Beta-adrenergic blocker therapy does not worsen intermittent claudication in subjects with peripheral arterial disease. A meta-analysis of randomised control trials. *Arch Intern Med.* 1991;151:1769-1776.
8. Kannel WB, McGhee DL. Update on some epidemiological features of intermittent claudication in subjects with peripheral vascular disease. *J Am Geriatr Soc.* 1985;22:13-18.
9. Anti-platelet Trialists Collaboration. Collaboration overview of randomised trials on anti-platelet therapy. 1. Prevention of death, myocardial infarction and stroke by prolonged anti-platelet therapy in various catagories of patients. *BMJ.* 1994;308:81-106.
10. CAPRIE Steering Committee. A randomised, blinded, trial of clopidogrel versus aspirin in patients at risk of ischaemic events (CAPRIE). *Lancet.* 1996;348:1328-1339.
11. Visseren FL, Eikelboom BC. Oral anticoagulant therapy in patients with peripheral artery disease. *Semin Vasc Med.* 2003;3(3):339-344.
12. Scandinavian Simvastatin Survival Group Study. Randomised trial of cholesterol lowering in 4444 patients with coronary heart disease: the Scandinavian Simvastatin Survival Study (4S). *Lancet.* 1994;344:1383-1389.
13. Sacks FM, Pfeffer MA, Moyle LA, et al. For the Cholesterol and Recurrent Events Trial Investigators. The effect of pravastatin on coronary events after myocardial infarction in patients with average cholesterol levels. *N Engl J Med.* 1996;335:1001-1009.
14. Cameron HA, Waller PC, Ramsey LE. Drug treatment of intermittent claudication: a critical analysis of the methods and findings of published clinical trials. *Br J Clin Pharmacol.* 1988;26:569-576.
15. Strandness DE, Dalman RL, Panian S, et al. Effect of cilostazol in patients with intermittent claudication: a randomized, double-blind, placebo-controlled study. *Vasc Endovasc Surg.* 2002;36(2):83-91.
16. Van der Zaag ES, Legemate DA, Nguyen T, et al. Aortoiliac reconstructive surgery based upon the results of duplex scanning. *Eur J Vasc Endovasc Surg.* 1998;16:383-389.
17. Catalano C, Fraioli F, Laghi A, et al. Infrarenal aortic and lower-limb arterial disease: diagnostic performance of multi-detector row CT angiography. *Radiology.* 2004;231:555-563.
18. Nicholson T, Downes M. Contrast nephrotoxicity and iso-osmolar contrast agents: implications of NEPHRIC. *Clin Radiol.* 2003;58:659-660.
19. Willmann JK, Wildermuth S, Pfammater T, et al. Aorto-iliac and renal arteries: prospective intraindervidual comparison of contrast-enhanced three-dimensional MR angiography and multidetector row CT angiography. *Radiology.* 2003;226:798-811.
20. Dormandy JA. Management of Peripheral Arterial Disease (PAD). TASC Working Group. TransAtlantic Inter-Society Consensus (TASC). *Eur J Endovasc Surg.* 2000;19(Suppl A): S1–S244.

21. Rutherford RB, Durham JA, Kumpe DA. Endovascular intervention for lower extremity ischaemia. In: Rutherford RB, ed. *Vascular Surgery*. 4th ed. Philadelphia: WB Saunders; 1995:858-874.

22. Nevelsteen A, Wouters L, Suy R. Aortofemoral Dacron reconstruction for aorto-iliac occlusive disease: a 25 year survey. *Eur J Vasc Surg*. 1991;5:179-186.

23. McCarthy MJ, Olojugba D, Loftus IM, et al. Lower limb surveillance following autologous vein bypass should be life long. *Br J Surg*. 1998;85:1369-1372.

24. Greenhalgh RM, Belch JJ, Brown LC, et al. The adjuvant benefit of angioplasty in patients with mild to moderate intermittent claudication (MIMIC) managed by supervised exercise, smoking cessation advice and best medical therapy: results from two randomised trials for stenotic femoropopliteal and aortoiliac arterial disease. *Eur J Vas Endovasc Surg*. 2008 (Dec);36(6):680-688.

25. Graham R. Case of obstructed aorta. Communicated by Sir G Blane. Medico-Chirurgical Transactions, London, 1814.

26. Leriche R. De la résection du carrefour aortico-iliaque avec double sympathectomie lombaire pour thrombose artéritique la l'aorte: le syndrome de l'oblitération termino-aortique par artérite. *La presse médicale, Paris*. 1940;48:601-607.

27. Ricco JB. Unilateral iliac artery occlusive disease; a randomised multi-centre trial examining direct revascularisation versus crossover bypass. *Ann Vasc Surg*. 1992;16:841-852.

28. Smeets L, de Borst GJ, Vries JP, et al. Remote iliac artery endarterectomy: seven year results of a less invesive technique for iliac artery occlusive disease. *J Vasc Surg*. 2003;38:1297-1304.

29. Loggia M, Javerliat I, DiCentra I, et al. Total laparoscopic bypass for aorto-iliac occlusive lesions: 93 case experience. *J Vasc Surg*. 2004;40:899-906.

30. Tetteroo E, van der Graff Y, Bosch JL, et al. Randomised comparison of primary stent placement versus primary angioplasty followed by selective stent placement in patients with iliac artery occlusive disease. *Lancet*. 1998;18:499-505.

31. Norgren L, Hiatt WR, Dormandy JA, et al. Inter-Society Consensus for the Management of Peripheral Arterial Disease (TASC II). *J Vasc Surg*. 2007;45(Suppl S):S5-S67. PMID 17223489.

Lower Limb Claudication Due to Bilateral Iliac Artery Occlusive Disease: The Case for Iliac Stenting and Femorofemoral Crossover Bypass

18

Jean-Baptiste Ricco and Olivier Page

A 54-year-old man presents to your clinic complaining of bilateral rest pain of the toes and a past medical history of cramping pain in his calves when he walks. The patient had a 30-pack year smoking history and remains an active smoker. Clinical examination revealed an absent left femoral pulse and a diminished right femoral pulse. Popliteal and pedal pulses were absent on both sides. Bilateral carotid bruits were noted. Palpation of the abdominal aorta was normal. The patient was also moderately breathless on minimal exertion and had a chronic productive cough. The ECG was normal, a chest x-ray showed evidence for chronic obstructive pulmonary disease (COPD). FEV1 was 950 mL not enhanced after inhalation of bronchodilators. The patient was currently taking medications for hypertension and elevated cholesterol.

The patient had a Duplex-scan with measurements of the ABI that was 0.40 on the right side and of 0.29 on the left. The Duplex showed an occlusion of the left external iliac artery and significant stenoses of the right common and external iliac arteries with occlusion of both superficial femoral arteries. The patient had also mild bilateral carotid artery stenosis.

The duplex scan was followed by digital percutaneous subtraction contrast angiography that showed an occlusion of the left external iliac artery and a significant stenosis of the right common and external iliac arteries. Severe occlusive lesions were also seen in both common femoral arteries (Figs. 18.1–18.3). The superficial femoral artery was occluded on both sides. Significant lesions of the crural arteries were also present (not shown).

J-B. Ricco (✉)
Section of Vascular Surgery and Vascular Intervention,
University of Poitiers Medical School, Poitiers, France

G. Geroulakos and B. Sumpio (eds.), *Vascular Surgery*,
DOI: 10.1007/978-1-84996-356-5_18, © Springer-Verlag London Limited 2011

Question 1

Before discussing any surgical options, what kind of cardiac evaluation would you consider as appropriate in this case?

A. ECG and transthoracic echocardiography
B. Stress echocardiography
C. Coronary computed tomography angiography (CCTA)
D. Coronary angiography

This patient had no previous myocardial infarction and no clinical sign of myocardial ischemia. The ECG and cardiac echography were considered as normal. No further cardiac evaluation was considered in this case. **[Q2-A]**

Question 2

Which of the following surgical options will you consider in this case?

A. Aortobifemoral bypass (ABF) with distal anastomosis on both profunda femoris arteries
B. Percutaneous bilateral iliac stenting with left external iliac recanalization
C. Bilateral iliac stenting with left external iliac recanalization and bilateral femoral bypass to the profunda
D. Right iliac stenting with right femoral bypass to the profunda and crossover femoro-femoral bypass to the left profunda
E. Right iliac stenting with a right femoral to profunda endarterectomy with patch plasty and crossover femorofemoral bypass to the left profunda

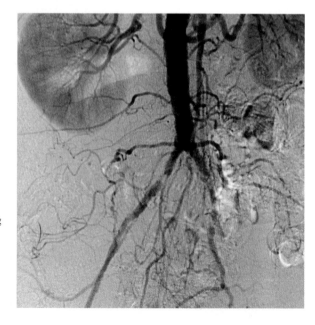

Fig. 18.1 Percutaneous angiography with brachial artery catheterization using the Seldinger technique. Early film sequence showing severe stenosis of the right common iliac artery, stenosis of the left common iliac artery and occlusion of the left external iliac and femoral arteries

Fig. 18.2 Percutaneous angiography showing a moderate stenosis of the right external iliac artery, that was found to be significant on color duplex with PSV > 3.5 m/s

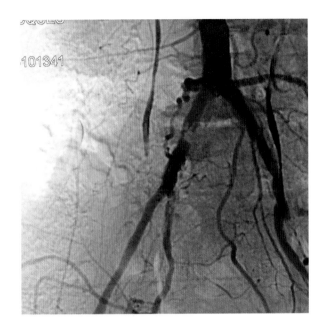

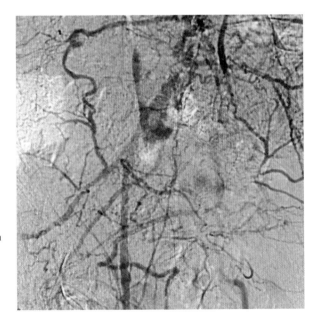

Fig. 18.3 Percutaneous angiography. Delayed film showing late revascularization of the profunda femoris arteries with occlusion of the right common femoral artery and significant disease of the left common iliac artery

An hybrid technique [Q3-D] was used in this case with stenting of the right common and external iliac arteries associated with a right bypass to the profunda and a cross-over femorofemoral bypass to the left profunda. Option [Q3-E] was also considered as an alternative, but not used in this case, considering the extensive lesions in the right profunda femoris artery. Option **[Q3-C]** was considered also as a possibility but impossible to achieve due to the extension of the iliac lesions into the left common femoral artery.

Question 3

Which of the following will be part of your follow-up management?

A. Prescription of aspirin
B. Prescription of statins
C. Enrolment of the patient in a supervised exercise program
D. Follow up at 6-month and then every year with a color duplex scan and ankle brachial index measurement
E. Smoking cessation advice with psychological and specific drug therapy if needed
F. All of the above

All of these options were offered to the patient who registered in a supervised exercise program but didn't quit smoking completely. Rest pain disappeared, mild claudication with a walking distance of 600 m was considered as acceptable by the patient and improved gradually further.

18.1
Commentary

This patient has a chronic critical limb ischaemia (CLI) caused by iliac and infrainguinal atherosclerotic disease. This most advanced form of peripheral arterial disease is associated with a high risk of cardiovascular events that include major limb loss, myocardial infarction and death.[1-4] In these cases, the 5 year life expectancy is approximately 50%.[5,6] Considering the high-risk nature of the CLI population, as well as the number of treatment options, precise risk evaluation is necessary in such a case.

18.2
Clinical Assessment

We used in this case, the PREVENT III CLI Risk Score[7,8] which is an easy to use risk stratification model developed to predict amputation free survival in patients with peripheral arterial disease. This relatively young patient (<75 years), who was not on dialysis, had no tissue loss and no clinical coronary disease was considered as a low risk case (Score <3) with a high probability to be alive at 1-year with intact lower limbs. In this case, cardiac evaluation was reduced to the minimum [**Q1: A**]. The main risk of this patient was the coexisting COPD. Preoperative preparation required in this case were (1) immediate smoking cessation, (2) inhaled bronchodilators, (3) deep breathing maneuvers.

18.3
Imaging Techniques

A color-duplex scan of the aortoiliac and limb arteries was done first to have a morphological and hemodynamic evaluation of the arterial lesions [**Q1:A**]. Duplex provides a remarkably complementary package of anatomic and physiologic information that is unrivaled by other modalities. As part of this evaluation, measurement of the ankle brachial index (ABI) is a simple and useful test that can be performed with a minimum of time. In this case an ABI of less than 0.5 with rest pain confirmed the diagnosis of CLI.

Current sophisticated duplex scanners provide three types of information: gray-scale B-mode imaging, color-flow imaging, and pulsed-Doppler spectral waveform analysis. Doppler velocity sampling is performed in all patent segments. The most widely recommended criterion for diagnosis of peripheral artery stenosis is a 100% peak systolic velocity step-up (velocity ratio ≥ 2) compared with a normal segment of artery proximal to the stenosis. Several investigators determined that this finding correlated closely with a 50% angiographic diameter reduction.[9]

CT-scan with contrast media (CTA) provides high quality images of the aorta, and iliac arteries. But calcified lesions are difficult to analyze with CTA and femoropopliteal or tibial arteries are not well analyzed by CTA. In addition, CTA exposes the patient to ionizing radiations and contrast-induced nephropathy.

Contrast-enhanced magnetic resonance angiography (MRA) can also image the aortoiliac and limb arteries with comparable results to CTA. Disadvantages of MRI are its lack of wide availability particularly in France due to Health care budget constraints, contraindication in patients with cardiac pacemakers, and artifacts from stainless-steel components.

In summary, CTA is used routinely in patients with aortoiliac lesions, but in such a situation with multilevel arterial occlusive disease as shown by duplex scanning, we preferred a percutaneous angiography to have high-quality images of the femoral arteries and distal run-off vessels.

18.4
Revascularization Options

Taking into account the patient's risk factors and the extent of arterial disease, the following options were available.

18.5
Aortobifemoral Bypass

ABF with distal anastomoses on to the profunda femoris arteries is an option for this rela-tively young patient with CLI. The patency rate of ABF is 85% to 90% at 5-year, and 70% at 10-year. ABF remains one of the most durable reconstruction in vascular surgery[10] and with proper patient selection, the operative mortality is an acceptable 2%. However this patient had severe COPD which is a leading cause of postoperative morbidity and mortal-ity in aortic surgery. A less aggressive alternative was therefore sought.

18.6
Iliac Angioplasty and Stenting

In this case, according to TASC II,[11] right common and external iliac artery lesions could be classified as category B and the occluded left external iliac artery as category D. In addi-tion, this patient had multiple stenoses involving the common femoral artery with an occlusion of the superficial femoral artery on both sides.

On the right side, we did the profunda revascularization first using an open technique, that will be described below. This bypass was followed by a primary stenting of the right common and external iliac arteries. In this case, the plaque on the right external iliac artery was not extending into the common femoral artery (CFA), leaving an area relatively free of disease with the distal endpoint of the stent being above the inguinal ligament. On the left side, the presence of a significant CFA/EIA disease was defined by an absent femoral pulse and a 3x peak systolic velocity step-up across the diseased CFA artery with more than 80% luminal narrowing (B-mode imaging) extending proximally in the EIA and dis-tally into the profunda. In this case, the distal endpoint of the iliac stent will have been located at the level of the CFA below the inguinal ligament with a potential risk of kinking. As for open surgery, an adequate femoral outflow is necessary for aortoiliac angioplasty. We considered therefore that left iliac stenting was not appropriate in this patient and decide to use a crossover femorofemoral bypass to the left profunda with stenting of the right common and external iliac arteries.

18.7
Iliac Stenting Combined with Profunda Femoris Artery Revascularization

Hybrid surgery with right iliac stenting and bilateral femoral revascularization appeared as the best solution in this case. The procedure was done in the operating room with the use of epidural anesthesia. On the right side, revascularization of the profunda was done first using an 8 mm diameter PTFE bypass (Fig. 18.4). Proximal anastomosis was done on the terminal portion of the external iliac artery, distal anastomosis was done on a non-diseased

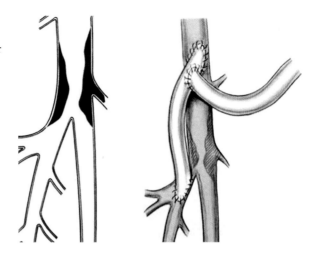

Fig. 18.4 Right iliofemoral bypass to the profunda femoris artery and crossover bypass

segment of the profunda femoris artery, 3 cm distal to its origin. This bypass procedure was followed by a primary stenting. The bypass was punctured with an 18-gauge needle, a 7F sheath was placed over the wire, through the bypass and iliac arteries. Stenting of the common and external iliac arteries was done using respectively a 8/60 mm stainless steel stent and a 7/60 mm nitinol stent.

Regarding the profunda femoris artery revascularization, a right CFA endarterectomy extending into the profunda is an alternative. In this case a longitudinal arteriotomy is created on the CFA and extended into the profunda. A standard endarterectomy is performed with the distal endarterectomy ending as a fine tapering of the CFA lesion into the profunda femoris artery, and the proximal endpoint cut just proximal to the inguinal ligament. The arteriotomy is then closed with a standard elliptical polyester patch and running sutured anastomosis.

Considering the extensive lesions on the right profunda, we preferred in this case the use of a PTFE bypass to the profunda with a distal anastomosis on a non-diseased segment without the risk of flap or residual stenosis.

The crossover femorofemoral bypass was then constructed between the right iliofemoral bypass and the distal left profunda using a 8 mm polyester graft. The follow-up was uneventful. The right ABI increased from 0.45 to 0.70, and the left ABI increased from 0.28 to 0.65 and remained stable 3 years after the procedure. A CTA (Fig. 18.5) showed the result of the procedure.

18.8
Rationale for Angioplasty of "Donor" Iliac Artery Prior to Femorofemoral Crossover Bypass

Successful femorofemoral crossover bypass is highly dependent on a hemodynamically satisfactory donor iliac arterial system. Endovascular intervention for selected iliac artery lesions provides excellent short- and long-term results in terms of hemodynamic improvement

Fig. 18.5 Contrast-enhanced
CT scan (*CTA*) showing a
patent right iliac stenting
with revascularization of the
right profunda femoris
artery and femorofemoral
crossover bypass to the left
profunda femoris artery

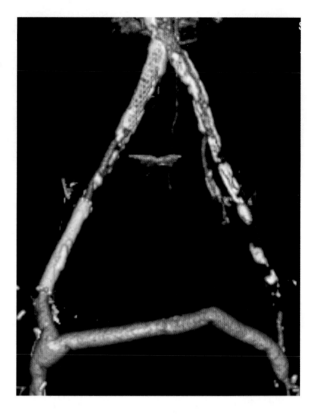

and patency. Several authors have now reported experience with transluminal balloon angio-plasty prior to or concomitant with femorofemoral bypass.[12,13] Results of these studies have supported the view that donor iliac artery balloon angioplasty with stenting in selected cases is associated with a satisfactory hemodynamic outcome and patency rate. The results of bal-loon angioplasty have probably improved since those initial prior studies were published. AbuRahma and colleagues have shown that the likelihood of success with this approach is substantially higher if the dilated donor iliac artery lesion is short and in the common iliac artery.[14] Ricco et al.[15] published the long-term results of a multicentre randomized study on direct bypass versus crossover bypass for unilateral iliac artery occlusive disease. The objec-tive of this trial was to compare late patency after direct and crossover bypass in 143 good-risk patients with unilateral iliac occlusive disease not amenable to angioplasty. These patients with unilateral iliac artery occlusive disease and disabling claudication were ran-domized into two surgical treatment groups, i.e., crossover bypass ($n=74$) or direct bypass ($n=69$). Iliac lesions TASC class [C in 87 (61%) patients and D in 56 (39%) patients], and superficial femoral artery (SFA) run-off were comparable in the two groups. Patients under-went yearly follow-up examinations using color flow duplex scanning with ankle-brachial systolic pressure index measurement. Median follow-up was 7.4 years. Primary endpoints were primary patency and assisted primary patency. Primary patency at 5 years (Fig. 18.6) was higher in the direct bypass group than in the crossover bypass group [$92.7\pm6.1\%$ vs.

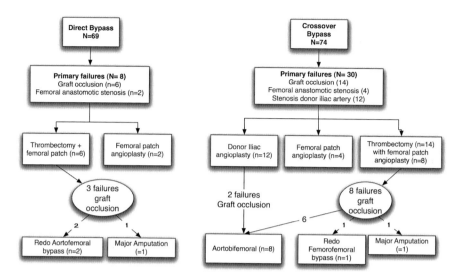

Fig. 18.6 Primary patency of 69 direct (*D*) and 74 crossover (*C*) bypass procedures analyzed according to the Kaplan-Meier method. The number of patients at risk in each group at various intervals is indicated at the bottom of the figure. Results are expressed as percentage with 95% confidence interval (95% CI). Primary patency rates at 5 and 10 years were $71.8\pm10\%$ and $55.6\pm12\%$ respectively in the crossover bypass group as compared to $92.7\pm6\%$ and $82.9\pm13\%$ respectively in the direct bypass group ($p=0.001$, hazard ratio: 4.1 with 95% CI: 1.8–6.7). (reprinted with permission from J.B. Ricco et al. J Vasc Surg. 2008;47:45-53.)

$73.2\pm10\%$, $p=0.001$]. Assisted primary patency and secondary patency at 5 years were also higher after direct bypass than crossover bypass [$92.7\pm6.1\%$ vs. $84.3\pm8.5\%$, $p=0.04$ and $97.0\pm3.0\%$ vs. $89.8\pm7.1\%$, $p=0.03$ respectively]. Patency at 5 years after crossover bypass was significantly higher in patients presenting no or low-grade SFA stenosis than in patients presenting high-grade ($\geq50\%$) stenosis or occlusion of the SFA [$74.0\pm12\%$ vs. $62.5\pm19\%$, $p=0.04$]. In both treatment groups, patency was comparable using PTFE and polyester grafts. Overall survival was $59.5\pm12\%$ at 10 years. This study showed that late patency was higher after direct bypass than crossover bypass in good-risk patients with unilateral iliac occlusive disease not amenable to angioplasty. This randomized study shows that determination of the status of the donor iliac artery was a key element for successful crossover bypass (Fig. 18.7). As early as 1973, Porter et al.[16] acknowledged the frequency of some degree of contralateral iliac disease in patients with extensive unilateral iliac disease and became one of the first groups to recommend use of donor iliac angioplasty in combination with crossover bypass. Not surprisingly use of endovascular techniques that can provide excellent long-term results in selected iliac artery lesions has improved the outcome of crossover bypass in patients with a suboptimal donor iliac artery.[17–20] The experience of several authors[21,22] has supported this view. In non-randomized studies comparing crossover femoral grafts with or without donor iliac balloon angioplasty, both Perler et al.[19] and Schneider et al.[20] concluded that patency of the crossover bypass in patients who underwent preliminary stenting of the iliac artery was comparable to that of patients whose donor iliac artery was normal. These findings clearly

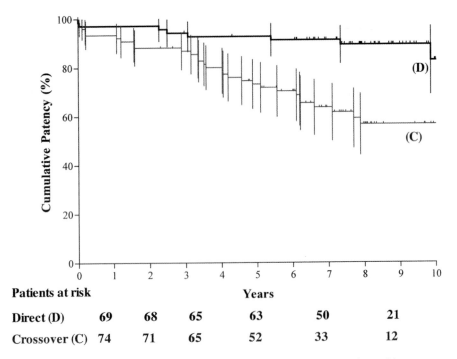

Fig. 18.7 Flowchart representing primary and secondary failures occurring in patients with crossover and direct bypass grafts. There were 30 primary failures of crossover bypass and eight primary failures of direct bypasses. Arterial flow was successfully maintained or restored by donor iliac angioplasty, thrombectomy, or femoral patch angioplasty in 20 failed crossover bypasses and in five failed primary direct bypasses. Secondary failures required ten aortobifemoral grafts and one new crossover femorofemoral graft. Two major amputations were required in patients with failed direct or crossover bypass and unreconstructable distal arterial disease. (reprinted with permission from J.B. Ricco et al. J Vasc Surg. 2008;47:45-53.)

support the use of angioplasty at the same time as crossover bypass in eligible patients with donor iliac lesions. Measurement of ABI also enabled us to compare hemodynamics after crossover and direct bypass. This comparison indicated that the hemodynamic results of the two procedures were comparable.

18.9
Occlusive Disease of the Common Femoral Artery, Profunda Orifice and Superficial Artery in Patients with Iliac Angioplasty

When the superficial femoral artery is occluded, iliac angioplasty is likely to succeed only if the profunda femoris artery is normal or revascularized and has developed collateral pathways to the popliteal artery with one or two tibial runoff. Construction of the crossover femorofemoral bypass was deemed necessary in this case because of the extensive left femoral artery lesions that render any attempt to left iliac endovascular recanalization quite hazardous with the distal end of the stent below the inguinal ligament. As said previously, it is important to have for both angioplasty and open surgery an adequate outflow. The use of such a combined approach to lower extremity revascularization is not new and many authors reported excellent long-term results after combined iliac angioplasty/stenting and profunda or distal revascularization.[24] [Q2:D]

18.10
Supervision and Follow-up of the Patient

A follow-up visit at yearly intervals with duplex evaluation and a structured or supervised walking program are essential in patients operated for CLI. Three concepts need to be explained to the patients: (1) A dedicated walking time should be tailored to each patient (e.g. 30–45 min, 3–5 days per week), (2) Walking instructions to walk at a comfortable pace and stop for a brief rest whenever leg pain becomes severe, (3) recording walking time, length and weight loss. This program should be associated with smoking cessation, use of statins and antiplatelet therapy.[25] [Q3:F]

References

1. Criqui MH, Langer RD, Fronek A, et al. Mortality over a period of 10 years in patients with peripheral arterial disease. *N Engl J Med*. 1992;326:381-386.
2. McKenna M, Wolfson S, Kuller L. The ratio of ankle and arm arterial pressure as an independent predictor of mortality. *Atherosclerosis*. 1991;87:119-128.
3. Murabito JM, Evans JC, Nieto K, Larson MG, Levy D, Wilson PW. Prevalence and clinical correlates of peripheral arterial disease in the Framingham Offspring Study. *Am Heart J*. 2002;143:961-965.
4. Howell MA, Colgan MP, Seeger RW, Ramsey DE, Sumner DS. Relationship of severity of lower limb peripheral vascular disease to mortality and morbidity: a six-year follow-up study. *J Vasc Surg*. 1989;9:691-696.
5. Adam DJ, Beard JD, Cleveland T, et al. Bypass versus angioplasty in severe ischaemia of the leg (BASIL): multicentre, randomised controlled trial. *Lancet*. 2005;366:1925-1934.
6. Stoyioglou A, Jaff MR. Medical treatment of peripheral arterial disease: a comprehensive review. *J Vasc Interv Radiol*. 2004;15:1197-1207.
7. Schanzer A, Mega J, Meadows J, Samson RH, Bandyk DF, Conte MS. Risk stratification in critical limb ischaemia: derivation and validation of a model to predict amputation-free survival using multicenter surgical outcomes data. *J Vasc Surg*. 2008;48:1464-1471.
8. Schanzer A, Goodney PP, YouFu L, et al. Validation of the PIII CLI Risk Score for the prediction of amputation-free survival in patients undergoing surgical bypass for critical limb ischaemia. *J Vasc Surg*. 2009;50:769-775.
9. Rose SC. Noninvasive vascular laboratory for evaluation of peripheral arterial occlusive disease. Part II. Clinical applications: chronic atherosclerotic, lower extremity ischaemia. *J Vasc Interv radiol*. 2000;11:1257-1275.

10. Brewster DC. Current controversies in the management of aortoiliac occlusive disease. *J Vasc Surg*. 1997;25:365-379.
11. Norgren L, Hiatt WR, Dormandy JA, Nehler MR, Harris KA. Fowkes FGR on behalf of the TASC II working group. Inter-Society Consensus for the Management of Peripheral Arterial Disease (TASC II). *Eur J Vasc Endovasc Surg*. 2007;33:S54-S57.
12. Pursell R, Sideso E, Magee TR, Galland RB. Critical appraisal of femorofemoral crossover grafts. *Br J Surg*. 2005;92:565-569.
13. Kim YW, Lee JH, Kim HG, Huh S. Factors affecting the long-term patency of crossover femorofemoral bypass graft. *Eur J Vasc Endovasc Surg*. 2005;30:376-380.
14. AbuRahma AF, Robinson PA, Cook CC, Hopkins ES. Selecting patients for combined femorofemoral bypass grafting and iliac balloon angioplasty and stenting for bilateral iliac disease. *J Vasc Surg*. 2001;33:S93-S99.
15. Ricco JB, Probst H, French University Surgeons Association. Long-term results of a multi-center randomized study on direct versus crossover bypass for unilateral iliac artery occlusive disease. *J Vasc Surg*. 2008;47:45-53.
16. Porter JM, Eidemiller LR, Dotter CT, Rosch J. Vetto RM. Combined arterial dilatation and femorofemoral bypass for limb salvage. *Surg Gynecol Obstet*. 1973;137:409-412.
17. Walker PJ, Harris JP. May J. Combined percutaneous transluminal angioplasty and extra-anatomic bypass for symptomatic unilateral iliac occlusion with contralateral iliac artery stenosis. *Ann Vasc Surg*. 1991;5:209-217.
18. Shah RM, Peer RM, Upson JF, Ricotta JJ. Donor iliac angioplasty and crossover femorofemoral bypass. *Am J Surg*. 1992;164:295-298.
19. Perler BA, Williams GM. Does donor iliac artery percutaneous transluminal angioplasty or stent placement influence the results of femorofemoral bypass. Analysis of 70 consecutive cases with long-term follow-up. *J Vasc Surg*. 1996;24:363-370.
20. Schneider JR, Besso SR, Walsh DB, Zwolack RM, Cronenwett JL. Femorofemoral versus aortofemoral bypass. Outcome and hemodynamic results. *J Vasc Surg*. 1994;19:43-57.
21. Criado E, Burnham SJ, Tinsley EA, Johnson G, Keagy BA. Femorofemoral bypass graft: analysis of patency and factors influencing long-term outcome. *J Vasc Surg*. 1993;18:495-505.
22. Brewster DC, Cambria RF, Darling RC, et al. Long-term results of combined iliac balloon angioplasty and distal surgical revascularization. *Ann Surg*. 1989;210:324-331.
23. Marin ML, Veith FJ, Sanchez LA, et al. Endovascular aortoiliac grafts in combination with standard infrainguinal arterial bypasses in the management of limb-threatening ischemia. *J Vasc Surg*. 1995;22:316-325.
24. Cynamon J, Marin ML, Veith FJ, et al. Stent-graft repair of aortoiliac occlusive disease coexisting with common femoral artery disease. *J Vasc Interv Radiol*. 1997;8:19-26.
25. Heart Protection Study Collaborative Group. Randomised trial of the effects of cholesterol-lowering with simvastatin on peripheral vascular and other major vascular outcomes in 20, 536 people with peripheral arterial disease and other high-risk conditions. *J Vasc Surg*. 2007;45:645-654.

Endovascular Management of Lower Limb Claudication due to Infra-Inguinal Disease

19

Daniel J. Reddy and Mitchell R. Weaver

An unemployed 56 year old man presents with several months duration of worsening left calf pain upon ambulation. After less than ½ block he must cease walking owing to the calf and foot pain which is relieved by rest. Occasionally he has nocturnal rest pain affecting his left foot. The patient must rely on walking for transportation and the activities of daily life. Past medical history is significant for 45 pack-years of tobacco cigarette smoking, bronchitis, hypertension, hyperlipidemia, previous poly-substance abuse and extensive varicose veins of both lower extremities. Serology is positive for syphilis and hepatitis C.

Physical exam: both femoral pulses are palpable as is the right popliteal pulse. The left popliteal and both dorsalis pedis and posterior tibial pulses are absent to palpation. The envelope of skin is intact and there is normal motor and sensory function of both lower extremities. Pertinent medications include clopidogrel, amlodipine and hydrochlorothiazide. The referring physician has initiated narcotic pain medicines for the rest pain. The serum creatinine is normal.

Question 1

Which of the following would be the optimal management plan?

A. Primary amputation of the left leg to control the rest pain and avoid relapse into narcotic addiction
B. Risk factor modification, lower extremity non-invasive arterial studies and plans for angiography
C. Smoking cessation clinic referral and follow up in 4–6 months
D. Initiate supervised exercise program and return in 6 months
E. A 6 week trial of pentoxifylline or cilostazol

D.J. Reddy (✉)
Department of Surgery, Wayne State University, Detroit, MI, USA

G. Geroulakos and B. Sumpio (eds.), *Vascular Surgery*,
DOI: 10.1007/978-1-84996-356-5_19, © Springer-Verlag London Limited 2011

The patient agrees to attend the smoking cessation clinic and will go to see the exercise therapist as well. You have applied for approval to prescribe pentoxifylline. Moreover, you have counseled the patient about the seriousness of his condition and the threat it poses to the viability of his left leg. After segmental arterial pressure studies are obtained, you discuss the pros and cons of diagnostic and possible interventional angiography and recommended it to him. He gives his informed consent.

Question 2

What do these lower extremities non-invasive segmental arterial studies demonstrate? (Fig . 19.1)

A. Moderate occlusive disease on the right and much more severe disease on the left
B. Normal study
C. Mild to moderate occlusive arterial disease on the left
D. Normal waveforms on the right and slight dampening of the waveforms on the left
E. Incompressibility consistent with diabetes mellitus and, therefore, not diagnostic

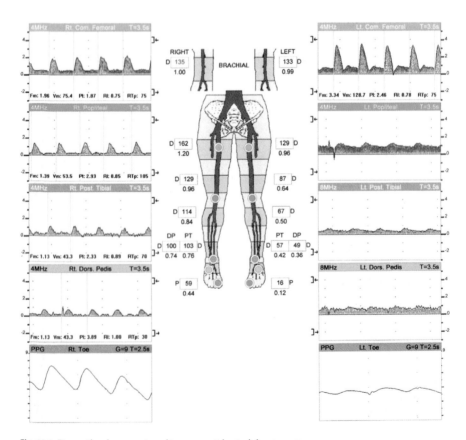

Fig. 19.1 Presenting lower extremity segmental arterial pressures

Question 3

Given the available information: history, pulse deficit pattern on physical exam and the non-invasive report what approach do you plan for the aortogram and runoff which you plan to perform in the interventional suite (hybrid OR suite unavailable)?

A. Percutaneous retrograde right femoral
B. Left transaxillary
C. Percutaneous retrograde left femoral
D. Translumbar
E. Right transaxillary

You proceed with ultrasound localization and micropunture (0.018) technique for percutaneous retrograde right common femoral puncture and, using Seldinger technique, experience no difficulty upsizing to a 5 F introducer sheath but do experience difficulty passing the 0.035 starter J wire into the aorta. You stop and inject contrast through the flush port of the 5F introducer sheath and obtain images. What does this image demonstrate? (Fig. 19.2)

Question 4

A. Perforation of the right common iliac artery and need for immediate transportation to the operating room for hemostasis
B. Normal appearing aorto-iliac system and the need to push harder on the wire
C. Extensive irregularities of the artery walls but no other significant findings

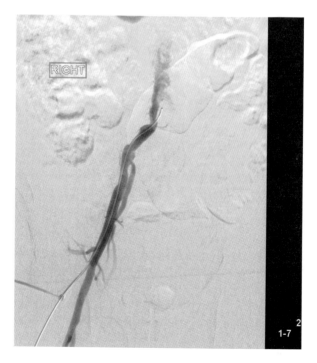

Fig. 19.2 Right iliac arteriogram

D. Dissection plane in the diseased artery wall at the distal aorta and common iliac with intravasation of contrast without perforation

E. Normal appearing aorto-iliac system but a minor dissection of no consequence

You are able to pass a hydrophilic guide wire into the aorta and obtain an aortogram which demonstrates extensive atherosclerotic plaque. Magnified views of the common iliac artery are included. You successfully deploy a self expanding bare metal stent spanning the area of artery narrowing and origin of the dissection plan. After touch up an angioplasty balloon catheter, what is your next step? (Figs. 19.3 and 19.4)

Question 5

A. Reposition the flush catheter just above the aortic bifurcation for injection and in order to obtain the planned runoff images of the femoral popliteal and infrapopliteal segments

B. Stop the procedure at this point, the patient has had enough

C. Stop the procedure at this point the surgeon has had enough

D. Go to the operating room. Only a femoral popliteal bypass is possible. The non-invasive study was enough information

E. Reconsider primary amputation

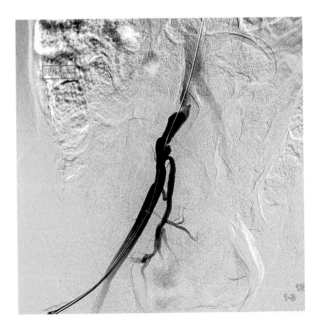

Fig. 19.3 Subsequent right iliac arteriogram

Fig. 19.4 Distal aorta and right iliac arteriogram

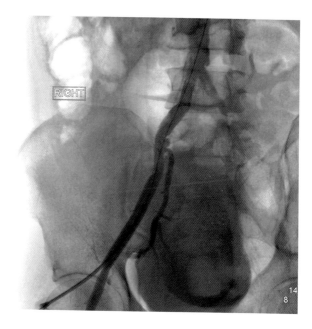

Question 6

You obtain the runoff images. What is demonstrated in these images? (Figs. 19.5 and 19.6)

A. There is a long segment occlusion of the left superficial femoral artery
B. The demonstrated occlusion is chronic

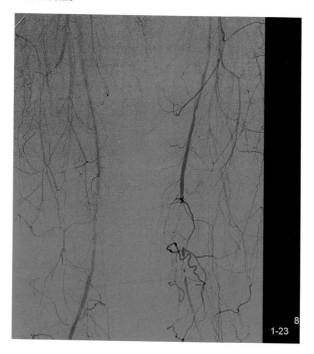

Fig. 19.5 Bilateral femoral arteriogram

Fig. 19.6 Bilateral popliteal arteriogram

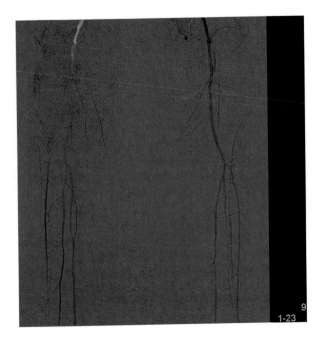

C. The deep femoral artery is open and provides collaterals which reconstitute the distal superficial femoral artery proximal to the popliteal artery
D. The proximal infrapopliteal arterial segments are open
E. All of the above (A, B, C, and D)
F. None of the above

You decide to proceed with endovascular reconstruction of the left superficial femoral artery. The following week you schedule this procedure in the operating room in the event circumstances prompt you to proceed with (open) bypass operation for limb salvage. In order to avoid crossing over the narrow and diseased aortic bifurcation from the right side you elect a (left) ipsilateral antegrade approach.

Question 7

What problem have you now encountered demonstrated in this image? (Fig. 19.7)

A. The proximal superficial femoral artery is now occluded
B. Your wire has passed into the deep femoral artery
C. The superficial femoral artery can be selected but the sheath needs to be pulled back into the common femoral artery first
D. The need for a stiffer wire to forcefully cross the occluded vessel
E. Both B and C

You manage to pass a wire into the superficial femoral artery above the occlusion as demonstrated in this image (Fig. 19.8).

Fig. 19.7 Left popliteal arteriogram

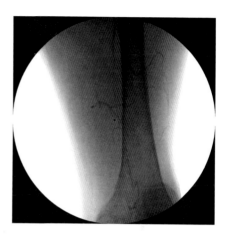

Question 8

What's your next move?

A. Call for a laser which is the only device that can cross a lesion of this length
B. Initiate long term catheter directed thrombolytic therapy and transfer to the Surgical Intensive Care Unit (SICU)
C. Using a soft tip wire, with back up stiffness, gently pass the wire through the chronic occlusion
D. Mechanical thrombolysis with a jet spray of tissue plasminogen activator
E. Mechanical thrombectomy with a rotating tip device

The wire passes and is securely "parked" in the infrapopliteal segment. There appears to be a small amount of extravasation of contrast originating from the occluded segment that was crossed (Fig. 19.9).

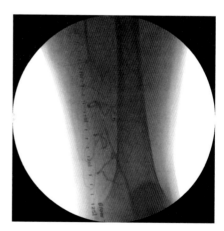

Fig. 19.8 Left distal femoral artery arteriogram

Fig. 19.9 Left distal femoral artery arteriogram

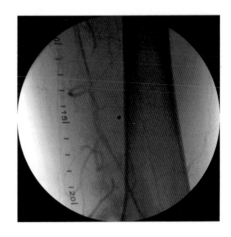

Question 9

What is your next move?

A. Immediately convert to open operation because of the extravasation
B. Deploy a bare metal stent across the occluded segment and balloon angioplasty it
C. Deploy a covered stent across the occluded segment and balloon angioplasty it
D. Use coil embolization to control the bleeding that might occur later that night
E. B or C

You successfully deploy a covered stent across the lesion and follow up with balloon angioplasty and completion images (Figs. 19.10–19.12). A pulse is now palpable behind the knee and there is a faintly palpated pulse in the foot and excellent Doppler derived arterial signal.

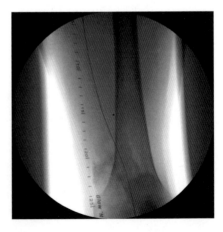

Fig. 19.10 Left femoral arteriogram

Fig. 19.11 Distal left femoral arteriogram

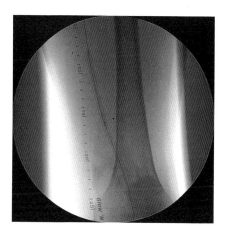

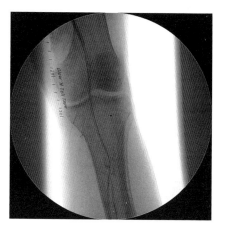

Fig. 19.12 Left popliteal arteriogram

Question 10

What do these post reconstruction lower extremities non-invasive segmental arterial studies, obtained a week later, demonstrate? (Fig. 19.13)

A. No improvement from preoperative study (Fig. 19.1)
B. Improved waveforms and ankle brachial index on the right
C. Improved waveforms and ankle brachial index on the left
D. Improved waveform and systolic pressure in the left hallux
E. B and C
F. B, C and D

After five months of satisfactory status, the patient became non-compliant with his daily clopidogrel 75 mg regime and abruptly stopped taking this antiplatelet inhibitor against medical advice. Five days later he developed rest pain his left foot and again sought medical attention. The following non-invasive testing (Fig. 19.14) and left lower extremity arteriogram images were obtained (Figs. 19.15 and 19.16).

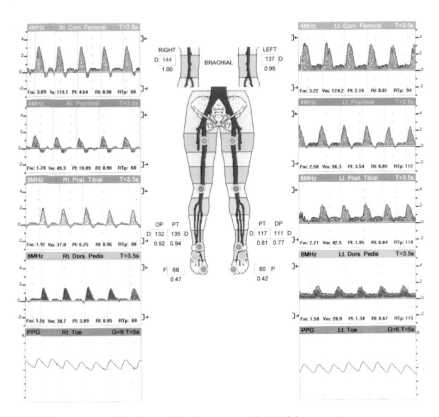

Fig. 19.13 Post reconstruction lower extremity segemental arteruial pressures

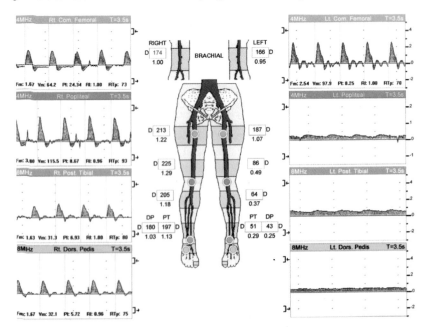

Fig. 19.14 Lower extremity segmental arterial presures when patient returned acutely symptomatic

Fig. 19.15 Subtracted left femoral arteriogram (AP) at the level of the mid and distal thigh

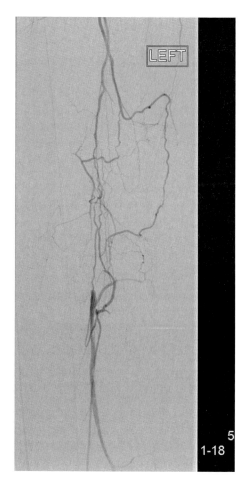

Question 11

What is your impression?

A. No change in his arterial status. The patient is exhibiting "drug-seeking" behavior
B. The superficial femoral artery stent graft is now occluded
C. There is debris in the tibial peroneal arterial trunk which may represent emboli
D. Normal non-invasive test result
E. Both B and C are correct

It is determined that open femoral to popliteal bypass graft is required for limb salvage. An exhaustive search in both upper and lower extremities does not reveal suitable autogenous vein for reconstructive arterial operation. You proceed with femoral to popliteal bypass graft employing synthetic arterial substitute as an alternative to major amputation of the limb and obtain an on-table completion angiogram (Fig. 19.17).

Fig. 19.16 Subtracted left popliteal arteriogram (AP magnified) at the level of the knee

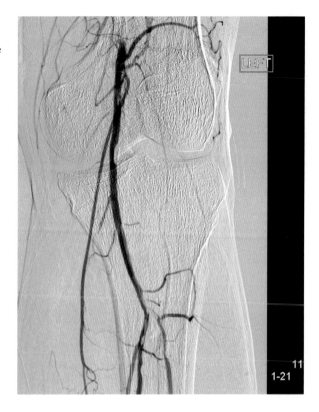

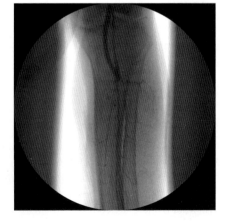

Fig. 19.17 On table completion arteriogram following arterial reconstruction by synthetic bypass grafting (AP) at the level of the left knee and leg

Question 12

Which statement is true about selection of graft material for femoral popliteal bypass for limb salvage?

A. Autogenous tissue is the preferred conduit
B. Composite autogenous tissue such as spliced together segments of cephalic vein is preferred over synthetic conduit
C. Vascular Surgeons should be very reluctant to employ synthetic prosthesis for femoral popliteal bypass and search diligently for autogenous conduits
D. Patients always prefer amputation over synthetic conduit
E. Surgeon self-esteem is more important than limb salvage for the patient
F. A, B and C are all correct

19.1
Commentary

The patient in this clinical scenario has multiple risk factors for atherosclerosis and co-morbidities complicating his clinical presentation. Identification of risk factors and steps to modify them are to the patient's benefit as is a program of supervised exercise. Nonetheless, this presentation warrants action beyond these measures as this patient will be at risk for limb loss in the near future when this condition progresses to tissue loss or even gangrene as is likely. Angiography is advised to plan intervention to avoid the natural history of this condition were it allowed to progress unchecked.[1,2] **[Q1: B]**

The segmental arterial pressure and waveform studies are consistent with the history and physical exam. They demonstrate alterations in the waveforms and pressure on both sides in multiple arterial segments both above and below the inguinal ligament. The problem is demonstrably worse on the left (indexes at the ankle of 0.42 and 0.36) than it is on the right (indexes of 0.74 and 0.76). Incompressible arteries such as seen in diabetes mellitus patients would have erroneous pressure in the 300 mmHg or greater.[1,3] **[Q2: A]**

Percutaneous transaxillary approaches have many useful applications. It is associated with a higher incidence of complications and manipulation for interventional work would only increase the risks.[4-6] There is no need to employ a transaxillary approach when both femoral pulses are palpable. The translumbar approach for angiography has a noble history and is still employed on occasion. There would be no opportunity for interventional work were it the selected approach and is not necessary with both femoral pulses present. Approaching from the right side has the potential benefit of allowing "up and over" crossing of the aortic bifurcation and potential antegrade balloon angioplasty or stenting for the symptomatic, left, side. **[Q3: A]**

Even with ultrasound localization and micropunture techniques to avoid puncture site complications, passage of wires in diseased arteries is not without hazards. Hydrophilic wires pass more easily but can undermine, dissect or even perforated atherosclerotic plaques. In this case a safer "J" wire dissected a plane in this very diseased vessel. The important maneuver when passage is difficult is to stop and obtain images and assess the situation thereby avoiding any substantial complications. **[Q4: D]**

With satisfactory appearance of the stented plaque that had been dissected there is no need to abandon the planned procedure. The pertinent diagnostic information is still lacking. Although a diagnostic angiogram can easily be obtained in the operating room and a decision is possible you already have a catheter positioned for necessary images and proceed. Transfer to the operating room for bypass or amputation is not needed or appropriate. **[Q5: A]**

The lesion demonstrated is a relatively long (several centimeters) chronic occlusion of the left superficial femoral artery. The occlusion is chronic because the collaterals are numerous, well developed and tortuous. It takes time for the muscular arteries to resound to the occlusion and manifest these characteristics. The distal superficial femoral is reconstituted by these collaterals originating from the deep femoral and the popliteal artery in turn patent as are the proximal infrapopliteal runoff arteries. **[Q6: E]**

The antegrade ipsilateral puncture of the common femoral artery is possible and it avoids the challenge in this patient of crossing a very diseased distal aorta that is configured in a narrow angle. One of the hazards is inadvertent passage of the guide wire into the deep femoral artery (demonstrated in this image, Fig. 19.6). The operator repositions the guide wire in to the superficial femoral artery and advances the introducer sheath over this wire. **[Q7: C]**

When a wire is successfully across a chronic total occlusion but is safely intra luminal beyond the lesion there are many options. Often times, traversing these lesions through the native lumen is not possible, but these lesions are able to be crossed through the subintimal plane, re-entering the true lumen in the distal target artery. The standard subintimal wire technique is most common, however if the distal target artery cannot readily be re-entered there are commercially available devices such as the Outback LTD Re-Entry Catheter (Cordis) that may be used to re-enter the true lumen. Once a wire is passed the lesion and in the true lumen many endovascular treatment techniques are available. Percutaneous subintimal angioplasty with selective stenting has been shown to be technically feasible and safe with satisfactory limb salvage rates. Long term durability is still a weakness of this therapy, but the durability of subintimal angioplasty is often reported better than that for prosthetic graft bypass.[7–9] Many argue that laser is not the best choice nor is atherectomy although this is debated.[10–12] In any case the rotating tip devices are for atherctomy, not thrombectomy. Mechanical thrombolysis would be ineffective were it attempted for chronic lesions that have organized and are the result of atherosclerotic plaques. Passing the wire is your and the patient's best bet. **[Q8: C]**

Minor extravasation is not worrisome as long as it is clearly demonstrated that the wire is in the distal arterial segment. There is no need to convert to an open operation at this time and no place or need for embolization. Vascular Surgeons debate bare metal stenting versus covered stents. In this case with the extravasation we would argue for a covered stent. Recent results appear to favor covered stenting from a longer term patency rate.[13–15] **[Q9: C]**

Objective follow up is a hallowed tradition and a necessary feature in vascular surgery. Non-invasive testing, particularly when there has been a pre-treatment study available for comparison, is convenient and cost effective.[1,2,16] This study, when compared with the pre treatment study demonstrates improved waveform and pressure indexes on the right (secondary to the bare metal stent placed in the right iliac). The pressure indexes and waveform on the left are greatly improved as are the hallux pressures and waveforms (secondary to the covered stent reconstruction of the left superficial femoral artery). **[Q10: F]**

Although clopidogrel can be an expensive medicine it is considered to be of patient benefit following stent grafting in the infrainguinal arterial segment following long segment subintimal arterial reconstruction. This patient's symptoms and non-invasive testing results are distinctly abnormal. The new lab test reveals limb arterial flow that has deteriorated from the initial post reconstruction study, obtained 5 months earlier to establish a surveillance baseline (Figs. 19.13 and 19.14). Ischemia to this degree of severity is frequently associated with rest pain. Matters seem to have been made worse by the obvious debris in the tibial peroneal trunk and origin of the anterior tibial artery (Fig. 19.16) not seen in the previous images (Figs. 19.6 and 19.12). It is likely that this represent a recent embolus from the more proximal segment that is now occluded (Fig. 19.15). **[Q11: E]**

There is no controversy that autogenous conduit is preferred for arterial reconstruction bypass operation, particularly when the target for the distal anastomosis is below the knee.[17,18] However, the authors believe that there are a few circumstances when vein depletion (for example from: multiple vein harvests for coronary artery bypass grafts, long standing chronic hemodialysis, extensive prior vein phlebectomies, long standing intravenous drug abuse, previous amputations, post phlebitis leg syndrome or congenital vascular anomalies) may make autogenous conduit use either impractical or impossible. A Utopian mindset on the part of an actual operating Vascular Surgeon seldom if ever serves the patient well. **[Q12: F]**

References

1. Norgren, et al. Inter-society consensus for the management of peripheral arterial disease (TASC II). *J Vasc Surg.* 2007;451S.
2. Hirsch At, Haskal ZJ, Hertzer NR, et al. Guidelines for the management of patients with peripheral arterial disease. *J AM Coll Cardiol.* 2006;47:1239-1312.
3. Brooks B, Dean R, Patel S, Wu B, Moyneaux L, Yue DK. TBI or not TBI: that is the question. Is it better to measure toe pressure than ankle pressure in diabetic patients? *Diabet Med.* 2001;18:528-532.
4. Grollman JH, Marcus R. Transbrachial arteriography: techniques and complications. *Cardiovasc Intervent Radiol.* 1988;11:32-35.
5. Watkinson AF, Hartnell GG. Complications of direct brachial artery puncture for arteriography: a comparison of techniques. *Clin Radiol.* 1991;44:189-191.
6. Heenan SD, Grubnic S, Buckenham TM, Belli AM. Transbrachial arteriography: indiations and complications. *Clin Radiol.* 1996;51:205-209.
7. Schmieder G, Richardson A, Scott E, Stokes G, Meier G, Panneton J. Selective stenting in subintimal angioplasty: analysis of primary stent outcomes. *J Vasc Surg.* 2008;48:1175-1181.

8. Treiman G, Treiman R, Whiting J. Results of percutaneous subintimal angioplasty using routine stenting. *J Vasc Surg*. 2006;43:513-519.
9. Scott E, Biuckians A, Light R, Burgess J, Meier G, Panneton J. Subintimal angioplasty: our experience in the treatment of 506 infrainguinal arterial occlusions. *J Vasc Surg*. 2008;48:878-884.
10. Sarac T, Altinel O, Bannazadeh M, Kashyap V, Lyden S, Clair D. MidTerm outcome predictors for lower extremity procedures. *J Vasc Surg*. 2008;48:885-890.
11. Chung SW, Sharafuddin MJ, Chigurupati R. Midterm patency following atherectomy for infrainguinal occlusive disease: a word of caution. *J Vasc Surg*. 2008;48:1634.
12. McCarthy WJ, Vogelzang RL, Nemcek AA, et al. Excimer-laser-assisted femoral angioplasty:Early results. *J Vasc Surg*. 1991;13:607-614.
13. Dearing D, Patel K, Compoginis J, Kamel M, Weaver F, Katz S. Primary stenting of the superficial femoral and popliteal artery. *J Vasc Surg*. 2009;3:542-547.
14. Surowiec SM, Davies MG, Eberly SW, et al. Percutaneous angioplasty and stenting of the superficial femoral artery. *J Vasc Surg*. 2005;2:269-278.
15. Dosluoglu HH, Cherr GS, Lall P, Harris L, Dryjski M. Stenting vs above knee olytetrafluoroethylene bypass for TransAlantic Inter-Society Consensus-II C and D superficial femoral artery disease. *J Vasc Surg*. 2008;5:1166-1174.
16. Ahn SS, Rutherford RB, Becker GJ, et al. Reporting standards for lower extremity arterial endovascular procedures. *J Vasc Surg*. 1993;17:1103.
17. Mills JL. P values may lack power: the choice of conduit for above-knee femoropopliteal bypass graft. *J Vasc Surg*. 2000;32:402-405.
18. Veith FJ, Gupta SK, Ascher E, White-Flores S, et al. Six-year prospective multicenter randomized comparison of autologous saphenous vein and expanded polytetrafluoroethylene grafts in infrainguinal arterial reconstructions. *J Vasc Surg*. 1986;3:104-114.

Endovascular Management of Non-Healing Leg Ulceration

Jean Starr and Patrick Vaccaro

A 72 year old non-smoking female with a past medical history of hypertension, well-controlled diabetes, and stable coronary artery disease, status post CABG with bilateral great saphenous vein harvests, presents to her podiatrist. She developed an ulcer over the right first metatarsal head after wearing a new pair of shoes approximately 4 months ago. The wound is gradually getting larger, despite appropriate local wound care and off-loading procedures. She is referred to you for evaluation for arterial insufficiency.

Physical examination reveals normal and equal bilateral femoral pulses with no palpable distal pulses. There are well-healed, bilateral medial thigh incisions. The toes are pink with brisk capillary refill. There is diminished sensation to fine touch bilaterally, but normal motor function is noted. The ulcer base is pale with fibrinous debris. There is no foul odor or obvious cellulitis.

Question 1

The best first step in her evaluation and/or management is:

A. Operative debridement to eliminate necrotic tissue and bone and initiation of oral antibiotics, based on culture results.
B. Lower extremity arterial Dopplers with waveforms.
C. MRA of the lower extremities.
D. Angiography with possible intervention.
E. Start Cilostazol and a walking program.

The ankle-brachial indices are greater than one and a digital brachial index is 0.6 bilaterally. Upper thigh waveforms are multiphasic; popliteal and pedal waveforms are monophasic. Exercise testing was not performed due to her inability to walk on a treadmill.

J. Starr (✉)
Division of Vascular Diseases and Surgery, The Ohio State University, Columbus, OH, USA

G. Geroulakos and B. Sumpio (eds.), *Vascular Surgery*,
DOI: 10.1007/978-1-84996-356-5_20, © Springer-Verlag London Limited 2011

Question 2

Which of the following is true?

A. ABIs correlate well with long-term survival in PAD patients.
B. DBIs are an unreliable measure of PAD in diabetic patients due to small vessel calcification.
C. A direct popliteal artery pressure measurement of greater than 50 mmHg helps to predict a positive outcome after angioplasty.
D. A pulsus tardus waveform on a lower extremity arterial duplex examination correlates with adequate arterial perfusion.

An aortogram with runoff was performed via the left femoral artery and showed a normal aortoiliac segment with a 20 cm left superficial femoral artery (SFA) occlusion and diffuse tibial stenoses with contiguous flow into the foot. The right superficial femoral artery showed three areas of focal stenosis with the proximal and mid lesions measuring 1 cm and the distal measuring 2 cm in length (Fig. 20.1). The most distal lesion ended proximal to the adductor canal. The popliteal artery had no significant stenosis. The right posterior tibial and peroneal arteries were totally occluded and did not provide any collateral flow into the foot (Fig. 20.2). The anterior tibial artery had several areas of distal stenoses, all proximal to the ankle. The most severe was just above the ankle joint (Fig. 20.3). There was no complete pedal arch, but abundant collateral flow in the foot was present.

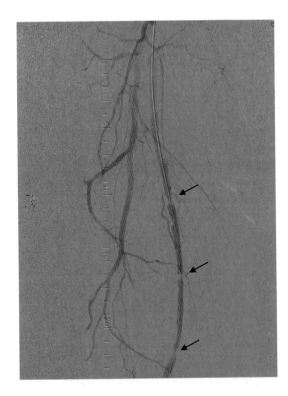

Fig. 20.1 Right SFA tandem stenoses

Fig. 20.2 Distal popliteal and
proximal tibial anatomy

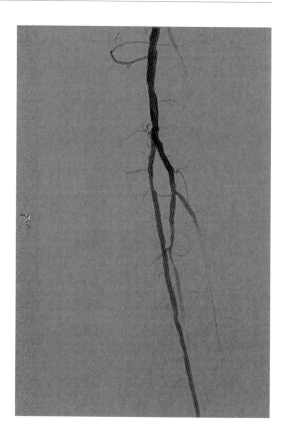

Question 3

The TASC (Trans-Atlantic Societal Classification) category of the superficial femoral
artery segment is best identified as:

A. TASC A
B. TASC B
C. TASC C
D. TASC D
E. TASC E

Question 4

The best treatment option for this patient is:

A. Medical management with Cilostazol, Clopidigrel, and referral to a wound care center.
B. Percutaneous revascularization of the femoral artery lesions, with distal synthetic
   popliteal to anterior tibial bypass at the ankle.

Fig. 20.3 Distal anterior tibial
stenoses

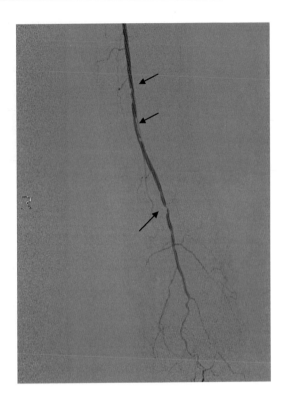

C. Percutaneous revascularization of the femoral and anterior tibial arteries.
D. Right femoral to anterior tibial composite bypass graft.

Discussion with the patient occurred pre-procedurally in the office setting. She was offered concomitant intervention if deemed appropriate at the time and informed consent was obtained. The patient was given appropriate sedation and anticoagulated with heparin. The diagnostic 5Fr sheath was exchanged for a 6Fr RDC angled guiding sheath. Cannulation of the contralateral common iliac was performed with the aid of a SOS catheter and 0.035 stiff hydrophilic guidewire under constant fluoroscopic guidance. The sheath was advanced to the right external iliac artery. Roadmap techniques and small amounts of contrast were used to cross the SFA lesions. An angled, hydrophilic coated 5Fr catheter was employed to assist in crossing the stenoses. The tip of the guidewire was placed in the distal popliteal artery. A 5 mm x 4 cm cryoplasty balloon was inflated at each diseased area with an adequate angiographic appearance and no evidence of dissection or other complication (Fig. 20.4).

Next, the 0.035 guidewire was exchanged for a 0.014 exchange length guidewire and the lesions in the anterior tibial artery were crossed. The stenoses were treated with a 2.5 mm × 5 cm balloon with good results and no complications (Fig. 20.5). The sheath was partially withdrawn and the left femoral artery was imaged. The access site was felt to be adequate for an arterial closure device which was placed without complication. The heparin was not reversed.

Following treatment, her post procedure anterior tibial ankle waveform was multiphasic. Her ulcer improved with a reduction in diameter, however the first metatarsal head was exposed. The patient underwent right first toe transmetatarsal amputation 2 weeks later

Fig. 20.4 Result after SFA cryoplasty with improvement in all three stenoses

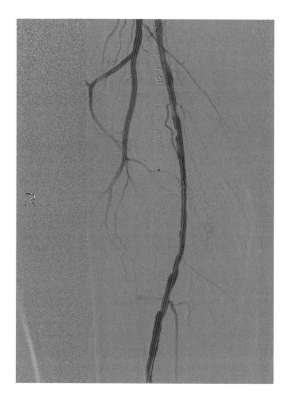

which healed nicely. Six months later, routine lower extremity arterial non-invasive testing showed a flat right ankle PVR. The patient denied new ulceration or rest pain.

Question 5

The patient should be offered:

A. Repeat angiogram and intervention if anatomically appropriate.
B. Operative revascularization.
C. Medical management with warfarin therapy and risk factor modification.
D. Risk factor modification and protective orthotics.

20.1
Commentary

Critical limb ischemia may include ischemic rest pain, non-healing ulcers, or gangrene, all of which may lead to limb loss if left untreated, and at the very least cause significant lifestyle changes. Initial evaluation should include lower extremity arterial dopplers with

Fig. 20.5 Results after PTA of distal anterior tibial artery

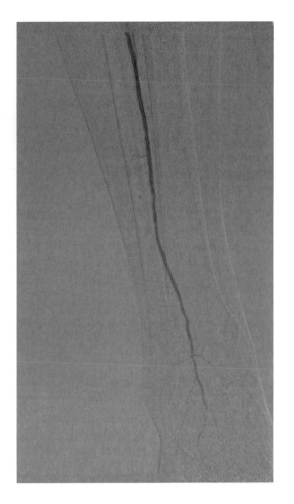

waveforms which serve to give an idea of disease distribution and severity. Testing is non-invasive, inexpensive, and widely available. Non-invasive vascular testing, especially duplex imaging, may help to rule out more proximal occlusive disease, and allow less contrast to be used during angiography and interventional procedures.[1] Adding arterial duplex imaging may also help plan an interventional procedure by identifying target lesions. Additionally, a baseline ankle-brachial index (ABI) or waveform may be utilized to assess the adequacy of an intervention and is one means of following a patient's vascular status over time, especially if there is a worsening in the clinical situation. **[Q1: B]**

Although magnetic resonance (MR) angiography may help delineate extent and location of disease, a pre-planned intervention obviously cannot be performed simultaneously. There are additional risks to patients with chronic kidney disease, related to Gadolinium administration. The most severe involves nephrogenic systemic fibrosis which is characterized by thickening and tightening of the skin and subcutaneous tissues and can involve the skeletal muscle, lung, liver, testes, or myocardium. The outcome can be fatal.[2] Adequate

MR vascular imaging equipment and software are not uniform, nor widely available. Interpretation, especially with total occlusions, may be subjective as well. Advantages may include the avoidance of an iodinated contrast study if an intervention is not feasible or indicated. Exposure to a radiation source is also avoided. The local complications of a percutaneous procedure, including pseudoaneurysm formation, hematoma, arterial occlusion, and bleeding, are averted.

Computed tomographic angiography (CTA) is sometimes used as a minimally invasive diagnostic tool for the evaluation of vascular disease. Drawbacks include the inability to perform a concomitant intervention, as with MRA, the need for iodinated contrast with the known inherent risks, and the use of radiation. CTA has the additional disadvantage of difficulty imaging accurately in the presence of heavily calcified lesions.[3]

ABI's have also been suggested for patients free from clinical signs and symptoms of vascular disease with other risk factors. They have been shown to correlate with long term survival. An ABI of<0.9 has been shown to have double the 10 year overall mortality, cardiovascular mortality, and major coronary event rate.[4] Digital-brachial waveforms may be more reliable than ABI's in patients with large vessel calcifications, such as is commonly found in diabetics.[5] Digital vessels are often spared calcification and therefore are compressible and allow non-invasive pressure measurements. Direct popliteal pressures may help predict the healing potential in patients undergoing below the knee amputation.[6] A pulsus tardus waveform indicates a more proximal obstruction and may arise due to a post-stenotic pressure drop or changes in post-stenotic vessel compliance. It is used most commonly for evaluation of renal artery stenosis.[7] [Q2: A]

The initial TASC recommendations, originally published in 2000,[8] were more recently revised in 2007 by representatives from 16 different societies and all concerned specialties.[9] In both TASC publications, anatomic criteria are grouped into four classifications as an effort to give clinical management guidelines based on severity of disease. Since the 2000 inception, more evidence has emerged in support of endovascular therapies and this has been incorporated into the latest recommendations. The level of available evidence reviewed (level A, B, or C) was also analyzed by content experts and applied. The 2007 femoral artery criteria are listed in Fig. 20.6. Recommendations for intervention are described in Table 20.1. There are separate categories for iliac artery atherosclerotic disease. No recommendations for tibial occlusive disease are currently available. This patient's SFA lesions are best categorized as TASC class B and an endovascular approach is recommended as the first line of treatment. There is no TASC class E category in any anatomic distribution. [Q3: B]

This patient's critical limb threatening ischemia warrants timely intervention in order to prevent further tissue and potential limb loss. Restoration of direct flow to the area of ischemia is ideal and may provide better healing rates.[10] She has limited autogenous vein available, with potentially short segments of great saphenous vein below the knee, small saphenous vein, and cephalic vein. Consideration should be given to obtaining non-invasive mapping of these venous segments. Distal tibial and pedal revascularization with prosthetic or composite grafts has poorer long term patency than autogenous bypasses, but there has been no direct comparison to endovascular intervention, solely for the infrapopliteal vascular bed. There is evidence that infrainguinal angioplasty may be a better first alternative for patients who are anatomically suitable and have a life expectancy less than 2 years, especially when autogenous vein is unavailable.[11] There may be a high restenosis

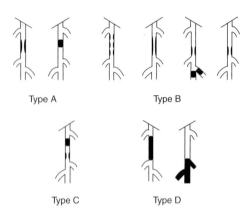

Fig. 20.6 TASC II infrainguinal classification

Lesion type	Description
A	Single stenosis ≤10 cm in length *Single occlusion ≤5 cm in length*
B	Multiple lesions (stenoses or occlusions), each ≤5 cm *Single stenosis or occlusion ≤15 cm not involving the infrageniculate popliteal artery* Single or multiple lesions in the absence of continous tibial vessels to improve inflow for a distal bypass *Heavily calcified occlusion ≤15 cm in length* Single popliteal stenosis
C	Multiple stenoses or occlusions totaling >15 cm with or without heavy calcification *Recurrent stenoses or occlusions that need treatment after two endovascular interventions*
D	Chronic total occlusions of CFA or SFA (>20 cm, involving the popliteal artery) *Chronic total occlusion of popliteal artery and proximal trifurcation vessels*

Table 20.1 Preferred options for treating femoropopliteal lesions

Type of lesion	Treatment recommendations
TASC A	Endovascular therapy is the treatment of choice
TASC B	Endovascular therapy is the preferred treatment
TASC C	Surgery is preferred for good risk patients
TASC D	Surgery is the treatment of choice

rate, but there is acceptable limb salvage rate in patients with limb threatening ischemia.[12,13] This patient has limited autogenous vein and an appropriate primary intervention is percutaneous revascularization. Options include balloon angioplasty, cryoplasty, stenting, and atherectomy, in addition to other techniques. **[Q4: C]**

Consensus does not exist regarding the type of endovascular management for atherosclerotic infrainguinal disease. Balloon angioplasty was the first modality introduced and is still advocated by some for short segment, uncomplicated lesions. Nitinol stenting has recently shown superiority over simple balloon angioplasty but debate continues.[14] Covered stent placement has also gained in popularity with improved outcomes.[15] Unfortunately, stent fractures with diminished patency rates have limited universal adaptation of these practices. Forces on the SFA at the adductor canal, including compression, expansion, torsion, and flexion, adversely impact metallic devices. Mechanical limitations of current stent designs have led to new, longer stent designs which may increase long term patency rates. Development of better drug eluting stent and balloon technology may also help to improve outcomes.

Restenosis of stented arterial beds creates a future problem regarding management of in-stent restenosis when it occurs. Plain and cutting balloon angioplasty, cryoplasty, and drug-eluting balloon technology may offer future solutions but currently only anecdotal data exist.[16] Research with bioabsorbable stent technology may lead to the elimination of long-term mechanical stent problems and may be a vector for drug delivery directly to diseased segments.[17]

Other areas of concern for infrainguinal interventions include the common femoral and popliteal arteries which lie at flexion points and the SFA origin where the major branch vessel, the profunda femoris, offers a significant source of collateral flow in cases of limb threatening ischemia. Laser, directional, and rotational atherectomy techniques have been devised as the primary procedure or for debulking diseased segments so that ballooning may be performed with fewer complications. Atherectomy may be a good adjunct in these problem areas and even in highly calcified segments where ballooning and stenting may not be feasible.

Patient treatment and management should not end at the completion of the interventional procedure. Risk factor modification, including diabetic and hypertensive control, statin therapy, smoking cessation, and addition of anti-platelet medication should be individualized for each patient. Personalized health care will continue to become an important aspect of vascular patient care, combining individual genomic information and clinical data with available health information technologies. More aggressive and earlier risk reduction may avert many of the late complications of vascular disease. Health care agencies have clearly begun to recognize the importance of individualized care.[18]

Optimal wound treatment should be instituted and healing status closely monitored. Patients should be educated about signs of deteriorating vascular status, including recurrent claudication or rest pain and development of new ulcerations. Non-invasive vascular testing may be a helpful addition to physical examination if there is a clinical change. Less circulation is needed to maintain intact skin, so once a wound heals, a decrease in arterial inflow may not necessarily require restoration. This patient is appropriately managed by close follow up, risk factor management, counseling, and protective orthotics. **[Q5: D]**

References

1. Hingorani A, Ascher E, Marks N. Preprocedural imaging: new options to reduce need for contrast angiography. *Semin Vasc Surg*. 2007 Mar;20(1):15-28.
2. Deo A, Fogel M, Cowper SE. Nephrogenic systemic fibrosis: a population study examining the relationship of disease development to gadolinium exposure. *Clin J Am Soc Nephrol*. 2007;2:264-267.

3. Ouwendijk R, Kock MC, van Dijk LC, et al. Vessel wall calcifications at multi-detector row CT angiography in patients with peripheral arterial disease: effect on clinical utility and clinical predictors. *Radiology*. 2006 Nov;241(2):603-608.
4. Fowkes FG, Murray GD, Butcher I, et al. Ankle brachial index combined with framingham risk score to predict cardiovascular events and mortality: a meta-analysis. *JAMA*. 2008 Jul 9;300(2):197-208.
5. Ramsey DE, Manke DA, Sumner DS. Toe blood pressure. A valuable adjunct to ankle pressure measurement for assessing peripheral arterial disease. *J Cardiovasc Surg*. 1983 Jan-Feb; 24(1):43-48.
6. Nicholas GG, Myers JL, DeMuth WE Jr. The role of vascular laboratory criteria in the selection of patients for lower extremity amputation. *Ann Surg*. 1982 Apr;195(4):469-473.
7. Deane CR, Needleman L. The cause of pulsus tardus in arterial stenosis. *Radiology*. 1995 Jan;194(1):28-30.
8. Dormandy JA, Rutherford RB. Management of Peripheral Arterial Disease (PAD). TASC Working Group. TransAtlantic Intersociety Concensus (TASC). *J Vasc Surg*. 2000 Jan;31 (1 part 2):S1-S296.
9. TASC II Working Group, Norgren L, Hiatt WR, et al. Inter-society consensus for the management of peripheral arterial disease (TASC II). *J Vasc Surg*. 2007 Jan;45(Suppl S):S5-S67.
10. Reichman W, Nichols B, Toner J, Jenvey W, Sobel M. Strategies in the treatment of major tissue loss and gangrene: results of 100 consecutive vascular reconstructions. *Ann Vasc Surg*. 1990 May;4(3):233-237.
11. BASIL trial participants, Adam DJ, Beard JD, Cleveland T, et al. Bypass versus angioplasty in severe ischemia of the leg (BASIL): multicenter, randomized controlled trial. *Lancet*. 2005 Dec;366(9501):1925-1934.
12. Haider SN, Kavanagh EG, Forlee M, et al. Two-year outcome with preferential use of infrainguinal angioplasty for critical ischemia. *J Vasc Surg*. 2006 Mar;43(3):504-512.
13. Giles KA, Pomposelli FB, Hamdan AD, et al. Infrapopliteal angioplasty for critical limb ischemia: relation of TransAtlantic InterSociety Consensus class to outcome in 176 limbs. *J Vasc Surg*. 2008 Jul;48(1):128-136.
14. Schillinger M, Sabeti S, Loewe C, et al. Balloon angioplasty versus implantation of nitinol stents in the superficial femoral artery. *NEJM*. 2006 May;354(18):1879-1888.
15. Saxon RR, Dake MD, Volgelzang RL, Katzen BT, Becker GJ. Randomized multi-center study comparing expanded polytetrafluoroethylene-covered endoprosthesis placement with percutaneous transluminal angioplasty in the treatment of superficial femoral occlusive disease. *J Vasc Interv Radiol*. 2008 Jun;19(6):823-832.
16. Shammas NW. Restenosis after lower extremity interventions: current status and future directions. *J Endovasc Ther*. 2009 Feb;16(Supp 1):170-182.
17. Brown DA, Lee EW, Loh CT, Kee ST. A new wave in the treatment of vascular occlusive disease: Biodegradable stents – animal experience and scientific principles. *J Vasc Interv Radiol*. 2009 Mar;20(3):315-324.
18. Personalized Health Care Expert Panel Meeting: Summary Report. Submitted to US Department of Health and Human Services by the Lewin Group, Inc. Sept. 10, 2007.

Bypass to the Popliteal Artery

21

Keith D. Calligaro and Matthew J. Dougherty

A 62-year-old overweight postal worker presented with complaints of cramps in his right calf. He stated that this reproducible pain occurred each time he walked 50 yards and resolved upon sitting down. He denied tissue loss or rest pain. His past medical history was significant for hypertension, hypercholesterolemia and tobacco use, as well as coronary revascularization.

On physical examination, he had bilateral carotid bruits, normal heart examination, and a strong right femoral pulse, but absent popliteal and pedal pulses. His left lower extremity had a saphenectomy scar. Both extremities had shiny, hairless skin without ulcerations or gangrene.

Question 1

Which of the following is not an indication for a bypass to the popliteal artery?

A. Mild to moderate intermittent claudication.
B. Non-healing toe ulcer with an ankle brachial index (ABI) of 0.30.
C. Rest pain.
D. Symptomatic popliteal aneurysm, entrapment syndrome, or adventitial cystic degeneration.

The patient's blood pressure and cholesterol levels were controlled well by medication. He lost excess weight, quit smoking, and initiated cilostazol therapy, but to no avail. His symptoms persisted and he was so incapacitated that he was unable to continue delivering the mail.

Arteriography was performed, demonstrating patency of the right iliac arteries but severe occlusive disease of the superficial femoral artery. There was reconstitution of the popliteal artery with two-vessel run-off. The patient consented to a femoropopliteal bypass procedure.

K.D. Calligaro (✉)
Section of Vascular Surgery and Endovascular Therapy, Vascular Surgery Fellowship,
Pennsylvania Hospital, Clinical Professor of Surgery,
University of Pennsylvania School of Medicine,
700 Spruce St - Suite 101, Philadelphia, PA 19106
e-mail: kcalligaro@aol.com

G. Geroulakos and B. Sumpio (eds.), *Vascular Surgery*,
DOI: 10.1007/978-1-84996-356-5_21, © Springer-Verlag London Limited 2011

Question 2

The conduit yielding the best long-term patency for this bypass is:

A. Dacron
C. Autologous vein
C. PTFE
D. Umbilical vein
E. Cryograft vein

Question 3

A distal cuff or patch is most likely worthwhile for which type of bypass?

A. Femoropopliteal above-knee reversed vein graft.
B. Femorotibial in situ vein graft.
C. Femoropopliteal above-knee PTFE.
D. Femorotibial PTFE.
E. Femoral-femoral PTFE cross-over graft.

Femoropopliteal bypass was performed with in situ greater saphenous vein to the below-knee popliteal artery. There was resolution of the patient´s claudication, and he was able to return to work. Unfortunately, he became lost to follow-up, and 2 years later he returned with complaints of recurrent claudication in his right lower extremity. Neither popliteal nor pedal pulses were palpable. Duplex ultrasonography and arteriography demonstrated several sites with elevated velocities, suggestive of two moderate focal stenoses in the proximal half of his bypass graft as well as a severe narrowing at the distal anastomosis.

Question 4

What are the treatment options for a failing graft?

A. Aspirin therapy
B. Percutaneous transluminal angioplasty (PTA)
C. Laser-assisted angioplasty and atherectomy
D. Amputation

The patient was taken to the operating room, where a longitudinal incision was made through the distal portion of his vein graft and popliteal artery. Under fluoroscopy, balloon angioplasty of the proximal moderate stenoses was performed, with excellent results. Using a small segment of autologous saphenous vein, patch angioplasty of the distal anastomosis was performed. Completion angiography revealed a widely patent graft, and his distal pulses were again appreciated on palpation. He was able to resume his usual activities and was seen routinely in the vascular clinic.

Question 5

The most useful serial postoperative test to assess graft patency and a possible failing graft is:

A. Arteriography
B. Pulse volume recordings
C. Duplex ultrasonography
D. Ankle brachial index
E. Magnetic resonance angiography (MRA)

21.1
Commentary

Mild to moderate intermittent claudication is not an indication for surgical bypass. Most (approximately 75%) patients presenting with only intermittent claudication have a benign course, remaining stable or improving with conservative measures, such as smoking cessation, weight loss and alteration in diet, graduated exercise programs, and medical treatment of risk factors (e.g. hypertension, hypercholesterolemia, diabetes). Claudication is a strong and independent predictor of mortality, however, and thus concomitant identification of comorbidities such as coronary and cerebrovascular atherosclerotic disease may have significant impact on survival.

Pharmacological therapy may be initiated with rheological agents such as pentoxifylline or cilostazol with variable effect. Antiplatelet therapy is frequently started to prevent cardiac or cerebrovascular complications. Only a minority (10–20%) of patients require surgical reconstruction, and few (3–6%) ultimately progress to major amputation.[1]

Revascularization is reserved for patients with disabling claudication or evidence of critical ischemia manifest as acute motor or sensory loss, chronic tissue loss or rest pain. Other less common etiologies for lower-extremity ischemia may cause femoropopliteal occlusion and are occasionally indications for surgical revascularization. **[Q1: A]**

Long-term patency rates are highest when autologous vein is used as conduit. If the greater saphenous vein is not available, then lesser saphenous vein, femoropopliteal vein, or upper-extremity veins may be acceptable alternatives. The advantages of in situ vein bypass grafting include the preservation of the vein's nutrient supply and the better size match of the proximal and distal artery to the proximal and distal vein. Using reversed vein grafts, however, avoids the endothelial trauma of valve lysis. Although at times somewhat conflicting, the literature does not support the superiority of one technique over the other for femoropopliteal bypasses.

The use of human umbilical vein[2] or cryopreserved vein has also been described with varying success. The latter may be a potential alternative to prosthetic grafts if autologous vein is unavailable, but in below-knee revascularization, cryopreserved vein has demonstrated the tendency for aneurysmal degeneration and poor long-term patency.[3]

Prosthetic grafts in the suprageniculate bypass have demonstrated patency rates that are comparable with those for autologous vein.[4] The type of prosthetic graft is less important than the age of the patient or the size of the conduit.[5] The patency of prosthetic grafts to infrageniculate arteries, however, is significantly worse than that of autologous vein. Further, the use of composite prosthetic and autologous vein does not seem to improve long-term patency compared with pure prosthetic grafts.[6]

Finally, there have been reports of endovascular treatment of femoropopliteal atherosclerotic disease, including percutaneously inserted covered stents[7] and prosthetic grafts introduced through a femoral arteriotomy and anchored distally with stent deployment.[8] Long-term patency with these techniques remains to be evaluated. **[Q2: B]**

Intimal hyperplasia occurs frequently at the distal anastomosis when a prosthetic graft is used for an infrainguinal bypass and compromises its survival. Modifications to improve long-term patency include various vein cuffs and patches. Using these techniques theoretically improves compliance match between the prosthetic material and the artery at the distal anastomosis. The reduction in turbulence minimizes the trauma to the arterial endothelium and decreases its proliferative response.

The Miller cuff was studied in a prospective randomized study to determine its potential benefit in improving the patency rate of distal supra- and infrageniculate femoropopliteal polytetrafluoroethylene (PTFE) grafts. Although no difference was noted in above-knee bypasses with or without vein cuff, a statistically significant improvement in patency was observed in below-knee procedures.[9] Similarly, the Taylor patch has been reported to improve patency of infrageniculate bypasses.[10] **[Q3: D]**

Salvage of a bypass graft in the early postoperative period may include strategies such as thrombectomy and revision of technical errors. These errors include graft kinks, retained valve leaflets, intimal flaps, and residual arteriovenous fistulas in an in situ graft.

Recently, percutaneous endovascular techniques such as balloon angioplasty have been utilized with increasing frequency but with equivocal results. Focal lesions (less than 20 mm) are more amenable to catheter-based techniques than are more diffuse stenoses, but even these favorable lesions may recur. Laser angioplasty and atherectomy, however, have not been shown to be beneficial in the preservation of failing grafts.

Thrombolysis may be considered for patients who present with sudden and recent onset of symptoms attributable to bypass graft occlusions. For patients with chronic graft occlusion, a new bypass graft provides improved clinical outcome, but in acute graft occlusion, thrombolysis may improve limb salvage and reduce the magnitude of the subsequent surgical procedure.[11]

For short-segment stenoses, patch angioplasty or interposition within an existing vein graft with autologous or prosthetic material may be performed to preserve a bypass to the popliteal artery. Although technically simpler and requiring less autologous material, patch angioplasty has inferior results when compared with interposition.[12] Longer-segment stenoses are preferably treated with interposition or jump graft around the area of narrowing. Failing these strategies, however, the creation of an entirely new bypass may be required.

Amputation is reserved for tissue loss or ischemic pain without possible vascular reconstruction. Long-term survival of patients requiring major amputation is poor. **[Q4: B]**

Early graft failure (i.e. within the first 30 postoperative days) is most likely the result of a technical error, hypercoagulability, poor distal run-off, or postoperative hypotension. In addition to avoidable technical errors, early graft failure may be secondary to endothelial trauma, the use of imperfect conduit, or poor surgical judgement with regard to the adequacy of inflow or outflow.

Graft failure within the first few years of surgery is usually attributable to intimal hyperplasia. Subsequent graft failure is most frequently secondary to progression of atherosclerotic disease.

It is vital to identify a failing graft before complete occlusion to preserve the patency of the graft. Lower-extremity revascularization can be salvaged with simple interventions if lesions leading to intimal hyperplasia and hemodynamic compromise can be identified before graft thrombosis. Revision of stenotic lesions in a failing but nonoccluded graft results in superior patency when compared with revision of similar lesions in an occluded graft. It also leads to fewer amputations and subsequent revisions. Additionally, the repair of a failing graft is less costly than emergent revision of a failed graft or of amputation.[13]

Postoperative duplex ultrasonography detects correctable abnormalities early, precludes the need for angiography in many cases, and markedly improves assisted primary patency of vein bypass grafts. Recommended surveillance includes initial ABI and duplex studies at 1 week, followed by evaluations at 3, 6, 9, 12, 18, and 24 months, then annually thereafter. High-grade stenoses can be identified and corrected before thrombosis occurs. Criteria for the diagnosis of a failing graft include monophasic signals, peak systolic velocity (PSV) less than 45 cm/s throughout the bypass, any PSV greater than 300 cm/s, or a PSV ratio across a stenosis of greater than 3.5.[14] **[Q5: C]**

References

1. Illig KA, Ouriel K. Nonoperative treatment of claudication. In: Cameron JL, ed. *Current surgical therapy*. 6th ed. St Louis: Mosby; 1998:767-770.
2. Aalders GJ, van Vroonhoven TJMV. Polytetrafluoroethylene versus human umbilical vein in above-knee femoropopliteal bypass: six-year results of a randomized clinical trial. *J Vasc Surg*. 1992;16:816-824.
3. Martin RS, Edwards WH, Mulherin JL, Edwards WH, Jenkins JM, Hoff SJ. Cryopreserved saphenous vein allografts for below-knee lower extremity revascularization. *Ann Surg*. 1994;219:664-672.
4. AbuRahma AF, Robinson PA, Holt SM. Prospective controlled study of polytetrafluoroethylene versus saphenous vein in claudicant patients with bilateral above knee femoropopliteal bypasses. *Surgery*. 1999;126:594-602.
5. Green RM, Abbott WM, Matsumoto T, et al. Prosthetic above-knee femoropopliteal bypass grafting: five-year results of a randomized trial. *J Vasc Surg*. 2000;31:417-425.
6. LaSalle AJ, Brewster DC, Corson JD, Darling RC. Femoropopliteal composite bypass grafts: current status. *Surgery*. 1982;92:36-39.
7. Henry M, Amor M, Ethevenot G, et al. Initial experience with the Cragg Endopro System 1 for intraluminal treatment of peripheral vascular disease. *J Endovasc Surg*. 1994;1:31-43.
8. Spoelstra H, Casselman F, Lesceu O. Balloon-expandable endobypass for femoropopliteal athero-sclerotic occlusive disease. *J Vasc Surg*. 1996;24:647-654.
9. Pappas PJ, Hobson RW, Meyers MG, et al. Patency of infrainguinal polyte-trafluoroethylene bypass grafts with distal interposition vein cuffs. *Cardiovasc Surg*. 1998;6:19-26.

10. Taylor RS, Loh A, McFarland RJ, Cox M, Chester JF. Improved technique for polytetrafluoroethylene bypass grafting: long-term results using anastomotic vein patches. *Br J Surg.* 1992;79:348-354.
11. Comerota AJ, Weaver FA, Hosking JD, et al. Results of a prospective, randomized trial of surgery versus thrombolysis for occluded lower extremity bypass grafts. *Am J Surg.* 1996;172:105-112.
12. Bandyk DF, Bergamini TM, Towne JB. Durability of vein graft revision: the outcome of secondary procedures. *J Vasc Surg.* 1991;13:200-210.
13. Wixon CL, Mills JL, Westerband A, Hughes JD, Ihnat DM. An economic appraisal of lower extremity bypass graft maintenance. *J Vasc Surg.* 2000;32:1-12.
14. Calligaro KD, Syrek JR, Dougherty MJ, et al. Selective use of duplex ultrasound to replace preoperative arteriography for failing arterial vein grafts. *J Vasc Surg.* 1998;27:89-95.

Bypass to the Infrapopliteal Arteries for Chronic Critical Limb Ischemia

22

Enrico Ascher and Anil P. Hingorani

An 85-year-old male with a history of diabetes, hypertension, hypercholesterolemia, coronary artery bypass, and active tobacco use presented with a gangrenous right first toe. The patient stated that he had no history of trauma to the area, and complained of rest pain in the foot. The patient had been in otherwise good health since his coronary artery bypass 12 years ago. On physical examination, the patient was in no physical distress. The patient had a well-healed median sternotomy scar. Auscultation of the heart revealed a regular rate without any murmurs. He was obese. Abdominal examination revealed no palpable masses. The patient had bilateral femoral and popliteal pulses but no pedal pulses. The patient had bilateral, well-healed scars from the greater saphenous vein harvest sites. The right gangrenous toe was dry without any evidence of infection.

Question 1

Which of the following statements regarding chronic lower-extremity ischemia are wrong?

A. If the patient refuses any intervention, then anticoagulation alone may be helpful
B. The contralateral asymptomatic lower extremity should also undergo angiography as there may be severe atherosclerotic disease there as well
C. The treatment options remain unchanged if the patient presents with only rest pain, ischemic ulcer or claudication
D. The patient cannot undergo revascularization without contrast arteriography as there are no other alternatives

The patient's arterial duplex demonstrated moderate distal right superficial femoral artery disease. The ankle brachial indices (ABIs) and pulse volume recordings demonstrated findings consistent with moderately decreased perfusion at the calf level and severely decreased perfusion at the ankle and transmetatarsal levels. The cardiac review of systems was unremarkable, and a persantine thallium obtained 6 months ago revealed no perfusion defects. Electrocardiogram (ECG), chest X-ray and routine preoperative blood tests were

E. Ascher (✉)
The Vascular Institute of New York, Brooklyn, NY, USA

G. Geroulakos and B. Sumpio (eds.), *Vascular Surgery*,
DOI: 10.1007/978-1-84996-356-5_22, © Springer-Verlag London Limited 2011

231

normal. Venous duplex mapping revealed inadequate veins (sclerotic and too small) in the bilateral upper and lower extremities.

Question 2

Preoperative medications/lifestyle changes that should be added to the patient's regimen to reduce his overall cardiovascular risk based upon randomized prospective data include:

A. Aspirin
B. A statin
C. Angiotensin-converting enzyme inhibitors
D. Tobacco cessation
E. A beta-blocker

Percutaneous angiogram of the right lower extremity demonstrated moderate right distal superficial femoral artery stenosis with distal occlusion. The popliteal appeared to be severely diseased with occlusion of the tibioperoneal artery and proximal anterior tibial artery. The mid-anterior tibial artery reconstituted and ran down to the dorsalis pedis artery. No other vessels appeared to be adequate.

Question 3

What type of options would you consider for this lower extremity?

A. Below-knee amputation
B. Digital amputation
C. Tibial bypass with expanded polytetrafluoroethylene (ePTFE) with a venous interposition or fistula
D. Tibial bypass with cadaveric vein
E. Sympathectomy
F. Chelation therapy
G. Subintimal angioplasty

The patient underwent a successful bypass with ePTFE to the anterior tibial artery and did stop smoking after the procedure. The patient's toe underwent autoamputation and the rest pain has resolved. He was followed up 2 years after the procedure with a patent bypass.

Question 4

What is the patient's long-term prognosis in terms of mortality, graft patency, and limb salvage after successful bypass?

A. The long-term mortality, patency, and limb salvage are about 20% and therefore are so poor that no intervention should be made.

B. The mortality and patency are 50% at 4–5 years. The limb salvage is 70% at 4 years. If the patient has a reasonable life expectancy and functional status, he should undergo the revascularization.

C. The mortality, patency, and limb salvage rates are irrelevant in this age group.

Question 5

Which patients would you consider to be inoperable? What treatment options may be offered to this subset of patients?

22.1
Commentary

Indications for revascularization to the tibial vessels are limited to ischemic ulcers, gangrene, and rest pain. The long-term patency of the bypass is affected directly by continued tobacco use, and the patient should be urged to stop smoking. Anticoagulation plays no role as the sole management of this patient. Even though the patient may have asymptomatic contralateral disease, there is no role for further investigation. Angiography may be used to visualize both inflow and outflow sites. In general, the most distal available inflow site is utilized to shorten the length of the graft. Time-delayed imaging may be required to visualize the calf and foot arteries because of reduced flow. The use of magnetic resonance angiography (MRA) has proven to be beneficial in identifying patent lower-extremity arteries, particularly in view of the recent advances in imaging software and hardware.[1–3] Finally, high resolution duplex imaging has now become a viable alternative for visualization of inflow and outflow sites with the added advantages of cost reduction, fewer complications associated with angiography, and the ability to identify the least calcified artery segment.[4–8] However, both MRA and duplex imaging should only be used as preoperative imaging modalities after they have been validated at each center. [Q1: A, B, C, D]

Increasing focus on the perioperative and long-term management of patients with peripheral arterial disease has identified that all the factors listed in Question 2 can significantly reduce the incidence of cardiovascular events in these patients. These data have been supported by large multicenter randomized prospective trials[9, 10] Therefore, it becomes incumbent on the vascular surgeon to also consider these as part of the treatment plan when evaluating a patient with peripheral arterial disease. [Q2: A, B, C, D, E]

Evolution of vascular surgery techniques in the past decade, combined with the availability of an adequate venous conduit, has permitted a liberal and aggressive approach to salvage ischemic limbs caused by advanced atherosclerosis. This approach is epitomized by the construction of arterial bypasses to the terminal branches of tibial vessels.[11] However, significant numbers of patients continue to face the threat of a major amputation because of insufficient vein necessary to perform a totally autogenous bypass to one of the infrapopliteal arteries. In these cases, less durable grafts made of prosthetic material must be used if limb salvage is to be attempted. Accordingly, several adjunctive techniques have been designed in an attempt to improve the poor patency results achieved with prosthetic bypasses. These include the administration of immediate and chronic anticoagulants,[12] the construction of a vein patch or cuff at the distal anastomosis to prevent occlusion by intimal hyperplasia,[13, 14] and the creation of an arteriovenous fistula to increase graft blood flow in high-outflow-resistance systems.[15, 16] Despite initial enthusiasm, the results using cadaveric vein have been poor and resulted in its very limited use.[17, 18] **[Q3: C]** If the popliteal artery had been not as diseased, an attempt at subintimal angioplasty with angiography or with duplex guidance may also be considered.[19, 20]

The expected long-term mortality of this patient is 24–50% at 4–5 years and is due mostly to myocardial ischemia.[21] The expected patency of these techniques is 50–60% at 3–4 years.[21-24] The expected limb salvage rates are 70–80% at 3–4 years.[21-24] **[Q4: B]**

Based on these data, we would suggest that there is no role for amputation or sympathectomy in this particular patient. However, if the patient had prohibitive cardiac risks, had nonreconstructable disease, or was already so neurologically impaired that the limb was not of any utility to the patient, then observation, primary amputation, hyperbaric oxygen therapy or perhaps experimental protocols involving angiogenesis factors may be in order. **[Q5]**

References

1. Carpenter JP, Owen RS, Baum RA, et al. Magnetic resonance angiography of peripheral runoff vessels. *J Vasc Surg.* 1992;16:807.
2. Cambria RP, Kaufman JA, L'Italien GJ, et al. Magnetic resonance angiography in the management of lower extremity arterial occlusive disease: a prospective study. *J Vasc Surg.* 1997;25: 380-389.
3. Hingorani A, Ascher E, Markevich N, et al. Magnetic resonance angiography versus duplex arteriography in patients undergoing lower extremity revascularization: which is the best replacement for contrast arteriography? *J Vasc Surg.* 2004;39(4):717-722.
4. Ascher E, Mazzariol F, Hingorani A, Salles-Cunha S, Gade P. The use of duplex ultrasound arterial mapping as an alternative to conventional arteriography for primary and secondary infrapopliteal bypasses. *Am J Surg.* 1999;178:162-165.
5. Mazzariol F, Ascher E, Salles-Cunha SX, Gade P, Hingorani A. Values and limitations of duplex ultrasonography as the sole imaging method of preoperative evaluation for popliteal and infrapopliteal bypasses. *Ann Vasc Surg.* 1999;13:1-10.
6. Mazzariol F, Ascher E, Hingorani A, Gunduz Y, Yorkovich W, Salles-Cunha S. Lower-extremity revascularisation without preoperative contrast arteriography in 185 cases: lessons learned with duplex ultrasound arterial mapping. *Eur J Vasc Endovasc Surg.* 2000;19:509-515.
7. Ascher E, Markevich N, Schutzer RW, et al. Duplex arteriography prior to femoral-popliteal reconstruction in claudicants: a proposal for a new shortened protocol. *Ann Vasc Surg.* 2004;18(5):544-551.
8. Ascher E, Hingorani A, Markevich N, Schutzer R, Kallakuri S. Acute lower limb ischemia: the value of duplex ultrasound arterial mapping (DUAM) as the sole preoperative imaging technique. *Ann Vasc Surg.* 2003;17(3):284-289.

9. Hackam DG. Cardiovascular risk prevention in peripheral artery disease. *J Vasc Surg*. 2005;41(6):1070-1073.

10. Yusuf S, Sleight P, Pogue J, Bosch J, Davies R, Dagenais G. Effects of an angiotensin-converting-enzyme inhibitor, ramipril, on cardiovascular events in high-risk patients. The Heart Outcomes Prevention Evaluation Study Investigators. *N Engl J Med*. 2000 Jan 20;342(3):145-153.

11. Ascer E, Veith FJ, Gupta SK. Bypasses to plantar arteries and other tibial branches: an extended approach to limb salvage. *J Vasc Surg*. 1988;8:434-441.

12. Flinn WR, Rohrer MJ, Yao JST, McCarthy WJ, Fahey VA, Bergan JJ. Improved long-term patency of infragenicular polytetrafluoroethylene grafts. *J Vasc Surg*. 1988;7:685.

13. Siegman FA. Use of the venous cuff for graft anastomosis. *Surg Gynecol Obstet*. 1979; 148:930.

14. Miller JH, Foreman RK, Ferguson L, Faris I. Interposition vein cuff for anastomosis of prosthesis to small artery. *Aust N Z J Surg*. 1984;54:283.

15. Dardik H, Sussman B, Ibrahim IM, et al. Distal arteriovenous fistula as an adjunct to maintain arterial and graft patency for limb salvage. *Surgery*. 1983;94:478.

16. Ascer E, Veith FJ, White-Flores SA, Morin L, Gupta SK, Lesser ML. Intraoperative outflow resistance as a predictor of late patency of femoropopliteal and infrapopliteal arterial bypasses. *J Vasc Surg*. 1987;5:820.

17. Albertini JN, Barral X, Branchereau A, et al. Long-term results of arterial allograft below-knee bypass grafts for limb salvage: a retrospective multicenter study. *J Vasc Surg*. 2000;31:426-435.

18. Harris L, O'Brien-Irr M, Ricotta JJ. Long-term assessment of cryopreserved vein bypass grafting success. *J Vasc Surg*. 2001;33:528-532.

19. Hingorani A, Ascher E, Markevich N, et al. The role of the endovascular surgeon for lower extremity ischemia. *Acta Chir Belg*. 2004;104(5):527-531.

20. Ascher E, Marks NA, Schutzer RW, Hingorani AP. Duplex-guided balloon angioplasty and stenting for arterial occlusive disease: an alternative in patients with renal insufficiency. *J Vasc Surg*. in press.

21. Neville RF, Dy B, Singh N, DeZee KJ. Distal vein patch with an arteriovenous fistula: a viable option for the patient without autogenous conduit and severe distal occlusive disease. *J Vasc Surg*. 2009 Jul;50(1):83-88.

22. Ascher E, Gennaro M, Pollina RM, et al. Complementary distal arteriovenous fistula and deep vein interposition: a five-year experience with a new technique to improve infrapopliteal prosthetic bypass patency. *J Vasc Surg*. 1996;24:134-143.

23. Kreienberg PB, Darling RC 3rd, Chang BB, Paty PS, Lloyd WE, Shah DM. Adjunctive techniques to improve patency of distal prosthetic bypass grafts: polytetrafluoroethylene with remote arteriovenous fistulae versus vein cuffs. *J Vasc Surg*. 2000;31:696.

24. Hingorani AP, Ascher E, Markevich N, et al. A ten-year experience with complementary distal arteriovenous fistula and deep vein interposition for infrapopliteal prosthetic bypasses. *Vasc Endovascular Surg*. 2005 Sep–Oct;39(5):401-409.

Popliteal Artery Entrapment

23

Luca di Marzo and Norman M. Rich

A 26-year-old female presented with a 6-year history of cold foot, paraesthesia and cramping in both legs after intensive physical training. She was a recreational body-builder and complained of her symptoms mostly after sporting activity. Symptoms subsequently became more severe, with cramping requiring 20 min to release after sport.

Question 1

What is the presentation of cases with popliteal artery entrapment?

A. The patient is often sporty with muscular calves.
B. The patient often complains of rest pain or necrosis.
C. The patient often complains of mild symptoms with paraesthesia, cold foot and cramping after intensive physical training.
D. Venous complains are often encountered.
E. Symptoms due to arterial embolisation are often present.

The patient smoked 20 cigarettes a day. Her past medical history included pancreatitis when she was 12 years old and tonsillectomy when she was 19 years old. On physical examination, she appeared healthy, with both legs appearing athletic. Lower-limb pulses were normal, but bilateral pedal pulse reduction was noted after calf muscle contraction. A popliteal artery entrapment (PAE) was therefore suspected, and the patient was sent for noninvasive vascular evaluation. Doppler and color Doppler showed normal posterior tibial and popliteal recordings, with signal disappearance on both legs during calf muscle contraction. Doppler examination was conducted with the patient supine recording the posterior tibial artery during maneuver (Fig. 23.1). Color Doppler was performed, with the patient prone, and the sample volume placed in the popliteal artery. Muscular contraction of the calves showed an arterial occlusion on color flow imaging (Fig. 23.2).

L. di Marzo (✉)
Department of Surgery P Valdoni, Sapienza University of Rome,
Rome, Italy

G. Geroulakos and B. Sumpio (eds.), *Vascular Surgery*,
DOI: 10.1007/978-1-84996-356-5_23, © Springer-Verlag London Limited 2011

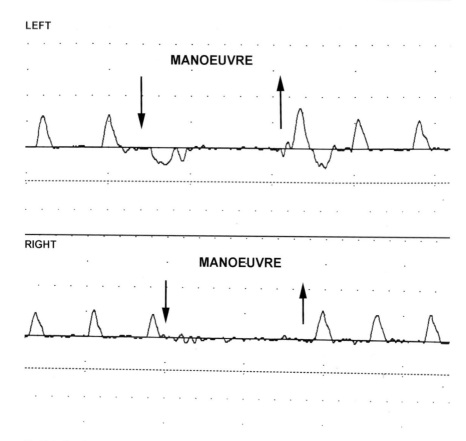

Fig. 23.1 Continuous-wave Doppler recording the posterior tibial artery during maneuver

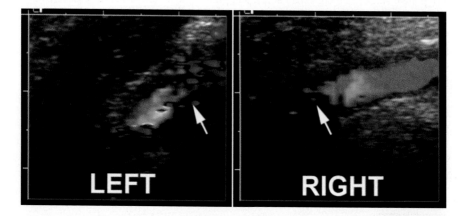

Fig. 23.2 Color Doppler during muscular contraction of the calves, showing arterial occlusion

Diagnosis of bilateral PAE was made. Arteriography was conducted to confirm the diagnosis: it showed normal popliteal arteries, with right severe stenosis and left occlusion during calf muscle contraction (Fig. 23.3). Magnetic resonance angiography (MRA) was attempted, which demonstrated bilateral popliteal occlusion during maneuver (Fig. 23.4).

Question 2

How will you make the diagnosis of PAE?

A. Doppler can detect PAE.
B. Arteriography is only carried out preoperatively to confirm results of ultrasound scans.
C. MRA may be diagnostic in the hands of an experienced practitioner.
D. Duplex scanning can detect PAE.
E. Angio-CT with last generation apparatus is able to detect PAE.

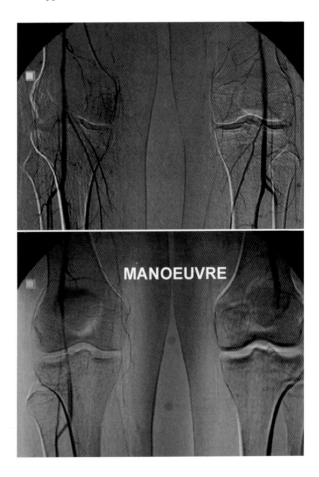

Fig. 23.3 Arteriography showing normal popliteal arteries, with right severe stenosis and left occlusion during calf muscle contraction

Fig. 23.4 MRA demonstrating bilateral popliteal occlusion during maneuver

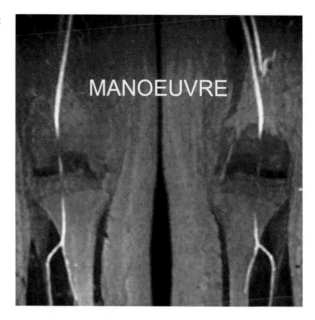

Question 3

Which of the following statements regarding angiograms of a patient with PAE are correct?

A. Normal angiograms at rest are often encountered in entrapments.
B. The angiograms show an occlusion or severe stenosis during calf muscles contractions.
C. Three-vessel run-off is often encountered in PAE.
D. An arterial occlusion is encountered in PAE diagnosed at a late stage.
E. A post-stenotic aneurysm may be encountered.

The patient was considered for bilateral surgical treatment. A posterior approach to the popliteal fossa was made through a Z-shaped incision. The medial gastrocnemius muscle had a large accessory head with a lateral and cranial insertion, causing bilateral compression of the popliteal artery and vein. This head was resected on both legs, without any need for muscular reconstruction.

Question 4

Which of the following statements regarding the treatment of PAE are correct?

A. Musculotendineous sectioning is the treatment of choice in patients with a normal popliteal artery.
B. Vascular reconstruction should be limited to cases with stable arterial impairment.
C. If vascular reconstruction is planned, then the use of autologous vein is mandatory.

D. The posterior approach is recommended to expose all the structures causing compression.

E. The structure causing PAE must be sectioned completely, as incomplete sectioning may cause recurrence.

Question 5

Which of the following statements regarding the incidence of entrapment are correct?

A. The medial gastrocnemius muscle is involved in almost 80% of cases of PAE.
B. Venous entrapment is described more often than arterial entrapment.
C. Venous entrapment is concomitant in 20% of cases of PAE.
D. More than one structure may be the cause of arterial entrapment.
E. Classification of arterial entrapment includes 12 different types.

The postoperative course was uneventful and the patient was discharged 5 days after surgery, returning back to normal activity after 3 weeks. Follow-up demonstrated complete regression of symptoms. Ultrasound examinations (Doppler and color Doppler) showed normal popliteal flow with negative response to PAE maneuvers 1 month after surgery. The patient is now doing sport (swimming) again without any further complaints.

23.1
Commentary

The first case of PAE was treated surgically in 1959 in a 12-year-old boy complaining of claudication after walking 300 m. At surgical exploration, Hamming[1] at Leyden University in The Netherlands found an occluded artery with an anomalous course medial to the medial gastrocnemius muscle. He transected the muscle and performed a successful popliteal artery thromboendarterectomy. A previous description of the disease was reported in 1879 by Stuart,[2] a medical student at the University of Edinburgh. During the dissection of an amputated leg of a 64-year-old man, he observed the popliteal artery coursing around the medial head of the gastrocnemius muscle and aneurysmal changes in the popliteal artery distal to the point of external muscular compression.

Since then, many case reports have been published. A few authors have published small series.[3-6] Unfortunately, the papers that were collected were missing details and showed poor patient follow-up[7]

In Rome in 1998, the Popliteal Vascular Entrapment Forum was founded. Surgeons from around the world with the greatest experience in this field world were invited as founding members of the forum. Great effort was addressed to collect different series with comparable criteria. The criteria established by the Society for Vascular Surgery (SVS) were reviewed and accepted, with some minor changes. Common opinion was to consider both arterial and venous entrapment as a common disease defined as vascular entrapment. The functional form of entrapment was discussed. This was first described by Rignault et al.[8] in 1985, and describes cases in which the anatomy of the popliteal fossa is normal. Symptoms are usually caused by hypertrophy of the muscles determining a compartment syndrome.[8, 9] Functional entrapment was included in the classification as type F (Table 23.1).

Popliteal artery entrapment is no longer a rare disease. It is encountered more and more often, particularly in young adults. Athletes practicing sports causing hypertrophy of the limb muscles are at higher risk due to an anomalous relationship of the popliteal artery and its surrounding musculotendineous structures. The artery is compressed each time the leg moves, causing peripheral ischaemia during intensive exercise. With time, this intermittent arterial trauma may give rise to stable arterial damage, with occlusion or post-stenotic aneurysm. Early diagnosis and treatment play an important role in limiting surgical treatment to the sectioning of the structure causing the arterial compression. **[Q1: A, C]**

The diagnosis of PAE is based primarily on ultrasound scanning. Both continuous-wave Doppler and color Doppler are able to detect the presence of an arterial compression due to entrapment. The maneuvers to be performed are well described and are able to detect suspected cases.[7] Great care should be taken to suspect early cases of PAE in patients complaining of minor symptoms (paraesthesia, cold foot and cramping after intensive physical training). Arteriography is limited to cases with positive ultrasound examinations, and it requires great care in repeating the maneuvers to confirm the popliteal compression. Both Angio-CT and MRA may be diagnostic, but they need latest-generation apparatus and the input of a radiologist with great experience in both the disease and the imaging method. **[Q2: A, B, C, D, E] [Q3: True A, B, C, D, E]**

Surgical treatment consists of sectioning the musculotendineous structure causing the entrapment. The anomalous structure needs to be sectioned entirely in order to avoid recurrence of the entrapment due to hypertrophy of the remaining anomalous muscle. It is important to remember that complete exposure of the popliteal fossa is obtained through a posterior approach. The medial approach limits the view of the medial gastrocnemius muscle. In our opinion, this exposure should be limited to cases in which the arterial impairment is extended to the tibial vessels and a distal reconstruction needs to be planned. However, early diagnosis allows surgical treatment to be limited to the muscle sectioning, which should be considered the first-choice treatment. When a popliteal severe stenosis, occlusion or aneurysm is present, then an arterial reconstruction is indicated. In this case, we recommend the use of autologous material to reconstruct the artery. This improves the

Table 23.1 Classification of popliteal vascular entrapment

Type features
I Popliteal artery running medial to the medial head of gastrocnemius
II Medial head of gastrocnemius attached laterally
III Accessory slip of gastrocnemius
IV Popliteal artery passing below popliteal muscle and medial head of gastrocnemius
V Primary venous involvement
VI Variants
F Functional entrapment

long-term patency rate. Great effort should be paid for alternative vein preparation when the saphenous vein is unavoidable. **[Q4: A, B, C, D, E]**

The medial gastrocnemius muscle is often the cause of compression. However, more than 20 different anatomical variants have been described, and sometimes multiple and complex structures may be associated with the medial gastrocnemius muscle in causing PAE. The popliteal vein is involved in the compression in 20% of cases affected by PAE. Moreover, isolated popliteal vein entrapment is described with increasing frequency in the literature. **[Q5: A, C, D]**

References

1. Hamming JJ. Intermittent claudication at an early age due to anomalous course of the popliteal artery. *Angiology*. 1959;10:369-370.
2. Stuart PTA. Note on a variation in the course of the popliteal artery. *J Anat Physiol*. 1879;13:162.
3. Bouhoutsos J, Daskalakis E. Muscular abnormalities affecting the popliteal vessels. *Br J Surg*. 1981;68:501-506.
4. Rich NM, Collins GJ, McDonald PT, Kozloff L, Claget PG, Collins JT. Popliteal vascular entrapment. Its increasing interest. *Arch Surg*. 1979;114:1377-1384.
5. Di Marzo L, Cavallaro A, Mingoli A, Sapienza P, Tedesco M, Stipa S. Popliteal artery entrapment syndrome: the role of early diagnosis and treatment. *Surgery*. 1997;122:26-31.
6. Levien L, Veller MG. Popliteal artery entrapment syndrome: more common than previously recognized. *J Vasc Surg*. 1999;30:587-598.
7. Di Marzo L, Cavallaro A, Sciacca V, Mingoli A, Stipa S. Natural history of entrapment of the popliteal artery. *J Am Coll Surg*. 1994;178:553-556.
8. Rignault DP, Pailler JL, Lunel F. The "functional" popliteal entrapment syndrome. *Int Angiol*. 1985;4:341-343.
9. Turnipseed WD, Pozniak M. Popliteal entrapment as a result of neurovascular compression by the soleus and plantaris muscles. *J Vasc Surg*. 1992;15:285-294.

Adventitial Cystic Disease of the Popliteal Artery

24

Bernard H. Nachbur and Jon Largiadèr

A 49-year-old female presented with a 3-week history of left calf intermittent claudication at 150 m, which had occurred suddenly and without preliminary herald signs. The patient was a nonsmoker and had no risk factors, such as hypertension, diabetes or hyperlipidaemia. She was engaged in regular sporting activity, playing tennis all year round and skiing in the winter. She thought at first that it might be a strained muscle and would subside spontaneously. This did not happen and she sought medical advice.

At clinical examination, the popliteal and pedal pulses of the left leg were barely palpable and were absent after exercise. Angiological examination of the right leg was normal. The ankle systolic pressure at the right side was 128 mm Hg with a slight rise to 132 mm Hg after exercise. On the left side, ankle systolic pressure at rest was 88 mm Hg with a post-exercise reduction to 58 mm Hg. On duplex sonography, a 5-cm long polycystic swelling surrounding the left popliteal artery was found to be the cause of occlusion of the popliteal artery. The superficial femoral artery and the infrapopliteal arteries showed no trace of atherosclerotic disease. Ultrasonography demonstrated that the content of the cyst was clear and homogeneous. No other cause for popliteal occlusion was found.

Question 1

What is the aetiology of this condition?
An angiogram (Fig. 24.1) showed a 3-cm long subtotal occlusion of the proximal popliteal artery suggesting medial compression, an eccentric form of occlusion reminiscent of an hourglass stenosis (scimitar sign). The top frame of the cross-section of the computed tomography (CT) scan performed at the same time shows an adventitial cyst of approximately 1.5 cm in diameter adjacent to the artery, actually within the arterial wall.

B.H. Nachbur (✉)
University of Berne, Berne, Switzerland

G. Geroulakos and B. Sumpio (eds.), *Vascular Surgery*,
DOI: 10.1007/978-1-84996-356-5_24, © Springer-Verlag London Limited 2011

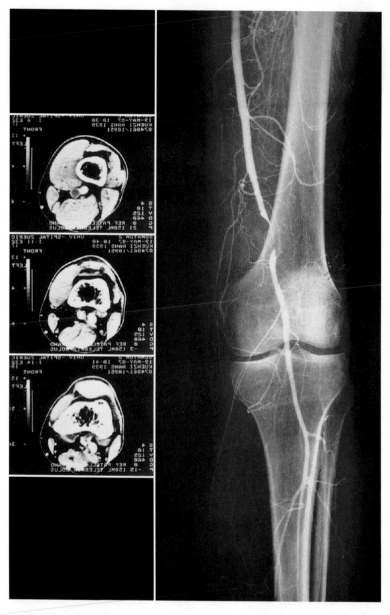

Fig. 24.1 Hourglass-shaped subtotal occlusion of the middle portion of the popliteal artery (scimitar sign) caused by compression by a cyst in the arterial wall, which can be seen in the top panel of the cross-section of the CT scans

Question 2

Which of the following statements regarding adventitial cystic disease are correct?

A. It affects only the popliteal artery.
B. It can occur elsewhere, such as in arteries near the hip, wrist or ankle joints.
C. It presents with initial signs of acute occlusive disease.
D. It usually begins with intermittent claudication.
E. It can be elicited by loss of pedal pulses during hyperextension of the leg.
F. The cyst is calcified and contains atheromatous material.
G. The cyst contains a viscous gelatinous fluid.

The popliteal artery was laid free posteriorly through a S-shaped popliteal incision. The arterial wall contained a cyst filled with a gelatinous mucoid yellowish substance. The occluded arterial segment was resected and replaced by interposition of a segment of saphenous vein. Figure 24.2 shows the popliteal artery before and after surgery with complete normalisation of patency.

A 49-year-old woman complained of sporadic episodes of intermittent claudication of varying intensity.[1] At times, she could walk freely; at other times, after physical exercise with bending of the knee, intermittent claudication would occur after walking distances of 200–300 m. Angiography revealed only discrete semilunar narrowing of the middle portion of the popliteal artery, as shown in Fig. 24.3 (scimitar sign). At the time of this examination, the patient had hardly any complaints.

Question 3

Adventitial cystic disease of the popliteal artery can be diagnosed reliably by:

A. Duplex coloured sonography.
B. Injection of indium[111] and scintigraphy.
C. The semilunar sign (scimitar sign) or hourglass sign at angiography.
D. A meniscus-shaped proximal occlusion at angiography.
E. T2-weighted magnetic resonance imaging (MRI).
F. Systolic bruit in the hollow of the knee.
G. Intravascular ultrasound imaging.
H. CT scanning.

Question 4

What are the treatment options?
The popliteal artery was laid free posteriorly through a popliteal incision. The arterial wall was surrounded by a 5-cm long polycystic tumour in the centre of which was a 3-mm wide stem that could be followed to the knee joint. A fine probe was introduced for injection of

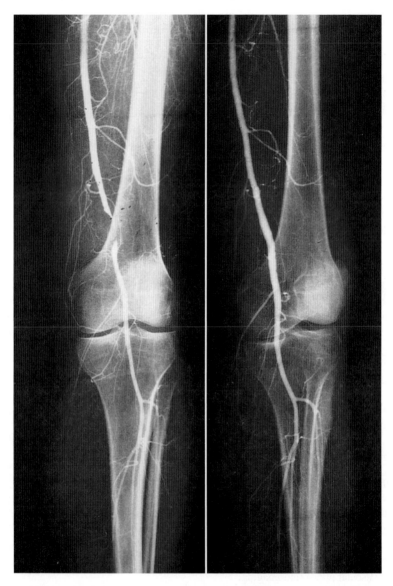

Fig. 24.2 Popliteal adventitial cyst before and after segmental resection and interposition of a segment of autologous vein

contrast medium. The cyst took the appearance of a Baker cyst, which was filled with a jelly-like yellowish mucoid substance. The cyst was found to be lying in the outer layers of the adventitia and was removed easily without causing any damage to the artery itself (Figs. 24.4 and 24.5).

Fig. 24.3 Angiography of the popliteal artery, with a discrete semilunar deformity (arrow pointing to the scimitar sign). At the time of this angiography, the patient was in momentary clinical remission

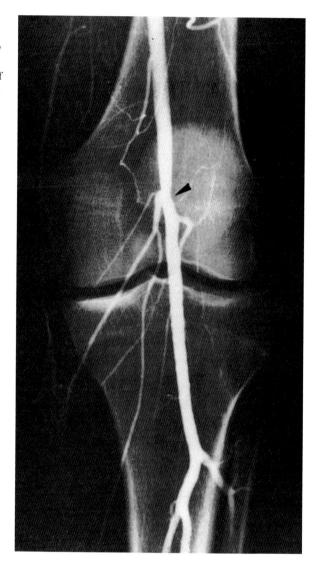

The varying clinical presentation of intermittent claudication in this case can be explained by pressure changes occurring within the cyst during different physical activity.[1] Histologically, the wall of the cyst consisted of collagenous connective tissue covered on the inside by a single interrupted or several layers of cuboid cells akin to synovial mesothelium[2] (Fig. 24.6). The stem connecting with the knee joint had a similar structure. The lumen of both cyst and stem contained viscous basophil fluid; they are therefore best likened to ganglions.

Fig. 24.4 (*Left*) The whole
extent of the 6-cm long cyst
surrounding the popliteal
artery

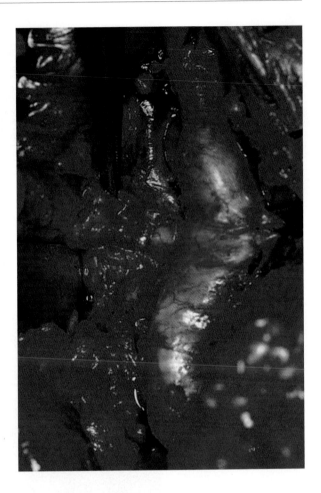

24.1
Commentary

Trauma has been ruled out overwhelmingly on the grounds that the disease would be seen
predominantly in people engaged in competitive sports: this is not the case. All cases of
adventitial cystic disease reported in the literature have occurred in nonaxial vessels during
limb differentiation and development. It is therefore postulated that during limb bud development, cell rests derived from condensations of mesenchymal tissue destined to form the
knee, hip, wrist or ankle joints are incorporated into the nearby and adjacent nonaxial vessels from vascular plexuses during the same stage of development, and in close proximity
to the adjacent condensing joint structures.[3] It is postulated further that these cell rests are
then responsible for the formation of adventitial cystic disease in adult life, when mucoid
material secreted results in a mass lesion within the arterial or venous wall.[3] Figure 24.7
shows a row of cross-sections of a resected and totally occluded popliteal segment. In this

Fig. 24.5 (*Right*) The perivascular cyst being resected, with the artery remaining intact

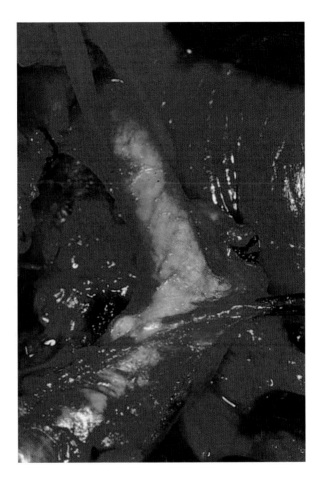

case, the cyst is clearly in the midst of the arterial wall and does not appear to be located in the adventitia.

According to the hypothesis of Levien and Benn,[3] popliteal adventitial cystic disease manifests itself in adults. Early cases manifest in the third decade, but most cases occur in the fourth and fifth decades; it occurs less frequently in later stages of life.[4] The male: female ratio is about 5:1. In summary, there is little doubt that popliteal cystic disease is congenital. **[Q1]**

Popliteal adventitial cysts are located mostly in outer levels, i.e. in the adventitia of the popliteal artery, but they may also occur in the common femoral artery adjacent to the hip joint along the iliofemoral axis, in locations near the elbow or the wrist, and in veins.[5] A total of 45 extrapopliteal localisations have been described. These extrapopliteal locations account for 20–25% of all cases of adventitial cystic disease. Carlsson et al.[6] have also observed adventitial cystic disease in the common femoral artery. **[Q2: B, D, G]**

Fig. 24.6 The wall of the cyst covered on the inside by a single interrupted or several layers of cuboid cells akin to synovial mesothelium

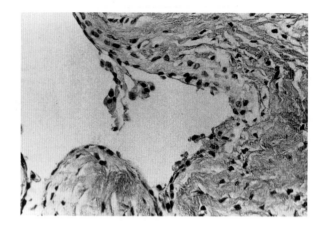

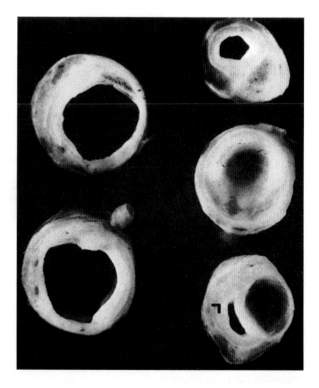

Fig. 24.7 Cross-section through an artery with a large adventitial cyst and compression of the arterial lumen of the resected popliteal artery

Because of the sometimes varying degree of intermittent claudication or occasional disappearance of symptoms, the disease can be mistaken for a popliteal entrapment syndrome. Noninvasive techniques have vastly improved diagnosis. Duplex coloured scanning followed by T2-weighted MRI now appear to be the best choice. Both methods are capable of visualising the cyst surrounding the popliteal artery and ruling out the popliteal entrapment syndrome.[4] Koppensteiner et al.[7] have shown that intravascular ultrasound imaging can reliably identify adventitial cystic disease as well. Digital subtraction angiography is necessary to define the degree of stenosis or the length of occlusion. Stenotic lesions have an hourglass appearance or present with a semilunar impression (the scimitar sign).[4] **[Q3: A, C, E, G, H]**

The treatment options depend on the degree of stenosis and whether the popliteal artery is occluded. In the case of total occlusion, most authors have resorted to total resection of the affected popliteal arterial segment with interposition either of autologous vein or ring-enforced polytetrafluoroethylene (PTFE) grafts. The initial success rate is reportedly almost 90%.[4]

If the cyst lies within the adventitia and surrounds and compresses the artery without having given rise to total occlusion, as in our second case, then the artery does not have to be resected if the cyst can be removed entirely.[1] Partial removal of the cyst is thought to bear the risk of recurrence.[1] If a connecting stem usually accompanied by a small collateral artery is present, then this should be resected at the level of the knee capsule to avoid recurrence.[2] The initial success rate in 68 cases treated accordingly is 94%[4]; in our own experience, it was successful in case 2 described above.[1]

There is the possibility of resecting only part of the artery, e.g. the medial vascular aspect that bears the cyst, and then replacing the wall defect with a vein patch. This approach has been used in a small number of patients, with success in three of four cases.[4] Percutaneous transluminal angioplasty (PTA) has been performed just once, and failed. PTA should therefore probably be discarded as an treatment option.

An interesting series of seven cases has been reported by Do et al.[8] They forwarded a 14-gauge needle with real-time ultrasonic guidance transcutaneously directly into the cyst and aspirated its contents in cases presenting with stenosis only (but not in the presence of total occlusion). This was carried out on an outpatient basis, with a 100% success rate. Follow-up colour duplex sonography performed between 1 and 32 months after the procedure showed no recurrent stenosis.[8]

While the method of percutaneous aspiration of a popliteal cyst guided by ultra-sonography is appealing because it can be done on an outpatient basis and mini-invasively, the question of recurrence is not settled since the cyst remains in place; hence the capacity to form mucinous substance remains and with it the possibility of recurrence. Although Do et al. know of no recurrence in their cases followed up for 1–32 months, there is a definite need for a more systematic long-term follow-up, which should be conducted in all cases in which the cyst has not been removed by resection.

There is the occasional report of percutaneous clot lysis of occluded popliteal arteries followed by aspiration of the contents of the cysts. This method was reported by Samson and Willis[9] to be successful, but its reliability has not been proven by others. There is hardly a valid contraindication against surgical removal of an occluded popliteal segment in the presence of occlusion, and this is probably the method of choice that offers the greatest chances for complete recovery.

Finally, there are reports of spontaneous resolution of the popliteal cysts.[10, 11] It must be assumed, therefore, that occasionally cysts can burst or their contents escape into the periarticular space. This mechanism has been surmised by Soury et al.[10]

In conclusion, the treatment of choice remains surgical resection, either of the cyst alone if it surrounds the artery or of the occluded segment if total occlusion and appositional thrombosis has occurred. In this case, vein graft interposition should be performed. In expert hands, percutaneous transluminal aspiration has been shown to be efficacious. **[Q4]**

Acknowledgement   Special thanks go to Professor Jon Largiadèr, who offered the documentation of the two patients operated on by him at the University Hospital of Zurich.

References

1. Largiadèr J, Leu HJ. Sogenannte zystische Adventitiadegeneration der Arteria poplitea mit Stielverbindung zum Kniegelenk. *Vasa*. 1984;13:267-272.
2. Leu HJ, Largiadèr J, Odermatt B. Pathogenesis of the so-called adventitial degeneration of peripheral blood vessels. *Virchow Arch A*. 1984;404:289-300.
3. Levien LJ, Benn CA. Adventitial cystic disease: a unifying hypothesis. *J Vasc Surg*. 2000;28:193-205.
4. Tsolakis IA, Walvatne CS, Caldwell MD. Cystic adventitial disease of the popliteal artery: diagnosis and treatment. *Eur J Vasc Endovasc Surg*. 1998;15:188-194.
5. Chakfe N, Beaufigeau M, Geny B, et al. Extra-popliteal localizations of adventitial cysts. Review of the literature. *J Mal Vas*. 1997;22:79-85.
6. Carlsson S, Sandermann J, Hansborg N. Adventitial cystic disease in the common femoral artery. *Ann Chir Gynaecol*. 2001;90:63-64.
7. Koppensteiner R, Katzenschlager R, Ahmadi A, et al. Demonstration of cystic adventitial disease by intravascular ultrasonic imaging. *J Vasc Surg*. 1996;23:534-536.
8. Do DD, Braunschweig M, Baumgartner I, Furrer M, Mahler F. Adventitial cystic disease of the popliteal artery: percutaneous guided aspiration. *Radiology*. 1997;2303:743-746.
9. Samson RH, Willis PD. Popliteal artery occlusion caused by cystic adventitial disease: successful by urokinase followed by non-resectional cystotomy. *J Vasc Surg*. 1990;12:591-593.
10. Soury P, Riviere J, Watelet J, Peillon C, Testart J. Spontaneous regression of a sub-adventitial cyst of the popliteal artery. *J Mal Vasc*. 1995;20:323-325.
11. Owen ER, Speechly-Dick EM, Kour NW, Wilkins RA, Lewis JD. Cystic adventitial disease of the popliteal artery – a case of spontaneous resolution. *Eur J Vasc Surg*. 1990;4:319-321.

The Obturator Foramen Bypass

25

Jørgen J. Jørgensen, Andries J. Kroese,
and Lars E. Staxrud

A 62-year-old man presented with a 2-week history of continuous pain in the left lower abdomen radiating to the groin. For several weeks, he had complained of general malaise, including tiredness and poor appetite, and diarrhoea once or twice per day. His general practitioner palpated a pulsating, tender mass in the left groin and referred him to the department of vascular surgery at the nearby university hospital. Three years previously, he had been operated upon with a Dacron aorto-bifemoral bypass for critical ischaemia and intermittent claudication in the left and right lower limbs, respectively. On admission, the patient was in a relatively good general condition, although his body temperature was 38.5°C, pulse rate was 96 bpm, and blood tests showed an elevated sedimentation rate, C-reactive protein (CRP) and leucocyte count. Palpation of the left iliac fossa was slightly painful. The inguinal swelling was covered by erythematous skin and was estimated to be approximately 4 cm in diameter.

Question 1

What is the most likely diagnosis at this stage?

A. False aneurysm/pseudoaneurysm
B. Infected Dacron graft
C. Lymphadenitis
D. Incarcerated inguinal or femoral hernia
E. Incarcerated obturator hernia
F. A-V fistula

Based on the clinical signs and symptoms, treatment with broad-spectrum antibiotics was started.

J.J. Jørgensen (✉)
Department of Vascular Surgery, Oslo University Hospital, Aker, Oslo, Norway

G. Geroulakos and B. Sumpio (eds.), *Vascular Surgery*,
DOI: 10.1007/978-1-84996-356-5_25, © Springer-Verlag London Limited 2011

Question 2

Which of the following investigations should be considered to confirm the diagnosis, and in what order?

A. Duplex scanning
B. Arteriography
C. Computed tomography (CT) scanning with aspiration of perigraft fluid for Gram staining and culture
D. Magnetic resonance imaging (MRI)
E. Leucocyte-labelled scintigraphy
F. Surgical exploration

Ultrasonography revealed that the Dacron graft and femoral arteries were not pathologically dilated but that the anastomotic site was surrounded by fluid. Some of this perigraft fluid was aspirated and was found to contain coagulase-negative staphylococci (CNS). Antibiotic treatment was adjusted accordingly.

Question 3

Vascular graft infection in the groin may be primary treated without resecting the graft itself when there is:

A. No signs of false aneurysm formation
B. An infected anastomosis, but without bleeding
C. A thrombosed graft
D. No septicaemia
E. An infected anastomosis with bleeding

MRI and CT scanning revealed that only the left limb of the bifurcation graft was infected, most likely only in the groin, involving the site of the anastomosis.

Question 4

What treatment options, in addition to antibiotics, are available for the management of an infected vascular graft in the groin?

A. Excision with or without a revascularisation procedure.
B. Repeated extensive wound debridement, and insertion of gentamicin mats.
C. Debridement, skin closure, and insertion of a closed irrigation system.
D. Debridement and muscle flap transposition.
E. None; use long-term antibiotic treatment only.

Since the proximal limit of graft infection could not be ascertained, it was decided to operate on the patient with a partial graft resection. Because the indication for primary operation had been critical ischaemia due to multilevel atherosclerotic disease, revascularisation was planned. Therefore, a preoperative angiography was performed, which showed signs of progressive atherosclerosis as compared with previous angiograms. The proximal part of the left superficial femoral artery was occluded, whereas the distal part was patent. Of the crural arteries, only the posterior tibial was patent. The profunda femoral artery was patent but peripherally stenotic. In the right lower extremity, the superficial femoral artery was occluded, but the profunda artery and three crural arteries were patent, although partially stenotic. Based on these findings, an obturator foramen bypass (OFB) on the left side was planned.

Under general anaesthesia, an 8-mm ring-reinforced polytetrafluoroethylene (PTFE) graft was implanted as an OFB between the proximal part of the limb of the previously implanted Y-graft and the distal superficial femoral artery. During the same operation, the distal part of the infected graft was resected.

Question 5

What is the most common indication for an OFB procedure?

A. Infected femoral (false) aneurysm
B. Revascularisation in cases with extensive local trauma
C. Tissue scarring in the groin subsequent to radical tumour surgery, radiation or burns
D. Sciatic artery aneurysm exclusion
E. Infection confined to the distal part of an aortofemoral bypass graft

Question 6

Describe briefly how you would perform an OFB procedure.

After a hypotensive period on the first postoperative day, the left lower limb showed clinical signs of increased ischaemia. Blood pressure at the ankle was 60 mmHg and the ankle brachial pressure index (ABPI) was 0.4 – slightly lower than preoperatively. Duplex scanning could not rule out a technical defect of the OFB, for example kinking. Therefore, an angiography via the right groin was performed, which did not show any major technical defects. Subsequently anticoagulation therapy was started.

Question 7

What is the least frequent complication of an OFB?

A. Urinary bladder injury
B. Injury of the obturator nerve and blood vessels
C. Kinking of the graft due to erroneous transmuscular tunnelling
D. Infection of the obturator graft
E. Bleeding, thrombosis
F. Injury of the internal iliac artery

The further postoperative course was uneventful. Two weeks later, the patient was discharged with complaints of claudication in the left lower extremity and a walking distance of approximately 50 yards. Oral antibiotics were to be continued for 3 months and anticoagulation indefinitely.

Question 8

What alternative revascularisation procedures after removal of an infected vascular graft in the groin may be considered?

A. Subintimal angioplasty of the native iliac artery
B. Semi-closed endarterectomy (ring-stripping) of the iliac artery
C. Axillofemoral bypass by lateral route
D. Subvulvular bypass
E. Subscrotal bypass
F. Bypass with autologous vein

25.1
Commentary

In patients with a vascular prosthesis anastomosed to the external iliac or common femoral artery, presenting with a painful tumor in the groin, the primary tentative diagnosis should be infected graft. Alternative diagnoses include non-infected false aneurysm, incarcerated inguinal, femoral or obturator hernia, lymphadenitis and A-V fistula. **[Q1: B]**

25.2
Preoperative Measures

Even though positive cultures may be lacking, treatment with intravenous broadspectrum antibiotics, including those against anaerobic microorganisms, are initiated on clinical suspicion of graft infection alone. Late vascular graft infections may be caused by CNS, low virulent bacteria that are often difficult to diagnose by standard techniques.[1]

Preoperatively, it is crucial to obtain as much information as possible about the extent of graft infection. Duplex scanning ultrasonography is an appropriate first modality to evaluate perigraft or other groin masses. CT scanning is more effective in the diagnosis of aortic graft infection, especially when combined with aspiration of perigraft fluid for Gram staining and aerobic and anaerobic cultures.[2] MRI can be even more reliable.[3] However, optimal diagnostic accuracy may be obtained by combining CT or MRI with indium-labelled leucocyte scintigraphy.[4] Duplex scanning and arteriography do not play significant roles in establishing the diagnosis of a vascular graft infection, but they are used for diagnosing graft occlusion, false aneurysm formation and anastomotic bleeding, and for planning the revascularisation procedure. In certain cases of inguinal graft infection, contrast sinography may be appropriate to investigate the extent of infection. Finally, when vascular graft infection is suspected despite negative diagnostic tests, surgical exploration of the graft is necessary to detect the presence of perigraft fluid or to confirm whether the graft is incorporated in tissue. It is generally accepted that firm in-growth of surrounding tissue into the vascular prosthesis excludes the presence of graft infection. Although CT scanning and MRI can be very helpful in delineating the boundaries of infection preoperatively, the final judgement concerning the extent of infection is usually made intraoperatively. [Q2: A, C, D, E, F]

If only the distal part of the graft is infected, there are several therapeutic options in addition to antibiotics. [Q3: A, B, D] If the proximal part of the graft is also infected, then it should be removed entirely. If a revascularisation procedure is warranted, then an extra-anatomic bi- or unilateral axillofemoral bypass may be established, preferably as a first-stage procedure before the entire infected graft is removed.

In the majority of cases, for example if the graft is occluded and the limb is viable, no vascular reconstruction is required.[5] In cases of limited infection, with no signs of anastomotic bleeding or septicaemia, then local treatment without graft resection may be attempted: wound debridement, irrigation, the use of gentamicincontaining collagen mats, and muscle transposition may be alternative ways of treating inguinal vascular graft infections.[6] [Q4: A, B, C, D]

If only the distal part of an aortofemoral prosthesis has to be removed, and revascularisation is necessary, then OFB is a very good alternative. It is not a common operation and comprises less than 0.5% of all arterial reconstructions.[7] Since Shaw and Baue[8] introduced this procedure, published results of OFB rarely comprise more than 10–15 patients.[7, 9–14] However, vascular surgeons should be familiar with its indications and technique when addressing challenging revascularisation problems in a hostile groin.

25.3
The Concept of the Obturator Foramen Bypass

The rationale behind this operation is based on creating an arterial conduit from the aortoiliac segment to the superficial femoral, popliteal or deep femoral artery, depending on run-off conditions, while avoiding contaminated, infected or destroyed tissues in the groin. By routing the vascular graft through the obturator foramen, dorsally to the hip joint, in a layer between the adductor magnus and longus muscles, the area of the femoral triangle is circumvented. Autologous saphenous vein has been shown to give satisfying results, reducing the danger of secondary graft infection.[15] However, since the saphenous vein may be too narrow and/or too short, in most cases an externally reinforced Dacron or PTFE graft is used, especially since these conduits offer greater resistance against compression and kinking. Under special circumstances, the obturator bypass can be performed as a cross-over ilioprofunda procedure using the contralateral iliac artery as the inflow site, the graft being routed through the prevesical space of Retzius.[16]

The main indication for this procedure (80% of cases) is infection confined to the distal iliac and inguinal part of an aortofemoral bypass graft.[1] Other indications include the need for a revascularisation procedure in cases of infected femoral aneurysm, extensive local trauma, tissue scarring in the groin subsequent to radical tumour surgery, and/or therapeutic radiation or burns.[18–20] Over the last years an increasing number of infected pseudoaneurysms in the groin among drug addicts are observed. In need of revascularisation OFB should be considered.[21] Further, as the number of endovascular procedures with percutaneous femoral access has also risen over the last decades an increasing number of groin complications may be even more common in the future.[14] The obturator bypass has also been used in rare cases for revascularisation of sciatic artery aneurysm exclusion.[22] **[Q5: A, E]**

25.4
Obturator Foramen Bypass Technique

The patient lies in the prone position, usually with the hip and knee joints slightly flexed, abducted and externally rotated. Some surgeons prefer to have the hip joint overextended a little to facilitate the tunnelling manoeuvre through the obturator foramen. The operation is usually performed under general anaesthesia, sometimes combined with epidural anesthesia to relieve postoperative pain. In all cases, a urinary catheter should be in place, since urinary bladder injury is a potential danger of this operation. **[Q7]**

If the indication for surgery is an infected prosthetic vascular graft in the groin, then it is an advantage to determine in advance whether a reconstruction is necessary. Thus, the sterile part of the operation, establishing a new vascular conduit, can be done first.[1] The infected groin is sealed off with occlusive drape. Through a longitudinal paramedian incision or a curved, transverse lower abdominal incision, the proximal part of the graft is approached transperitoneally or retroperitoneally, respectively. Retroperitoneal access is a good alternative if one is certain that the infection is limited to the inguinal area. The involved graft limb is dissected proximally, close to the bifurcation. Firm incorporation of the graft in the surrounding tissue and a negative Gram stain of perigraft fluid indicate that the proximal part of the graft can be preserved.[23] The graft limb is then transected, and the distal part is closed by sutures and pushed down towards the inguinal ligament. The overlying peritoneum is oversewn to separate the proximal graft from the infectious area. A ringed PTFE graft of diameter 6 or 8 mm is anastomosed in an end-to-end (Fig. 25.1) or end-to-side fashion to the proximal limb of the bifurcation graft. By careful blunt and sharp dissection, and with the aid of a large-blade self-retaining retractor, the ureter and bladder are identified. The pelvic organs are pushed gently towards the midline, rendering access to the obturator foramen. The sharp edge of the opening in the obturator fascia is usually identified easily by digital palpation on the anteromedial aspect of the foramen. This opening is dilated with long, slim grasping forceps with a blunt tip, taking care not to damage the obturator artery, vein and nerve that curve around the posterolateral edge of the foramen. Alternatively, other designs of blunt tunnellers can be used. It is therefore prudent to lead the forceps through the foramen bimanually, palpating where the tip of the forceps is to meet the fascial opening. We prefer tunnelling through the obturator foramen

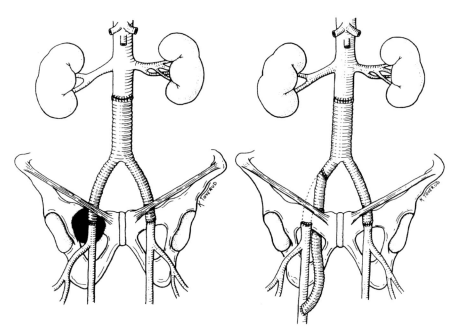

Fig. 25.1 The principle of OFB (Reprinted from Kroese AJ and Rosen L[1] © 1996, with permission from Elsevier)

from below, in a plane anteriorly to the adductor magnus muscle and posteriorly to the pectineus, adductor longus and brevis muscles. Some surgeons choose to do this manoeuvre from the retroperitoneal space downwards.[11] The PTFE graft may be irrigated retrogradely with heparinised saline to ensure unrestricted flow.

Through an incision in the thigh, medial to the sartorius muscle, the femoropopliteal or profunda femoral artery is exposed for the distal anastomosis, which is usually performed in an end-to-side fashion. The profunda femoral artery is situated anteriorly to the adductor magnus and brevis muscles, covered partially by the adductor longus muscle. By retracting the superficial femoral vessels and the vastus medialis muscle laterally, a dense fascia between the adductor longus and the vastus medialis is exposed. This fascia is incised, thereby severing the attachment of the adductor longus to expose the profunda vessels. The overlying profunda vein is often divided and ligated to simplify the approach towards the profunda artery.[24, 25] Rudich et al. report a case of postoperative thigh necrosis which may illustrate that ligation of the proximal popliteal artery above the distal anastomosis should be avoided in fear of insufficient collateral circulation.[26]

After closing the abdominal and thigh incisions, the patient is redraped and the infected groin is exposed. Swabs are taken for bacterial culture. Necessary debridement is performed, the infected anastomosis is excised, and the femoral artery is closed with a running monofilament suture. The infected graft is removed by withdrawing it under the inguinal ligament from the retroperitoneal space. Finally, the wound is irrigated lavishly before closing it over a suction catheter.

Perioperative complications occur in approximately 7% of cases.[8, 12, 27] Bleeding from obturator vessels can be prevented by adhering to sound surgical principles.

Perforation of the urinary bladder, vagina or sigmoid colon by faulty tunnelling of the graft is a serious complication that may lead ultimately to loss of limb.[28, 29]

Since the obturator bypass is threatened by infection, long-term postoperative antibiotic treatment is advised. Although the duration is debatable, a period of 6–12 weeks can usually be agreed upon. Graft thrombosis may lead to severe ischaemic symptoms, and may even threaten the viability of the lower limb, since important collateral vessels in the inguinal region may have been sacrificed during the previous operation. Gluteus muscle necrosis may also compound this critical situation. Therefore, thrombectomy or thrombolysis of the thrombosed OFB graft should be attempted without delay. **[Q7: F]**

The obturator bypass in the management of infected vascular grafts seems to be a valuable procedure.[12, 30] However, long-term results with this operation in terms of patency, limb salvage and survival rates are difficult to evaluate because the studies are usually small and include cases with different indications for obturator bypass. However, the majority of patients suffer from symptomatic peripheral arterial disease. In a review of the literature, perioperative mortality rates varied between zero and 14%. Survival rates after 1 and 5 years were 81% and 61%, respectively. Secondary patency rates for PTFE prostheses at 1 and 5 years were 71% and 52%, respectively. Short-term limb salvage rates up to 76–85%[1] and a 5-year salvage rate of 55% could be achieved.[12] Patel et al. report a graft patency of 80% and limb salvage rate of 60% at 5 years.[14] The results depend on the indication for operation and are better in patients without atherosclerosis. In patients with atherosclerosis, graft patency depends on factors such as run-off conditions and the progression of the underlying atherosclerosis.

There are several other options for revascularisation after the removal of an infected vascular graft in the groin, including semi-closed endarterectomy (ringstripping) or balloon angioplasty of the native iliac artery, axillofemoral bypass by lateral route avoiding the infected groin,[31, 32] and subscrotal bypass.[33] However, the OFB gives better results than bypass through these alternative extraanatomical routes. If the groin is not grossly infected, then an autologous bypass of saphenous[34] or femoral vein[35] or thrombectomised femoral or iliac artery may be placed in situ without causing major problems, although the danger of future graft rupture is always present.[36] In addition, in situ revascularisation with a rifampicin-impregnated graft may give satisfactory results.[37] **[Q8: A, B, C, E, F]**

Although the obturator bypass procedure is not used frequently, it should be a part of the vascular surgeon's armamentarium. It may be effective in solving a difficult revascularisation problem in the groin, if performed appropriately.

References

1. Kroese AJ, Rosen L. What is the optimal treatment for the infected vascular graft? In: Greenhalgh RM, Fowkes FGR, eds. *Trials and tribulations in vascular surgery*. London: WB Saunders; 1996:17-34.

2. Low RN, Wall SD, Jeffrey RB Jr, Sollitto RA, Reilly LM, Tierney LM Jr. Aorto-enteric fistula and perigraft infection: evaluation with computed tomography. *Radiology.* 1990;175:157-162.

3. Spartera C, Morettini G, Petrassi C, et al. The role of MRI in the evaluation of aortic graft healing, perigraft fluid collection and graft infection. *Eur J Vasc Surg.* 1990;4:69-73.

4. Prats E, Banzo J, Abos MD, et al. Diagnosis of prosthetic vascular graft infection by technetium-labelled leukocytes. *J Nucl Med.* 1994;35:1303-1307.

5. Lorentzen JE, Nielsen OM, Arendrup H, et al. Vascular graft infection: an analysis of 62 graft infections in 2411 consecutively implanted synthetic vascular grafts. *Surgery.* 1985;98: 81-86.

6. Kretschmer G, Niederle B, Huk I, et al. Groin infections following vascular surgery: obturator bypass versus biologic coverage – a comparative analysis. *Eur J Vasc Surg.* 1989;3:25-29.

7. Sautner T, Niederle B, Herbst F, et al. The value of obturator bypass. A review. *Arch Surg.* 1994;129:718-722.

8. Shaw RS, Baue AE. Management of sepsis complicating arterial reconstructive surgery. *Surgery.* 1963;53:75-86.

9. Prenner KV, Rendl KH. Indications and techniques of obturator bypass. In: Greenhalgh RM, ed. *Extra-anatomic and secondary arterial reconstructions.* London: Pitman Books; 1982:201-221.

10. Erath HG Jr, Gale SS, Smith BM, Dean RH. Obturator foramen grafts: the preferable alternate route? *Ann Surg.* 1982;48:65-69.

11. Pearce WH, Ricco JB, Yao JS, Flinn WR, Bergan JJ. Modified technique of obturator bypass in failed or infected grafts. *Ann Surg.* 1983;197:344-347.

12. Nevelsteen A, Mees U, Deleersnijder J, Suy R. Obturator bypass: a sixteen year experience with 55 cases. *Ann Vasc Surg.* 1987;1:558-563.

13. Geroulakos G, Parvin SD, Bell PRF. Obturator foramen bypass, the alternative route for sepsis in the femoral triangle. *Acta Chir Scand.* 1988;154:111-112.

14. Patel A, Taylor SM, Langan EM, et al. Obturator Bypass: A Classic Approach for the Treatment of Contemporary Groin Infection. *Am Surg.* 2002;68:653-658.

15. Panetta T, Sottiurai VS, Batson RC. Obturator bypass with nonreversed translocated saphenous vein. *Ann Vasc Surg.* 1989;3:56-62.

16. Atnip RG. Crossover ilioprofunda reconstruction: an expanded role for obturator foramen bypass. *Surgery.* 1991;110:106-108.

17. Stain SC, Weaver FA, Yellin AE. Extra-anatomic bypass of failed traumatic arterial repairs. *J Trauma.* 1991;31:575-578.

18. Donahoe PK, Froio RA, Nabseth DC. Obturator bypass graft in radical excision of inguinal neoplasm. *Ann Surg.* 1967;166:147-149.

19. Wood RFM. Arterial grafting through the obturator foramen in secondary haemorrhage from the femoral vessels. *Angiology.* 1982;33:385-392.

20. Ferreira U, Reis LO, Ikari LY, et al. Extra-anatomical transobturator bypass graft for femoral artery involvement by metastatic carcinoma of the penis: report of five patients. *Worl J Urol.* 2008;26:489-491.

21. Matoussevitch V, Aleksic M, Gawenda m, Brunkwall J. Primary extraanatomical revascularization for groin infections in drug addicts. *VASA.* 2007;36:210-214.

22. Urayama H, Tamura M, Ohtake H, Watanabe Y. Exclusion of a sciatic artery aneurysm and an obturator bypass. *J Vasc Surg.* 1997;26:697-699.

23. Padberg FT, Smith SM, Eng RHK. Accuracy of disincorporation for identification of vascular graft infection. *Arch Surg.* 1995;130:183-187.

24. Nunez AA, Veith FJ, Collier P, Ascer E, Flores SW, Gupta SK. Direct approaches to the distal portions of the deep femoral artery for limb salvage bypasses. *J Vasc Surg.* 1988;8:576-581.

25. Millis JM, Ahn SS. Transobturator aorto-profunda femoral artery bypass using the direct medial thigh approach. *Ann Vasc Surg.* 1993;7:384-390.

26. Rudich M, Gutierrez IZ, Gage AA. Obturator Foramen Bypass in the Management of Infected Vascular Prostheses. *Am J Surg*. 1979;137:657-660.

27. Det RF, Brands LC. The obturator foramen bypass: an alternative procedure in iliofemoral artery revascularisation. *Surgery*. 1981;89:543-547.

28. Sheiner NM, Sigman H, Stilman A. An unusual complication of obturator foramen arterial bypass. *J Cardiovasc Surg*. 1969;10:303-314.

29. Szilagyi DE, Smith RF, Elliott JP, Vrandecic MP. Infection in arterial reconstruction with synthetic grafts. *Ann Surg*. 1972;176:321-326.

30. Lai TMD, Huber D, Hogg J. Obturator foramen bypass in the management of infected prosthetic vascular grafts. *Aust N Z J Surg*. 1993;63:811-814.

31. Leather RP, Karmody AM. A lateral route for extra-anatomical bypass of the femoral artery. *Surgery*. 1977;81:307-309.

32. Trout HH, Smith CA. Lateral iliopopliteal arterial bypass as an alternative to obturator bypass. *Ann Surg*. 1982;48:63-64.

33. Baird RN. Subscrotal bypass for the infected groin. In: Greenhalgh RM, ed. *Vascular and endovascular techniques*. London: WB Saunders; 1994:257-259.

34. Scriven MW, Oshodi TO, Lane IF. Saphenous vein grafting in aortic graft infection: a new answer to and old challenge. *Eur J Vasc Endovasc Surg*. 1995;10:258-260.

35. Nevelsteen A, Lacroix H, Suy R. Autogenous reconstruction with the lower extremity deep veins: an alternative treatment of prosthetic infection after reconstructive surgery for aortoiliac disease. *J Vasc Surg*. 1995;22:129-134.

36. Ehrenfeld WK, Wilbur BG, Olcott CN, Stoney RJ. Autogenous tissue reconstruction in the management of infected prosthetic grafts. *Surgery*. 1979;85:82-92.

37. Young RM, Cherry KJ Jr, Davis PM, et al. The results of in situ prosthetic replacement for infected aortic grafts. *Am J Surg*. 1999;178:136-140.

Diabetic Foot

26

Mauri J.A. Lepäntalo, Milla Kallio, and Anders Albäck

A 54-year-old smoker with type 2 diabetes of 7 years duration had a minor abrasion to the lateral aspect of the left fifth toe. The patient was known to have hypertension, nephropathy and retinopathy, and he was overweight. His glycaemic control was good following recent addition of insulin to his oral medication. The superficial ulcer did not bother the patient, and it was initially followed up in his local healthcare centre. Two months later, the patient was referred to a community hospital because of infection and suspicion of osteomyelitis. He now had an infected ulcer lateral to the head of the fifth metatarsal, with a discharge. Plain X-ray films showed suspected osteomyelitis. Dorsalis pedis and posterior tibial pulses were reported to be present. The C-reactive protein (CRP) level was 31 mg/L, leucocytes 14.8×10^9/L, and blood glucose 12 mmol/L.

Question 1

What condition(s) are likely to be responsible for the foot problem?

A. Infection
B. Atherosclerotic macroangiopathy
C. Diabetic microangiopathy
D. Neuropathy

Question 2

What is the simplest tool available in the surgery or outpatient clinic to detect osteomyelitis?

A. Plain X-ray films.
B. Clinical examination with blunt nasal probe.
C. Magnetic resonance imaging.
D. Computer tomography.

M.J.A. Lepäntalo (✉)
Department of Vascular Surgery, Helsinki University Central Hospital, Helsinki, Finland

G. Geroulakos and B. Sumpio (eds.), *Vascular Surgery*,
DOI: 10.1007/978-1-84996-356-5_26, © Springer-Verlag London Limited 2011

Question 3

What simple tools are available in the surgical outpatient clinic to assess angiopathy?

A. Palpation of foot arterial pulses.
B. Examination of audible signal with hand-held continuous wave Doppler.
C. Ankle pressure measurement.
D. Duplex scanning of lower extremity arteries.

Question 4

What simple tools are available in the surgery or outpatient clinic to assess neuropathy?

A. Monofilament sensation testing.
B. Achilles tendon reflex.
C. Tuning fork testing.
D. Electroneuromyography (ENMG).

The patient was admitted to the medical ward for treatment of his infected foot. Despite the administration of intravenous antibiotic treatment, later modified according to the results of bacterial cultures, the infection progressed. One week after admission, lateral and superficial plantar compartments were drained operatively on the lateral side of the fifth metatarsal head and between the fourth and fifth metatarsal heads. Abundant pus was obtained, and the fifth metatarsal head was observed to be soft. The operative wound was left open. The infection seemed to subside, and the patient was discharged after a 16-day admission with oral clindamycin treatment and local wound care.

Question 5

What major problems were neglected at this point?

A. Presence of osteomyelitis.
B. Presence of ischaemia.
C. The wound was left without coverage with split thickness skin grafting.
D. The weight-bearing wound area of the foot was not protected with a cast.

Despite continuous antibiotic treatment and local treatment of the open lesion on the lateral aspect of the foot, the situation worsened over the next 2 months and the patient was readmitted to the hospital. The patient had fever and his CRP level was 123 mg/l. The serum creatinine was 1.6 mg/dL. An immediate wound debridement and amputation of the fourth toe was performed, after which the patient was admitted to a vascular surgical unit (Fig. 26.1). There was a faint popliteal pulse with no other pulses palpated distally. Ankle brachial indices (ABIs) were 1.35 and 1.21. The patient could not feel the

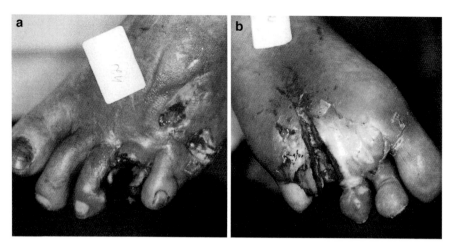

Fig. 26.1 Foot at the time of admission to the vascular unit

touch of the monofilament on the plantar surface of the great toe or the first and fifth metatarsal heads.

Question 6

How would you further examine the circulation non-invasively or invasively?

A. Toe pressure measurement.
B. Ankle pressure measurements and pulse wave recordings.
C. Treadmill test with pressure measurements.
D. Duplex scanning of distal arteries.
E. Magnetic resonance angiography.
F. Digital subtraction angiography.

The toe pressures were 73 mm Hg on the right side and 29 mm Hg on the left side. A selective angiography was obtained the next day (Fig. 26.2).

Question 7

What angiographic findings typical of diabetes can you see?

A. Normal aortoiliac segments.
B. Haemodynamically non-significant occlusive disease of crural vessels.
C. Significant occlusive disease of crural vessels.
D. Severe occlusive disease of all foot vessels.
E. Patent foot vessel.

Fig. 26.2 Angiography of the left lower limb

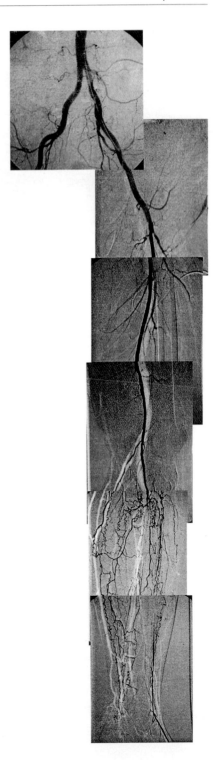

Question 8

What treatment strategy would you prefer?

A. No possibilities for reconstruction. Choose the best medical treatment, then wait and see.
B. No possibilities for reconstruction. Foot-level amputation up to bleeding tissue.
C. Below-knee amputation.
D. Possible acute debridement, reconstruction to pedal artery, and further wound excision later.
E. No wound excision and reconstruction to pedal artery until the wounds are clean.

Question 9

If you consider vascular reconstruction, what would be your preferred inflow site in this patient?

A. Common femoral artery.
B. Superficial femoral artery.
C. Popliteal artery.

A popliteopedal reconstruction was made 5 days after admission to the vascular surgical unit. The great saphenous vein was used in situ with the supragenicular popliteal artery as an inflow vessel. Despite achieving an acceptable initial flow of 51 mL/min, the graft thrombosed the next day and a thrombectomy and a revision of the graft was made. A narrow segment below the knee was replaced with a reversed proximal great saphenous vein under angioscopic control. A flow of 110 mL/min was measured with transit time flowmetry.

Question 10

Which of the following methods are adequate for intraoperative control?

A. Angiography alone.
B. Doppler alone.
C. Flowmetry alone.
D. Flowmetry with a method giving morphological information.
E. Intraoperative duplex scanning alone.

The postoperative ABI was 0.97. Wound excision and three-ray amputation of the lateral toes were performed 2 days after revascularisation. The patient was discharged 2 weeks after admission and transferred to the community hospital. Split thickness skin grafting was performed there. The patient was discharged home with a heel-sandal (an offloading shoe in which the body weight is borne only by the heel), antibiotic treatment for one more week, and local wound care. The healing of the wound progressed well. Six weeks after the vascular reconstruction, the patient was prescribed insoles. He also used a silicon piece correcting the position of the second toe (Fig. 26.3).

Fig. 26.3 Foot at 1-year follow-up

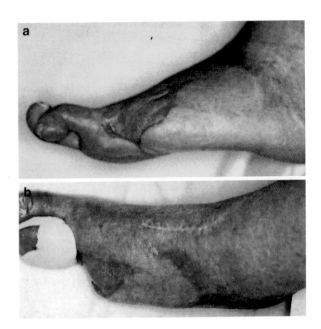

At 1-year follow-up, ABI was greater than 1.3/0.91 and toe pressures were 65/55 mm Hg. Duplex surveillance findings indicated a possible vein graft stenosis.

Question 11

What are the findings indicating vein graft stenosis in the duplex examination?

A. Midgraft peak systolic velocity (PSV) of less than 45 cm/s.
B. V2/V1 ratio greater than 3 (V2, PSV at the site of the maximum stenosis; V1, PSV in the normal graft adjacent to the stenosis).
C. Maximum PSV greater than 300 cm/s.
D. End-diastolic flow velocity (EDV) greater than 20 cm/s.

A control angiography was performed, but no severe stenosis was found (Fig. 26.4).

26.1
Commentary

This case illustrates the problems related to delayed diagnosis and treatment of diabetic neuroischaemic foot. The aetiology of diabetic foot ulceration and infection is multifactorial. Our patient evidently had infection and also neuropathy. Neuropathy often abolishes sensation, and an unpleasant odour and discharge may be the first signs of infection to the

Fig. 26.4 Control angiography after 1-year follow-up

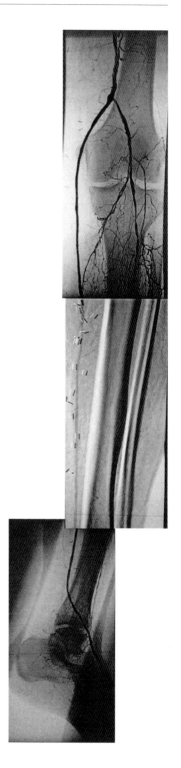

Table 26.1 Classification of diabetic foot lesions by grading and staging according to the depth of the lesion and the presence of infection and ischaemia, as proposed by Armstrong et al.2 Updated

Depth
Grade 0: pre- or post-ulcerative site which has healed
Grade I: superficial wound through the epidermis or epidermis and dermis which does not penetrate to tendon, capsule or bone
Grade II: wound which penetrates to tendon or capsule
Grade III: wound which penetrates to bone or joint
Infection and ischaemia
Stage A: clean wound
Stage B: non-ischaemic infected wound
Stage C: ischaemic non-infected wound
Stage D: ischaemic infected wound to tendon, capsule or bone

patient, especially if the lesion is situated on the plantar aspect of the foot. The role of microangiopathy in diabetic foot is not confirmed, but ischaemia due to atherothrombotic disease often plays a major role.[1] **[Q1: A, B, D]**

The simplest method is to examine the ulcer with a blunt nasal probe. If it hits the bone, then osteomyelitis is most likely. The diabetic wounds should be classified systematically according to a precise system, such as the Armstrong classification (Table **26.1**), which takes into account both the depth of the lesions and the presence of ischaemia and infection.[2] Plain X-ray films are of limited value and magnetic resonance imaging (MRI) is the most reliable tool for diagnosis of osteomyelitis.[3] **[Q2: B]**

The patient was reported to have palpable distal pulses at one time but not at another time. Furthermore, the popliteal pulse was reported to be palpable and ABI to be normal. Palpation of foot pulses is not a fully reproducible observation, and they may be considered normal if both tibialis posterior and dorsalis pedis pulses are clearly felt.[4] If either is not palpated, non-invasive evaluation is necessary. It is far more difficult to palpate the popliteal pulse, and it has been suggested that if an inexperienced palpator feels the popliteal pulse, this indicates an aneurysm. Systolic pressure measurements taken at the level of the ankle by a Doppler device are the most common non-invasive method for assessment of atherothrombotic disease. However, the results may be biased due to the presence of mediasclerosis, which is present in 15–40% of diabetics.[5] Incompressible arteries may allow the signal to be heard in cuff pressures as high as the patient tolerates. In patients with mediasclerosis, the ABI typically exceeds 1.15.[6] The audible Doppler signals may help the examiner, as an open inflow channel gives high-pitched biphasic signals but collateral flow around an occlusion usually gives only a low-pitched monophasic murmur. **[Q3: A, B, C]**

Symptoms of neuropathy include loss of sensation, hyperaesthesia and burning, and aching pain, which are often worse at night.[7] Many patients with severe neuropathy are asymptomatic. Achilles tendon reflex, monofilament sensation testing and 128-Hz tuning fork testing are other recommended clinical tests.[8] **[Q4: A, B, C]**

The primary diagnostic work-up in this case was clearly deficient. The patient obviously had osteomyelitis, which would have necessitated prompt drainage and amputation. Furthermore, the role of ischaemia should also have been evaluated and corrected within 3–5 days after proper drainage. **[Q5: A, B]**

The Doppler-derived pressures were clearly pseudohypertensive due to the arterial wall stiffness. Pseudohypertension affects digital arteries far less frequently, and therefore toe pressures are more reliable. A pulse volume recording at the ankle can also help to detect mediasclerosis. Another method is to measure systolic blood pressure at the ankle with Doppler but without an occluding cuff – the pole test.[9] The examiner listens to the Doppler signals of the supine patient while the foot is elevated gradually until the signals disappear. The scale in the pole gives the pressure at the ankle ($0.75 \times$ pressure (cm) equals the pressure (mm Hg)). In centres where duplex scanning of distal arteries can be done by trained validated examiners this method would preferably be the next investigation. Magnetic resonance angiography is also a method of choice if high-quality images are available and especially when the patient suffers from marked nephropathy. On the other hand in centres where technically demanding endovascular procedures can be done during diagnostic contrast angiography this is – as in our case – the primary imaging technique. **[Q6: A, B, D, E, F]**

Atherosclerotic changes in diabetes are typically situated in femoral and crural arteries, or only in crural arteries, in contrast to non-diabetic patients who tend to have the first symptoms from the obliteration of the aortic bifurcation. Despite proximal crural artery occlusion, the pedal arteries may be patent, as was the dorsalis pedis artery in this patient. **[Q7: A, C, E]**

The treatment strategy is affected strongly by the presence and severity of infection. A superficial ulceration may be only the tip of the iceberg. There may be penetration, hidden to the eye, into deep tissues. Vigorous debridement must be carried out to establish the degree of penetration and to remove all necrotic tissue.[3] Fulminant infection may necessitate guillotine amputation. The bypass can often be performed 3–5 days after debridement. If ischaemia plays a major role and the infection is quiescent, then revascularisation can, in selected cases, be performed first. Vascular reconstruction can be performed in as many as 90% of diabetic patients with peripheral arterial disease.[10] The best outflow vessel in continuity with the foot should be selected.[11] Diabetes is not considered to affect the outcome of graft patency, although female diabetic patients are reported to have worse outcome regarding patency and leg salvage.[12] In limbs with large tissue defects, a microvascular free muscle flap transfer can be used for defect coverage in conjunction with long bypass.[13] **[Q8: D]**

Short bypasses do well if the inflow artery is not compromised, as in our patient. Although the above-knee popliteal artery gave better results as the inflow vessel than the below-knee popliteal artery in our own series,[14] the question is not settled. **[Q9: C]**

Angiography is the gold standard for intraoperative monitoring. The accuracy of flowmetry is affected strongly by the reproducibility of the method. In contrast to older methods, transit-time flowmetry, which does not require information on the diameter of the vessels, has proven to be very accurate.[15] Despite this, it gives only flow values and does not inform about the morphology. The present case clearly shows how the typically narrow segment of the great saphenous vein below the knee was missed despite good flow during the initial hyperaemia. In this area, there was an intimal tear caused by the valvulectomy catheter. Unfortunately, an angioscope was not used in the first operation. An angioscope visualises the inner surface of the vessel, whereas intravascular ultrasound is better for detecting changes within the vessel wall. Doppler and duplex may be used for intraoperative monitoring as well. Doppler gives only haemodynamic information, whereas duplex gives a combination of anatomical and haemodynamic information. There is no best method for intraoperative monitoring, but the optimal method would be to have both hae-modynamic and morphological information. **[Q10: A, D, E]**

As there is a 30% risk of developing neointimal hyperplasia and graft stenosis within the first postoperative year, duplex surveillance is considered an essential part of postoperative care. All the suggested duplex criteria are indicative of vein graft stenosis, but none of them can be 100% sensitive in detecting stenosis.[16] Our case demonstrates that using liberal duplex criteria, false positive findings are easily encountered as the angiography was deemed normal. **[Q11: A, B, C, D]**

References

1. LoGerfo FW, Coffman JD. Vascular and microvascular disease in the diabetic foot: implications for foot care. *N Engl J Med.* 1984;311:1615-1619.
2. Armstrong DG, Lavery LA, Harkless LB. Validation of a diabetic wound classification system. *Diabetes Care.* 1998;21:855-859.
3. Levin ME, O'Neal LW. *The Diabetic Foot.* St Louis: Mosby; 1983.
4. Lundin M, Wiksten JP, Peräkylä T, et al. Distal pulse palpation: is it reliable? *World J Surg.* 1999;23:252-255.
5. Lehto S, Niskanen L, Suhonen M, Rönnemaa T, Laakso M. Medial artery calcification. A neglected harbinger of cardiovascular complications in non-insulin-dependent diabetes mellitus. *Arterioscler Thromb Vasc Biol.* 1996;16:978-983.
6. Takolander R, Rauwerda JA. The use of non-invasive vascular assessment in diabetic patients with foot lesions. *Diabet Med.* 1996;13:S39-42.
7. Veves A, Sarnow MR. Diagnosis, classification and treatment of diabetic peripheral neuropathy. *Clin Pod Med Surg.* 1995;12:19-30.
8. International Working Group on the Diabetic Foot. International consensus on the diabetic foot. Netherlands: International Working Group on the Diabetic Foot, 1999.
9. Smith FCT, Shearman CP, Simms MH, Gwynn BR. Falsely elevated ankle pressures in severe leg ischaemia: the pole test – an alternative approach. *Eur J Vasc Surg.* 1994;8:408-412.
10. Reiber GE, Lipsky BA, Gibbons GW. The burden of diabetic foot ulcers. *Am J Surg.* 1998;176(2A):5S-10S.
11. LoGerfo FW, Gibbons GW, Pomposelli FB, et al. Trends in the care of the diabetic foot. expanded role of arterial reconstruction. *Arch Surg.* 1992;127:617-621.
12. Lepäntalo M, Tukiainen E. Combined vascular reconstruction and microvascular muscle flap transfer for salvage of ischaemic legs with major tissue loss and wound complications. *Eur J Vasc Endovasc Surg.* 1996;12:1-5.
13. Luther M, Lepäntalo M. Femorotibial reconstructions for chronic critical leg ischaemia: influence on outcome by diabetes, gender and age. *Eur J Vasc Endovasc Surg.* 1997;13:569-577.
14. Biancari F, Kantonen I, Albäck A, Ihlberg L, Lehtola A, Lepäntalo M. Popliteo-to-distal bypass grafts for leg ischaemia. *J Cardiovasc Surg.* 2000;41:281-286.
15. Albäck A, Mäkisalo H, Nordin A, Lepäntalo M. Validity and reproducibility of transit time flowmetry. *Ann Chir Gynaecol.* 1996;85:325-331.
16. Sladen JG, Reid JD, Cooperberg PL, et al. Color flow duplex screening of infrainguinal grafts combining low and high velocity criteria. *Am J Surg.* 1989;158:107-112.

Part IV

Surgery of the Major Branches of the Infradiaphragmatic Aorta

Chronic Visceral Ischemia

27

George Geroulakos and William Smead

A 68-year-old woman presented with a 19-month history of generalized abdominal pain. Initially, she experienced the pain following meals, but subsequently the pain became persistent. Over this period of time, she lost 12 kg in weight. For the last few months before admission, she started having diarrhea once to twice per day. There was no blood or mucus in the stool. Her past medical history included partial gastrectomy 17 years earlier for benign disease. On examination, the patient looked cachectic. Her abdomen was slightly distended, and the bowel sounds were increased. There was a high-pitched epigastric bruit. Routine blood tests were normal.

Question 1

Which is the likely diagnosis for our patient on the basis of the available information so far?

A. Cancer of the pancreas
B. Peptic ulcer
C. Subacute intestinal obstruction secondary to adhesions
D. Mesenteric angina
E. Cancer of the large bowel

Fecal fat measurement was 17.6 g/day (normal value <6 g/day). Gastroscopy was performed, which showed features compatible with atrophic gastritis. This was followed by computed tomography (CT) scanning of the abdomen, which reported that the pancreas could not be defined well as a result of paucity of retroperitoneal fat. In addition, CT showed non-specific thickening of the small-bowel loops. Endoscopic retrograde cholecystopangreatography (ERCP) was performed, which ruled out pancreatic pathology. A small-bowel enema did not demonstrate any significant findings. A colonoscopy was performed, which showed two isolated ulcers in the ascending colon (Fig. 27.1) and raised the possibility of ischaemic colitis. Figure 27.2 shows the lateral aortogram of our patient, and demonstrates an occlusion of the coeliac artery and 95% stenosis of the superior mesenteric artery. A diagnosis of chronic visceral ischaemia was made.

G. Geroulakos (✉)
Imperial College of Science Technology and Medicine,
Charing Cross Hospital, and Ealing Hospital, London, UK

G. Geroulakos and B. Sumpio (eds.), *Vascular Surgery*,
DOI: 10.1007/978-1-84996-356-5_27, © Springer-Verlag London Limited 2011

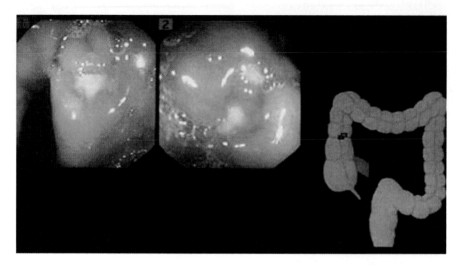

Fig. 27.1 Colonoscopic view of an isolated ulcer in the ascending colon in a patient with chronic visceral ischemia

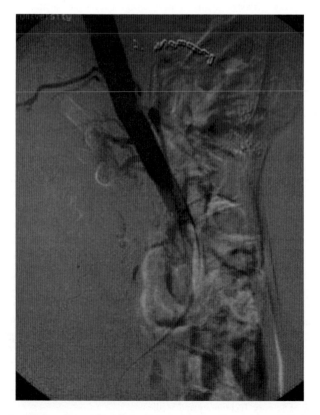

Fig. 27.2 Lateral aortogram demonstrating occlusion of the coeliac artery and a 95% stenosis of the superior mesenteric artery

Question 2

Which of the following statements regarding chronic visceral ischaemia is correct?

A. It has a marked male preponderance.
B. As described in our patient, it usually takes more than 1 year from the first presentation of the symptoms until the final diagnosis is made.
C. It presents clinically as an undiagnosed malignancy.
D. Symptoms occur when at least one of the three visceral arteries has significant disease.
E. It may cause malabsorption.

The patient underwent antegrade revascularisation, via a ninth rib extraperitoneal thoracoabdominal approach, of the coeliac artery and the revascularisation, superior mesenteric artery. An 8-mm Dacron graft was used approach, as a conduit.

Question 3

Which of the following statements regarding the management of this patient are false?

A. The best patency can be achieved using a venous conduit.
B. Revascularisation of the coeliac artery was unnecessary, and equally good results could have been achieved with revascularisation of only the superior mesenteric artery.
C. Surgical revascularisation should not have been considered in this elderly, frail patient because it has an excessive mortality rate of about 30% in most series.
D. Percutaneous transluminal angioplasty (PTA) should have been the method of choice.

The postoperative recovery of the patient was uneventful. She was discharged home on the eighth postoperative day. Six months later, she was asymptomatic and had gained 5 kg in weight. However, at 12 months the patient presented to the outpatient clinic with recurrent postprandial abdominal pain. A duplex examination showed that the graft to superior mesenteric artery anastomosis had more than 60% stenosis and the graft to coeliac artery anastomosis was occluded.

Question 4

What would you advise your patient?

A. Reoperation aiming to revascularise the coeliac artery and place a patch on the graft to superior mesenteric artery anastomosis.
B. Angioplasty and stenting of the graft to superior mesenteric artery anastomosis.
C. Conservative management advising the patient to take small and frequent meals.
D. Start the patient on Cilostazol 100 mg twice per day.

The patient underwent angioplasty and stenting of the graft to superior mesenteric artery anastomosis with an excellent technical and clinical result. Twenty-four months following this procedure the patient remains asymptomatic.

27.1
Commentary

As described in our patient, the clinical picture of chronic visceral ischaemia includes abdominal pain with or without diarrhea and weight loss. The diagnosis of chronic visceral ischaemia is in doubt if the patient has no significant decrease in total body mass. The abdominal pain occasionally radiates to the back. The pain of visceral ischaemia has similarities to that of carcinoma of the stomach, pancreatic carcinoma and peptic ulceration. Diarrhea may be explained by the increased motility of the bowel induced by the ischaemia; it may also be secondary to malabsorption. [Q1: A, B, D, E]

Other symptoms that may be seen include nausea and vomiting, which have been associated with gastric motility disorders caused by ischaemia.[1] An epigastric bruit may or may not be present. Our group and others have reported a marked female patient distribution of this condition.[2-4] The reason for this peculiar sex distribution remains undetermined. However, it has been suggested that it could be the result of the inclusion of cases of Takayasu's aortitis in reports of atherosclerotic chronic visceral ischaemia.[5] Takayasu's aortitis closely mimics atherosclerosis of the abdominal aorta and has a marked female predominance. The time from the onset of symptoms to diagnosis is usually more than 12 months.[6] The diagnosis of chronic visceral ischaemia is a clinical one. As shown clearly in our case, contrast studies, abdominal ultrasound, endoscopy and CT are not essential to the diagnosis but will prove important in eliminating other sources of abdominal discomfort. In all instances, lateral views of biplane aortography demonstrate visceral occlusive lesions compatible with the diagnosis. As a result of an abundant network of collateral vessels, clinical symptoms are present when at least two of the three visceral arteries have significant disease. There are known asymptomatic cases with all three visceral arteries thrombosed, thus emphasizing the fact that chronic visceral ischaemia cannot be diagnosed exclusively on the basis of X-rays. [Q2: B, C, E]

Techniques of revascularisation include transection and reimplantation, bypass grafting, endarterectomy and balloon angioplasty with or without stent placement. There is no consensus regarding the best surgical approach for the treatment of chronic visceral ischaemia. This condition is encountered infrequently, and it is unlikely that a single center can treat enough patients and accumulate sufficient experience to develop principles of treatment by demonstrating significant differences between the various mesenteric revascularisation strategies. Bypass grafting is the most common type of visceral revascularisation performed; it may originate from several different locations, including the supracoeliac aorta, the infrarenal aorta and the common iliac arteries. Regardless of the bypass technique used, the status of the donor artery is critical to success.[7] The distal thoracic aorta is usually free of atherosclerotic disease and is an excellent origin of a short antegrade bypass to the superior mesenteric artery. The bypass is placed in the direction of normal blood flow, thus reducing anastomotic turbulence. In addition, this design eliminates the possibility of kinking and thrombosis by compression or traction from the overlying intestinal mesentery, which may be observed with retrograde grafts originating from the infrarenal aorta or the iliac arteries. The distal portion of the thoracic aorta may be approached from the abdomen through division of the crura.[8]

There is no uniform agreement about the graft material of choice. In early reports, vein grafts had patency rates inferior to synthetic grafts.[9,10] More recent reports described the use of either autogenous veins or prosthetic grafts with excellent long-term function and no difference in patency rates.[11,12] In our case, we used synthetic Dacron bypass because it is always available, spares the patient from the morbidity of one or more incisions for the harvesting of the vein, and provides good early and long-term results. Aorto-superior mesenteric artery bypass alone is usually sufficient to provide good symptomatic relief as a result of the extensive collateral circulation, even when all three visceral arteries are occluded. Hollier et al.[13] have shown that complete revascularisation in multivessel disease resulted in a late recurrence of 11%, while when one of three stenotic vessels was revascularised the recurrence rate was 50%. They concluded that it is preferable to revascularise as many vessels as possible to provide the best chance of long-term relief. Most recent series report an acceptable operative mortality rate ranging from 3% to 8%. Our patient could have been considered for angioplasty of the superior mesenteric artery. In a recent large series of patients ($n = 51$) who had angioplasty and stenting as first choice treatment for the management of chronic visceral ischaemia the initial technical success rate was 93%. No 30-day mortality was observed. During a median follow up of 25 months, two patients died of mesenteric ischemia and the 2 year primary patency rate dropped to 60%.[14] A recent review comparing surgical and endovascular revascularization for chronic mesenteric ischaemia concluded that surgical treatment has superior long-term patency and requires fewer reinterventions. However it is more invasive with greater morbidity and mortality compared to endovascular treatment. Endovascular techniques may be preferable in patients with significant co-morbidities, concomitant aortic disease or indeterminate problems.[15] [Q3: False A, B, C, D]

Recurrent visceral ischaemia is not uncommon after primary visceral revascularisation for chronic visceral ischaemia. In a large series of 109 patients who underwent primary visceral revascularisation at the University of California, San Francisco over a period of 38 years, 19 patients had recurrent visceral ischemia, 12 (11%) patients had recurrent chronic visceral ischemia, and seven (6.4%) had acute visceral ischemia.[16] The minimally invasive nature of the endovascular techniques and the increased complication rate of reoperations renders the endovascular approach a reasonable first option in properly selected patients with recurrent symptoms.[17] [Q4: B]

References

1. Babu SC, Shah PM. Celiac territory ischemic syndrome in visceral artery occlusion. *Am J Surg.* 1993;166:227-230.
2. Geroulakos G, Tober JC, Anderson L, Smead WL. Antegrade visceral revascularisation via a thoracoabdominal approach for chronic visceral ischaemia. *Eur J Vasc Endovasc Surg.* 1999;17:56-59.
3. Zelenock G, Graham LM, Whitehouse WM, et al. Splanchnic arteriosclerotic disease and intestinal angina. *Arch Surg.* 1990;115:497-501.
4. Geelkerken RH, van Bockel JH, De Ross WK, Hermans J, Terpstra JL. Chronic mesenteric vascular syndrome. Results of reconstructive surgery. *Arch Surg.* 1991;126:1101-1106.

5. Lande A. Abdominal Takayasu's aortitis, the middle aortic syndrome and atherosclerosis. *Int Angiol.* 1998;17:1-9.
6. Schneider PA, Ehrenfeld WK, Cunningham CG, Reilly LM, Goldstone J, Stoney RJ. Recurrent chronic visceral ischaemia. *J Vasc Surg.* 1992;15:237.
7. Rheudasil JM, Stewart MT, Schellack JV, Smith RB, Salam AA, Perdue GD. Surgical treatment of chronic mesenteric arterial insufficiency. *J Vasc Surg.* 1988;8:495-500.
8. Kazmers A. Operative management of chronic mesenteric ischaemia. *Ann Vasc Surg.* 1998;12:299-308.
9. Rob C. Surgical diseases of the celiac and mesenteric arteries. *Arch Surg.* 1966;93:21-30.
10. Stoney RJ, Ehrenfeld WK, Wylie EJ. Revascularization methods in chronic visceral ischaemia caused by atherosclerosis. *Ann Surg.* 1977;186:468-476.
11. Bauer GM, Millay DJ, Taylor LM, Porter JM. Treatment of chronic visceral ischaemia. *Am J Surg.* 1984;148:138-144.
12. McMillan WD, McCarthy WJ, Bresticker MR, et al. Mesenteric artery bypass: objective patency determination. *J Vasc Surg.* 1995;21:729-741.
13. Hollier LH, Bernatz PE, Pairolero PC, Spencer Payne W, Osmundon PJ. Surgical management of chronic intestinal ischaemia. A reappraisal. *Surgery.* 1981;90:940-946.
14. Fioole B, van de Rest HJ, van Leersum M, et al. Percutaneous transluminal angioplasty and stenting as first-choice treatment in patients with chronic mesenteric ischaemia. *J Vasc Surg.* 2010;15:386-391.
15. Biebl M, Oldenburg WA, Paz-Fumagalli R, McKinney JM, Hakaim AG. Surgical and interventional visceral revascularization for the treatment of chronic mesenteric iscahemia- when to prefer which? *World J Surg.* 2007;31:562-568.
16. Schneider DB, Schneider PA, Reilly LM, Ehrenfeld WK, Messina LM, Stoney RJ. Reoperation for recurrent chronic visceral ischaemia. *J Vasc Surg.* 1998;27:276-286.
17. Robless P, Belli AM, Geroulakos G. Endovascular versus surgical reconstruction for the management of chronic visceral ischaemia: a comparative analysis. In: Geroulakos G, Cherry K, eds. *Diseases of the Visceral Circulation.* London: Arnold; 2002:108-118.

Acute Mesenteric Ischemia

28

Jonathan S. Refson and John H.N. Wolfe

A 78-year-old woman presented to the emergency department with a 12-h history of sudden-onset abdominal pain. She had vomited after the pain started, and she had also had two episodes of diarrhoea. Until this time, she had been well, although she was known to be in atrial fibrillation and took digoxin 125 mg daily.

On examination, she was distressed and obviously in pain. Baseline observations revealed a pulse of 110 bpm, irregularly irregular, blood pressure of 95/60 mm Hg, respiratory rate of 28 breaths/min, and temperature of 37.3°C. Her chest was clear, heart sounds were normal (irregular rhythm), and the jugular venous pressure was not elevated. Abdominal examination was unremarkable, with a soft abdomen and minimal tenderness despite severe pain, and normal bowel sounds.

The investigations shown in Table 28.1 were performed by the admitting surgeon.

Electrocardiogram (ECG) revealed atrial fibrillation with no other acute changes. Erect chest X-ray revealed normal lung fields and no free gas under the diaphragm. Abdominal radiography was unremarkable except for minimal small-bowel distension.

Question 1

Which of the following is the most unlikely diagnosis?

A. Acute ulcerative colitis
B. Pancreatitis
C. Mesenteric venous thrombosis (MVT)
D. Acute mesenteric ischaemia (AMI)
E. Diabetic ketoacidosis

J.S. Refson (✉)
Department of Vascular Surgery, Princess Alexandra Hospital, Harlow, UK

G. Geroulakos and B. Sumpio (eds.), *Vascular Surgery*,
DOI: 10.1007/978-1-84996-356-5_28, © Springer-Verlag London Limited 2011

Table 28.1 Investigations performed by the admitting surgeon Updated

Investigation	Finding
Urinalysis	No abnormality
Biochemistry	Na⁺ 139 mmol/l
	K⁺ 4.6 mmol/l
	Creatinine 112 mmol/l
	Glucose 6.1 mmol/l
	Amylase 2000 IU/l
Haematology	Haemoglobin 12.3 g/dl
	White cell count 27,000
	Platelets 235,000
Arterial blood gas	pH 7.21
	pCO$_2$ 3.2 kPa
	pO2 9.4 kPa
	HCO$_3^-$ 17 mmol/l
	Base excess -8

Question 2

What are the most common causes of AMI?

A. Renal failure
B. Atrial fibrillation
C. Multi-organ failure
D. Anti-phospholipid syndrome
E. Atherosclerotic disease

Question 3

Which of the following tests are of use in the acute management of a patient with AMI?

A. Echocardiography
B. Lateral-view mesenteric angiography
C. Thyroid function tests (TFTs)
D. Non-contrast computed tomography (CT) scanning
E. Mesenteric vessel duplex Doppler

At this point, the patient was taken to the high-dependency unit, where the following measures were undertaken: high-flow oxygen therapy by mask (15 L/min), continuous ECG monitoring, central venous pressure (CVP) monitoring, urinary catheter inserted to monitor urinary flow hourly, and infusion of 4 L of fluid resuscitation. Intravenous broad-spectrum antibiotics and an anticoagulant dose of intravenous heparin were also given. After 2 h of resuscitation, the patient's blood pressure was 130/85 mm Hg, pulse 100 bpm and CVP +8 cm water. She was still in a lot of pain despite 10 mg of diamorphine, and she was still tachypnoeic. Repeat blood gas and blood count investigations were as in Table 28.2.

Because the patient was persistently acidotic with an elevated white count and in severe pain, she was taken to the operating theatre for an emergency laparotomy. Almost the

Table 28.2 Repeat blood gas and blood count investigations. Updated

Investigation	Finding
Haematology	Haemoglobin 10.2 g/dL White cell count 37,000 × 10⁹/L Platelets 235 × 10⁹/L
Arterial blood gas	pH 7.19 pCO_2 3.1 kPa pO_2 49.4 kPa HCO_3^- 11 mmol/L Base excess −15

entire small bowel and most of the large bowel were found to be ischaemic but viable. There was a pulse in the proximal superior mesenteric artery (SMA) but nothing was palpable beyond the origin of the middle colic vessel.

Question 4

What operative options are available to achieve restoration of flow to the bowel?

A. Full heparinisation
B. Catheter thrombectomy
C. Axillofemoral bypass
D. Mesenteric bypass with a vein graft
E. Mesenteric bypass with prosthetic graft

Clot was removed successfully from the SMA. However, despite the majority of the bowel receiving a good blood supply, several areas remained dusky in appearance.

Question 5

What features of the bowel's appearance determine whether it is viable?

A. The presence of peristalsis
B. Lack of foul odour from the peritoneal cavity
C. Serosal sheen
D. Mesenteric pulsation
E. Active bleeding from the cut surface of the bowel at the time of resection

Question 6

Having determined that an area of the bowel is non-viable, what action should you take?

A. Revascularise the bowel, then remove that which is non-viable
B. Remove the non-viable bowel, then revascularise the remaining bowel

C. Resect all non-viable bowel and primarily anastomose ends; then close the abdomen
D. Close the abdomen and start the patient on an intravenous infusion of diamorphine
E. Resect all non-viable bowel and exteriorise viable ends; plan relook laparotomy

28.1
Commentary

The incidence of AMI is approximately 1/100,000 in the UK and USA.[1,2] AMI is a life-threatening vascular emergency. It accounts for 0.1% of emergency admissions,[3] and based on several large series it has a mortality of between 60% and 100%.[3-7] Females are affected twice as often as males, and the median age at presentation is 70 years.[6]

The clinical presentation is often not as clear-cut as described in the case above. However, some if not all of the described features will be present. One must have a high index of clinical suspicion in anyone aged over 55 years who presents with abdominal pain out of proportion to the physical signs elicited on abdominal examination.[8] The diagnosis should also be considered in patients with known peripheral arterial disease and abdominal pain. The triad of abdominal pain, a cardiac source of embolus and gut emptying, as described by Klass,[9] make AMI the most likely diagnosis. In addition to this triad, the finding of a marked leucocytosis, metabolic acidosis and hyperamylasaemia are also suggestive of AMI. It is also not unusual for there to have been a history of previous embolic events.[8] Pancreatitis can be difficult to differentiate from AMI, and laparotomy is indicated if suspicion of AMI is aroused. **[Q1: E]**

Defining the aetiology of AMI is important as the different causes have different treatments. The most common presentation, as described in our case, is of superior mesenteric embolus; this accounts for about 50% of all cases.[3,5-7] The usual source for these clots is the atria in patients in atrial fibrillation or the ventricle if the patient has recently sustained a myocardial infarction. Another potential source of emboli is atheroma from the aortic wall following radiological procedures in which catheters and guidewires have been passed up the aorta. The consequence of such an event can be catastrophic, as the mesenteric circulation has not had time to develop a collateral circulation.

The next most frequent aetiology is SMA thrombosis, which accounts for between 25% and 50% of cases.[3,5-7] This results from progression of atheromatous disease at the origin of the SMA. It is important to note that a long-standing stenosis may have caused symptoms of chronic mesenteric ischaemia in the months before its ultimate occlusion.[10] Therefore, in a patient with pre-existing symptoms of mesenteric ischaemia, sudden onset of abdominal pain should be regarded as AMI until proven otherwise.

Non-occlusive mesenteric ischaemia (NOMI), first described by Ende in 1958,[11] is the next most frequently encountered condition, occurring in about 20% of cases.[3,5,6] In this situation, the patient is often critically ill from another cause and the mesenteric ischaemia is due to vasoconstriction leading to reduced flow in the splanchnic circulation. This may be due to cardiogenic shock, hypovolaemia or vasoconstricting inotropes. Even after reversal of shock, mesenteric hypoperfusion may persist for several hours.[12,13]

MVT is the least common cause and accounts for about 5% of AMI.[14–16] The thrombotic process is thought to start in the superior mesenteric vein and spreads to the portal vein; the inferior mesenteric vein is usually spared. The onset of symptoms is more insidious and may have a history of several days. It is caused by the same provoking factors that one finds in any thrombotic situation: sluggish flow, clotting abnormality and vessel wall damage (Virchow's triad). It is associated most commonly with hypercoagulable states, abdominal trauma or intra-abdominal sepsis.[17–20] The diagnosis is often made at laparotomy and encompasses a spectrum of severity from segmental mesenteric venous thrombosis to the entire portal vein being thrombosed. **[Q2: B, E]**

Diagnostic confirmation of AMI poses a dilemma. Should one delay in order to confirm a suspicion and risk converting a salvageable situation into a non-salvageable one?[21] There is little evidence on which to base sound advice. However, if the patient is cardiovascularly stable with minimal symptoms, and one has prompt access to angiography, then this provides accurate diagnosis (Fig. 28.1). Some authors recommend colour-flow duplex at the bedside during the resuscitation phase[22, 23]; this procedure is less time-consuming than angiography, but it requires considerable skill that is not always available. Furthermore, good views are often hampered by obesity and/or overlying bowel gas.

Transthoracic echocardiography is useful in identifying a cardiac source for emboli and may help in making the decision regarding postoperative anticoagulation. However, it is not as sensitive as transesophageal echo in searching for left atrial emboli and may waste valuable time.

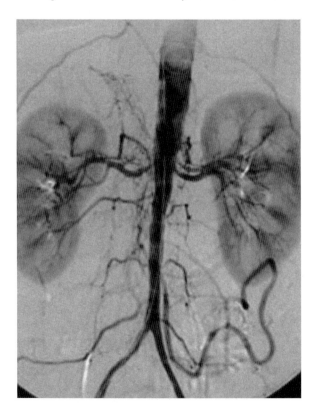

Fig. 28.1 Narrowed atherosclerotic aorta with no coeliac or superior mesenteric filling

Contrast-enhanced CT may be of use in identifying mesenteric venous thrombosis.[24] This will not prevent laparotomy as bowel resection may well be necessary. If there is clear evidence of peritonism and a high index of suspicion for AMI, then the patient should be resuscitated rapidly and this should be followed by urgent laparotomy. **[Q3: B, E]**

In order to answer Question 4, one has to be confident of the aetiology of AMI. In our case, there is embolus in the SMA. The abdomen should be approached through a long midline incision, which will afford excellent exposure. Having entered the abdomen, a quick survey of the viscera and extent of ischaemia should give some information on the aetiology of the AMI (see below). At this point, the main aim of surgery is to restore flow to the ischaemic viscera if viable. In order to do this, the transverse mesocolon is elevated and the ligament of Treitz identified and the fourth part of the duodenum mobilised. The root of the mesentery is palpated to feel for the SMA pulse. If, as in our case, the AMI is due to an embolic event, then a proximal SMA pulse should be palpable and the duodenojejunal flexure and proximal few centimetres of jejunum should be viable. The emboli usually lodge at a variable site 3–8 cm from the origin of the SMA, usually at the point where the middle colic artery arises[6,8,21] (Fig. 28.2a, b).

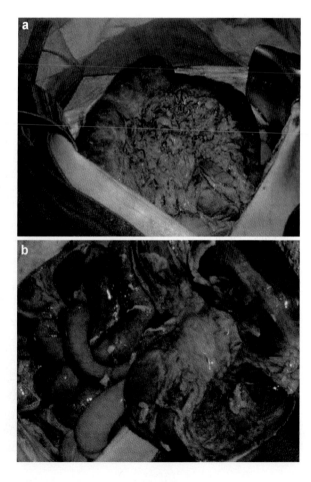

Fig. 28.2 (**a, b**) Patchy mid-gut infarction due to atherosclerotic occlusion of superior mesenteric artery (SMA)

In order to expose the SMA, the inferior leaflet of the mesocolon is entered along the course of the vessel and a 5-cm section of artery is dissected out and slung with Silastic sloops. At this point, if the patient has not been heparinised previously, then they should be given an intravenous dose of 5000 units of unfractionated heparin. A longitudinal arteriotomy is made in the cleared SMA (on the left margin of the vessel, to permit easier graft placement, should a bypass be necessary),[21] and a size 3 or 4 Fogarty embolectomy catheter is passed up and down the vessel to retrieve the embolus. Once adequate backward and forward flow has been achieved, the vessel should be flushed with heparinised saline; the arteriotomy can then be closed primarily or with a patch (depending on size), using a 6/0 or 7/0 Prolene suture.

At this point, the anaesthetist should be warned that you are about to reperfuse the viscera. Metabolites that have accumulated in the ischaemic viscera will pass rapidly from the mesenteric venous circulation into the systemic circulation, which can precipitate circulatory collapse and, over several hours, result in the development of systemic inflammatory response syndrome (SIRS). There is no point in revascularising dead bowel; indeed, this is dangerous. Irrefutably dead bowel should be removed before revascularisation. It is important to note that if, on opening the abdomen, the entire small bowel is black and irreversibly ischaemic, then the most appropriate thing to do is close the abdomen and keep the patient comfortable with morphine: death will usually follow within a matter of hours.

In the event that there is no pulse palpable at the SMA origin, then the revascularisation strategies are similar to those for chronic visceral ischaemia (see Chapter 24). In this case, attempts at thrombectomy will fail as the catheter will not cross the occlusion. The options available are retrograde bypass from the infrarenal aorta to the SMA, antegrade bypass from the supracoeliac aorta (with concomitant revascularisation of the coeliac trunk if it is occluded), aortomesenteric endarterectomy, or side-to-side anastomosis between the SMA and aorta. Prosthetic material should be avoided since transmural migration of bacteria is likely to contaminate the graft. Also, if the lower aorta and iliac systems are heavily calcified, then it may be better to select the supracoeliac aorta for the inflow site of the bypass. The use of a temporary shunt for immediate reperfusion while the bypass is being constructed seems sensible.[21]

At this point in the procedure, the viscera need to be inspected again and any dubiously viable bowel resected. If the patient is otherwise young and fit, then it may be better to resect all the necrotic bowel, exteriorise the remaining ends, and consider long-term total parenteral nutrition or small-bowel transplantation. If there is no evidence of arterial compromise and a pulse is palpable in the SMA, then one should suspect either NOMI or MVT.

NOMI usually results in widespread patchy ischaemia. Treatment entails resection of obviously non-viable bowel, attempting to be as conservative as possible. The remaining bowel must be inspected at a second-look laparotomy 24–48 h later. During surgery, several strategies have been described to improve mesenteric flow: a combination of systemic dopamine and an opiate epidural,[25] papaverine infusion (30–60 mg/h) into the SMA either via direct puncture fine bore or angiographically placed catheter.[13,26,27] At relook laparotomy, the extent of the ischaemia should be reassessed; treatment may need to be abandoned if the gangrene is progressing. Mortality of this condition is depressingly high at 70–80% despite the therapeutic measures outlined above.[13]

The classic laparotomy findings in MVT are ascites and swollen omentum with bowel infarction. Like NOMI, MVT is managed by resection of non-viable bowel, which is most frequently sharply demarcated and found in the mid-small bowel. Again, second-look laparotomy is mandatory. Anticoagulation with heparin and then warfarin is mandatory in view of the high incidence of recurrent MVT. Investigation of any underlying prothrombotic disorder along with long-term anti-coagulation improves survival.[28,29]

Thrombolysis has been used successfully in MVT in two studies where the diagnosis had been established by non-invasive means and peritoneal signs had not developed.[30,31] Venous thrombectomy has also been reported to be successful in a handful of cases.[19,32-34] This procedure is likely to be difficult, as the peritoneum is usually oedematous. **[Q4: B, D]**

The classic features of ischaemia are oedema, loss of peristalsis, loss of surface sheen, staining of the serosa, absent mesenteric pulsation, or frank gangrene with or without perforation (Fig. 28.3). The decision at surgery is, after revascularisation (providing it was appropriate or feasible), how much small bowel to resect. Once there is good flow to the viscera, then reversibly ischaemic segments should declare themselves viable and the rest will need to be resected. Other adjuncts to inspection and palpation are continuous-wave Doppler, pulse oximetry and fluorescein dye.[35] The next question is whether to exteriorise or anastomose the open ends of the bowel. The arguments against exteriorising are that many stomata may be necessary and they do not guarantee that the intervening segments may not subsequently become ischaemic; however, this is extremely safe and avoids the complication of a necrotic anastomosis. Performing primary anastomoses and leaving the abdomen open and covering it with a see-through bag (a cut-open bag of saline)[36] allows direct visualisation of the viscera at all times; second-look laparotomy can then be planned on the appearance of the gut.[36] If all looks well by 72 h and the patient's condition is stabilising, then they can be returned to theatre for planned abdominal closure. **[Q5: A, C, E], [Q6: B, E]**

The short-term management of these cases is demanding on staff and time, but if best results are to be achieved, then no short cuts can be taken.

AMI is a treatable vascular emergency. It requires a high index of clinical suspicion, rapid aggressive resuscitation and diagnostic manoeuvres to determine the specific underlying cause. This will allow a prompt, directed revascularisation procedure after optimisation

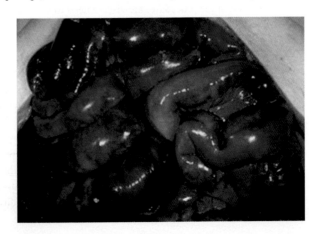

Fig. 28.3 Gut showing features of fixed staining

of cardiac performance, or correction of a hypercoagulable state. This effort is directed at maximising the amount of salvageable bowel. These strategies are the cornerstones for a successful outcome in this life-threatening vascular catastrophe.

References

1. Marston A. Diagnosis and management of intestinal ischaemia. *Ann R Coll Surg Engl.* 1972;50:29-44.
2. Stemmer EA, Connolly JE. Mesenteric vascular insufficiency. Identification and management. *Calif Med.* 1973;118:18-29.
3. Stoney RJ, Cunningham CG. Acute mesenteric ischemia. *Surgery.* 1993;114:489-490.
4. Klempnauer J, Grothues F, Bektas H, Pichlmayr R. Long-term results after surgery for acute mesenteric ischemia. *Surgery.* 1997;121:239-2343.
5. Montgomery RA, Venbrux AC, Bulkley GB. Mesenteric vascular insufficiency. *Curr Probl Surg.* 1997;34:941-1025.
6. McKinsey JF, Gewertz BL. Acute mesenteric ischemia. *Surg Clin North Am.* 1997;77:307-318.
7. Schoots IG, Koffeman GI, Legemate DA, Levi M, van Gulik TM. Systematic review of survival after acute mesenteric ischaemia according to disease aetiology. *Br J Surg.* 2004;91(1):17-27.
8. Bergan JJ. Diagnosis of acute intestinal ischaemia. *Semin Vasc Surg.* 1990;3:143-148.
9. Klass AA. Embolectomy in acute mesenteric ischaemia. *Ann Surg.* 1951;134:913-917.
10. Dunphy JE. Abdominal pain of vascular origin. *Am J Med Sci.* 1936;192:109-112.
11. Ende N. Infarction of the bowel in cardiac failure. *N Engl J Med.* 1958;258:879-881.
12. Fry RE, Huber PJ, Ramsey KL, Fry WJ. Infrarenal aortic occlusion, colonic blood flow, and the effect of nitroglycerin afterload reduction. *Surgery.* 1984;95:479-486.
13. Boley SJ, Sprayregan S, Siegelman SS, Veith FJ. Initial results from an aggressive roentgeno-logical and surgical approach to acute mesenteric ischemia. *Surgery.* 1977;82:848-855.
14. Rhee RY, Gloviczki P. Mesenteric venous thrombosis. *Surg Clin North Am.* 1997;77:327-338.
15. Bassiouney HS. Non-occlusive mesenteric ischaemia. *Surg Clin North Am.* 1997;77:319-326.
16. Krupski WC, Selzman CH, Whitehill TA. Unusual causes of mesenteric ischaemia. *Surg Clin North Am.* 1997;77:471-502.
17. Clavien PA, Durig M, Harder F. Venous mesenteric infarction: a particular entity. *Br J Surg.* 1988;75:252-255.
18. Grewal HP, Barrie WW. Congenital antithrombin III deficiency causing mesenteric venous infarction: a lesson to remember – a case history. *Angiology.* 1992;43:618-620.
19. Vates P, Cumber PM, Sanderson S, Harrison BJ. Mesenteric venous thrombosis due to protein C deficiency. *Clin Lab Haematol.* 1991;13:137-139.
20. Tossou H, Iglicki F, Casadevall N, Delamarre J, Dupas JL, Capron JP. Superior mesenteric vein thrombosis as a manifestation of a latent myeloproliferative disorder. *J Clin Gastroenterol.* 1991;13:597-598.
21. Whitehill TA, Rutherford RB. Acute intestinal ischaemia caused by arterial occlusions: opti-mal management to improve survival. *Semin Vasc Surg.* 1990;3:149-156.
22. Nicoloff AD, Williamson WK, Moneta GL, Taylor LM, Porter JM. Duplex ultrasonography in evaluation of splanchnic artery stenosis. *Surg Clin North Am.* 1997;77:339-355.
23. Jager K, Bollinger A, Valli C, Ammann R. Measurement of mesenteric blood flow by duplex scanning. *J Vasc Surg.* 1986;3:462-469.

24. Clavien PA, Huber O, Mirescu D, Rohner A. Contrast enhanced CT scan as a diagnostic proce-
    dure in mesenteric ischaemia due to mesenteric venous thrombosis. *Br J Surg.* 1989;76:93-94.
25. Lundberg J, Lundberg D, Norgren L, Ribbe E, Thorne J, Werner O. Intestinal hemodynamics
    during laparotomy: effects of thoracic epidural anesthesia and dopamine in humans. *Anesth
    Analg.* 1990;71:9-15.
26. Aldrete JS, Han SY, Laws HL, Kirklin JW. Intestinal infarction complicating low cardiac
    output states. *Surg Gynecol Obstet.* 1977;144:371-375.
27. Rivers SP. Acute non-occlusive intestinal ischaemia. *Semin Vasc Surg.* 1990;3:172-175.
28. Jona J, Cummius GM, Head MB, Govostis MC. Recurrent primary mesenteric venous throm-
    bosis. *JAMA.* 1974;227:1033-1035.
29. Matthews JE, White RR. Primary mesenteric venous occlusive disease. *Am J Surg.*
    1971;122:579-583.
30. Al Karawi MA, Quaiz M, Clark D, Hilali A, Mohamed AE, Jawdat M. Mesenteric vein throm-
    bosis, non-invasive diagnosis and follow-up (US + MRI), and non-invasive therapy by strep-
    tokinase and anticoagulants. *Hepatogastroenterology.* 1990;37:507-509.
31. Robin P, Gruel Y, Lang M, Lagarrigue F, Scotto JM. Complete thrombolysis of mesenteric
    vein occlusion with recombinant tissue-type plasminogen activator. *Lancet.* 1988;1:1391.
32. Inahara T. Acute superior mesenteric venous thrombosis: treatment by thrombectomy. *Ann
    Surg.* 1971;174:956-961.
33. Mergenthaler FW, Harris MN. Superior mesenteric vein thrombosis complicating pancre-
    atoduodenectomy: successful treatment by thrombectomy. *Ann Surg.* 1968;167:106-111.
34. Daune B, Batt M, Graglia JC, et al. Mesenteric ischemia of venous origin. The value of early
    computed tomography. *Phlebologie.* 1990;43:615-618.
35. Tollefson DF, Wright DJ, Reddy DJ, Kintanar EB. Intraoperative determination of intestinal
    viability by pulse oximetry. *Ann Vasc Surg.* 1995;9:357-360.
36. Agrawal T, Refson J, Gould S. Telly Tubby Tummy, a novel approach to the management of
    laparostomy. *Ann R Coll Surg.* 2001;83(6):440.
37. Hanisch E, Schmandra TC, Encke A. Surgical strategies – anastomosis or stoma, a second
    look – when and why? *Langenbecks Arch Surg.* 1999;384:239-242.

Renovascular Hypertension

29

Constantina Chrysochou and Philip A. Kalra

A 55-year-old male is referred for investigation of lower limb claudication pains. His past medical history includes long standing hypertension and a previous myocardial infarction 3 years previously with subsequent coronary angioplasty and stenting. He is a life long smoker, but rarely takes any alcohol. His symptomatic claudication arises after walking for approximately 200 m on the level. He is receiving an angiotensin converting enzyme inhibitor (ACE-I), which, according to the General Practitioner's letter, was commenced about 2 months before referral, and he also receives a diuretic and a calcium antagonist at full dosage to optimize his blood pressure. On examination he is noted to have bilateral ilio-femoral bruits but palpable pedal pulses. His blood pressure remains sub-optimally controlled at 170/90 mmHg. He is commenced on an alpha-blocker (Doxazosin).

Following the clinic visit you review his blood results and notice that there has been a deterioration in his renal function with the serum creatinine increasing from 120 to 180 µmol/L and estimated glomerular filtration rate (eGFR) decreasing from 58 to 36 mL/min since the time of referral.

Question 1

Which of the following statements support your suspicion that the patient has renovascular disease contributing to his poorly controlled blood pressure?

A. Longstanding hypertension

B. There is difficulty in controlling the blood pressure with three different anti-hypertensive drugs

C. There was a relatively rapid deterioration of renal function between the time of referral and the first clinic visit

D. He is an arteriopath with symptoms of lower limb claudication pains

C. Chrysochou (✉)
Department of Renal Medicine, Salford Royal Hospital and University of Manchester, Manchester, UK

G. Geroulakos and B. Sumpio (eds.), *Vascular Surgery*,
DOI: 10.1007/978-1-84996-356-5_29, © Springer-Verlag London Limited 2011

Question 2

What would be the most appropriate investigation(s) to decide whether the hypertension has a renovascular origin?

A. Direct intra-arterial angiography
B. Renography with captopril provocation
C. Magnetic resonance angiography (MRA)
D. Computerized tomography angiogram (CTA)
E. Duplex ultrasound of the renal arteries

In this patient, magnetic resonance imaging showed diffuse aorto-iliac disease. There was a 90% stenosis with post stenotic dilatation at the ostium of the left renal artery and the kidney was 10 cm in length. On the right hand side there were two renal arteries, the smaller of these exhibited a 50% renal artery stenosis (RAS). The kidney measured 11 cm in length.

In view of the deterioration in renal function and the poorly controlled hypertension it is decided to stop the ACE-inhibitor and to proceed to intervention.

Question 3

What is the most appropriate revascularization approach for the renal artery stenosis?

A. Aortorenal bypass
B. Thromboendarterectomy
C. Percutaneous transluminal angioplasty (PTA) with stent
D. PTA alone
E. Nephrectomy

Question 4

Which are the most frequent serious complications seen after renal artery PTA?

A. Arterial rupture
B. Occlusion
C. Cholesterol microembolisation
D. Contrast-related Acute kidney injury
E. Groin haematoma

The patient underwent percutaneous angioplasty with bare-metal stent placement in the left renal artery. The right renal artery was not amenable to endovascular intervention. The procedure progressed without complications and the patient was sent home the day after treatment in good condition.

He was reviewed again after 2 weeks at which stage his creatinine had improved to 140 μmol/L (eGFR 49 mL/min). His blood pressure (165/90) control had improved to some extent.

Question 5

Which of the following would be most appropriate for his future management?

A. Regular clinic review with attention to medical control of blood pressure, and vasculo-protective therapy

B. Repeat renal artery imaging with possible repeat left renal artery stenting

C. Right renal artery PTA and stenting

D. Surgical revascularization of the left kidney

29.1
Commentary

Renovascular disease is common, and atheromatous renovascular disease (ARVD) accounts for 90% of renal artery stenosis (RAS) in western populations. The remainder is mainly due to fibromuscular disease (FMD) which usually presents as hypertension in younger patients.

There has been a steady increase in the number of patients diagnosed with ARVD in the last 2 decades.[1] ARVD is a disease of ageing just as is the case with other traditional macrovascular atheromatous diseases, and it is strongly associated with coronary artery disease (CAD), congestive cardiac failure, aorto-iliac and more distal peripheral vascular disease (PVD) and cerebrovascular disease. The finding of ARVD during investigation and management of one of these other vascular diseases can be of detrimental prognostic importance.[2,3] For example, 15–30% of patients with CAD have evidence of ARVD, with RAS>50% detectable in about 5%.[4] A close relationship exists between the number of diseased CAD vessels and severity of RAS.[4] In turn, prospective observational studies have shown that the presence and severity of RAS confer a negative impact upon survival in these CAD patients.[5] Due to anatomic proximity, aorto-iliac disease is very frequently associated with ARVD, most studies showing that around 40–45% of patients referred for investigation of PVD have the disease.[6]

ARVD can be identified in about 2% of selected hypertensive populations.[7] Conversely, around 90% of patients with ARVD have hypertension, but whether this hypertension is the direct result of ARVD, rather than simply an association, is often difficult to determine. A strict definition of "renovascular hypertension" necessitates that the hypertension is cured or substantially improved following correction of the RAS (usually with revascularization). Renovascular hypertension has been listed as the primary cause of end stage renal disease(ESRD) in 5.2%[8] of the US dialysis population. With an increasingly ageing population, the incidence of ARVD is likely to continue to rise, as will the related cardiological and renal burden on the healthcare system.

Clinical features which would lead a clinician to suspect ARVD include:

- Patients with cardiovascular risk factors, e.g., smokers, type 2 diabetics, evidence of atheroma in other vascular beds
- Rapid onset of hypertension in young people (FMD)
- Rapid deterioration of previously well-controlled essential hypertension
- Malignant/accelerated hypertension or hypertensive crises
- Three-drug- (or more) resistant hypertension
- Hypertension and deteriorated renal function
- Impaired renal function on commencement of renin angiotensin blocking (RAB) therapy (ACE inhibitors, angiotensin receptor blockers or renin inhibitors)
- Flash pulmonary oedema
- Epigastric, flank or back bruit
- Discrepancy of >1.5 cm between kidney sizes on imaging

In our patient, the presence of concomitant vascular disease and marked smoking history provided a higher suspicion for ARVD. The sudden deterioration in renal function with RAB and poorly controlled hypertension supported investigation for renovascular hypertension. [Q1: B, C, D]

Many radiological techniques have been used to investigate the presence of RAS. All these methods have their advantages and disadvantages. The three most commonly used radiological methods are magnetic resonance angiography (MRA), computerized tomography angiography (CTA) and duplex sonography as they are non-invasive and they can provide a reasonable estimation of the degree of RAS. The most appropriate radiological method will depend on availability, and the patient's level of kidney function – due to the risks posed by nephrogenic systemic fibrosis (NSF) and contrast induced nephropathy in those with severe renal dysfunction (see below). The various investigational methods are briefly considered below:

29.2
MRA

Advantages: Contrast enhanced MRA with gadolinium (Gd) provides a non-invasive, rapid and accurate investigation of the degree of RAS[9–11] with high specificity and sensitivity (Fig. 29.1). MR imaging (MRI) has the potential to assess the functional and morphological characteristics within the renal parenchyma.

Disadvantages: Gd-enhanced MRI has been implicated in causing cases of NSF in patients with moderate to severe renal impairment,[12,13] the condition being characterized by skin thickening, systemic fibrosis and even death. Guidance from the UK Commission on Human Medicines recommends that certain types of Gd containing agents should not be used in patients with advanced CKD with the result that MRA is now performed with

Fig. 29.1 Magnetic resonance angiography image showing a tight stenosis on the left side (*white arrow*) and a shrunken kidney downstream to the stenosis

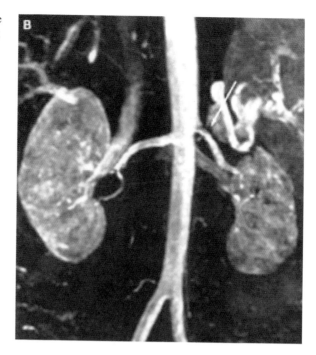

major caution in patients in CKD stages 4 and 5.[14] Other contraindications to MR imaging include patients with metallic implants such as pacemakers, and claustrophobia.

29.3
CTA

Advantages: CTA can acquire a large amount of data in a relatively short time. It has similar sensitivity/specificity to MRA for detection of RAS (Fig. 29.2).

Disadvantages: The disadvantages of CTA are the need to use significant amounts of potentially nephrotoxic iodinated contrast which may result in contrast nephropathy in those with low GFR. Patients are also exposed to relatively high doses of ionizing radiation, and the presence and degree of RAS can often be obscured by heavily calcified vessels.

29.4
Intra-arterial Angiography

Advantages: Accurate assessment of the degree of RAS. Usually only employed to confirm the presence of RAS at a renal angioplasty procedure.

Disadvantages: This is an invasive procedure and the most costly investigative method for ARVD. It provides only 2-D images and also poses a risk of contrast nephropathy.

Fig. 29.2 CTA with red arrow
indicating area of stenosis
(Courtesy of Dr. Alistair
Cowie, Radiology
Department, Salford Royal
Hospital)

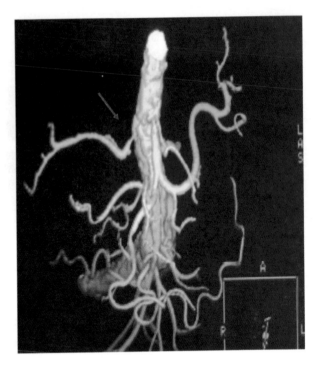

29.5
Duplex Ultrasonography (DU)

Advantages: DU is sensitive for the detection of RAS and the doppler waveforms obtained can provide an indication of distal and intra-renal arteriosclerosis. Color or power Doppler and the use of ultrasonic contrast agents are more promising in functional assessment, but are still experimental innovations.

Disadvantages: Studies are time consuming, operator dependent and have been shown to be subject to wide intra- and inter-observer variations.

Intra-arterial Doppler: allows assessment of distal vascular disease using intra-renal blood flow velocity measurements.[15] However, it is an invasive procedure which is not generally applicable in clinical practice.

Captopril renography: is now an outdated technique rarely used to detect functionally significant RAS except in true renovascular hypertension with normal renal function. Its diagnostic usefulness is limited in CKD. Captopril renography has been shown to be inferior to CTA and MRA in detecting RAS in meta-analyses of these techniques.[16]

The most appropriate radiological techniques for **Question 2 would be options C, D or E**. Our patient underwent an MRA.

29.6
Treatment

One of the major priorities in the management of ARVD is to improve blood pressure to reduce cardiovascular burden and prevent renal decline. However, the treatment of ARVD has been the subject of much debate in recent years, particularly because of the possibility that renal revascularization therapy might improve patient outcomes. In the past there has been limited high-quality evidence regarding outcomes after revascularization, but in the latter part of 2009 the initial results of the ASTRAL trial were published, a study which recruited over 800 patients.[17]

29.6.1
Medical Treatment

ARVD is part of a diffuse vascular disease process and extra-renal vascular pathology is the major contributor to poor outcome. Cardiovascular protection forms the mainstay of treatment. Lifestyle changes include smoking cessation. Patients should receive an anti-platelet agent and a statin.[18] Anti-hypertensive medication should be titrated aiming for a blood pressure of <130/80, although this can be a hard target to achieve given the long-standing nature of the hypertension and arterial stiffness seen in some cases. Patients often require combinations of several antihypertensive drugs for effective blood pressure control. Where possible, the addition of RAB is recommended. This may appear controversial as guidelines recommend caution with ACE-I/ARB use in patients with bilateral RAS or a solitary functioning kidney with RAS because potentially an acute reduction in GFR may occur due to an ACE-I/ARB – induced reduction of glomerular hydrostatic pressure. However, with careful titration of doses and checking of renal function (7–10 days post ACE-I/ARB introduction and after each dose increment), such serious complications can be detected early. An increase of creatinine of >25% over baseline would be regarded as a reason to stop the drugs. Revascularization is emerging a means of allowing continuation of these beneficial drugs when renal functional deterioration is observed, although studies are still awaited in this regard. Other benefits to RAB include reduction of proteinuria[19] and left ventricular hypertrophy,[20] both significant independent predictors of mortality in ARVD (as in patients with other causes of CKD).

29.6.2
Revascularization

Renal revascularization procedures are performed in 16% of newly diagnosed ARVD cases.[1] Over the course of the last 2 decades the availability of endovascular techniques has increased accessibility of patients to revascularization, and now <2% of all procedures are surgical (compared to 35% in 1992[21]). There are certain indications for renal revascularization procedures which have a wide consensus of support (albeit, non-evidence-based). These include:

- Prevention or treatment of life threatening flash pulmonary oedema[22–24]
- Relief of critical stenosis in order to preserve renal mass
- Acute occlusion that has resulted in acute kidney injury (AKI)[25,26] (Fig. 29.3a and b)
- Renovascular hypertension resistant to multiple medications[27]

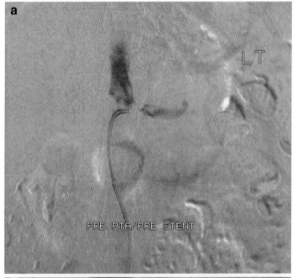

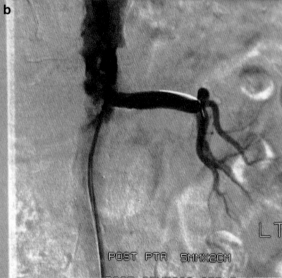

Fig. 29.3 (a) Left main renal artery pre-revascularization. (b) Post-angioplasty/stent insertion with restoration of renal artery patency and flow (Courtesy of Dr. Nicholas Chalmers, Radiology Department, Manchester Royal Infirmary)

Outside of these indications, studies have shown a variable benefit of revascularization over conservative medical management, in terms of hypertension control and especially renal functional outcome. Until recently there has been a lack of adequately powered randomized controlled trials to detect a difference, and in other studies the patient phenotype has been inconsistent. The Angioplasty and Stent for Renal Arterial Lesions (ASTRAL) [17]trial reported its initial findings in 2009, it being the largest randomized control trial to date comparing medical treatment to revascularization with medical therapy in 806 patients with anatomically significant ARVD. Over an average follow-up period of 34 months, no renal functional (the primary end-point), systolic or diastolic blood pressure, cardiovascular event or mortality benefit was provided by revascularization with medical therapy, compared to medical therapy alone, in a clinically relevant, but relatively asymptomatic ARVD population. Within this population there is no doubt that some patients will have shown improvements in renal function and blood pressure control, and further analyses will be directed at assessing whether a series of clinical and investigational characteristics would reliably identify this subgroup. The minority of patients who do improve in this way after revascularization are classed as having a "functionally significant" RAS, but also, importantly, they have renal parenchyma which has not been irretrievably damaged by prior ischaemic and hypertensive stresses.

Our patient underwent percutaneous left renal artery angioplasty and stenting. **[Q3: C]** Currently, stent supported angioplasty has widely replaced plain balloon angioplasty of RAS because of the superior short and long term angiographic results of stenting,[25,28–30] especially with far lower rates of re-stenosis seen in atherosclerotic ostial lesions, which might occur because of elastic recoil or plaque resistance. Other benefits include a reduction in renin and angiotensin production[30] and larger luminal dilatation. Furthermore, endovascular techniques reduce the operative morbidity and mortality of open surgical repair.[31] Technical developments such as drug eluting stents,[32] and distal protection devices (e.g., a balloon or filter placed distally during intervention to capture atheromatous and thrombotic debris before it reaches the renal capillary bed), may increase the safety and effectiveness of revascularization. Patients receiving both glycoprotein IIb/IIIa inhibitors and embolic protection devices have less occurrence of platelet-rich emboli in distally placed filters.[33] These measures are not widely used, and deterioration in renal function may still continue despite their use.[34]

Even endovascular revascularization is a procedure which may carry significant risk. Complications may occur in up to 25% of patients,[35] most of which are minor, such as groin bruising and haematoma over the percutaneous wound entry site, or temporary deterioration of renal function, presumably due to contrast-induced injury. However, in ASTRAL 6.8% of patients suffered serious complications of revascularization including major renal arterial abnormailities (peudoaneurysm formation, thrombosis and occlusion, renal artery dissection), cholesterol emboliztion and even death. **[Q4: D, E]**

A range of surgical options are available to treat RAS and these include aortic graft and renal bypass, aorto-renal bypass, aorto-renal endarterectomy and extra-anatomical bypass. At least 70% of patients who undergo surgical repair have concomitant aortic disease, and most clinicians would now recommend surgery for RAS when this is accompanied by more complex aorto-renal disease. The results after surgical revascularization are uncertain because of positive reporting bias and the presence of many relatively small case series in the literature. Nevertheless, one retrospective study of 222 patients from 1974 to 1987, encompassing a mean follow-up of 7.4 years, showed an operative mortality of 2.2%, hypertension improvement in 72.4% and preservation of renal function in 71.3%.[36]

29.7
Prognosis

The presence of ARVD is associated with a guarded prognosis. The strong presence of other co-morbid cardiovascular disease is reflected in the high incidence of cardiovascular events[37,38] and death. In fact, the risk of death is almost *six times greater* than that of progressing onto renal replacement therapy (RRT).[1] Patients who do require RRT have a poor life expectancy.[8,39] However, with improvement in management (e.g., blood pressure control and statin use), the natural tendency of RAS lesions to progress over time is controllable.[18] In the ASTRAL study, insights were provided that suggest that cardiovascular risk management is having an effect upon reducing mortality in ARVD. The annual mortality in ASTRAL was around 8% for all patients (mean age 70 years), which is half that of the 16.3% noted in the previous largest epidemiological cohort of ARVD patients (a 5% random sample of the US Medicare population involving patients aged >67 years) who had been studied in 2001–2002.[1] About 85% of ASTRAL patients were receiving a statin at 1 year follow-up, and 80% were receiving anti-platelet therapy. The focus of management during follow up of this patient would include lifestyle modification advice, control of blood pressure and monitoring of renal function. [Q5: A]

References

1. Kalra PA, Guo H, Kausz AT, et al. Atherosclerotic renovascular disease in United States patients aged 67 years or older: risk factors, revascularization, and prognosis. *Kidney Int.* 2005;68(1):293-301.
2. Gray BH, Olin JW, Childs MB, Sullivan TM, Bacharach JM. Clinical benefit of renal artery angioplasty with stenting for the control of recurrent and refractory congestive heart failure. *Vasc Med.* 2002;7(4):275-279.
3. Zeller T, Muller C, Frank U, et al. Survival after stenting of severe atherosclerotic ostial renal artery stenoses. *J Endovasc Ther.* 2003;10(3):539-545.
4. Harding MB, Smith LR, Himmelstein SI, et al. Renal artery stenosis: prevalence and associated risk factors in patients undergoing routine cardiac catheterization. *J Am Soc Nephrol.* 1992;2(11):1608-1616.
5. Conlon PJ, Little MA, Pieper K, Mark DB. Severity of renal vascular disease predicts mortality in patients undergoing coronary angiography. *Kidney Int.* 2001;60(4):1490-1497.
6. Missouris CG, Buckenham T, Cappuccio FP, MacGregor GA. Renal artery stenosis: a common and important problem in patients with peripheral vascular disease. *Am J Med.* 1994;96(1):10-14.
7. Derkx FH, Schalekamp MA. Renal artery stenosis and hypertension. *Lancet.* 1994;344(8917):237-239.

8. Guo H, Kalra PA, Gilbertson DT, et al. Atherosclerotic renovascular disease in older US patients starting dialysis, 1996 to 2001. *Circulation.* 2007;115(1):50-58.

9. van den Dool SW, Wasser MN, de Fijter JW, Hoekstra J, van der Geest RJ. Functional renal volume: quantitative analysis at gadolinium-enhanced MR angiography – feasibility study in healthy potential kidney donors. *Radiology.* 2005;236(1):189-195.

10. Bakker J, Olree M, Kaatee R, et al. Renal volume measurements: accuracy and repeatability of US compared with that of MR imaging. *Radiology.* 1999;211(3):623-628.

11. Coulam CH, Bouley DM, Sommer FG. Measurement of renal volumes with contrast-enhanced MRI. *J Magn Reson Imaging.* 2002;15(2):174-179.

12. Grobner T. Gadolinium – a specific trigger for the development of nephrogenic fibrosing dermopathy and nephrogenic systemic fibrosis? *Nephrol Dial Transplant.* 2006;21(4): 1104-1108.

13. Marckmann P, Skov L, Rossen K, Heaf JG, Thomsen HS. Case-control study of gadodiamide-related nephrogenic systemic fibrosis. *Nephrol Dial Transplant.* 2007;22(11):3174-3178.

14. Commission on Human Medicines. Nephrogenic systemic fibrosis (NSF) with gadolinium-containing magnetic resonance imaging (MRI) contrast agents: update. Medicines and Healthcare Products Regulatory Agency Web site. Available at: http://www.mhra.gov.uk/Safetyinformation/Safetywarningsalertsandrecalls/Safetywarningsandmessagesformedicines/CON2030229. Accessed February 1, 2010. 26-7-0007. Ref Type: Internet Communication.

15. Mounier-Vehier C, Cocheteux B, Haulon S, et al. Changes in renal blood flow reserve after angioplasty of renal artery stenosis in hypertensive patients. *Kidney Int.* 2004;65(1): 245-250.

16. Vasbinder GB, Nelemans PJ, Kessels AG, Kroon AA, de Leeuw PW, van Engelshoven JM. Diagnostic tests for renal artery stenosis in patients suspected of having renovascular hypertension: a meta-analysis. *Ann Intern Med.* 2001;135(6):401-411.

17. Wheatley K, Ives N, Gray R, et al. Revascularization versus medical therapy for renal-artery stenosis. *N Engl J Med.* 2009;361(20):1953-1962.

18. Cheung CM, Patel A, Shaheen N, et al. The effects of statins on the progression of atherosclerotic renovascular disease. *Nephron Clin Pract.* 2007;107(2):c35-c42.

19. Treatment of adults and children with renal failure: standards and audit measures. 3rd edn. London: RCP London and the Renal Ass, 2002. 2007. Ref Type: Generic.

20. Shekelle PG, Rich MW, Morton SC, et al. Efficacy of angiotensin-converting enzyme inhibitors and beta-blockers in the management of left ventricular systolic dysfunction according to race, gender, and diabetic status: a meta-analysis of major clinical trials. *J Am Coll Cardiol.* 2003;41(9):1529-1538.

21. Kalra PA, Guo H, Gilbertson DT, et al. Atherosclerotic renovascular disease in the United States. *Kidney Int.* 2010;77(1):37-43.

22. Bloch MJ, Trost DW, Pickering TG, Sos TA, August P. Prevention of recurrent pulmonary edema in patients with bilateral renovascular disease through renal artery stent placement. *Am J Hypertens.* 1999;12(1 Pt 1):1-7.

23. Pickering TG, Herman L, Devereux RB, et al. Recurrent pulmonary oedema in hypertension due to bilateral renal artery stenosis: treatment by angioplasty or surgical revascularisation. *Lancet.* 1988;2(8610):551-552.

24. Messina LM, Zelenock GB, Yao KA, Stanley JC. Renal revascularization for recurrent pulmonary edema in patients with poorly controlled hypertension and renal insufficiency: a distinct subgroup of patients with arteriosclerotic renal artery occlusive disease. *J Vasc Surg.* 1992;15(1):73-80.

25. Harden PN, MacLeod MJ, Rodger RS, et al. Effect of renal-artery stenting on progression of renovascular renal failure. *Lancet.* 1997;349(9059):1133-1136.

26. Scoble JE. Atherosclerotic nephropathy. *Kidney Int Suppl.* 1999;71:S106-S109.

27. Goldsmith DJ, Reidy J, Scoble J. Renal arterial intervention and angiotensin blockade in atherosclerotic nephropathy. *Am J Kidney Dis.* 2000;36(4):837-843.

28. Van de Ven PJ, Kaatee R, Beutler JJ, et al. Arterial stenting and balloon angioplasty in ostial atherosclerotic renovascular disease: a randomised trial. *Lancet.* 1999;353(9149):282-286.

29. Iannone LA, Underwood PL, Nath A, Tannenbaum MA, Ghali MG, Clevenger LD. Effect of primary balloon expandable renal artery stents on long-term patency, renal function, and blood pressure in hypertensive and renal insufficient patients with renal artery stenosis. *Cathet Cardiovasc Diagn.* 1996;37(3):243-250.

30. Zeller T, Frank U, Muller C, et al. Predictors of improved renal function after percutaneous stent-supported angioplasty of severe atherosclerotic ostial renal artery stenosis. *Circulation.* 2003;108(18):2244-2249.

31. Alhadad A, Ahle M, Ivancev K, Gottsater A, Lindblad B. Percutaneous transluminal renal angioplasty (PTRA) and surgical revascularisation in renovascular disease – a retrospective comparison of results, complications, and mortality. *Eur J Vasc Endovasc Surg.* 2004;27(2):151-156.

32. Granillo GA, van Dijk LC, McFadden EP, Serruys PW. Percutaneous radial intervention for complex bilateral renal artery stenosis using paclitaxel eluting stents. *Catheter Cardiovasc Interv.* 2005;64(1):23-27.

33. Cooper CJ, Haller ST, Colyer W, et al. Embolic protection and platelet inhibition during renal artery stenting. *Circulation.* 2008;117(21):2752-2760.

34. Holden A, Hill A. Renal angioplasty and stenting with distal protection of the main renal artery in ischemic nephropathy: early experience. *J Vasc Surg.* 2003;38(5):962-968.

35. Tan J, Filobbos R, Raghunathan G, et al. Efficacy of renal artery angioplasty and stenting in a solitary functioning kidney. *Nephrol Dial Transplant.* 2007;22(7):1916-1919.

36. Steinbach F, Novick AC, Campbell S, Dykstra D. Long-term survival after surgical revascularization for atherosclerotic renal artery disease. *J Urol.* 1997;158(1):38-41.

37. Edwards MS, Craven TE, Burke GL, Dean RH, Hansen KJ. Renovascular disease and the risk of adverse coronary events in the elderly: a prospective, population-based study. *Arch Intern Med.* 2005;165(2):207-213.

38. Wright JR, Shurrab AE, Cheung C, et al. A prospective study of the determinants of renal functional outcome and mortality in atherosclerotic renovascular disease. *Am J Kidney Dis.* 2002;39(6):1153-1161.

39. Conlon PJ, Athirakul K, Kovalik E, et al. Survival in renal vascular disease. *J Am Soc Nephrol.* 1998;9(2):252-256.

Midaortic Syndrome

30

James C. Stanley and Jonathan L. Eliason

A 15-year-old boy with neurofibromatosis-1 (NF-1) was recognized to have severe hypertension when being screened for a school athletic team. His blood pressure was 225/110 mmHg. His only complaint was lower extremity fatigue with modest physical activity. A continuous systolic bruit that did not vary with respiration was noted in his epigastrium. There was a femoral-radial artery pulse delay. He had palpable pedal pulses, with good capillary fill in his toes. The left border of cardiac dullness was 8 cm to the left of the mid-sternal line with a sustained apical impulse. There were no cardiac murmurs. An electrocardiogram documented mild left ventricular hypertrophy. His chest film revealed a slightly enlarged heart. There was no rib-notching to suggest collateral vessels due to a thoracic aortic coarctation. His basic blood chemistries and urinalysis were normal. Prior to his referral to our hospital he had undergone an attempted percutaneous transluminal angioplasty (PTA) of the right renal artery. Failure of the renal PTA and refractory hypertension led to his admission for further study and therapy.

Question 1

What would be the definitive manner of imaging his aorta and its branches?

A. Ultrasonography
B. Computed tomographic arteriography (CTA)
C. Magnetic resonance angiography (MRA)
D. Conventional arteriography (Digital subtraction angiography)

Conventional aortography was chosen to best define his vascular anatomy because of its greater definition of small arteries. It documented an abdominal aortic narrowing beginning at the CA level and extending below the renal arteries, as well as ostial narrowings of both renal arteries, the celiac artery (CA) and superior mesenteric artery (SMA) (Fig. 30.1).

J.C. Stanley (✉)
Section of Vascular Surgery, Department of Surgery, University of Michigan Cardiovascular
Centre, University of Michigan Medical School, Ann Arbor, MI, USA

G. Geroulakos and B. Sumpio (eds.), *Vascular Surgery*,
DOI: 10.1007/978-1-84996-356-5_30, © Springer-Verlag London Limited 2011

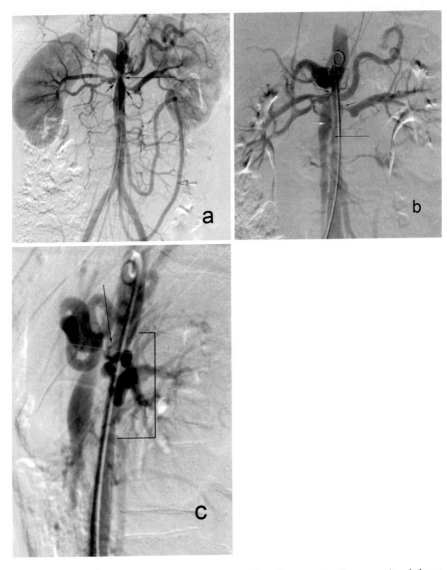

Fig. 30.1 Angiographic images suggesting (**a**) suprarenal aortic narrowing (*long arrow*) and abnormal proximal renal arteries (*short arrows*), with a large mesocolic vessel (*hollow arrow*) suggesting either SMA or aortic narrowing or both. Magnification images (**b**) define bilateral renal artery ostial stenoses (short arrows) with irregular mural aneurysms, a midabdominal aortic narrowing (*long arrow*) and a proximal SMA dilation (*white arrow*), presumed to be poststenotic. Lateral aortography (**c**) confirmed the narrowing of the aorta (bracket) and proximal SMA stenosis (*arrow*)

Deep abdominal ultrasonography prior to his referral had documented abnormal mid-abdominal aortic, bilateral renal artery, CA, and SMA velocities, all of which exceeded 300 cm/s, compared to a 125 cm/s velocity in the infrarenal aorta. The anatomic detail of the splanchnic and renal circulation revealed by ultrasonography was limited. Similarly, an MRA obtained before the failed PTA did not clearly delineate the suspected anatomic extent of his aortic branch narrowings.

Question 2

What are the preferred treatment options in managing this patient's aortic disease?

A. Thoracoabdominal bypass
B. Patch aortoplasty
C. Aggressive medical therapy with a polypharmacy including ACE inhibitors and diuretics
D. Percutaneous ballon angioplasty with stenting
E. A thoracoabdominal bypass was performed with a 16 mm ePTFE graft.

Question 3

How would you treat the bilateral renal and splanchnic arterial stenotic disease in this patient?

A. Aortic implantation of the normal renal and mesenteric arteries beyond their stenotic segments
B. Renal or mesenteric bypasses with an internal artery graft
C. Renal or mesenteric bypasses with a vein graft
D. Balloon angioplasty

The left renal artery and SMA distal to their proximal stenotic segments were transected, spatulated, and reimplanted onto the adjacent infrarenal aorta. The right renal artery was reconstructed with an iliorenal bypass.

Question 4

How would you treat the renal and splanchnic arterial disease?

A. At the same time the aortic coarctation is being repaired?
B. At a different time than the aortic repair?
C. BWith anti-inflammatory agents (immunosuppressants)?
D. With anti-thrombotic agents (ASA, clopidogrel)?

Treatment of the renal artery and SMA narrowings occurred at the same time as the aortic repair.

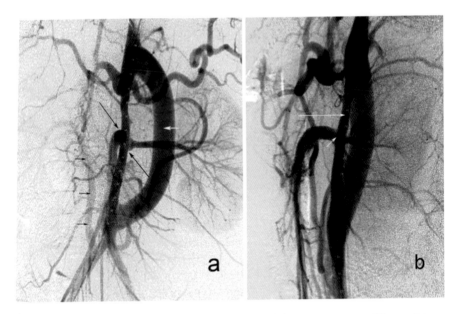

Fig. 30.2 Postoperative AP aortography (**a**) documenting satisfactory appearance of thoracoabdominal bypass (*white arrow*), aortic implantations of the SMA (*long arrow*) and left renal artery (*long arrow*), as well as a right iliorenal bypass (short arrows). Lateral aortography (**b**) confirmed satisfactory implantation of the SMA (*short arrow*) onto the hypoplastic segment of the midabdominal aorta (*long arrow*)

Question 5

What are appropriate follow-up studies after the aortic coarctation repair?

A. Ultrasonography and exercise ankle brachial indices
B. CTA
C. MRA
D. Conventional catheter-based arteriography

The patient underwent a conventional aortogram prior to discharge on postoperative day 6, to confirm the reconstruction's adequacy (Fig. 30.2). His abnormal preoperative lower extremity perfusion pressures (bilateral ABI of 0.75) became normal postoperatively (bilateral ABI of 1.1).

30.1
Commentary

Coarctation of the abdominal aorta is a rare disease causing hypertension and encompassing many different etiologies and diverse methods of treatment.[1-22] Given that essential hypertension in childhood for all practical purposes is nonexistent, evidence of sustained blood pressure elevations refractory to simple drug interventions should raise the suspicion of a secondary form of hypertension. Furthermore, the presence of NF-1 and its known association with arterial stenoses would raise a suspicion of the midaortic syndrome. These later patients often have coexisting splanchnic and renal artery occlusive disease.

Aortic Coarctation Character: An earlier collective review of 119 patients identified suprarenal coarctations in 11%, intrarenal coarctations in 54%, infrarenal coarctations in 25%, and diffuse aortic hypoplasia in 12%.[8] A contemporary series of 53 patients from the University of Michigan, revealed 69% suprarenal, 23% intrarenal, and 8% infrarenal abdominal aortic coarctations. The latter reflects a more contemporary classification of aortic coarctation, based upon the most superior level of the narrowing.[17] Indeed, it is the most cephalic extent of the disease that defines the complexity of the aortic reconstruction, with considerable differences if the CA and SMA are involved, compared to the renal arteries alone. Most aortic coarctations are diminutive vessels, often with an hour-glass narrowing representing a lack of growth in developmental lesions or circumferential contraction in cases of an inflammatory aortitis. Such morphologic changes are best identified by detailed imaging. **[Q1]**

Associated Renal and Splanchnic Arterial Disease: Nearly 80% of patients with abdominal aortic developmental lesions have been reported to have renal artery stenoses,[8] a finding consistent with the recent Michigan series in which 87% had renal artery narrowings or occlusions.[17] Splanchnic arterial occlusive disease has been previously reported to affect 22% of patients with abdominal aortic coarctations.[8] The true incidence of splanchnic arterial involvement may be much greater, in that lateral aortograms were not routinely obtained in evaluating many of these patients. The more complete imaging in the recent Michigan series revealed 62% to have CA or SMA stenoses and occlusions, with both vessels involved in 82% of these cases.[17] Suprarenal or infrarenal coarctations, when distant from the CA and SMA, are less likely to be associated with stenotic branch disease, compared to more centrally located abdominal aortic coarctations. Presence of these branch narrowings are best defined by detailed imaging. **[Q1]**

Pathogenesis: Many abdominal aortic coarctations appear related to events occurring around the 25th day of fetal development. At that time the two embryonic dorsal aortas fuse and lose their intervening wall to form a single vessel. Overfusion of the two embryonic dorsal aortae or their failure to fuse with subsequent obliteration of one of these vessels would predictably result in an aortic narrowing.[23] Developmental overfusion of the two primitive dorsal aortas receives support in patients with decreased aortic diameters who have single origins of the lumbar arteries.[17,24]

Multiple renal arteries to one or both kidneys in nearly half of the patients exhibiting suprarenal and intrarenal abdominal aortic coarctations exceeds the 25–35% observed in the general population and also supports a developmental etiology of these narrowings.[8,16] Normal aortic development occurs at approximately the same embryonic time that the multiple metanephric arteries involute, leaving a single renal artery. Dominance of this single renal artery is alleged to result from its obligate hemodynamic advantage over adjacent metanephric vessels. It is likely that if aortic narrowings exist, flow disturbances will occur in the vicinity of this principle renal artery and diminish its hemodynamic advantage, allowing persistence of adjacent metanephric channels. The fact that aortic narrowings distant from the renal arteries are less likely to be associated with multiple renal arteries lends further credence to this developmental hypothesis.[8,16,17,25]

Viral-mediated events may impede transition of fetal mesenchymal tissue to vascular smooth muscle or alter its organization and growth in utero, and also result in developmental aortic narrowings. Certain viruses, including rubella, are cytocidal and inhibitory to cell replication, with intimal fibroplasia and aortic hypoplasia occurring as a consequence.[26–29] In fact, fibroproliferative intimal disorders have been documented in the aorta and large elastic arteries of 16.5% of patients exhibiting the congenital rubella syndrome.[28]

Patients with NF-1 exhibit an unusually high frequency of arterial abnormalities, including developmental abdominal aortic coarctations and renal artery stenoses.[30] Because of the protean nature of NF-1 and infrequent genetic analyses of patients with abdominal aortic coarctation, the exact frequency of this disease among these individuals is unknown. Nevertheless, 29% of the recent Michigan series' patients carried a diagnosis of NF-1.[17] The primary vascular pathology in neurofibromatosis appears to be related to abnormal smooth muscle growth, not entrapment or invasion of the arterial wall by neural elements.[31,32] Similar events may affect patients with the Alagille syndrome,[33] and Williams' syndrome.[34]

Panaortitis with adventitial or periadventitial fibrosis and associated inflammatory cell infiltrates, suggesting an active or chronic aortitis, is another well recognized cause of abdominal aortic coarctations. The proposition that most abdominal aortic coarctations are a variant of an inflammatory aortitis like Takayasu's disease is quite controversial and not supported by histological findings.[21,35] This cause of aortic narrowings, suspected in only 8% of the recent Michigan series,[17] is encountered much more often in the subcontinent populations of Asia and South America.

Clinical Manifestations: Most patients with midaortic syndrome present with uncontrolled hypertension due to suprarenal or intrarenal aortic coarctations, and coexisting renal artery stenoses in many cases. Changes in pulsatile flow and pressure across renal stenoses or aortic narrowings are responsible for renin-angiotensin system activation and subsequent blood pressure elevations. This form of renovascular hypertension is usually resistant to simple pharmacologic control. An occasional patient reports exercise-related lower extremity fatigue, but true claudication is rare. Associated splanchnic arterial occlusive disease affects a majority of those aortic narrowings, yet symptomatic intestinal ischemia is very uncommon.[17,36] In the recent Michigan series, more than half the patients manifest splanchnic occlusive lesions, yet only 6% experienced intestinal angina.[17]

Abdominal aortic coarctations usually cause signs or symptoms during the first or second decade of life, yet an earlier review noted that patients had reached a mean age of 22 years before the diagnosis was actually confirmed.[8] Untreated, this entity has been associated with stroke, progressive left ventricular hypertrophy with congestive heart failure and flash pulmonary edema, and less often with renal insufficiency.[37] In one review, 55% of untreated patients died at a mean age of 34 years.[8]

Clear anatomic imaging is essential to establishing a correct diagnosis of midaortic syndrome. [Q1] Deep abdominal ultrasonography may provide evidence of narrowed vessels with documented increases in velocity blood flow. Ultrasonography may useful for screening, but it is inadequate at providing precise information about the character and location of stenotic disease in small arteries. [Q1: A] MRA is noninvasive and may give an accurate accounting of aortic and aortic branch disease. However, a severe stenosis may be suggested by MRA when such is not present, because of the phase-drop out phenomenon associated with turbulent blood flow. This often occurs in the face of arterial tortuosity, without the presence of an actual arterial narrowing. **[Q1: C]** Thus, either multi-slice CTA or catheter-related conventional digital subtraction arteriography are the favored examinations when assessing the disease pattern in patients with midaortic syndrome. **[Q1: B, D]**

Treatment Options: The two procedures most commonly performed in treating aortic coarctations remain open interventions.[17] *Patch aortoplasty*, when technically feasible has recently become a common means of treating isolated abdominal aortic coarctations. **[Q2: B]** *Thoracoabdominal bypass* may be favored in certain patients having too narrow or too lengthy of a coarctation segment to allow easy placement of a patch, as well as in certain patients having complex disease affecting the renal and splanchnic arteries. **[Q2: A]**

Thoracoabdominal bypass grafts usually originate from the distal thoracic aorta above the diaphragm or from the supraceliac aorta at the diaphragmatic hiatus, being passed behind the left kidney to the distal aorta.[17] In some patients, aortic exposure may be facilitated by a thoracoabdominal incision through the left sixth or seventh intercostals space extending from the posterior axillary line across the costal margin, onto the abdomen, in either an oblique fashion to the right of the umbilicus or as a midline incision to just above the pubis. In younger children and adolescents, a transverse supraumbilical abdominal incision has been used most often, extending laterally to the posterior axillary lines, combined with medial rotation of the viscera, allowing access to the abdominal aorta from its supraceliac level at the aortic hiatus to the origin of the iliac arteries. **[Q2: A]**

Dacron graft knitted or woven thoracoabdominal grafts have been used in the distant past, with expanded Teflon grafts used more often in recent years because of their greater stability regarding postimplantation dilatation.[17] Graft diameter should be chosen to be as big as possible, short of being so large that excessive luminal thrombus would accumulate. In children, the intent is to oversize grafts compared to the aorta, with anticipated growth otherwise resulting in a graft too small to maintain normal distal pressures and flow. In the ideal circumstance, one should use a graft whose size would not represent a kinetic energy-consuming constriction as the patient grows into maturity. This means having a conduit at least 60% or 70% the size of the adult aorta. This translates into using 8–12 mm grafts in young children, 12–16 mm grafts for early adolescents, and 14–20 mm grafts in late adolescents and adults.[17] In the very young child, use of large conduits may not be possible. Graft length is considered a non-issue in older children and adolescents, with axial growth from the diaphragm to pelvis being minimal after age 9 or 10 in late childhood. **[Q2: A]**

Patch aortoplasty is usually undertaken when the coarctation segment is short and has a large enough diameter to allow completion of an anastomosis without an overlap of sutures from the opposing sides of the patch.[17] Whenever possible, patches in children should be made sufficiently large enough, similar to thoracoabdominal graft sizing, so as to not be constrictive with growth into adulthood, yet not so generous as to risk development of an extensive lining of unstable thrombus. Expanded Teflon graft material is again favored over-fabricated Dacron graft material, because of the latter's propensity for dilatation years after implantation. **[Q2: B]**

Endoluminal stenting of select abdominal aortic coarctations may be considered in some patients. **[Q2: C]** Current endovascular technologies appear to allow the safe treatment of focal stenoses, excluding tight fibrotic narrowings, remote from the CA, SMA, and renal arteries. Percutaneous transluminal angioplasty of an abdominal aortic coarctation was first reported in 1983.[13] Subsequent case reports described the transition to stenting in these cases.[1,6] In fact, early and late failures of balloon angioplasty alone suggest that stent placement is necessary to overcome the significant recoil of these often hypoplastic and highly fibrotic aortic narrowings.[7,10,17,38] The authors remain cautious at accepting the long-term benefits of endoluminal treatment of abdominal aortic coarctation in any patient, except adults with very focal narrowings distant from their renal arteries. Given the high frequency with which the renal and splanchnic arteries are affected in abdominal aortic coarctation, especially in the younger-growing patient, the number of lesions amenable to endovascular repair may be limited. **[Q2: C]**

Reoperations after repairs of abdominal aortic coarctation are infrequent, but may be required for anastomotic narrowings or if a patient outgrows the adequacy of the primary procedure. The fact that nearly 10% of the currently reported cases in the Michigan series required late secondary operations supports the importance of life-long follow-up of these patients.[17] Aneurysmal aortic deterioration in the region of a patch in one of the patients in that series, many years after the initial reconstruction and 2 years after she completed her only pregnancy, deserves note. The effect of gestational hormones and blood pressure increases during pregnancy may be relevant, in that pregnancy-related aortic diameter increases of 1.5 cm or more have been observed at the site of thoracic aortic coarctation repairs in nearly 10% of those undergoing such an inteyvervention.[39] Although this finding may not be directly extrapolated to abdominal aortic coarctation repairs, it does justify close surveillance of those patients who subsequently become pregnant. **[Q5]**

Division and reimplantation of the normal renal artery beyond an ostial stenosis onto the adjacent aorta become an important means of renal revascularization in these patients.[17,37] **[Q3: A]** In these circumstances, the transected renal artery is usually spatulated anteriorly and posteriorly to create a generous anastomotic orifice. An oval aortotomy is best made with an aortic punch, being a little more than twice the diameter of the renal artery being implanted. This will provide a sufficiently large anastomosis so an anastomotic narrowing would not evolve as the child grows. These anastomoses are usually performed using interrupted monofilament sutures in young patients. However, a continuous suture is often used in older adolescents with large renal arteries. Most implantations of the renal artery are into a normal infrarenal segment of the aorta. Medial mobilization of the kidney may be necessary to ensure that there is no tension on the implanted renal artery. Implantation of a renal artery branch or accessory renal artery into a nondiseased adjacent main or segmental renal artery also involves spatulation of the segmental vessel and completion of the anastomosis using monofilament sutures. Implantation of a renal artery into the superior mesenteric artery may be undertaken when implantation elsewhere is deemed hazardous. **[Q3: A]**

Aortorenal bypass with the internal iliac artery used as a free graft has become preferred when a bypass is required.[17,37] **[Q3: B]** The excised internal iliac artery usually includes its inferior branches, which are incised to create a large common orifice for the aortic anastomosis. Distal anastomoses from the renal artery to the graft are completed after spatulation of both the iliac artery and renal artery to increase the anastomotic circumference. Such ovoid anastomoses were less likely to develop late strictures and are usually completed with interrupted sutures in very young children, although a continuous suture may be used in reconstructing larger renal arteries. Aortorenal bypasses with vein grafts were standard during the first decade of this experience, but because more than half these conduits undergo aneurysmal deterioration, they have not been favored during the past 25 years.[17,36] However, when no other alternative exists vein grafts may be used with a knitted Dacron sleeve placed about them so as to limit the expected graft expansion. [Q3: C]

Irreparable renal disease is often the reason for performance of a nephrectomy. Nonsalvageable kidneys exist when radionuclide renal imaging confirms marked loss of renal function to less than 10% of total renal function, associated with diminutive-sized kidneys 2–3 cm in length due to loss of parenchymal tissue. Irreparable renal disease also includes kidney's exhibiting multiple intrarenal aneurysms not amenable to any form of open reconstruction, in situ or ex vivo. In the aforenoted circumstances, and in the presence of a normal contralateral kidney, nephrectomy is reasonable.

The role of PTA in treating pediatric renovascular hypertension remains controversial. Failure after PTA for developmental disease might be anticipated, given the excessive elastic tissue in many stenoses, which would predictably contribute to early post-dilation recoil, as well as the minute caliber of these diseased vessels that might lead to their disruption.[37] Nevertheless, a small number of recent reports suggest success with catheter-based interventions.[20] It is of note that if the disease being treated is a quiescent inflammatory aortoarteritis, then more salutary outcomes might follow PTA than would be the case if developmentally hypoplastic renal arteries are being treated. However, even in the former setting, recurrent stenoses are frequent. [Q3: D]

Simultaneous or staged aortic and visceral artery reconstructions depend on the clinical relevance of the nonaortic disease as well as the proximity of the aortic reconstruction to the affected aortic branches. [Q4] Certainly, renal artery stenoses and secondary renovascular hypertension justify an aggressive reconstructive approach. A mandate to reconstruct the CA or SMA applies only to symptomatic cases. Nevertheless, a relative indication to prophylactically reconstruct these vessels exists when performance of an aortoplasty or renal revascularization would make a subsequent CA or SMA revascularization exceedingly difficult. [Q4: A] When the aortic reconstruction was distant from the CA or SMA, such as with thoracoabdominal bypass, a concomitant splanchnic revascularization is less likely to be performed. [Q4: B]

Long-term follow-up of patients undergoing surgical treatment of their abdominal aortic coarctation is warranted. At a minimum, noninvasive assessments of lower extremity blood flow with exercise ankle-brachial indices are recommended. [Q5: A] Imaging with MRA studies or CTA should be obtained if any evidence of diminished blood flow exists. [Q5: B, C] More detailed imaging with conventional arteriography is appropriate if blood pressure increases occur in those who have undergone concomitant renal artery reconstructions or whose renal blood flow is dependent upon their aortic reconstruction. [Q5: D]

Abdominal aortic coarctation represents a complex vascular disease, often complicated by coexisting renal and splanchnic arterial disease. Individualized treatment is dependent on the pattern of the anatomic lesions, patient age, and anticipated growth potential. Salutary outcomes following carefully performed operative therapy are anticipated in more than 90% of patients.

References

1. Ballweg J, Liniger R, Rocchini A, Gajarski R. Use of palmaz stents in a newborn with congenital aneurysms and coarctation of the abdominal aorta. *Catheter Cardiovasc Interv.* 2006;68:648-652.
2. Bergamini TM, Bernard JD, Mavroudis C, Backer CL, Muster AJ, Richardson JD. Coarctation of the abdominal aorta. *Ann Vasc Surg.* 1995;9:352-356.
3. Connolly JE, Wilson SE, Lawrence PL, Fujitani RM. Middle aortic syndrome: distal thoracic and abdominal coarctation, a disorder with multiple etiologies. *J Am Coll Surg.* 2002;194:774-781.
4. DeBakey ME, Garrett HE, Howell JF, Howell JF, Morris GC Jr. Coarctation of the abdominal aorta with renal arterial stenosis: surgical considerations. *Ann Surg.* 1967;165:830-843.
5. Delis KT, Gloviczki P. Middle aortic syndrome: from presentation to contemporary open surgical and endovascular treatment (Editorial comment by JC Stanley included). *Persp Vasc Surg Endovasc Ther.* 2005;17:187-206.
6. Eliason JL, Passman MA, Guzman RJ, Naslund TC. Durability of percutaneous angioplasty and stent implantation for the treatment of abdominal aortic coarctation: a case report. *Vasc Surg.* 2001;35:397-401.
7. Fava MP, Foradori GB, Garcia CB, Cruz FO, Aguilar JG, Kramer JG, Valdés FE. Percutaneous transluminal angioplasty in patients with Takayasu Arteritis: five year experience. *J Vasc Interv Radiol.* 1993;4:649-652.
8. Graham LM, Zelenock GB, Erlandson EE, Coran AG, Lindenaeur SM, Stanley JC. Abdominal aortic coarctation and segmental hypoplasia. *Surgery.* 1979;86:519-529.
9. Hallett JW Jr, Brewster DC, Darling RC, O'Hara PJ. Coarctation of the abdominal aorta: current options in surgical management. *Ann Surg.* 1980;191:430-437.
10. Lin Y-J, Hwang B, Lee P-C, Yang L-Y, Meng CCL. Mid-aortic syndrome: a case report and review of the literature. *Int J Cardiol.* 2007;123:348-352.
11. Messina LM, Reilly LM, Goldstone J, Ehrenfeld WK, Ferrell LD, Stoney RJ. Middle aortic syndrome. Effectiveness and durability of complex arterial revascularization techniques. *Ann Surg.* 1986;204:331-339.
12. Mickley V, Fleiter T. Coarctations of descending and abdominal aorta: long-term results of surgical therapy. *J Vasc Surg.* 1998;28:206-214.
13. Nanni GS, Hawkins IF, Alexander JA. Percutaneous transluminal angioplasty of an abdominal aortic coarctation. *AJR Am J Roentgenol.* 1983;140:1239-1241.
14. Schechter C, Angelini P, Treistman B. Percutaneous balloon catheter angioplasty of coarctation of the abdominal aorta: report of two cases. *Cathet Cardiovasc Diagn.* 1985;11:401-407.
15. Stadlmaier E, Spary A, Tillich M, Pilger E. Midaortic syndrome and celiac disease: a case of local vasculitis. *Clin Rheumatol.* 2005;24:301-304.
16. Stanley JC, Graham LM, Whitehouse WM Jr, Zelenock GB, Eriandson EE, Gronenwell IL, Lindenauer SM. Developmental occlusive disease of the abdominal aorta and the splanchnic and renal arteries. *Am J Surg.* 1981;142:190-196.
17. Stanley JC, Criado E, Eliason JL, Upchurch GR Jr, Berguer R, Rectenwald JE. Abdominal aortic coarctation: surgical treatment of 53 patients with a thoracoabdominal patch aortoplasty, or interposition aortoaortic graft. *J Vasc Surg.* 2008;48:1073-1082.
18. Stiller B, Weng Y, Berger F. Images in cardiology. Mid aortic syndrome: a rare cause of reversible cardiomyopathy. *Heart.* 2006;92:640.
19. Terramani TT, Salim A, Hood DB, Rowe VL, Weaver FA. Hypoplasia of the descending thoracic and abdominal aorta: a report of two cases and review of the literature. *J Vasc Surg.* 2002;36:844-848.
20. Tummolo A, Marks SD, Stadermann M, Roebuck DJ, McLaren CA, Hamilton G, Dillon MJ, Tullus K. Mid-aortic syndrome: long-term outcome of 36 children. *Pediatr Nephrol.* 2009;241:2225-2232.

21. Vaccaro PS, Myers JC, Smead WL. Surgical correction of abdominal aortic coarctation and hypertension. *J Vasc Surg.* 1986;3:643-648.

22. Wada J, Kazui T. Long-term results of thoracoabdominal bypass graft for atypical coarctation of the aorta. *World J Surg.* 1978;2:891-896.

23. Wd'A M. Congenital stenosis of the abdominal aorta. *Am Heart J.* 1937;13:633-646.

24. Arnot RS, Louw JH. The anatomy of the posterior wall of the abdominal aorta. Its significance with regard to hypoplasia of the distal aorta. *S Afr Med J.* 1973;47:899-902.

25. Stanley JC, Zelenock GB, Messina LM, Wakefield TW. Pediatric renovascular hypertension: a thirty-year experience of operative treatment. *J Vasc Surg.* 1995;21:212-227.

26. Esterly JR, Oppenheimer EM. Vascular lesions in infants with congenital rubella. *Circulation.* 1967;36:544-554.

27. Siassi B, Glyman G, Emmanouilides GC. Hypoplasia of the abdominal aorta associated with the rubella syndrome. *Am J Dis Child.* 1970;120:476-479.

28. Singer DB, Rudolph AJ, Rosenberg HS, Rawls WE, Boniuk M. Pathology of the congenital rubella syndrome. *J Pediatr.* 1967;71:665-675.

29. Stewart DR, Price RA, Nebesar R, Schuster SR. Progressive peripheral fibromuscular hyperplasia in an infant: a possible manifestation of the rubella syndrome. *Surgery.* 1973;73: 374-380.

30. Halperin M, Currarino G. Vascular lesions causing hypertension in neurofibromatosis. *N Engl J Med.* 1965;273:248-252.

31. Finley JL, Dabbs DJ. Renal vascular smooth muscle proliferation in neurofibromatosis. *Human Pathol.* 1988;19:107-110.

32. Greene JF, Fitzwater JE, Burgess J. Arterial lesions associated with neurofibromatosis. *Am J Clin Pathol.* 1974;62:481-487.

33. Quek SC, Tan L, Quek ST, Yip W, Aw M, Quak SH. Abdominal coarctation and Alagille syndrome. *Pediatrics.* 2000;106:e9.

34. Radford DJ, Pohlner PG. The middle aortic syndrome: an important feature of Williams' syndrome. *Cardiol Young.* 2000;10:597-602.

35. Lande A. Takayasu's arteritis and congenital coarctation of the descending thoracic and abdominal aorta: a critical review. *AJR Am J Roentgenol.* 1976;127:227-233.

36. Upchurch GR Jr, Henke PK, Eagleton MJ, Grigoryants V, Sullivan VV, Wakefield TW, Jacobs LA, Greenfield LJ, Stanley JC. Pediatric splanchnic arterial occlusive disease: clinical relevance and operative treatment. *J Vasc Surg.* 2002;35:860-867.

37. Stanley JC, Criado E, Upchurch GR Jr, Brophy PD, Cho KJ, Rectenwald JE. Pediatric renovascular hypertension: 132 primary and 30 secondary operations in 97 children. *J Vasc Surg.* 2006;44:1219-1229.

38. Siwik ES, Perry SB, Lock JE. Endovascular stent implantation in patients with stenotic aortoarteriopathies: early and medium-term results. *Catheter Cardiovasc Interv.* 2003;59: 380-386.

39. Vriend WJ, Drenthen W, Pieper PG, Ross-Hesselink JW, Winderman AN, vanVeldhulsen DS, Mulder, BJM. Outcome of pregnancy in patients after repair of aortic coarctation. *Eur Heart J.* 2005;26:2173-2178.

Part V

Management of Portal Hypertension

Management of Portal Hypertension

31

Yolanda Y. L. Yang and J. Michael Henderson

A 37-year-old woman with a history of hepatitis C, cirrhosis, and esophageal varices presented with hematemesis and melena. The patient had a history of a prior esophageal variceal bleeding episode 7 years ago, which required transfusion of four units of packed red blood cells (PRBC) and had been treated with endoscopic sclerotherapy. She was placed on nadolol at that time.

Question 1

If the patient had been found to have varices before any bleeding episode, she would benefit from which of the following?

A. Endoscopic treatment: sclerotherapy or band ligation.
B. Transjugular intrahepatic portal systemic shunt (TIPS).
C. Non-cardioselective beta-blocker.
D. A surgical shunt.

The patient re-presents one year prior to her current admission with a further variceal bleed documented at endoscopy, which required five units of PRBC. The acute episode of bleeding was managed with variceal banding, and the patient underwent a course of banding on an outpatient basis. She had no encephalopathy at that time, but did develop some ascites for a short period that responded to salt restriction, Aldactone, and Lasix. Over this past year, her liver function tests have been stable with her bilirubin at 1.0, albumin at 3.5, and a normal prothrombin time.

J.M. Henderson (✉)
Division of Surgery, Cleveland Clinic Foundation, Cleveland, OH, USA

G. Geroulakos and B. Sumpio (eds.), *Vascular Surgery*,
DOI: 10.1007/978-1-84996-356-5_31, © Springer-Verlag London Limited 2011

Question 2

An episode of acute variceal bleeding usually requires which of the following?

A. ICU admission with hemodynamic monitoring, blood, blood products, and fluid resuscitation.
B. An emergency portacaval shunt.
C. A transjugular intrahepatic portal systemic shunt.
D. Endoscopic therapy with sclerosis and/or band ligation.
E. Pharmacologic therapy.

At the present admission the patient is alert and oriented with no evidence of encephalopathy. She has well-preserved muscle mass on examination and is not clinically jaundiced. Her abdomen shows minimal ascites, with no hepatomegaly, but evidence of splenomegaly. Her laboratory studies showed a hemoglobin of 7 g/dL, AST 24, alkaline phosphatase 84, albumin 2.6, bilirubin 3.4, and international normalized ratio (INR) 1.6. She was receiving blood transfusion when examined and octreotide infusion at 50 μg/h. Esophagogastroduodenoscopy showed clot over an esophageal varix with evidence of other non-bleeding varices in both the distal esophagus and gastric fundus.

Question 3

Which of the following studies are important in evaluation and management decisions?

A. Calculation of Child's score.
B. Calculation of MELD score.
C. Endoscopy.
D. Doppler ultrasound.
E. Angiography.

Question 4

Which of the following statements are accurate in prevention of recurrent variceal bleeding?

A. All patients require portal decompression.
B. First-line treatment is with endoscopic band ligation and a beta-blocker.
C. Variceal decompression can only be achieved with a surgical shunt.
D. Liver transplant is good treatment for variceal bleeding in patients with end-stage liver disease.

Question 5

Decompression of gastroesophageal varices:

A. Can be achieved equally well with surgical shunt or TIPS.
B. Should only be used for patients who have failed endoscopic and pharmacologic therapy for bleeding varices.
C. Improves survival in patients with bleeding varices when compared to endoscopic therapy.
D. Is best achieved by liver transplant for all patients with variceal bleeding.

The patient presented in this case had recurring bleeding episodes through first-line treatment and was therefore a candidate for decompression. Evaluation with angiography and ultrasound showed patent splenic and portal veins and a normal left renal vein (Figs. 31.1–31.4). The patient had an elective distal splenorenal shunt (DSRS) for variceal decompression. She was in hospital for 7 days, and was discharged following shunt catheterization (Fig. 31.5) and documentation of patency. Follow-up over the next 4 years showed some progression of her hepatitis C, but no further episodes of variceal bleeding.

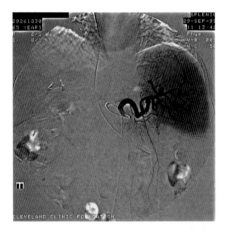

Fig. 31.1 Splenic artery injection. The catheter is in the splentic artery and is injected with contrast

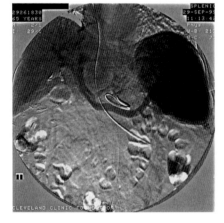

Fig. 31.2 Splenic vein. The contrast is followed as it flows out of the splenic vein and then cephalad in the portal vein. There is a significant umbilical vein (double shadow with the portal vein) and a small left gastric vein (off the splenic vein) filling on this study. The second, more caudal catheter is positioned within the left renal vein to aid preoperative determination of the spatial relationship between the splenic and left renal veins

Fig. 31.3 Normal left renal vein. This study has been performed via the right jugular vein, and demonstrates the left renal vein as it heads cephalad towards the inferior vena cava

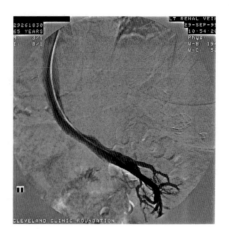

Fig. 31.4 Circumaortic left renal vein. A circumaortic left renal vein, present in 20% of the population, does not prevent construction of a DSRS. The superior and anterior component is always larger and can be used for the shunt. More problematic is a totally retroaortic vein, found in 4% of the population, which runs transversely and is more fixed in the retroperitoneum, making exposure of the anastomosis more difficult. These patients are better served with a splenocaval shunt

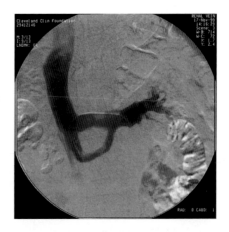

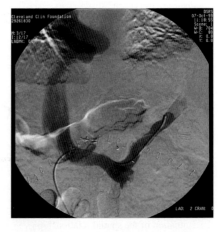

Fig. 31.5 Postoperative catheterization of the distal splenorenal shunt (DSRS). The tip of the catheter lies within the mobilized splenic vein, and the first bend marks the splenorenal anastomosis. The skin staples mark the extended left subcostal incision

31.1
Commentary

The case presented illustrates several important points:

- Prophylactic management of gastroesophageal varices, strictly speaking, is prior to the first bleeding episode. The risk of bleeding in a patient with cirrhosis is approximately 30%. Once they have had one bleeding episode, the risk of rebleeding rises to 75% without active therapy. Non-cardioselective beta-blockade with propranolol or nadolol is the preferred treatment for true prophylaxis for medium or large size varices. **[Q1: C]**
- Acute variceal bleeding is an emergency situation with a high mortality if not appropriately managed. Appropriate monitoring, pharmacologic therapy, and endoscopic diagnosis and treatment are the mainstays of treatment of an acute bleeding episode. It is a very small percentage of patients who do not have their bleeding controlled with the above measures and come to an emergency decompression. **[Q2: A, D]**
- The evaluation of the patient after an acute bleeding episode should assess the varices (endoscopy), the vascular anatomy (ultrasound and angiography) (Figs 31.1–31.4), and the liver disease (Child's class and MELD score). **[Q3: A, B, C, D, E]**
- When a patient has had an acute bleeding episode, their risk of rebleeding is over 70% if they have no specific treatment. The initial approach to treatment is to reduce the portal hypertension with a non-cardioselective beta-blocker, and to deal with the bleeding varices directly with endoscopic therapy. The majority of patients do not need variceal decompression at this stage. If the patient obviously has advanced to end-stage liver disease, a transplant evaluation is in order, and appropriate candidates should move forward with that treatment **[Q4: B, D]**
- When patients have recurrent bleeding through first-line treatment they may need decompression of their gastroesophageal varices. Surgical therapy will do this well in 95% of patients, while the success rates of radiologic shunts in the literature are not this high. Decompression of varices does not improve the survival of patients compared to other first-line treatment options. Liver transplant provides excellent variceal decompression, but its use is dictated by end-stage disease rather than variceal bleeding. **[Q5: B]**

31.2
General Considerations

The major complications of portal hypertension are variceal bleeding, ascites, and progressive hepatic dysfunction. Ascites and encephalopathy are signs of decompensation, and as a general guideline, are only effectively managed by liver transplant. Not all patients with these clinical endpoints may be suitable candidates for transplant. In contrast, variceal bleeding can occur in patients who have well-preserved liver function and therefore have a wider range of treatment options available.

The etiology of portal hypertension may be presinusoidal, as in portal vein thrombosis; sinusoidal, as in cirrhosis; and rarely, post sinusoidal, as in Budd-Chiari syndrome. Much the most common etiology in the USA and Europe is cirrhosis, with approximately 90% of patients having this etiology. The evaluation of the patient with suspected portal hypertension includes an endoscopy to assess size and extent of varices with risk factors for bleeding. Larger varices with red color signs are at increased risk of bleeding or of rebleeding. Laboratory tests should assess liver function, and overall disease status. Non-specific tests include bilirubin, prothrombin time, albumin, and liver enzymes. Recently documented is the importance of serum creatinine in assessing overall severity of disease and prognosis. The two standard methods for assessing this are the Child–Pugh score (Table 31.1), and the Model for Endstage Liver Disease (MELD score – Table 31.2). Other laboratory studies that are important relate to the etiology with hepatitis panels, alpha-fetoprotein as a marker for hepatocellular carcinoma, and specific markers for metabolic diseases such as hemochromatosis and Wilson's disease.

Imaging studies are important in evaluation, with ultrasound used to assess the liver morphology, and Doppler evaluation for liver vasculature. Patency of the main vessels and direction of flow can be assessed well with Doppler ultrasound. Angiography is still indicated for patients being considered for surgery. Accurate assessment of the splenic, portal, and left renal veins is important for DSRS, and may further elucidate details that are not seen on ultrasound. Liver biopsy is occasionally indicated in some patients for clarification of etiology and to delineate the activity of the liver disease process.

Table 31.1 Child–Pugh classification

Parameter	1 Point	2 Points	3 Points
Serum bilirubin (mg/dL)	<2	2–3	>3
Albumin (g/dL)	>3.5	2.8–3.5	<2.8
Prothrombin time (↑s)	1–3	4–6	>6
(INR)	<1.7	1.71–2.24	>2.25
Ascites	None	Controlled medically	Controlled poorly or uncontrolled
Encephalopathy	None	1–2	3–4

Classification: A, 5–6 points; B, 7–9 points; C, 10–15 points
INR international normalized ratio

Table 31.2 MELD score for stratification of liver disease severity

Score = $0.957 \times \log_e$ creatinine (mg/dL)

$+ 0.378 \times \log_e$ bilirubin (mg/dL)
$+ 1.120 \times \log_e$ INR

INR international normalized ratio

Management of portal hypertension falls in to three broad groups:

- Prophylactic treatment.
- Management of an acute variceal bleed.
- Prevention of recurrent variceal bleeding.

Prophylactic treatment is indicated for moderate or large size varices to reduce the risk of an initial bleed. Varices are present in 30–60% of patients with cirrhosis. Thirty percent of patients with varices will bleed from them. After an initial bleed, 20–50% will rebleed in the first week, and 75–80% will rebleed within a year. The mortality of an acute bleeding episode is approximately 25%. To reduce the risk of this initial bleed, the goal is to reduce portal pressure to <12 mm Hg or by 20% from the baseline. This is best achieved with a non-cardioselective beta-blocker (propranolol, nadolol).[1] Other treatments, such as endoscopic therapy, TIPS, or surgical shunt are not indicated for prophylaxis. There are currently further ongoing trials looking at band ligation for patients with large varices where this might be an appropriate method for prophylaxis.[2] **[Q1: C]**

Management of an acute variceal bleed involves resuscitation, pharmacologic reduction of variceal pressure, and endoscopic therapy.[3] Resuscitation requires careful monitoring and enough blood volume and transfusion to maintain blood pressure, but not over-transfuse and precipitate a vicious cycle of further bleeding. Octreotide is the drug of choice for pharmacologic pressure reduction and is given as a continuous infusion of 50 µg/h. Endoscopic therapy is combined with endoscopic evaluation and it best done with banding of varices if visibility is adequate. Occasionally, direct sclerotherapy injection may be required to stop acute bleeding. In the <10% of patients who do not have their acute bleeding controlled with such measures, or in whom early significant rebleeding occurs, early decompression is occasionally required. This can best be achieved with TIPS at the current time.

Prevention of recurrent variceal bleeding has to take in to account the risk of rebleeding, and the underlying liver disease. First-line treatment to prevent rebleeding is with a course of endoscopic banding in conjunction with pharmacologic therapy to reduce portal pressure with non-cardioselective beta-blocker.[3] This combination will reduce the risk of rebleeding to approximately 20%. Banding has been shown to be considerably better than sclerotherapy in terms of bleeding control and fewer complications. However, mortality is not significantly different in the randomized trials that compared banding to sclerotherapy. Concurrent with this first-line treatment, assessment and management of the underlying liver disease is important. At this time, assessment as to whether the patient is headed for transplant now or in the foreseeable future is important. If this is the case, more invasive therapies are precluded, transplant evaluation should be completed, and the patient should be appropriately listed. In this population, transplant has significantly improved the outcome of patients with Child's class C cirrhosis who have end-stage disease, and have variceal bleeding.

For better-risk patients who have recurrent bleeding through first-line treatment, variceal decompression may be indicated. The current options are with a radiologic shunt (TIPS).[4] or with a surgical shunt such as a DSRS,[5] or some type of portacaval shunt. The literature data indicates that the rebleeding rate with TIPS is in the 15–20% range.

Rebleeding with surgical shunts is in the 5% range. However, TIPS can be achieved in a much less invasive fashion compared to the major surgery required for a surgical shunt. Two randomized trials have compared TIPS to surgical shunt. Rosemurgy et al.[6] compared TIPS to an 8-mm H-graft interposition portacaval shunt. They showed notably lower rebleeding in the surgical shunt group, significantly less need for transplant, but no difference in mortality. They concluded that surgical shunt was preferable to TIPS. Henderson et al.[7] have compared TIPS to DSRS in Child's class A and B patients. They showed no significant difference in rebleeding between DSRS (6%) and TIPS (9%) in this trial; however, the TIPS group had an 82% reintervention rate to maintain decompression and this excellent control of bleeding. The encephalopathy rates were not significantly different in the two groups, and neither was survival. The conclusion from this trial is that bleeding can be equally efficaciously managed with TIPS or DSRS with no difference in survival or encephalopathy; however, significantly more reintervention is required in patients managed with TIPS. This trial is summarized in Table 31.3.

Have covered stents improved TIPS outcome? A multicenter prospective randomized trial in Europe[8] has shown a significantly lower dysfunction with covered stents, with a particular advantage in control of ascites in that trial. Survival was not significantly different with covered or uncovered TIPS stents (Table 31.4).

Table 31.3 Data for DSRS versus TIPS randomized trial[7]

Results	DSRS $n = 73$	TIPS $n = 67$	p
Rebleeding	4 (5.5%)	6 (9%)	NS
Reintervention	8 (11%)	55 (82%)	<0.0001
Encephalopathy			
Single event	36 (50%)	34 (50%)	NS
Multiple events	18 (25%)	17 (25%)	NS
Survival			
2-year	81%	88%	NS
5-year	64%	60%	NS

TIPS Transjugular intrahepatic portal systemic shunt, *DSRS* distal splenorenal shunt

Table 31.4 Data for covered versus uncovered TIPS – European trial[8]

Results	PTFE	Uncovered	p
"Dysfunction"	5 (15%)	18 (44%)	<0.001
Bleeding	2/19 (11%)	4/29 (14%)	NS
Ascites	1/20 (5%)	8/12 (67%)	<0.05
Reintervention	6/39 (15%)	22/41 (54%)	<0.05
Survival	27/39 (69%)	22/41 (54%)	NS

TIPS Transjugular intrahepatic portal systemic shunt

The data at this time would therefore indicate the following:

- Patients with cirrhosis and moderate to large varices should receive prophylactic therapy with non-cardioselective beta-blocker prior to the initial bleed.
- Patients with acute variceal bleeding should be managed in an intensive care unit with careful monitoring, adequate transfusion, pharmacologic and endoscopic therapy.
- Patients with recurrent variceal bleeding should be managed with endoscopic banding and a non-cardioselective beta-blocker. Only those patients who have well-preserved liver function, and rebleed through first-line treatment, should be considered for decompression. This can be achieved with either a surgical shunt or TIPS. Patients with end-stage liver disease need to be evaluated for their suitability for transplant and transplanted if appropriate. **[Q5: B]**

References

1. Schepke M, Kleber G, Nurnberg D, et al. Ligation versus propanolol for the primary prophylaxis of variceal bleeding in cirrhosis. *Hepatology*. 2004;40:65-72.
2. Sarin SK, Lamba GS, Kumar M, Murthy NS. Comparison of endoscopic ligation and propanolol for the primary prevention of variceal bleeding. *N Engl J Med*. 1999;340:988-993.
3. Grace ND, Groszmann RJ, Garcia-Tsao G, et al. Portal hypertension and variceal bleeding: an AASLD single topic symposium. *Hepatology*. 1998;28:868-880.
4. Boyer TD, Haskal ZJ. The role of transjugular intrahepatic portosystemic shunt in management of portal hypertension. *AASLD Pract Guidel Hepatology*. 2005;41:386-400.
5. Henderson JM. Distal splenorenal shunt. In: Blumgart LH, ed. *Surgery if the Liver, Biliary Tract, and Pancreas*, 4th ed.; Sect XV, Chap 98. 2005; in press.
6. Rosemurgy AS, Serafini FM, Zweibel BR, et al. Transjugular intrahepatic portosystemeic shunt vs. small-diameter prosthetic H-graft portacaval shunt: extended follow-up of an expanded randomized prospective trial. *J Gastrointest Surg*. 2000;4:589-597.
7. Henderson JM, Boyer TD, Kutner MH et al. and the DIVERT study group. DSRS vs. TIPS for refractory variceal bleeding: a prospective randomized controlled trial. *Gastroenterology*. 2006;130:1643-1651.
8. Bureau C, Garcia-Pagan JC, Otal P, et al. Improved clinical outcome using PTFE coated stents for TIPS: results of a randomized study. *Gastroenterology*. 2004;126:469.

Part VI

Management of Extracranial Cerebrovascular Disease

Management of Carotid Bifurication Disease

32

Wesley S. Moore

A 72-year-old white male was referred for evaluation and management following the finding of an asymptomatic carotid bruit, picked up on routine physical examination by his primary-care physician. The patient was asymptomatic with respect to ocular or hemispheric ischaemic events. His risk factors included a 30-year history of smoking one pack of cigarettes a day, which he quit a year ago. He had hypertension that was controlled well by two drugs. He had no history of coronary artery disease, diabetes mellitus, or symptoms of peripheral vascular disease. On physical examination, his temporal pulses were equal. His carotid pulses were full and equal, but there was a loud bruit over the right carotid bifurcation. His femoral, popliteal, dorsalis paedis and posterior tibial pulses were normally palpable bilaterally.

Question 1

What should the next step in this patient's evaluation be?

A. Counseling with respect to the nature of carotid territory ischaemic attacks
B. Start the patient on an antiplatelet drug, such as aspirin, and a statin
C. Counsel the patient with respect to the importance of refraining from cigarette smoking and careful control of blood pressure
D. Obtain bilateral carotid duplex scanning
E. All of the above

The patient underwent a bilateral carotid duplex scan. **[Q1: D]** The scan demonstrated a category 60–79% right carotid bulb stenosis. The plaque characteristic was one of mixed consistency, a mildly irregular surface, and minimal calcification. The left carotid bulb showed a category 20–59% stenosis. Both vertebral arteries were imaged with normal antegrade flow velocities.

W.S. Moore
Division of Vascular Surgery, UCLA, Los Angeles, CA, USA

G. Geroulakos and B. Sumpio (eds.), *Vascular Surgery*,
DOI: 10.1007/978-1-84996-356-5_32, © Springer-Verlag London Limited 2011

Question 2

What would be appropriate management for this patient?

A. Elective carotid endarterectomy
B. Full Coumadin anticoagulation
C. Aspirin antiplatelet management, a statin, and risk factor control

The patient was placed on aspirin antiplatelet therapy, begun on a statin,[9] counseled regarding the importance of good blood pressure control including the use of a beta blocker or ACE inhibitor, and given an appointment for a return visit in 6 months time for a repeat carotid duplex scan to see whether there was any evidence of progression. The patient was also counseled regarding the importance of calling the vascular service should he develop ocular or hemispheric transient ischaemic attacks within the 6-month interval before his return appointment. **[Q2: C]**

The patient did quite well for the next 4 months; then one afternoon, he noted the onset of an episode of numbness and weakness of his left hand. The hand was not totally paralyzed, but it was clearly numb, weak and uncoordinated. This cleared completely within a period of 10 min. The patient thought that this might have been related to his arm position and chose to do nothing further until the next day, when the same event occurred. At this point, he called his physician and was advised to return immediately. An emergent carotid duplex scan was ordered. The scan now showed progression to a category 80–99% stenosis with plaque once again of mixed consistency.

Question 3

What is the best management for this patient?

A. Clopidogrel antiplatelet therapy
B. Full Coumadin anticoagulation
C. Schedule elective carotid endarterectomy 1 month from now
D. Urgent right carotid endarterectomy

The patient now had two clear indications for proceeding with carotid endarterectomy: the onset of symptoms in the territory of the carotid lesion, and progression of the lesion to an 80–99% stenosis. Two additional decisions also had to be considered: the timing of operation and whether brain imaging was indicated. In view of the fact that the patient had an appropriate carotid artery lesion, and the symptoms were typical for hemispheric transient ischaemic events in the distribution of the carotid lesion, information gained from brain imaging such as computed tomography (CT) or magnetic resonance imaging (MRI) would be of limited value. Therefore, the cost/benefit ratio for brain imaging was clearly unfavorable. The timing of carotid endarterectomy was urgent. The patient had a new onset of transient ischaemic attacks and evidence of plaque progression. Therefore, the patient was now at highest risk of a hemispheric stroke. The optimum management for this patient would be emergent admission to the hospital and rapid evaluation for operation, including the patient's cardiac status.[10,11]

While this was taking place, it would be appropriate to start the patient on intravenous heparin anticoagulation. Once cleared from a cardiac standpoint, plans should be made to proceed with operation either that day or the next morning. **[Q3: D]**

The patient was admitted as an emergency to the hospital and started on intravenous heparin with a loading dose of 5,000 units and a continuing dose of 1,000 units/h. He was seen in cardiology consultation, an electrocardiogram (ECG) was obtained and a stress-echo study was performed. In the absence of any symptoms of coronary disease, a relatively normal ECG, and a stress-echo study showing a 55% ejection fraction, the patient was cleared for operation.

Question 4

What should the next step in this patient's management be?

A. Aortic arch angiogram with selected carotid arteriograms
B. Magnetic resonance angiogram (MRA)
C. CT angiogram
D. Proceed with operation on the basis of a duplex scan of diagnostic quality in an accredited laboratory

The patient was taken to the operating room the next morning. Before this, EEG electrodes were placed for intraoperative monitoring. An arterial line was placed for blood pressure monitoring, and general anaesthesia was administered. A vertical incision along the anterior border of the sternomastoid muscle was made. The facial vein was divided, and the common carotid, carotid bifurcation, internal and external carotid arteries were fully mobilized. There was a posterior plaque present in the common carotid artery, which was non-occlusive. The major plaque build-up was in the bulb of the internal carotid artery, which went a short distance beyond the bulb into the internal carotid artery distally. Beyond this point, the vessel was circumferentially soft. The distal internal carotid artery was somewhat collapsed, and no distal pulse was noted. Since the patient had experienced only transient symptoms and not a completed stroke, it was our plan to use an internal shunt only if there were electroencephalogram (EEG) changes with trial clamping. A bolus of 5,000 units of heparin was administered, and the internal, external and common carotid arteries were clamped. The EEG was observed: there were no changes. The amplitude and frequency of the EEG wave form were maintained. A longitudinal arteriotomy was made in the common carotid artery and extended through a very tight carotid stenosis. The plaque within the carotid bulb showed evidence of recent intraplaque haemorrhage. As we passed through the plaque, we emerged into an unencumbered internal carotid artery distally. A bifurcation endarterectomy was then performed with clean endpoints in the internal, external and common carotid arteries. The intimectomised surface was then irrigated with heparinised saline, and small bits of medial debris were removed carefully. The intimal endpoint was adherent to the media. Once we were satisfied that there was no evidence of intimal flap and all of the loose bits of medial debris were removed, attention was turned to closure.

Question 5

Closure of the arteriotomy should be:

A. A primary, carefully placed closure with 6–0 prolene
B. Closure with a patch angioplasty

The patient's arteriotomy was closed with a patch angioplasty using a collagenimpreg-nated knitted Dacron patch that was cut to length and beveled at each end. Upon comple-tion of the closure, blood flow was begun first to the external then to the internal carotid artery. Excellent pulsation in all vessels was noted. We then carried out a completion angiogram by placing a small needle in the patch and injecting contrast into the carotid bifurcation using a portable cine-fluoro unit. The carotid bifurcation was imaged, and there was an excellent technical result with no evidence of residual stenosis or intimal flap. Intracranial imaging was also carried out, and excellent flow into the carotid siphon and the anterior and middle cerebral arteries was confirmed. After meticulous haemosta-sis was achieved, a 7.0-mm Jackson Pratt drain was placed in the wound and brought out through a separate stab wound. The platysmal layer was closed with an absorbable suture, and the skin was closed with a subcuticular absorbable suture. An adhesive plastic dress-ing was applied directly to the skin, and the patient was returned to the recovery room. The patient awoke at his neurological baseline with no evidence of cerebral or cranial nerve deficit. His blood pressure was monitored carefully and was noted to be stable at 150/80 mmHg.

Question 6

After an appropriate stay in the recovery room, to where should the patient be transferred?

A. An intensive care unit with continual monitoring overnight
B. A step-down unit with 3 : 1 nursing coverage and monitoring capability
C. The patient should be left in the recovery room overnight
D. A regular hospital room

Since the patient was neurologically intact and was maintaining his normal blood pressure, he was transferred to a regular hospital room for routine overnight care. The patient spent an uneventful night in a regular hospital room. The following morning, we removed the dressing and drain. The patient was ambulatory and on a regular diet and was discharged home on the first postoperative day.[1] This management is typical of the so-called "fast-track" management of carotid bifurcation disease. Patients are usually admitted electively on the morning of operation, undergo carotid endarterectomy, spend a period of 2–3 h of observation in the recovery room, transfer to a regular hospital room, and are discharged the following morning. Thus, carotid endarterectomy has become extremely cost-effective in the overall medical economic environment. The patient was instructed to return for a routine visit in 3 weeks. At that time, we obtained a right carotid duplex scan to confirm the result of carotid endarterectomy and to establish a new baseline for future comparison. The next visit will be in 6 months, at which time a bilateral carotid duplex scan will be performed. The objective will be to look for evidence of intimal hyperplasia and recurrent stenosis on the side of operation as well as to document whether there is any progression of disease on the contra lateral, nonoperative side. If that test is unremarkable, then the next study will be at the 1-year anniversary. We will then see the patient on a yearly basis and obtain a bilateral carotid duplex scan as a part of that visit.

32.1
Commentary

Many decisions concerning recommendation to perform carotid endarterectomy are based upon the symptomatic status of the patient and the degree of stenosis, as measured by a percentage, in the carotid artery. The NASCET and ECST trials have clearly demonstrated the value of carotid endarterectomy over medical management in symptomatic patients with hemodynamically significant carotid stenoses. It is also well documented that the risk of stroke is greatest within the immediate time frame following the onset of hemispheric TIAs, and gradually diminishes during the course of a year. For this reason, patients and their physicians should be advised to consider the onset of TIAs as an urgent if not emergent indication for workup and intervention. All of the randomized trials have reported their data and have established a baseline threshold stenosis as an appropriate indication for carotid endarterectomy. While this would appear to be a very tangible and straightforward method of quantifying a carotid stenosis, confusion has developed because there are at least two different techniques for measuring percent of carotid stenosis: the North American method and the European method. The North American method was first described in a publication by Hass et al. as part of the Extracranial Arterial Occlusive Disease Study of the 1960s.[2] This method was used in the Veterans Administration Asymptomatic Carotid Stenosis trial and the Asymptomatic Carotid Atherosclerosis Study (ACAS), and was subsequently adopted by North American Carotid Endarterectomy Trial (NASCET) as their method of measurement. The North American method utilizes the following formula: percentage stenosis $= 1 - R/D$, where R is the minimal residual lumen diameter in millimeters, and D is the diameter of the normal internal carotid artery, distal to the bulb, where the walls of the artery become parallel. In contrast, the European method, which has been used in European trials, including the European Carotid Surgery Trial (ECST) trial, uses the following formula: percentage stenosis $= 1 - R/B$, where R again is the minimal residual lumen diameter in millimeters, and B is the projected diameter of the carotid bulb. Since the bulb is not visualized on a carotid arteriogram of a patient with carotid stenosis, a theoretical line is drawn outlining the bulb, emphasising the atheromatous burden within the bulb. Because of these two different methods, percentage stenoses as expressed in the European literature are not equal to percentage stenosis as measured by the North American method. For example, a 60% stenosis European is equal to an 18% stenosis North American; 70% stenosis European equals 40% stenosis North American; 80% stenosis European equals 61% stenosis North American; and 90% stenosis European equals 80% stenosis North American. Thus, when reading a specific article relating to carotid stenosis, it is important to determine which method of measurement is used in order to appropriately follow the recommendations made by the authors. The conservative management of an asymptomatic patient with moderate carotid stenosis includes the use of a statin and either an ACE inhibitor or a Beta blocker. The SPARCL study has clearly demonstrated the role of medical management in the primary prevention of stroke.

The management of patients with asymptomatic high-grade carotid stenosis has been controversial. However, following publication of ACAS and subsequent validation in the ACST study, the approach to management of patients who are asymptomatic has received more universal acceptance. The findings of the ACAS trial demonstrated that there was a 53% relative risk reduction of stroke in patients who underwent carotid endarterectomy for lesions producing at least a 60% diameter-reducing stenosis, by angiography, when compared with medical management alone.[3] It was also pointed out that a 60% diameter-reducing stenosis by angiography is not the same as a 60% stenosis as measured by duplex scan, since the duplex scan criteria for stenosis are concerned with carotid bulb measurement rather than a stenosis as compared with the diameter of the distal internal carotid artery. It is generally accepted that a 60% diameter-reducing stenosis of the internal carotid artery, by angiography, usually corresponds to a duplex scan finding of an 80–99% stenosis.[3] The ACST study performed in the UK found almost identical results.[4] One of the emerging issues concerning the management of asymptomatic patients with hemodynamically significant stenoses has been the improvement in medical management of these patients with the use of statin drugs. While statins were available during the later part of the ACAS trial and during the ACST trial, their use was not mandated as a part of medical management for either the control or the intervention group. Statins in combination with beta blockers or ACE inhibitors have clearly been shown to have a beneficial effect in reducing stroke morbidity and mortality in patients with carotid bifurcation disease who are treated medically alone or who undergo operation. While a post hoc analysis in the ACST trial failed to show any difference in result between those who were and were not on statins with respect to the benefit of carotid endarterectomy, there is clearly the need to repeat the asymptomatic trials in which modern medical management is used in both the control and intervention groups. However and until there are new trial data available, the level 1 evidence still supports the preferential use of carotid endarterectomy in well selected patients with asymptomatic, hemodynamically significant carotid stenosis for the primary prevention of stroke. While this approach will result in many patients receiving CEA who may never have had a stroke, there is still no reliable way to differentiate in advance those patients who will and those who will not have a stroke in the future. Clearly this information needs to be discussed with the patient and the treatment plan selected on the basis of preference and comfort level of the individual patient.

Patients with carotid artery disease who develop symptoms of hemispheric or monocular transient ischaemic events, or who have had a stroke with good recovery, are clearly good candidates for carotid endarterectomy providing that they have a diameter-reducing stenosis of 50% or greater by angiography. This is now accepted uniformly and has been well established by prospective randomized trials in both North America and the UK.[1,5,6]

The work-up of patients with carotid bifurcation disease for operation used to require the performance of a contrast angiogram to confirm the lesion, establish the degree of stenosis, and evaluate the intracranial circulation for other pathology, such as a stenosis of the carotid siphon or an aneurysm of the intracranial branches. As the quality and accuracy of carotid duplex scanning has improved in accredited laboratories throughout the world, the practice of using carotid duplex scan data as the sole imaging requirement before endarterectomy has proliferated. Most centers also require a confirmatory study such as an MRA or CTA before proceeding with operation. In our own unit, the accuracy of carotid duplex scanning in our laboratory is continually compared with the operative findings at the time of carotid endarterectomy. Initially, the carotid duplex scan data were compared with angiography. As our level of comfort with carotid duplex scanning has increased, contrast angiography has essentially been eliminated in our protocol. The only time we resort to additional contrast imaging is when the carotid duplex scan data and the clinical picture fail to correlate.

If the patient has equal upper-extremity blood pressures, as well as good and equal quality pulses in the carotid artery bilaterally, then the likelihood of the patient harboring a lesion at the level of the aortic arch is quite small. The only other pathology that might be missed in the absence of a contrast carotid angiogram is the rare occurrence of an intracranial lesion. It has been our practice to carry out completion angiography following carotid endarterectomy on the operating table. When the completion study is performed, we always make an effort to examine the intracranial circulation as well. To date, after many hundreds of carotid endarterectomy without angiography, there have only been two instances in which significant intracranial arterial pathology has been found. One was a small intracranial aneurysm measuring less than 10 mm; the other was a siphon stenosis, which, had it been known preoperatively, would not have changed the indication for carotid endarterectomy. Based upon this experience, we routinely carry out carotid endarterectomy on the basis of duplex scan alone. However, this duplex scan must be performed in our own laboratory, as we are unwilling to accept data from other laboratories as the sole basis for proceeding with operation. While there are many excellent laboratories that provide reliable data, we routinely cross-check data from outside laboratories with a test in our own laboratory. Since duplex scanning is relatively inexpensive, and since it has become a substitute for expensive studies associated with morbidity and mortality, such as contrast angiography, it is our opinion that this additional cost is money well spent.[7] Contrast angiography, while a longstanding gold standard, is expensive, promotes patient anxiety, and is associated with neurological morbidity and mortality. In the ACAS, where angiography was required before carotid endarterectomy, the risk of the angiogram with respect to stroke morbidity and mortality was equal to the risk of the operation itself.[1] MRA, while noninvasive, tends to be less accurate than a well-performed carotid duplex scan. MRA of the carotid bifurcation will frequently overestimate the percentage of stenosis and will lead to unnecessary operation in many instances. CT angiography, while more accurate, requires a large intravenous contrast bolus to perform the study. [Q4: D]

Another controversy in the management of patients with carotid bifurcation disease concerns the question of whether a carotid arteriotomy should be closed primarily or with a patch angioplasty. For many years, we routinely closed arteriotomies primarily when the vessel appeared to be of good calibre. A retrospective review of our data suggested that this had been a good practice in that our incidence of restenosis had been quite low. Many retrospective comparisons as well as prospective trials have shown inconclusive data concerning the merit of patch angioplasty versus primary closure. However, recently, a prospective trial in patients scheduled for staged bilateral carotid endarterectomy in whom one side was primarily closed and the second side closed with patch angioplasty conclusively demonstrated that those sides closed with patch angioplasty were associated with a statistically lower incidence of restenosis and complication. Based upon these convincing data, it is now our practice to routinely close all arteriotomies with a patch angioplasty.[8] **[Q5: B]**

Other surgeons have modified their surgical practice to perform the operation using eversion endarterectomy, thus avoiding a longitudinal arteriotomy. For those surgeons who are experienced with this technique, and in properly selected patients, this also appears to be a satisfactory alternative. The postoperative monitoring of the patients is important in ensuring the best outcome for these patients. In the past, it had been our practice to monitor patients routinely in the intensive care unit. However, with a retrospective review of our experience, the likelihood of having an untoward event requiring intensive-care nursing in a patient who was neurologically intact and with a normal blood pressure was extremely low. Therefore the cost/benefit advantage of intensive care unit utilization was clearly not there. We now routinely send patients to a regular hospital room. To date, there have been no untoward incidents that have led us to regret this policy. **[Q6: D]**

References

1. Moore WS, Barnett HJ, Beebe HG, et al. Guidelines for carotid endarterectomy: a multidisciplinary consensus statement from the ad hoc committee, American Heart Association. *Stroke.* 1995;26:188-201.
2. Hass WK, Fields WS, et al. Joint study of extracranial arterial occlusion. II. Arteriography, techniques, sites, and complications. *JAMA.* 1968;203(11):961-968.
3. Executive Committee for the Asymptomatic Carotid Atherosclerosis Study (ACAS). Endarterectomy for asymptomatic carotid artery stenosis. *JAMA.* 1995;273:1421-1428.
4. Asymptomatic Carotid Surgery Trial Collaborators. The MRC Asymptomatic Carotid Surgery Trial(ACST): carotid endarterectomy prevents disabling and fatal carotid territory strokes. *Lancet.* 2004;363:1491-1502.
5. North American Symptomatic Carotid Endarterectomy Trial Collaborators. Benefit of carotid endarterectomy in patients with symptomatic moderate or severe stenosis. *N Engl J Med.* 1998;339:1415-1425.
6. European Carotid Surgery Trialists Collaborative Group. Randomized trial of endarterectomy for recently symptomatic carotid stenosis: final results of the MRC European Carotid Surgery Trial. *Lancet.* 1998;351:1379-1387.
7. Chervu A, Moore WS. Carotid endarterectomy without arteriography. Personal series and review of the literature. *Ann Vasc Surg.* 1994;8:296-302.
8. AbuRahma AF, Robinson PA, Saiedy S, Richmond BK, Khan J. Prospective randomized trial of bilateral carotid endarterectomies: primary closure versus patching. *Stroke.* 1999;30:1185-1189.
9. Goldstein LB, Amarenco P, Lamonte M, et al. Relative effects of statin therapy on stroke and cardiovascular events in men and women: secondary analysis of the Stroke Prevention by Aggressive Reduction in Cholesterol Levels (SPARCL) study. *Stroke.* 2008;39(9):2444-2448.
10. Johnston SC. Transient ischemic attack: a dangerous harbinger and an opportunity to intervene. *Semin Neurol.* 2005;25:362-370.
11. Rothwell PM, Giles MF, Flossmann E, et al. simple score(ABCD) to identify individuals at high early risk of stroke after transient ischaemic attack. *Lancet.* 2005;366:29-36.

The Carotid Body Tumor

33

Mark-Paul F.M. Vrancken Peeters, Johanna M. Hendriks, Ellen V. Rouwet,
Marc R.H.M.van Sambeek, Hero van Urk, and Hence J.M. Verhagen

A 63-year old female was referred to our hospital because she had a mass on the right side of the neck. The swelling had slowly progressed in a couple of months. Besides problems with swallowing there were no other complaints. Her previous medical history was unremarkable and she could not remember any family members with similar lesions. Physical examination showed a non-tender mass with a diameter of around 6 cm located just anterior of the sternocleidomastoid muscle in the anterior triangle of the neck. The mass was mobile in a back-forward direction but could not be moved in a cranial-caudal direction. No signs of cranial nerve deficits were detected. An ultrasound examination showed a highly vascularized structure in the bifurcation between the internal and external carotid artery (Fig. 33.1).

Question 1

What is the most likely diagnosis that caused the swelling in the neck?

A. Enlarged lymph mode
B. Paraganglioma
C. Aneurysm of the carotid artery
D. Goitre of the right thyroid lobe
E. Cystic neck lesion

H.J.M. Verhagen (✉)
Department of Vascular Surgery, H-810, Erasmus University Medical Center, Rotterdam,
The Netherlands

G. Geroulakos and B. Sumpio (eds.), *Vascular Surgery*,
DOI: 10.1007/978-1-84996-356-5_33, © Springer-Verlag London Limited 2011

Fig. 33.1 An ultrasound of a carotid body tumor

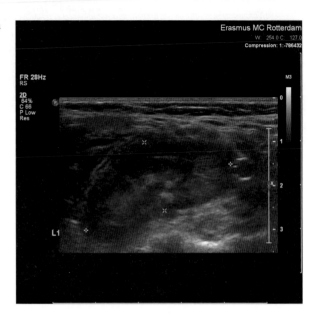

Question 2

Which of the following examinations is preferable to confirm the diagnosis? Rank in order of which is the best method.

A. Needle biopsy
B. Magnetic Resonance Imaging (MRI)
C. Contrast-enhanced angiography
D. Somatostatin receptor scintigraphy (SMS-scan)
E. Angiography

The diagnosis of carotid body tumor was confirmed by MRI (Fig. 33.2) and SMS-scan (Fig. 33.3). The lesion in the neck was measured 5.3 by 4.4 by 4.1 cm. The scans also revealed a similar vascularized mass near the aortic arch and one in the tympanic space of the middle ear. Because of the size of the tumor and the difficulty with swallowing, we decided to treat the patient.

Question 3

What are the possible complications due to the surgical excision of such a large mass in this area?

A. Horner's syndrome
B. Vocal cord paralysis
C. Paresis of the mandibular branch of the trigeminal nerve
D. Ipsilateral tongue paresis
E. All of the above

Fig. 33.2 A magnetic resonance imaging of a carotid body tumor, measuring 5.3 by 4.4 cm. Note the angulation of the carotid arteries due to the mass in between the bifurcation

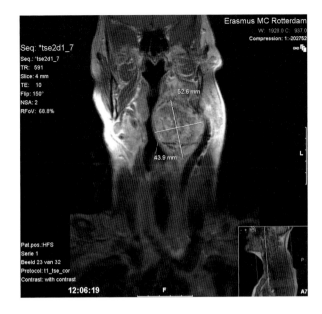

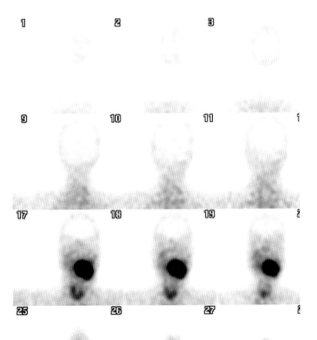

Fig. 33.3 A somatostatin receptor scintigraphy. Abnormally high uptake is monitored in the head and neck region indicating the presence of a carotid body tumor

Question 4

Which of the following statements is correct?

A. A Shamblin I tumor can always be removed without cranial nerve damage
B. A Shamblin III tumor can never be removed without cranial nerve damage
C. When the carotid body tumor is growing, encasement of the carotid arteries takes place
D. When a Shamblin III tumor is removed, the carotid bifurcation needs to be replaced
E. The chances of cranial nerve damage is not dependent of the size of the carotid body tumor

Question 5

What could be the best treatment option in this particular case?

A. Surgical excision
B. Selective embolization
C. Radiation therapy
D. Chemotherapy
E. Combination of these treatment modalities

The risk of complications with the surgical excision of such a large carotid body tumor is relatively high. Therefore, we first embolized the side branches of the external carotid artery and the thyrocervical trunk that feed the carotid body tumor, to let the tumor shrink in size (Fig. 33.4). After 1 year, the carotid body tumor had decreased in size to 4 by 3.5 by 3 cm. The smaller the size of the tumor, the more likely that resection of the tumor can be performed with minimal morbidity.

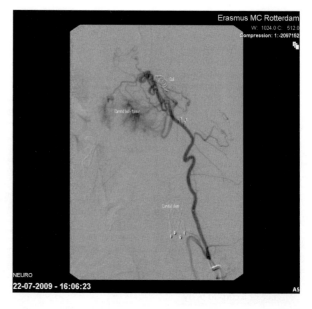

Fig. 33.4 Contrast angiography of the procedure, in which the feeding vessels to the carotid body tumor were coiled and a covered stent was placed in the common and internal carotid artery. In this way, the tumor was abolished from having access to the blood supply

33.1
Commentary

Paragangliomas are usually benign tumors from a collection of anatomically dispersed neuroendocrine organs associated with the autonomic nervous system and characterized by morphologically and cytochemically similar neurosecretory cells derived from the neural crest.[1] The paraganglia play an important role in homeostasis, either by acting directly as chemical sensors or indirectly by secreting catecholamines in response to stress. The paragangliomas are generally divided into two groups, those occurring in the head and neck region and those occurring elsewhere, with the adrenal medulla being the most frequent site. The most common locations of paraganglia in the head and neck region are the carotid bifurcation, the vagal nerve, the jugular foramen, and the tympanic space of the middle ear. The carotid body tumors (glomus caroticum), tumors in the carotid bifurcation, are the most common type of head and neck paraganglioma.

The carotid body is a small highly vascularized, ellipsoid structure located in the adventitia of the bifurcation of the common carotid artery.[2] The carotid body functions as an oxygen sensor and stimulates the cardiopulmonary system in hypoxia through afferent input by way of the glossopharyngeal nerve to the medullary reticular formation.[3] Carotid body tumors can develop spontaneously and can be induced by chronic hypoxia. The latter includes living at high altitudes and certain medical conditions (patients with chronic obstructive pulmonary disease, cyanotic heart diseases).[4-6] Familial cases are frequently bilateral or multifocal and have an earlier age of detection.[7] The inheritance pattern of paraganglioma is autosomal dominant modified by maternal genomic imprinting.[8] Five genetic loci have been identified.[8-12] The majority of the tumors are benign but local expansion can cause cranial nerve deficits and invasion of local structures such as the skull base and the parapharyngeal space. Malignancy is observed in about 5% of cases.[13] Malignancy cannot be defined on the basis of unique histological criteria of the tumor itself, but only by the presence of metastases, mostly in regional lymph nodes.[14]

33.2
Clinical Presentation

Carotid body tumors can be distinguished from other diseases, such as enlarged lymph nodes, aneurysms of the carotid artery, goitre of the right thyroid lobe, and cystic neck lesions by a detailed history and physical examination. Although carotid body tumors can occur at any age, they typically present themselves between the third and sixth decades of life.[15] The presence of an asymptomatic palpable mass, slowly growing in the anterior triangle of the neck, must raise suspicion for this diagnosis. In addition to this mass, the patient may present with cranial nerve deficit like hoarseness, tongue paresis, and dysphagia. Hormone production, like catecholamine secretion by the tumor, is generally present in only 5% of patients[13] and can cause hypertension.

On physical examination, the pulsatile mass can be moved laterally, but not vertically because of adherence to the carotid artery. A bruit may be heard over the mass, but this is a rare condition. Special attention should be made to the two most damaged cranial nerves in the case of a carotid body tumor: Paresis of the hypoglossal nerve causes tongue dysfunction and paresis of the vagal nerve causes hoarseness. **[Q1: B]**

A duplex ultrasound is usually performed to differentiate between a carotid body tumor and other possible diseases (Fig. 33.1). For further investigation magnetic resonance imaging (MRI) is the preferred method to visualize the circumscript mass at or above the carotid bifurcation (Fig. 33.2). Also, other locations of paraganglioma in the head and neck region can be identified with this imaging technique. **[Q2; B, D]** Use of contrast material usually shows a "salt and pepper" appearance caused by vessels with signal-voids within the tumor tissue. This shows the marked vascularization of the tumor which may help to differentiate them from other tumors with less vessels. If a paraganglioma is present, at least at one occasion the plasma and urine levels of catecholamines should be checked.

A somatostatine receptor scintigraphy (Fig. 33.4) is a nuclear scan that uses an injected radiolabeled somatostatin analogue octreotide. Somatostatin receptor scintigraphy can be used to detect paragangliomas as they contain somatostatin receptor carrying tissue. The patient receives an intravenous injection of this substance and imaging takes place after 24 and 48 h. Somatostatin receptor scintigraphy has a much higher sensitivity for paraganglioma than a MIBG scan[16] **[Q2: B, D]** If a carotid body tumor is suspected, fine needle aspiration should not be performed and certainly an incision biopsy should be avoided in all cases. The diagnosis of a carotid body tumor is difficult to make on fine needle aspiration and both procedures can give rise to unnecessary complications such as massive bleeding.

33.3
Treatment

The preferred treatment for carotid body tumors is either conservative or surgical. Excision is the preferred definitive treatment, although the postoperative morbidity rate as quoted in the literature is rather high. Morbidity includes cranial nerve dysfunction, mostly of nerves X and XII, but also other nerves can be damaged like the glossopharyngeal nerve, the facial nerve or the sympathetic nervous system. **[Q3: E]** Tumor size is important as larger tumors have a higher incidence of complications.[17] Postoperative mortality should not exceed 2–5% and occurs only in large tumors, while mortality is negligible in small tumors. Damage to the wall of the carotid artery, especially in the bifurcation, which is difficult to repair because the vessel wall is very thin as a result of dissection in the subadventitial space, may force the surgeon to clamp the internal carotid artery, sometimes leading to ischaemic stroke and death.

In 1972, Shamblin proposed a surgical classification for carotid body tumors based on their tendency to encase the carotid arteries. Shamblin group I are small tumors with minimal attachments to the carotid vessels. Surgical excision can be performed without difficulty and the percentage of cranial nerve damage is very low. Shamblin group II tumors are larger and partially encase the carotid arteries, while Shamblin group III tumors are very large tumors that completely encase the carotid arteries. The percentage of cranial nerve damage in Shamblin II tumors is around 7%.[17] In Shamblin III tumors, it is sometimes even necessary to sacrifice the carotid bifurcation to be replaced by a venous or synthetic interposition graft in order to reconstruct the carotid artery.[18] **[Q4: C]**

Embolization of the feeding branches of the external carotid artery or other main arteries can be performed a few days prior to surgery with the intention to decrease blood loss during operation. Although, this is an area of continuing controversy, some groups claim that embolization decreases blood loss during the operation.[19-21] Others have not found the embolization procedure helpful and they warn of the increased risk of stroke caused by emboli to the brain through collateral pathways.[22,23] Embolization has also been used in the past as an alternative treatment option in very high-risk patients who probably would not tolerate surgical excision.[24] In our patient, 1 year after the embolization procedure the tumor was still shrinking in size and we still have not operated this patient and resected the carotid body tumor. The risk of waiting even longer is the ability of these tumors to recruit new vessels so that perfusion and size will increase after a while. We are very hesitant to believe that embolization alone will be a definitive solution for these kind of tumors. **[Q5: 5]**

Radiation therapy is infrequently used as a treatment option for carotid body tumors. Radiotherapy is, however, a good alternative to surgery, especially for large, fast growing tumors, which are not eligible for surgery. Radiotherapy is effective in arresting growth, but it normally does not result in complete eradication of the tumor.[25] There is no evidence showing that chemotherapy might be effective against carotid body tumors.

33.4
Summary

Paragangliomas are slowly growing, benign tumors. The carotid body tumor is the most common type in the head and neck region. The diagnosis is suspected from the patient's history and physical examination. Ultrasound and MRI can usually confirm the diagnosis, while a somatostatin receptor scintigraphy is a reliable method for detecting multiple tumors and tumors at others locations. If the carotid body tumor is small and there is no documented growth, a wait-and-see policy is justified. A fast growing or large tumor should be treated surgically, cranial nerve dysfunction being the most common postoperative complication.

References

1. Lack EE. *Pathology of Adrenal and Extra-Adrenal Paraganglia*. Philadelphia: WB Saunders; 1994.
2. Netterville JL, Reilly KM, Robertson D, Reiber ME, Armstrong WB, Childs P. Carotid body tumors: a review of 30 patients with 46 tumors. *Laryngoscope*. 1995;105(2):115-126.

3. Pryse-Davies J, Dawsom IMP, Westbury G. Some morphologic, histochemical, and chemical observations on chemodectomas and the normal carotid body, including a study of the chromaffin reaction and possible ganglion cell elements. *Cancer.* 1964;17:185-202.

4. Edwards C, Heath D, Harris P, Castillo Y, Kruger H, Arias-Stella J. The carotid body in animals at high altitude. *J Pathol.* 1971;104(4):231-238.

5. Lack EE, Perez-Atayde AR, Young JB. Carotid body hyperplasia in cystic fibrosis and cyanotic heart disease. A combined morphometric, ultrastructural, and biochemical study. *Am J Pathol.* 1985;119(2):301-314.

6. Roncoroni AJ, Montiel GC, Semeniuk GB. Bilateral carotid body paraganglioma and central alveolar hypoventilation. *Respiration.* 1993;60(4):243-246.

7. McCaffrey TV, Meyer FB, Michels VV, Piepgras DG, Marion MS. Familial paragangliomas of the head and neck. *Arch Otolaryngol Head Neck Surg.* 1994;120(11):1211-1216.

8. Van der Mey AG, Maaswinkel-Mooy PD, Cornelisse CJ, Schmidt PH, van de Kamp JJ. Genomic imprinting in hereditary glomus tumours: evidence for new genetic theory. *Lancet.* 1989;2:1291-1294.

9. Astuti D, Latif F, Dallol A, et al. Gene mutations in the succinate dehydrogenase subunit SDHB cause susceptibility to familial pheochromocytoma and to familial paraganglioma. *Am J Hum Genet.* 2001;69(1):49-54.

10. Baysal BE, Ferrell RE, Willett-Brozick JE, et al. Mutations in SDHD, a mitochondrial complex II gene, in hereditary paraganglioma. *Science.* 2000;287(5454):848-851.

11. Niemann S, Muller U. Mutations in SDHC cause autosomal dominant paraganglioma, type 3. *Nat Genet.* 2000;26(3):268-270.

12. Huai-Xiang H, Khalimonchuk O, Schraders M, et al. SDH5, a gene required for flavination of succinate dehydrogenase, is mutated in paraganglioma. *Science.* 2009;325:1139-1142.

13. Manolidis S, Shohet JA, Jackson CG, Glasscock ME III. Malignant glomus tumors. *Laryngoscope.* 1999;109(1):30-34.

14. Lee JH, Barich F, Karnell LH, et al. National cancer data base report on malignant paragangliomas of the head and neck. *Cancer.* 2002;94(3):730-737.

15. Ward PH, Jenkins HA, Hanafee WN. Diagnosis and treatment of carotid body tumors. *Ann Otol Rhinol Laryngol.* 1978;87(5 Pt 1):614-621.

16. Kwekkeboom DJ, van Urk H, Pauw BKH, et al. Octreotide scintigraphy for the detection of paragangliomas. *J Nucl Med.* 1993;34:873-878.

17. van der Bogt KE, Vrancken Peeters MP, van Baalen JM, Hamming JF. Resection of carotid body tumors: results of an evolving surgical technique. *Ann Surg.* 2008;247:877-884.

18. Shamblin WR, ReMine WH, Sheps SG, Harrison EG Jr. Carotid body tumor (chemodectoma). clinicopathologic analysis of ninety cases. *Am J Surg.* 1971;122(6):732-739.

19. LaMuraglia GM, Fabian RL, Brewster DC, et al. The current surgical management of carotid body paragangliomas. *J Vasc Surg.* 1992;15(6):1038-1044.

20. Muhm M, Polterauer P, Gstottner W, et al. Diagnostic and therapeutic approaches to carotid body tumors. Review of 24 patients. *Arch Surg.* 1997;132(3):279-284.

21. Wang SJ, Wang MB, Barauskas TM, Calcaterra TC. Surgical management of carotid body tumors. *Otolaryngol Head Neck Surg.* 2000;123(3):202-206.

22. Leonetti JP, Donzelli JJ, Littooy FN, Farrell BP. Perioperative strategies in the management of carotid body tumors. *Otolaryngol Head Neck Surg.* 1997;117(1):111-115.

23. Litle VR, Reilly LM, Ramos TK. Preoperative embolization of carotid body tumors: when is it appropriate? *Ann Vasc Surg.* 1996;10(5):464-468.

24. Tasar M, Yetiser S. Glomus tumors: therapeutic role of selective embolization. *J Craniofac Surg.* 2004;15:497-505.

25. Hinerman RW, Amdur RJ, Morris CG, Kirwan J, Mendenhall WM. Definitive radiotherapy in the management of paragangliomas arising in the head and neck: a 35-year experience. *Head Neck.* 2008;30:1431-1438.

Vertebrobasilar Ischemia: Embolic and Low-Flow Mechanisms

34

Ramon Berguer

A 51-year-old male experienced over a period of 6 months a major stroke and several transient ischemic attacks (TIAs) of vertebrobasilar distribution. The original episode consisted of loss of balance, loss of coordination, and loss of the left visual field while driving a bus, which resulted in a road accident. Since then, he had experienced four additional episodes of aphasia and paraparesis lasting for 4–5 h. A diagnosis of vertebral artery dissection was made at the local hospital and he was placed on Coumadin. Concomitant diagnoses were hypertension, non-insulin-dependent diabetes, and hypercholesterolemia. In spite of adequate international normalized ratio (INR) levels, his symptoms continued and he was referred to us.

On admission, magnetic resonance imaging (MRI) showed right occipital and left cerebellar infarctions (Fig. 34.1).

Question 1

The work-up of this patient presenting with symptoms of vertebrobasilar ischemia and MR evidence of infarction in the posterior circulation territory must include:

A. CT scan of the brain
B. Carotid-vertebral duplex
C. Electroencephalogram (EEG)
D. Arteriogram
E. Echocardiogram

R. Berguer
Cardiovascular Center, The University of Michigan, Ann Arbor, MI, USA

G. Geroulakos and B. Sumpio (eds.), *Vascular Surgery*,
DOI: 10.1007/978-1-84996-356-5_34, © Springer-Verlag London Limited 2011

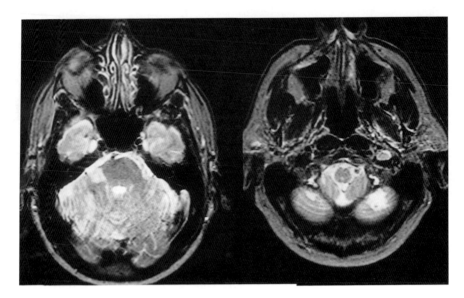

Fig. 34.1 MRI showing cerebellar and brainstem infarctions

Question 2

The etiology of infarction in the posterior circulation territory is:

A. Distal embolization of atheromatous material from vertebral or basilar artery lesions
B. Arrhythmia
C. Bilateral carotid disease in patients with absent vertebral arteries
D. Traumatic or spontaneous dissection of the vertebral artery
E. Transient drop in central aortic pressure in a patient with severe bilateral stenoses of both vertebral arteries

An arteriogram showed a 60% stenosis in the fourth portion of the right vertebral artery, and a tenuous, incomplete (dissected) left vertebral artery, which, at the level of C1, became a normal artery and, higher up, joined with the opposite vertebral artery (Fig. 34.2). A diagnosis of embolizing dissection of the left vertebral artery was made. Because the dissection was not responsive to medical therapy, the patient underwent a bypass from the left internal carotid to the left (suboccipital) vertebral artery using a saphenous vein.[1] The proximal vertebral site of the embolizing dissection was ligated above C1, immediately below the distal anastomosis of the carotid-vertebral bypass (Fig. 34.3). The patient did well from this operation and stopped having symptoms. His anticoagulation was discontinued. He remains asymptomatic after 5 years of follow-up.

Question 3

Once the objective diagnosis of vertebral artery dissection is made in a patient with vertebrobasilar symptoms the next step is:

Fig. 34.2 Arteriogram: dissection of the left vertebral artery, which is occluded from its origin to C4 (*lower arrow*), dissected and partially occluded from C4 to C1 (*between arrows*), and normal distal to C1 (Reprinted from Berguer[1], © 1999, with permission from The Society for Vascular Surgery)

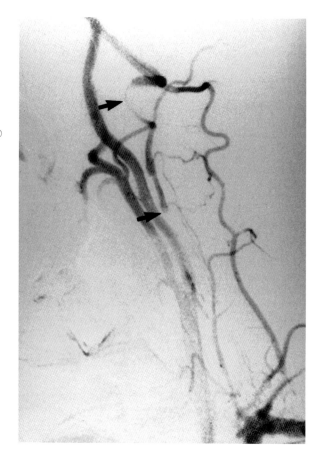

A. Anticoagulation with heparin, then Coumadin
B. Stenting of the dissection followed by antiplatelet therapy
C. Surgical bypass of the dissected segment with ligation of the proximal vertebral artery

34.1
Commentary

Dissection of the vertebral artery may occur spontaneously or result from trauma.[2-6] The traumatic event is usually an exaggerated extension or rotation of the neck as may occur during sports and deceleration injuries. Clinical presentation of dissection of the vertebral artery starts with pain over the posterolateral aspect of the neck irradiating to the nuchal area. There may be an interval of several days between the initial pain, announcing the dissection, and the development of clinical symptoms. The latter are ischemic manifestations of the dissection and appear in 60–90% of patients after an interval of several days, usually 1–2 weeks. In order to visualize the lesion, a carotid-vertebral duplex would not provide a discriminating datum to help in the decision on the management of our patient because it could only detect a concomitant carotid atheroma, which

Fig. 34.3 Postoperative carotid arteriogram showing a saphenous vein bypass from the distal cervical internal carotid to the vertebral artery beyond C1 (Reprinted from Berguer[1], © 1999, with permission from The Society for Vascular Surgery)

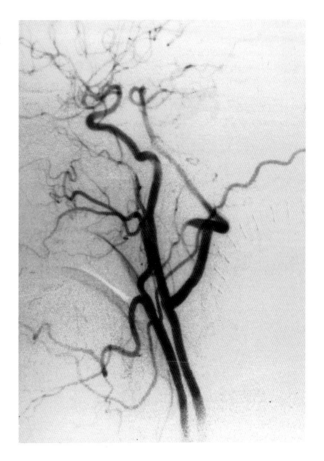

has never been shown to be the source of infarction in the cerebellum or brain stem. The dissected segment of the artery can be visualized by MRA, CTA or arteriography. The latter will provide in addition the information about the carotid arteries that you would have derived from the carotid-vertebral duplex. **[Q1: D, E] [Q2: A, D]** The visualization of the target territories (brain stem, cerebellum and often occipital lobes) is best done with MRI. The dense bone surrounding the brain stem creates resolution artifacts in the CT scan.

The treatment of symptomatic vertebral artery dissection is empirical with systemic anticoagulation. Patients with posterior fossa symptoms should undergo MRI before starting anticoagulation to rule out a subarachnoid hemorrhage. The latter may occur following dissection and rupture of the fourth (intracranial) segment of the vertebral artery.

Anticoagulation is empirically used for the treatment of symptomatic dissection because the ischemia that follows is usually the consequence of embolization from the double channel, not a low-flow effect. The fear of distal extension of the dissection with anticoagulants has prompted some leading experts to give antiplatelet therapy to patients with local symptoms (pain) and evidence of dissection but without central manifestations of ischemia (central nervous system deficits or MR evidence of infarction). Patients with massive infarction are not anticoagulated to avoid intraparenchymal bleeding. There is no indication for wire-catheter-stent manipulation of a dissected vertebral. In patients who are anticoagulated appropriately and continue to have intermittent symptoms, the dissected vertebral artery is considered to be the source of emboli. **[Q3: A]** In these circumstances, and if technically feasible, the dissected segment is excluded and bypassed.[7,8]

34.2
Vertebrobasilar Ischemia: Low-Flow Mechanism

A 62-year-old woman with a healthy lifestyle presented with a history of dimming of the visual field and passing out when she turned her head to the extreme right. Three months before, she had been evaluated elsewhere with a history suggestive of amaurosis fugax and bouts of imbalance and vertigo when she turned her head to the right. A carotid endarterectomy had been performed at another institution.

She continued to have severe vertebrobasilar symptoms with head turning. She had a myocardial revascularization 20 years ago, at which point she stopped smoking.

On examination, the patient appeared healthy, with normal and equal (124/80 mmHg) blood pressure in both brachial arteries. Neurological examination under resting conditions was normal. Her neck was silent. When her head was turned to the right, the patient developed dimming of vision, loss of balance, and a sensation of passing out. The arteriogram available from the previous operation carried out elsewhere showed a clearly dominant large left vertebral artery, but we could not see clearly the distal segment of the vessel. The right vertebral artery was small and diseased severely to a preocclusive level throughout its second segment. There was no evidence of posterior communicating arteries. Because the symptoms were repetitive and induced posturally, the patient was scheduled for a dynamic arteriogram. First, we obtained a view with a selective subclavian injection of the dominant left vertebral in the neutral position, which was normal. Following this, the patient's head was turned to the right; when she became symptomatic, the contrast injection was repeated (Fig. 34.4). This revealed a severe compression of the vertebral artery as it crossed over the posterior lamina of C1, the segment known as the *pars atlantica*.

The patient underwent exploration of the suboccipital space with dissection and exposure of the vertebral artery where it crossed the lamina of C1. The compression mechanism was between the sharp upper edge of the lamina and the occipital bone. A laminectomy was carried out to provide space for the artery to pass from the exit of the transverse foramen of C1 to the foramen magnum without bony compression (Fig. 34.5). The artery was examined by palpation and direct duplex interrogation; we could find no element of plaque or stenosis in the lumen once the artery was freed and the laminectomy completed. The patient became asymptomatic. Full-range motion of the neck no longer caused syncope or vertigo.

Fig. 34.4 Selective injection of a left
subclavian artery while the patient is
experiencing symptoms with her head
turned to the right. The single, dominant
vertebral artery is severely compressed
above C1 in its pars atlantica

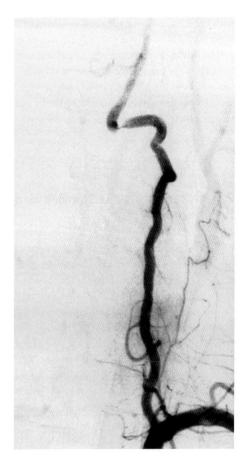

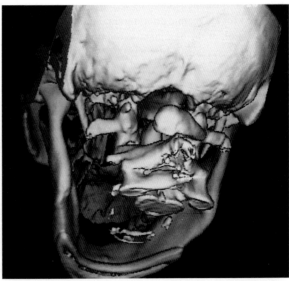

Fig. 34.5 Three-dimensional
reconstruction of a CT scan
of the craniocervical
junction. The lamina of C1
has been removed

Question 1

Which of the following statements regarding posturally induced symptoms is true?

A. The mechanism for ischemia is the restriction of flow by external compression of the artery.

B. The mechanism for ischemia is embolization from the damaged wall (dissection) or thrombus overlying the endothelial lining of the artery at the site of trauma.

C. Both mechanisms may exist.

Question 2

Which of the following statements are correct?

A. When dynamic symptomatic compression of the vertebral artery is demonstrated, angioplasty (with or without stent) is never indicated.

B. Angioplasty of a stenosed or dissected vertebral artery at the suboccipital level is likely to result in rupture of the artery or formation of an arteriovenous fistula.

C. Angioplasty and stenting of the distal vertebral artery is successful in stenosing lesions caused by external compression.

34.3
Commentary

In patients with low-flow ischemia secondary to extrinsic compression of the artery, the clinical picture is repetitive and can be induced by manipulating the patient's head in the trigger position. Those patients who develop vertigo and nystagmus immediately as the head is moved to a particular trigger position should be considered as having Benign Positional Vertigo caused by an osteolith displaced in one of the semicircular canals.[9] Patients with symptoms occurring with head rotation or extension generally experience symptoms a few seconds after inducing the trigger posture should have a dynamic arteriogram to show the anatomic lesion (extrinsic compression) at the same time as the patient experiences symptoms. Patients with low-flow symptoms (repetitive) and no evidence of embolization (negative MRI) may show deformity/compression of one vertebral artery but a normal contralateral vertebral artery during head rotation or extension. If the contralateral, undisturbed artery is of normal size and empties normally into the basilar artery, then the role of the compression of one vertebral artery causing the symptoms is doubtful. The suboccipital approach permits access to the vertebral artery from the transverse process of C2 to the foramen magnum. The techniques used to relieve compression at the suboccipital level are laminectomy, or laminectomy plus bypass. Vertebrobasilar ischemia of postural origin is generally the consequence of mechanical compression of the vertebral artery by osteophytes (and occasionally ligaments) in its extracranial trajectory. The mechanism for symptoms is generally low flow in a dominant vertebral artery that cannot be compensated for by flow from a contralateral hypoplastic or absent vertebral artery. This compression is seen very rarely in the first segment (origin–C6) caused by the tendon of the longus colli. External compression by vertebral osteophytes is usually observed in the second and third segments of the artery. In the second segment (C6–C2), the artery is usually compressed by osteophytes, and the symptoms generally appear with rotation of the neck. In the third segment (C2–C0), the compression occurs in the *pars atlantica* of the artery between C1 and the foramen magnum. The artery is compressed between the sharp upper edge of the lamina of C1 below and the occipital ridge above when the head is rotated in hyperextension. **[Q1: C]**

The ischemic symptoms are usually the consequences of low flow through a dominant vertebral artery because of complete or near-complete occlusion at the latter by compressing osteophyte. Less frequently, the ischemic effects may be embolic from the mural thrombi that develop at the site of repetitive trauma on the artery by the offending osteophyte. In other cases, the artery may dissect at the point of repetitive traumatic compression, which may result in occlusion and/or distal embolization. Symptoms in patients with vertebrobasilar ischemia from the low-flow mechanism are repetitive and can be reproduced every time the neck is brought to the trigger position. Patients with vertebrobasilar ischemia of embolic origin usually present with a clinical stroke or TIA in different areas. MRI in the low-flow group is usually normal, but in the embolic group it may show cerebellar, brainstem or occipital infarctions. An arteriogram is needed to outline precisely the point of compression and to discern the possibility of a dissection and/or tandem lesions. It is also important to outline the entire course of the opposite vertebral artery to establish whether it is complete, normal or hypoplastic, and whether at the time of the provocative dynamic arteriogram the opposite vertebral artery fills the basilar artery normally while the patient has symptoms. The latter would suggest that the mechanism of symptoms is not low flow.

There is no role for angioplasty, with or without stent, in the treatment of extrinsic compression of the vertebral artery. Balloon dilation of the thin-walled vertebral artery against the hard bony prominence of an osteophyte is likely to result in the rupture of the arterial wall and the formation of a false aneurysm or an arteriovenous fistula. If the compression of the vertebral artery is limited to the V2 segment (C6–C2), then the single or multiple elements of compression are bypassed by reconstructing the artery to the level of C1. This is done through an anterior approach.[8] In dynamic compression at the suboccipital level, the approach is posterior[1] and the treatment consists of a laminectomy, with or without bypass. If a bypass is chosen at this level its inflow is obtained from the high cervical carotid. The latter is exposed by moving aside the cranial nerves that block access to the internal carotid when approached posteriorly. **[Q2: A, B]**

References

1. Berguer R. Suboccipital approach to the distal vertebral artery. *J Vasc Surg*. 1999;30:344-349.
2. Mas JL, Bousse M-G, Harbourn D, Laplanc D. Extracranial vertebral artery dissection: a review of 13 cases. *Stroke*. 1987;18:1037-1047.
3. Mokri B, Houser OW, Sandok BA, Peipgzas DG. Spontaneous dissection of the vertebral arteries. *Neurology*. 1988;38:880-885.

4. Chiras J, Marciano S, Vega Molina J, Touboul J, Poirier B, Bories J. Spontaneous dissecting aneurysm of the extracranial vertebral artery (20 cases). *Neuroradiology*. 1985;27:327-333.
5. Ringel SP, Harrison SH, Noremberg MD, Austin JH. Fibromuscular dysplasia: multiple "spontaneous" dissecting aneurysms of the major cervical arteries. *Ann Neurol*. 1977;1:301-304.
6. Noelle B, Clavier I, Berson G, Hommel M. Cervicocephalic arterial dissections related to skiing. *Stroke*. 1994;24:526-527.
7. Caplan L. *Posterior Circulation Disease*. Cambridge: Blackwell; 1996:257.
8. Berguer R, Morasch MD, Kline RA. A review of 100 consecutive reconstructions of the distal vertebral artery for embolic and hemodynamic symptoms. *J Vasc Surg*. 1998;27:852-859.
9. Heidenreich KD, et al. Strategies to distinguish benign paroxysmal positional vertigo from rotational vertebrobasilar ischemia. *Ann Vasc Surg*. DOI: 10.1016/j.avsg.2009.09.018.

Takayasu's Arteritis Associated with Cerebrovascular Ischemia

35

Duk-Kyung Kim and Young-Wook Kim

A 12-year old Korean girl was presented with neck pain and transiently dimmed vision. One year before presenting, the patient developed fever, malaise and bilateral neck pain followed by right leg claudication. More recently, she experienced dimming of the visual field in both eyes, aggravated when facing upwards. She did not have episodes of imbalance, loss of coordination, diplopia or vertigo. She did not complain of dyspnoea, angina or abdominal angina. Her right arm blood pressure (BP) was 99/54 mmHg but the left arm BP was not checkable. A cardiac examination was normal. Both carotid pulses and the right brachial pulse were weak. The left brachial pulse, right popliteal and right dorsalis pedis pulses were not palpable. Bruit was audible over both carotid arteries and in the supraclavicular, infraclavicular and epigastric area. Neurology disclosed no abnormalities. Basal laboratory examinations revealed a white blood count of $9,700 \times 10^3/\mu L$, erythrocyte sedimentation rate (ESR) 66 mm/h, high sensitivity C-reactive protein (hsCRP) 1.19 mg/dL, protein/albumin 7.3/3.8 g/dL, creatinine 0.53 mg/dL and pro-brain-type natriuretic peptide (proBNP) 18.3 pg/mL.

Question 1

Which of the patient's findings does not fulfill diagnostic criteria of Takayasu's arteritis (TA)?

A. Age at disease onset <40 years
B. Claudication of extremities
C. Elevated ESR and CRP
D. Systolic blood pressure (SBP) difference >10 mmHg between arms
E. Bruit over subclavian arteries

Based on her clinical findings, she was diagnosed with Takayasu arteritis.

D.-K. Kim and Y.-W. Kim (✉)
Division of Cardiology, Department of Medicine, Samsung Medical Center, Sungkyunkwan University School of Medicine, Seoul, Korea and
Division of Vascular Surgery, Department of Surgery, Samsung Medical Center, Sungkyunkwan University School of Medicine, Seoul, Korea
e-mail: dkkim@skku.edu; ywkim@skku.edu

G. Geroulakos and B. Sumpio (eds.), *Vascular Surgery*,
DOI: 10.1007/978-1-84996-356-5_35, © Springer-Verlag London Limited 2011

Question 2

The work-up of this patient presenting with TA must include:

A. Conventional angiography
B. Duplex ultrasonography of the carotid artery and lower limb arteries
C. Computed tomography (CT) angiography of the aorta
D. Magnetic resonance imaging (MRI) and magnetic resonance (MR) angiography of the brain

Carotid duplex ultrasonography showed diffuse wall thickening (Fig. 35.1) and severe segmental stenosis of both common carotid arteries. There were diffuse 30% stenosis of the right innominate artery, occlusion of the distal portion of the right subclavian artery, 70% stenosis of the proximal portion of the left subclavian artery and total occlusion after the origin of the left vertebral artery. Duplex ultrasonography of the lower extremity arteries revealed long segmental occlusion of the right superficial femoral artery and the right anterior tibial artery. CT angiography of the thoracoabdominal aorta disclosed wall thickening of the aortic arch and proximal supratruncal branches, total occlusion of the superior mesenteric artery and well-developed collaterals from the inferior mesenteric artery. Brain MRI demonstrated no findings of acute infarction. MR angiography disclosed further findings with stenosis of proximal portion of the right internal carotid artery (Fig. 35.2).

Question 3

Which of the following statements is <u>false</u> regarding BP of the patient?

A. The patient's true BP is 99/54 mmHg.
B. In patient with TA, BP should be measured in all four extremities.
C. Renovascular hypertension is the most common cause of hypertension in patients with TA.
D. Atypical coarctation of the aorta can be a cause of high BP of the upper extremities.

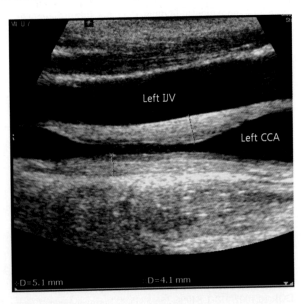

Fig. 35.1 Duplex ultrasonography showing long, smooth, homogenous concentric thickening of the proximal portion of the left common carotid artery. IJV; internal jugular vein, CCA; common carotid artery

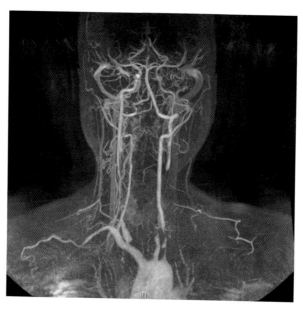

Fig. 35.2 Magnetic resonance (MR) angiography showing vascular involvement in the aortic arch branches. There were total middle occlusion of the right subclavian artery, focal osteal stenosis with post-stenotic dilatation and diffuse long segmental severe stenosis of the right common carotid artery. There were irregular margins of the proximal portion and near total occlusion of the mid portion of the left common carotid artery. The patient also had severe proximal stenosis and total occlusion of the left subclavian artery after the origin of the left vertebral artery and severe proximal stenosis of the left vertebral artery

Measurements of BP in the four extremities by Doppler plethysmography were as follows: right arm SBP 73 mmHg, left arm SBP 58 mmHg, right ankle SBP 82 mmHg and left ankle SBP 139 mmHg. In our patient, both subclavian arteries are occluded and the right superficial femoral artery is occluded as well. No significant stenosis was present in the descending thoracic and abdominal aorta. Only left ankle BP reflects true SBP, which means she is normotensive.

Question 4

In patients with TA involving arch vessels, intervention is indicated in the case of:

A. Severe stenosis of the left subclavian artery without subclavian steal syndrome
B. Severe symptomatic stenosis
C. Frequent episodes of visual dimming
D. Recurrent episodes of transient ischaemic attack (TIA)
E. Severe dizziness

Because of her neurologic symptoms suggesting amaurosis fugax, and severe narrowing of all three cervical arteries, intervention to restore cerebral circulation was planned to lessen her cerebral ischaemic symptoms. Disease activity affects the long-term patency of any bypass or angioplasty procedure. Evaluation of disease activity of TA was performed.

Question 5

In patients with TA, disease activity can be assessed by:

A. Presence of constitutional symptoms such as fever, malaise, arthralgia
B. Elevation of ESR or CRP level
C. Carotid tenderness (carotodynia)
D. Wall thickening or mural enhancement seen by CT or MR angiography
E. Increased uptake on positron emission tomography (PET)

In addition to the patient's systemic symptoms of fever and malaise, both the ESR and CRP level were high and carotodynia was present. Carotid CT angiography showed concentric diffuse wall thickening, hyperenhancement of mural wall and a hypoattenuating inner ring of the artery (Fig. 35.3). An (^{18}F) fluorodeoxyglucose (F-18 FDG) PET-CT scan

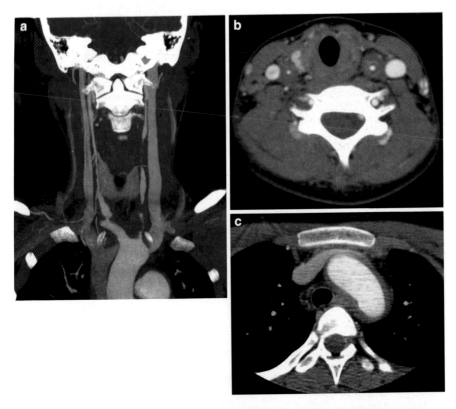

Fig. 35.3 Computed tomographic (CT) angiography. (**a**) Focal osteal stenosis is shown with post-stenotic dilatation and diffuse long segmental severe stenosis of the right common carotid artery. There were irregular margins of the proximal portion and skipped lesions of near total occlusion of the proximal and mid-portion of the left common carotid artery. (**b**) Concentric wall thickening of both common carotid arteries with mural enhancement and low attenuation of the inner concentric ring. This probably represents low attenuation of the intima between the enhanced outer wall of the aorta and intraluminal opacified blood. (**c**) Thickened wall of the aortic arch

showed moderate increase of uptake in the right proximal common carotid artery, left proximal and mid-common carotid artery and the aortic arch (Fig. 35.4). After prescription of prednisolone (0.5mg/kg/day) and aspirin (100 mg/day), her systemic symptom improved. After 6 months of steroid therapy, ESR and CRP dropped to 23 mm/h and 0.37 mg/dL, respectively. Her neck pain had disappeared. However, she experienced more frequent and severe visual dimming, which limited her daily activities. Dimming of the visual field made her walk looking downwards and sunlight exaggerated the amaurosis fugax. Follow-up CT angiography of the carotid arteries showed progression of stenosis of the left common carotid artery and the proximal left vertebral artery. She had severe long segmental lesions of three cervical arteries with a narrowed right innominate artery supplying the patent right vertebral artery (Figs. 35.5 and 35.6a).

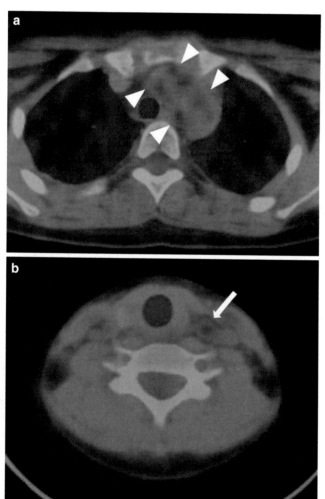

Fig. 35.4 Positron emission tomography (PET) scanning utilizing radioactively labelled (^{18}F) fluorodeoxyglucose (F-18 FDG)-CT showing mild FDG uptake of (**a**) the aortic arch wall (SUVmax = 2.7) (*arrow heads*) and (**b**) the left common carotid artery (SUVmax = 2.7) (*arrow*)

Fig. 35.5 Diagram showing lesions in the aortic
arch and aortic arch branches of the patient

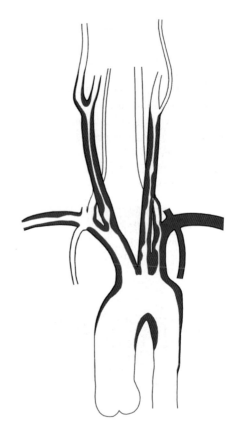

Question 6

In this stage, what kind of intervention do you recommend?

A. Anti-coagulation with heparin, then warfarin
B. Balloon angioplasty of the left vertebral artery
C. Stenting of both common carotid arteries followed by dual anti-platelet therapy
D. Bypass surgery to restore the cerebral blood flow
E. Carotid endarterectomy

We decided to perform bypass surgery for the revascularization of arch vessels with diffuse involvements.

Question 7

What surgical treatment would you recommend for this patient?

A. Ascending aorta-to-left carotid bypass
B. Ascending aorta-to-bicarotid bypass

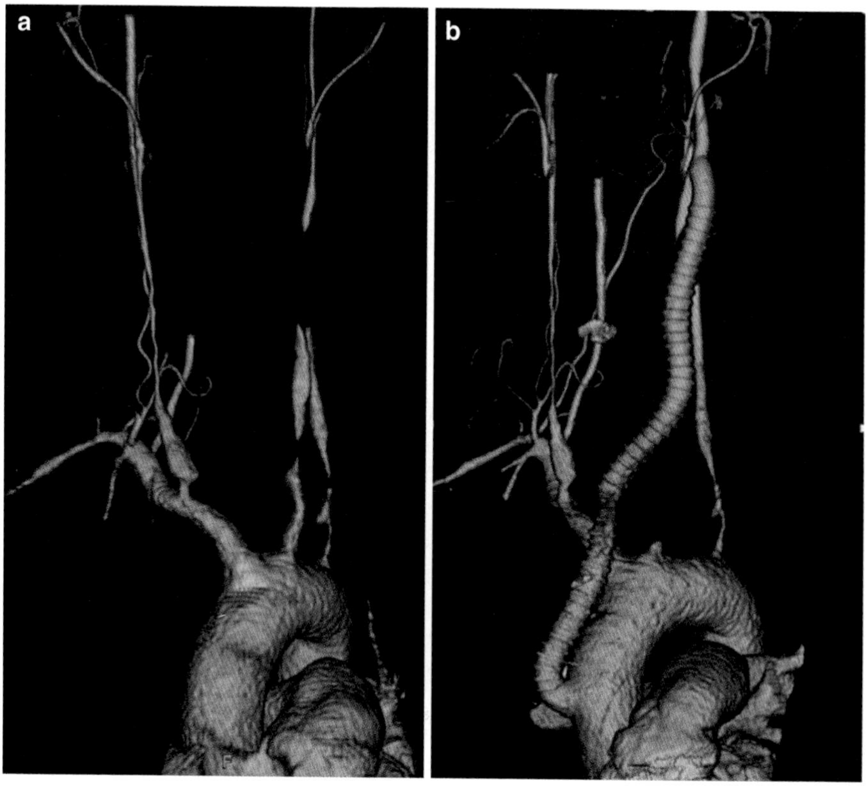

Fig. 35.6 Three-dimensional volume-rendered CT angiography image showing (**a**) pre-operative and (**b**) post-operative findings of aortic arch branches. The external ring-supported polytetrafluoroethylene (PTFE) graft from the ascending aorta to the left internal carotid artery is shown

C. Descending thoracic aorta-to-left carotid bypass
D. Right axillary-to-left carotid bypass

In this patient, the ascending aorta did not show FDG uptake on 18-FDG PET scans whereas CT angiography and duplex ultrasonography showed intimomedial thickening of the right proximal internal carotid artery. We decided to perform ascending aorta-to-left-carotid bypass using an external ring-supported polytetrafluoroethylene (PTFE) graft (Fig. 35.6b).

Question 8

What complications can occur after carotid reconstructive surgery in this patient?

A. Intracranial hemorrhage
B. Anastomotic restenosis
C. Anastomotic aneurysm
D. All of above

The patient's post-operative course was uneventful and she had complete resolution of the visual symptom. She reported considerable improvement in her daily activities. Six months later, a follow-up CT angiography revealed patency of the aorto–monocarotid bypass. She was placed on prednisolone (15 mg/day), methotrexate (15 mg/week) and clopidogrel (75 mg/day) postoperativerly. Her ESR/CRP values remained within upper normal limits. Patency of the bypass was confirmed by CT angiography during a 2-year follow-up.

35.1
Commentary

TA is a chronic vasculitis of the aorta and its major branches, with unknown aetiology. Women are affected in 80–90% of cases, with an age of onset usually between 10 and 40 years. It is common in Asia and Mexico but rare in Europe and North America. The rarity of the disease results in low clinical awareness in Western countries. The American College of Rheumatology has established diagnostic criteria for TA (Table 35.1).[1] **[Q1]** Our patient's clinical findings fulfill five out of six diagnostic criteria. The early diagnosis of TA can be difficult because early symptoms such as fatigue, malaise, weight loss, arthralgia and low-grade fever are non-specific. However, careful examination of the arteries at an early stage can detect a weak pulse, BP discrepancy between the arms, or bruits over the neck, supraclavicular and infraclavicular areas, or the abdomen. This early systemic phase is followed by a late chronic ischaemic phase in which vascular lesions progress slowly over years or decades (Fig. 35.7) with the development of collateral circulation. The incidence of ischaemic symptoms is relatively low compared with arteriosclerosis, despite the extensive steno-occlusive vasculopathy. Detection of bruits or decreased pulses

Table 35.1 American College of Rheumatology (1990) criteria for the diagnosis of Takayasu's arteritis

1. Age at disease onset <40 years:Development of symptoms or findings related to TA at age <40 years
2. Claudication of extremities:Development and worsening of fatigue and discomfort in muscles of one or more extremity while in use, especially the upper extremities
3. Decreased brachial artery pulse:Decreased pulsation of one or both brachial arteries
4. BP difference >10 mmHg:Difference of >10 mmHg in systolic BP between arms
5. Bruit over the subclavian arteries or aorta:Bruit audible on auscultation over one or both subclavian arteries or the abdominal aorta
6. Arteriogram abnormalities:Arteriographic narrowing or occlusion of the entire aorta, its primary branches or large arteries in the proximal upper or lower extremities, not caused by arteriosclerosis, fibromuscular dysplasia or similar causes; the changes are usually focal or segmental

For purposes of classification, a patient shall be said to have TA if at least three of these six criteria are present. The presence of any three or more criteria yields a sensitivity of 90.5% and a specificity of 97.8%. (Adapted from Ref. [1].)

BP, blood pressure (systolic; difference between arms).

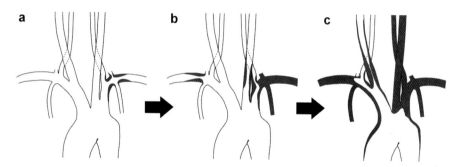

Fig. 35.7 Diagram showing progression of vascular lesions in the aortic arch branches in patients with Takayasu arteritis. (**a**) The initial vascular lesions frequently occur in the left middle or proximal subclavian artery. (**b, c**) As the disease progresses, the left common carotid, vertebral, brachiocephalic, right middle or proximal subclavian artery, right carotid and vertebral arteries and aorta might also be affected (Adapted from Ref. 26)

in a young woman narrows the differential diagnosis to TA. The differential diagnosis includes giant cell arteritis, atherosclerosis and fibromuscular dysplasia. **[Q1]**

Clinical manifestations of TA include systemic symptoms such as fatigue, weight loss and low-grade fever, myalgia and arthralgia. Vascular inflammation may lead to pain such as carotodynia. Most symptoms, however, are the result of ischaemia to organs supplied by stenotic vessels. Patients may have TIAs or strokes, visual aberration, symptoms of vertebrobasilar insufficiency, limb claudication, angina or renovascular hypertension, among others.[2] TA should be ruled out in young female patients with hypertension. Aortic regurgitation, prevalent in Korea and Japan, is often associated with aortic root dilation.[3]

Laboratory results reflect the underlying inflammatory process but are mostly non-specific. A normochromic normocytic anaemia suggestive of a chronic disease is present in most patients. The white blood cell count is usually normal or mildly elevated. Acute phase reactants, such as an elevated ESR and increased serum CRP, are a reflection of the inflammatory process. Although the blood tests are not always precise or reliable indicators of disease activity, they are most frequently used blood test to assess disease activity of TA. **[Q1: C]**

With contrast angiography, primary arteriographic abnormalities are smooth-walled, tapered, focal or narrowed areas with some areas of dilation. Collateral circulation is often prominent because of the chronic nature of the disease. Arteriography can define the location and appearance of the arterial lesion and might also allow a subsequent therapeutic approach through the same arterial puncture **[Q2: A]**. However, it does not evaluate mural changes and is an invasive test associated with some risks. Therefore, if a therapeutic intervention is not anticipated, a less invasive imaging technique may be preferred. CT angiography or MRI of the aorta can reveal the mural changes as well as luminal changes in evaluating large arteries.[4,5] At present, CT or MRI scans appear to be definitive for most patients **[Q2: C, D]**. When diagnosing or evaluating TA, we start with duplex ultrasonography of the carotid artery because duplex scan is non-invasive, has no risk and could disclose luminal and mural changes of the aortic arch branches. **[Q2: B]** Duplex ultrasonography is particularly useful for the assessment of the common carotid arteries, displaying a resolution of 0.1–0.2 mm.[6] In patients with TA, the typical lesion identified by ultrasonography is a long, smooth, homogenous concentric thickening of the arterial wall in contrast to an atherosclerotic plaque shown to be non-homogenous, often calcified and associated with an irregular wall.[7]

Although imaging is optimal at the common carotid and vertebral arteries, assessment of the proximal subclavian and distal internal carotid arteries is limited by overlying tissues.

Underlying systemic hypertension is often missed, as the BP measured in the upper extremities may underestimate the true BP, as a consequence of the subclavian/axillary artery involvements. [Q3: A] It is important to measure BP in all four extremities. [Q3: B] Hypertension develops in more than one half of cases because of renovascular hypertension caused by the narrowing of the renal artery, and by narrowing and decreased elasticity of the aorta and branches [Q3: C]. In the case of atypical coarctation of the aorta, the upper arm BP is elevated. [Q3: D] In rare patients with TA, BP measurements from all four extremities are falsely low because of stenosis or occlusion of extremity arteries combined with atypical coarctation. In such patients, adequate control of BP could be judged by the absence of left ventricular hypertrophy or hypertensive retinopathy. If such a patient has a mitral regurgitation, left ventricular systolic pressure (equal to aortic systolic pressure) can be estimated by mitral regurgitant Doppler flow.

TA usually involves the proximal neck vessels with diversion of the distal flow or collateral filling of distal vessels. Changes in cerebral haemodynamics in relation to occlusive cerebral vascular lesions are not fully understood. Visual disturbances, such as blurring or visual dimming, occur in 8–13% of patients with TA. Permanent loss of vision is unusual in this disease. Stroke and TIAs occur in 5% and 20% of cases, respectively.[8] Carotid stenosis and occlusion are frequently asymptomatic, and isolated subclavian stenosis seldom requires revascularization because of the general adequacy of the collateral circulation. [Q4: A] Therefore, it is uncertain when it might be appropriate to revascularize any stenosis of the arch vessels. Our indications of supra-aortic artery revascularizations are symptomatic stenosis >70%, severe dizziness or ocular symptom, episodes of stroke or TIA. [Q4: B, C, D, E] Occlusive lesions of all four cervical arteries usually have disabling symptoms. Only a minority of patients needs intervention in arch vessels. In the Mayo Clinic, over 27 years, 6% of all patients with TA (16/251) required a bypass of the arch vessels for cerebral ischaemia.[9] For the last 15 years in our institute, 7% of patients with TA (15/205) needed arch vessel bypass operations.

Ideally, interventions should be performed when the disease is inactive to minimize the risks of restenosis or anastomotic dehiscence. A recent study using serial angiography found that intervention performed on patients with stable disease and post-interventional treatment with immunosuppressive drugs were independent variables determining the maintenance of arterial patency.[10] Therefore, controlling disease activity is important before performing any revascularization. However it is not always possible to follow the principle due to urgency of intervention.

Clinical, laboratory and imaging findings of the patient suggested that she has moderately active arteritis. In the early active phase, arterial stenosis might reverse and ischaemic symptoms can improve in response to immunosuppressive therapy. Evaluation of disease activity in patients with TA is challenging. Clinical features do not correlate with acute-phase reactants in ~50% of cases. Imaging modalities do not always correlate with clinical and laboratory parameters. Up to 45% of patients in clinical remission have histological evidence of active disease. Lesions progress with regard to further stenosis or dilatation even in the absence of active disease. The most commonly used criteria of disease activity are NIH criteria (Table 35.2).[11] **[Q5]** However, NIH criteria are not validated. Surgical biopsy specimens from clinically inactive patients showed histologically active disease in 44% of patients. The hsCRP level and mural changes evaluated by CT and MRI were not included in the criteria. Recently, mural changes in CT or MRI have been reported to predict disease activity and response to immunosuppressive therapy. The mural changes indicative of an active TA lesion in CT angiography are a thickened arterial wall with mural enhancement and a poorly attenuated ring on delayed phase images.[12,13] MRI also has the potential to offer a means for assessment of disease activity. Contrast-enhanced MRI showing arterial wall thickening or mural enhancement indicates disease activity.[14] Vascular wall oedema demonstrated by T2-weighted MRI, in the absence of other clinical evidence of active disease, does not appear to be an indicator of active disease.[15] However, CT or MRI application to evaluate disease activity in patients with TA needs to be further explored in prospective studies, with data to date limited. **[Q5: D]** F-18 FDG PET can now be used to image the aorta and great vessels.[16] F-18 FDG PET might be useful in the early diagnosis of TA, as well as for the assessment of disease activity and response to medical treatment. F-18 FDG PET when co-registered with CT better localizes inflammatory activity in the vessel wall of patients with TA showing weak F-18 FDG accumulation.[17] **[Q5: E]**

Percutaneous transluminal angioplasty or bypass grafts might be considered in late cases when irreversible arterial stenosis has occurred and significant ischaemic symptoms are present. Angioplasty is preferable when the lesions are amenable to catheter-based therapy. However, percutaneous intervention is less likely to be successful because TA lesions of the cervical arteries are characteristically long, typically fibrotic and non-compliant, which needs higher balloon inflation pressure with increased risk of rupture and dissection. Angioplasty is more useful to dilate focal discrete lesions of coronary or renal arterial stenosis. **[Q6: B]** Even in this case, balloon angioplasty was preferable than stenting because of the higher restenosis rate when there is continued inflammation of a dilated lesion. **[Q6: C]** Restenosis is less likely following bypass surgery than angioplasty when performed after initiation of treatment, or if revascularization is followed by anti-inflammatory therapy. In this patient, we decided to perform bypass surgery for the revascularization of arch vessels with diffuse involvements. **[Q6: D]**

Endarterectomy or patch angioplasty is not usually selected because of the long segment involvement of the disease and technical difficulties of these procedures for patients with TA. **[Q6: E]** Therefore, arterial bypass is commonly recommended for patients with

Table 35.2 The NIH criteria for the definition of active disease in patients with Takayasu's arteritis

1. Systemic features such as fever, arthralgia (no other causes)
2. Increased erythrocyte sedimentation rate (men ≥ 15 mm/h, women ≥ 20 mm/h)
3. Features of vascular ischaemia or inflammation, such as claudication, diminished or absent pulse, bruit, vascular pain (carotodynia), asymmetric BP in either upper or lower limbs
4. Typical angiographic features

New onset or worsening of two or more features indicates "active disease."
BP, blood pressure (Adapted from Ref.[11].)

cerebrovascular insufficiency caused by TA. Two key points in carotid artery revascularization surgery for TA are the need to perform surgery in a quiescent phase of the disease, and selecting disease-free segments for anastomosis. Accordingly, it is important to determine the degree of activity of the vasculitis and co-existing morbidities such as renovascular hypertension. The clinician must select the target artery(s) to be revascularized, and determine the optimal site for the inflow artery for the bypass surgery and bypass conduit before the operation. In patients with co-existing severe uncontrolled renovascular hypertension caused by co-existing renal artery stenosis, we recommend renal artery intervention first before carotid artery reconstruction, to avoid cerebral hyperperfusion syndrome after carotid surgery. For this purpose, renal artery angioplasty is often recommended.

In patients with bilateral common carotid artery occlusion, some prefer to perform unilateral carotid reconstruction while others recommend bilateral carotid revascularizations. The proponents of unilateral carotid revascularization for patients with bilateral common carotid occlusion argue for the hypothetical advantage of a lower risk of cerebral hyperperfusion syndrome compared with bilateral carotid revascularization. [Q7: A] Proponents of bilateral carotid reconstruction argue for the expected advantages of greater cerebral blood flow after surgery compared with unilateral carotid reconstruction and a lower risk of recurrent cerebrovascular insufficiency when one of the grafts is occluded. [Q7: B] However, there has been no comparative study between unilateral and bilateral carotid artery reconstructions in patients with TA.

To select an optimal site of the proximal anastomosis free of an active lesion, easy access and the risk of late progression of the disease should be considered in patients with TA. Operative findings and pre-operative imaging studies (contrast-enhanced CT, contrast angiography, ultrasonography, MRI and PET scans) are used for the selection of the disease-free inflow artery.

The ascending aorta is often selected as an inflow artery during carotid artery reconstruction because involvement of disease is relatively uncommon at this segment of the aorta, and the risk of late development of anastomotic stenosis is lower than in cases using an aortic branch (e.g., the subclavian or axillary artery) as an inflow artery. [Q7: C, D] However, in patients with critical brain ischaemia, partial clamping of the ascending aorta can further compromise cerebral blood flow. To avoid this potential risk, the descending aorta can be selected as an inflow site for carotid revascularization surgery.[18] Regarding the bypass conduit, some recommend autogenous vein grafts,[19,20] while others prefer to use prosthetic grafts.[21,22]

Two categories of complication can develop after carotid artery reconstruction in patients with TA. One involves neurologic complications, which can occur during the operation or early post-operative period. The other category of late complications which are associated with the graft material, anastomosis site or progression of vasculitis. Most patients who undergo carotid revascularization have multiple and extensive extracranial carotid and vertebral artery occlusive lesions. During the operation, further ischaemia of brain can develop from neck tilting and aortic and carotid artery clamping. However, most patients can tolerate the surgery owing to extensive collateral circulation in the neck.

Cerebral hyperperfusion syndrome (CHS) can develop after carotid artery reconstruction in patients with severe brain ischaemia. It is believed that CHS results from a sudden increase of cerebral blood flow in conditions of impaired cerebral autoregulation, to maintain constant intracranial pressure. Symptoms of CHS may occur up to several weeks after revascularization but usually occur within the first few days. Clinically, patients with CHS present with an ipsilateral headache, convulsion, a neurological deficit (hemiparesis, hemiplegia, dysarthria or visual disturbance) or a facial oedema. The most catastrophic event of CHS is intracerebral haemorrhage. In patients who are undergoing carotid endarterectomy, longstanding hypertension, diabetes mellitus and severe brain ischaemia are known as risk factors of CHS.[23] To prevent CHS, pre- and post-operative BP control is extremely important. According to Tada et al.,[19] there was a lower incidence of cerebral hyperperfusion syndrome after using autogenous pantaloon vein grafts. **[Q8: A]**

As late complications, anastomotic restenosis, graft thrombosis, anastomotic false aneurysms and graft infections can occur. **[Q8: B, C]** Among these, an anastomotic aneurysm is one of the well-known complications after surgical treatment of patients with TA. Miyata et al.[24] reported that anastomotic aneurysms can occur at any time after operations for TA. They reported that the mean time before developing an anastomotic aneurysm was 9.8 years (range 1.6–30 years) and that the cumulative incidence was 6%, 12% and 19% at 10, 20 and 30 years after various forms of bypass surgery among patients with TA, respectively. They found that the only risk factor for the development of anastomotic aneurysms was the presence of an aneurismal lesion at the time of surgery. They recommended life-long follow-up for patients with TA who undergo arterial surgery. However, most (18/22) of the aneurysms occurred in an early series in which silk suturing was used for the arterial anastomosis. In recent series, anastomotic false aneurysms developed in only 1.8% and 3.5% of patients at 10 and 20 years, respectively. To prevent this complication, some authors have recommended reinforcement of the anastomotic suture line with the use of a Teflon felt strip.[25] We do not use any adjuvant surgical procedure to prevent anastomotic aneurysms. However, we consider that the post-operative monitoring of disease activity and pharmacologic treatment of active disease are very important for all patients with TA who undergo surgical intervention. **[Q8: C]**

References

1. Arend WP, Michel BA, Bloch DA, et al. The American College of Rheumatology 1990 criteria for the classification of Takayasu arteritis. *Arthritis Rheum.* 1990;33:1129-1134.
2. Liang P, Hoffman GS. Advances in the medical and surgical treatment of Takayasu arteritis. *Curr Opin Rheumatol.* 2005;17:16-24.
3. Matsuura K, Ogino H, Kobayashi J, et al. Surgical treatment of aortic regurgitation due to Takayasu arteritis: long-term morbidity and mortality. *Circulation.* 2005;112:3707-3712.
4. Park JH, Chung JW, Im JG, Kim SK, Park YB, Han MC. Takayasu arteritis: evaluation of mural changes in the aorta and pulmonary artery with CT angiography. *Radiology.* 1995;196: 89-93.
5. Choe YH, Kim DK, Koh EM, Do YS, Lee WR. Takayasu arteritis: diagnosis with MR imaging and MR angiography in acute and chronic active stages. *J Magn Reson Imaging.* 1999;10:751-757.
6. Kissin EY, Merkel PA. Diagnostic imaging in Takayasu arteritis. *Curr Opin Rheumatol.* 2004;16:31-37.

7. Andrew J, Mason JC. Takayasu's arteritis – recent advances in imaging offer promise. *Rheumtology (Oxford)*. 2007;46:6-15.
8. Maksimowicz-McKinnon K, Hoffman GS. Takayasu arteritis: what is the long-term prognosis? *Rleum Dis Clin North Am*. 2007;33:777-786. vi.
9. FieldsCE, Bower TC, Cooper LT, et al. Takayasu's arteritis: operative results and influence of disease activity. *J Vasc Surg*. 2006;43:64-71.
10. Park MC, Lee SW, Park YB, Lee SK, Choi D, Shim WH. Post-interventional immunosuppressive treatment and vascular restenosis in Takayasu's arteritis. *Rheumatology (Oxford)*. 2006;45:600-605.
11. Kerr GS, Hallahan CW, Giordano J, et al. Takayasu arteritis. *Ann Intern Med*. 1994;120:919-929.
12. Park JH, Chung JW, Im JG, Kim SK, Park YB, Han MC. Takayasu arteritis: evaluation of mural changes in the aorta and pulmonary artery with CT angiography. *Radiology*. 1995;196:89-93.
13. Park JH, Chung JW, Lee KW, Park YB, Han MC. CT angiography of Takayasu arteritis: comparison with conventional angiography. *J Vasc Interv Radiol*. 1997;8:393-400.
14. Choe YH, Han BK, Koh EM, Kim DK, Do YS, Lee WR. Takayasu's arteritis: assessment of disease activity with contrast-enhanced MR imaging. *AJR Am J Roentgenol*. 2000;175:505-511.
15. Tso E, Flamm SD, White RD, Schvartzman PR, Mascha E, Hoffman GS. Takayasu arteritis: utility and limitations of magnetic resonance imaging in diagnosis and treatment. *Arthritis Rheum*. 2002;46:1634-1642.
16. Andrews J, Al-Nahhas A, Pennell DJ, et al. Non-invasive imaging in the diagnosis and management of Takayasu's arteritis. *Ann Rheum Dis*. 2004;63:995-1000.
17. Kobayashi Y, Ishii K, Oda K, et al. Aortic wall inflammation due to Takayasu arteritis imaged with 18F-FDG PET coregistered with enhanced CT. *J Nucl Med*. 2005;46:917-922.
18. Shiiya N, Matsuzaki K, Watanabe T, Kuroda S, Yasuda K. Descending aorta to carotid bypass for takayasu arteritis as a redo operation. *Ann Thorac Surg*. 2003;76:283-285.
19. Tada Y, Sato O, Ohshima A, Miyata T, Shindo S. Surgical treatment of Takayasu arteritis. *Heart Vessels*. 1992;7:159-167.
20. Tada Y, Kamiya K, Shindo S, et al. Carotid artery reconstruction for Takayasu's arteritis the necessity of all-autogenous-vein graft policy and development of a new operation. *Int Angiol*. 2000;19:242-249.
21. Tann OR, Tulloh RM, Hamilton MC. Takayasu's disease: a review. *Cardiol Young*. 2008;18:250-259.
22. Rockman CB, Riles TS, Landis R, et al. Redo carotid surgery: An analysis of materials and configurations used in carotid reoperations and their influence on perioperative stroke and subsequent recurrent stenosis. *J Vasc Surg*. 1999;29:72-80. discussion 80–81.
23. Moulakakis KG, Mylonas SN, Sfyroeras GS, Andrikopoulos V. Hyperperfusion syndrome after carotid revascularization. *J Vasc Surg*. 2009;49:1060-1068.
24. Miyata T, Sato O, Deguchi J, et al. Anastomotic aneurysms after surgical treatment of Takayasu's arteritis: a 40-year experience. *J Vasc Surg*. 1998;27:438-445.
25. Erdogan A, Gilgil E, Oz N, Türk T, Demircan A. PTFE patching to prevent anastomotic aneurysm formation in Takayasu's arteritis. *Eur J Vasc Endovasc Surg*. 2003;25:478-480.
26. Ishikawa K. Diagnostic approach and proposed criteria for the clinical diagnosis of Takayasu's arteriopathy. *J Am Coll Cardiol*. 1988;12:964-972.

Part VII

Neurovascular Conditions of the Upper Extremity

Neurogenic Thoracic Outlet Syndrome and Pectoralis Minor Syndrome

36

Richard J. Sanders

A 30-year-old woman presented with complaints of pain in her neck, right shoulder, right trapezius, right anterior chest wall, right axilla, right arm, elbow, and forearm; occipital headaches every other day; numbness and tingling in all fingers of the right hand, worse in the fourth and fifth fingers; aggravation of her symptoms when elevating her arms, especially to comb or blow dry her hair or drive a car; weakness of her right hand and dropping coffee cups; and coldness and color changes in her right hand. The symptoms had been present for 1 year and began following a rear-end collision.

Her history began 1 year ago when her automobile was sitting still at a traffic light and another vehicle hit her from the rear. She wore a seat belt and recalled going forward and backward, but did not recall what happened to her neck at the time of the accident. She had no immediate symptoms. On the next day she awoke with a sore neck and pain above her shoulder blades. A few days later, she began noticing headaches in the back of her head that radiated forward to behind her eyes, and the neck soreness became progressively painful. Two or 3 weeks later, pain developed in the right shoulder area and down the right arm. Several weeks later, numbness and tingling developed in the fingers of the right hand, more noticeable in the ring and baby fingers. Because of severe, persistent right shoulder pain, arthroscopic repair of the right shoulder had been performed 6 months ago with partial improvement of her shoulder pain, but no change in any of her other symptoms.

Her occupation was a legal secretary. Since the accident, although she had been able to return to work, she was now able to work only 4 h a day. She could not type for more than 10 min, because the pain and numbness in her right hand was too uncomfortable. At home she could do light housework only. She could not vacuum, wash windows or floors, or lift heavy laundry baskets. Diagnostic studies to date included cervical spine X-rays, which were normal, and an electromyography/nerve conduction velocity (EMG/NCV) study, which revealed very mild nonspecific changes in the ulnar nerve distribution, but was close to normal.

Treatment to date included 6 months of physical therapy with the following modalities: heat, massage, ultrasound, neck stretching exercises, and posture.

R.J. Sanders
Department of Surgery, University of Colorado Health Science Center, Aurora, CO, USA

G. Geroulakos and B. Sumpio (eds.), *Vascular Surgery*,
DOI: 10.1007/978-1-84996-356-5_36, © Springer-Verlag London Limited 2011

Question 1

What is the most common cause of neurogenic thoracic outlet syndrome (TOS)?

A. Neck trauma
B. Cervical rib
C. Anomalous bands
D. Abnormal first rib
E. All of the above

On physical examination there was supraclavicular tenderness over the right scalene muscles but no tenderness over the left scalenes; tenderness over the right chest wall just below the right clavicle and in the right axilla but no such tenderness on the left side; a positive Tinel's sign over the right brachial plexus and a negative sign over the left; and reproduction of arm and hand symptoms with pressure over the right scalene muscles, but no such symptoms with pressure over the left scalene muscles. Head rotation and head tilting each caused pain in the contralateral hand and arm when turning and tilting to the left side. This did not occur when rotating and tilting to the right side.

Abducting the arms to 90° in external rotation (AER position) reproduced the right arm and hand symptoms within 15 s while no symptoms developed on the left side. The upper limb tension test (ULTT), modified from Elvey, was positive on the right side in the first position with symptoms worse in the second and third positions. The ULTT was negative on the left side.

Pectoralis minor muscle block, injecting 4 ml of 1% lidocaine into the right pectoralis minor muscle 3 cm below the clavicle, resulted in partial improvement of symptoms at rest, loss of tenderness over the right chest wall and in the right axilla. The ULTT was improved, but she still had some symptoms, partially reduced.

Scalene muscle block, injecting 4 mL of 1% lidocaine into the right anterior scalene muscle, resulted in further significant improvement in most of her physical findings.

Question 2

The diagnostic criteria for neurogenic TOS (NTOS) include which of the following?

A. History of neck trauma.
B. Paresthesia in the hand involving all five fingers, more frequently in the fourth and fifth.
C. Pain in the neck, shoulder, and upper extremity.
D. Occipital headaches.
E. Scalene muscle tenderness and duplication of symptoms in the 90° AER position.
F. Cut-off of the radial pulse on Adson's or 90° AER positioning.
G. Positive response to the scalene muscle block.
H. The ULTT is comparable to straight leg raising in the lower extremity and is an excellent test for TOS.

Question 3

The diagnostic criteria for neurogenic pectoralis minor syndrome (NPMS) include which of the following?

A. History of tenderness or pain in the anterior chest wall below the clavicle
B. Tenderness in the right axilla and below the right clavicle
C. Occipital headaches
D. Paresthesia in the hand involving the thumb, index and middle fingers
E. Severe weakness in the right arm

She was continuing neck stretching exercises at home on a daily basis emphasizing doing each stretch slowly, holding each stretch for a minimum of 15 s, and performing no more than three repeats at each session. She also was performing pectoralis minor stretches in an open doorway, holding her hand on each door jam as she dropped her body forward. In spite of this treatment, there was no improvement in her symptoms.

Question 4

Which of the following conditions can coexist with NTOS or require differentiation from it?

A. Carpal tunnel syndrome
B. Biceps/rotator cuff tendinitis or impingement syndrome
C. Cervical spine disease-disc, arthritis, spinal stenosis, cervical spine strain,Detc
D. Ulnar nerve entrapment at the elbow (cubital tunnel syndrome)
E. Pectoralis minor syndrome
F. Fibromyalgia
G. Brachial plexus injury
H. Brain tumor

Question 5

The indications for surgical decompression of the thoracic outlet areas are:

A. Failure of conservative treatment after a trial of at least 3 months
B. All other associated conditions have been recognized and treated as completely as possible
C. Symptoms are interfering with work, sleep, recreation, or activities of daily living
D. All of the above

Because of persistent symptoms in spite of adequate conservative therapy, and because she was partially disabled at work and at home, a supraclavicular anterior and middle scalenectomy, brachial plexus neurolysis, and first rib resection were performed along with a pectoralis minor tenotomy via a separate incision in the axilla.

Question 6

Which surgical procedures are acceptable to decompress the thoracic outlet area?

A. Transaxillary first rib resection
B. Supraclavicular anterior and middle scalenectomy with brachial plexus neurolysis
C. Supraclavicular anterior scalenectomy with or without brachial plexus neurolysis
D. Supraclavicular anterior and middle scalenectomy, first rib resection, and brachial plexus neurolysis
E. All of the above

Question 7

What are the major complications of TOS surgery?

A. Brachial plexus traction injury
B. Phrenic nerve injury
C. Subclavian artery injury
D. Subclavian vein injury
E. Long thoracic nerve injury
F. Second intercostal brachial cutaneous nerve injury (transaxillary approach only)
G. Thoracic duct injury (left side, supraclavicular approach only)
H. Supraclavicular nerve injury (supraclavicular approach only)
I. Horner's syndrome (supraclavicular approach only)
J. Pneumothorax
K. All of the above

She tolerated surgery well, had no postoperative complications, and was discharged from the hospital on the second postoperative day. After 4 weeks of convalescence at home, she returned to work, 4 h a day. After 1 month she was able to resume her job on a full-time basis. While most of her symptoms had improved, she still noticed occasional paresthesia in her hand and pain in her right shoulder when working for long periods. Her headaches were completely gone. She was pleased with her improvement from surgery even though she was not back to normal.

Question 8

What are the long-term results of surgical decompression of the thoracic outlet area?

A. 90% success
B. 75% success
C. 60% success
D. 40% success
E. None of the above

36.1
Commentary

There are three types of thoracic outlet syndrome (TOS): arterial, venous, and neurogenic.

NTOS comprises more than 95% of all TOS cases and is the most difficult to diagnose and treat. The etiology of NTOS in most patients is either a hyperextension neck injury or repetitive stress at work. The mechanism of neck injury from repetitive stress is a little obscure, but it probably comes from the worker's hands being occupied in one place so that the worker is constantly rotating his/her neck back and forth to perform the job or talk to people. Holding a telephone between ear and shoulder while typing is also a common form of neck strain. While some TOS patients have cervical ribs or congenital cervical bands, these are regarded as predisposing conditions and seldom are the primary cause. These patients usually do not develop symptoms until they experience some form of neck trauma.

Although first rib resection has become a standard form of therapy for neurogenic TOS, the first rib is rarely the cause of the symptoms. The pathology is tightness and scarring of the scalene muscles.[1] Rib resection is successful because the anterior and middle scalene muscles must be divided in order to remove the rib. Thus, by necessity, first rib resection includes scalenotomy and it is probably the latter that relieves the symptoms. **[Q1: A]**

The diagnosis of neurogenic TOS is by history and physical examination. This is not a diagnosis of exclusion. The typical history includes some type of neck trauma, although the patient does not always remember the incident, especially if there was no litigation involved. It is the job of the examiner to thoroughly ask about neck trauma. The symptoms usually include pain, paresthesia, and weakness in the upper extremity, but over 75% of patients also complain of neck pain and occipital headaches. The latter symptoms are not the result of brachial plexus compression; rather, they result from stretch injuries to the scalene muscles and referred pain to the back of the head. Most commonly paresthesia involves all five fingers of the hand, although it tends to involve the ulnar side of the hand and forearm more often than the radial side. The significant physical findings are scalene muscle tenderness, a positive Tinel's and positive Spurling's sign over the scalene muscles, and duplication of symptoms with the arms in the 90° AER position. A cut-off of the radial pulse in either the Adson's or 90° AER position is not a reliable sign in establishing a diagnosis. Up to 60% of normal people cut off their pulses in these dynamic positions while most NTOS patients do not cut off their pulses.[2] Not every patient will exhibit all of these criteria, but a diagnosis can be established if the majority of these criteria have been met.[3] The upper limb tension test (ULTT) is comparable to straight leg raising in the lower extremity. It is performed by having the patient abduct the arms to 90° with elbows extended, then dorsi-flex the wrists, followed by tilting the head, ear to shoulder, to each side. A positive response is onset of pain and paresthesia in the hand and arm.[4] **[Q2: A, B, C, D, E, G, H]**

Pectoralis minor syndrome was described over 60 years ago but was forgotten by most clinicians. Its recognition has recently been revived and it appears to be present in the majority of patients being seen for NTOS. It's symptoms of paresthesia and pain in the upper extremity are similar to those of NTOS. However, neck pain and occipital headaches are not due to pectoralis minor compression. Important signs on physical examination are tenderness over the pectoralis minor muscle just below the clavicle and tenderness in the axilla. In contrast from NTOS, patients with NPMS usually don't have much arm weakness, have very little neck pain, and more often have paresthesia in the first three fingers, although all five can be involved. NPMS frequently accompanies NTOS as a form of double crush syndrome.[5] Surgery for the two conditions can be performed together.[6,7] **[Q3: A, B, D]**

All symptoms of NTOS are nonspecific. Other conditions that also exhibit similar symptoms include abnormalities of the shoulder, elbow, wrist, and parascapular muscles. It is quite common for NTOS to coexist with some of these other conditions. **[Q4: A, B, C, D, E, F, G]**

In less than 1% of patients with NTOS, atrophy of hand muscles supplied by the ulnar nerve exists. In these patients, EMG studies demonstrate typical findings of ulnar neuropathy.[8] Otherwise, EMG and NCV studies are either normal or reveal nonspecific changes. Unfortunately, once atrophy develops, it is usually nonreversible.[9] At this stage, surgery can relieve pain and paresthesia, but not weakness.

Conservative therapy is always indicated first and is effective in the majority of patients.[10] Surgery should be regarded as a last resort. There are a variety of modalities of therapy for NTOS patients, the most important being home exercises, including neck stretching, abdominal breathing, and posture correction. After being instructed by a physical therapist the patient carries out the program on a daily basis at home. Hands-on therapy by a physical therapist is indicated for some of the associated diagnoses that coexist with TOS. Because neck traction, weights, resistance exercises, and strengthening exercises tend to make TOS symptoms worse, we do not recommend them for NTOS patients.

Some patients are refractory to all forms of physical therapy. If there is no improvement after several months of exercises, the patient's options are to either live with the symptoms or consider surgical decompression of the thoracic outlet. To be a candidate for surgery, in addition to failing conservative therapy after a trial of several months, the patient should have had all associated diagnoses treated and the symptoms should be partially or totally disabling. **[Q5: D]**

That there is more than one acceptable surgical procedure from which to choose indicates that no one operation has proved itself to be greatly superior to any other.

In 1972, after performing transaxillary first rib resection[11] for several years, we were disappointed to find the long-term success rate was just under 70%. We then changed to supraclavicular anterior and middle scalenectomy with brachial plexus neurolysis but were again disappointed to discover the success rate was identical to transaxillary first rib resection. The next choice of procedure was supraclavicular anterior and middle scalenectomy plus first rib resection through the same supraclavicular incision.[12,13] With this combined operation our early results were a few percentage points better than the first two operations, but the difference was not statistically significant. Other observers who have compared scalenectomy alone to scalenectomy with first rib resection have also not noted statistically significant differences between the two.[14–16] Finally, some surgeons still perform just anterior scalenectomy with neurolysis and report results that are similar to the more extensive procedures.[17,18] **[Q6: E]**

Major complications occur from all operations to decompress the thoracic outlet area regardless of the surgical approach. Injury to the subclavian artery and vein, brachial plexus, phrenic nerve, and long thoracic nerve are the most common serious complications. Less common are injuries to the thoracic duct and cervical sympathetic chain. Injuries to cutaneous nerves from either transaxillary or supraclavicular approaches are common. Plexus injury occurs from excessive traction, which at the time may not seem excessive. Plexus injury can also occur when a clamp on the subclavian artery to control bleeding accidentally includes a nerve of the plexus.

Plexus injury makes symptoms worse in 1% of patients. The incidence of temporary phrenic nerve injury during supraclavicular approaches is 10% because the phrenic nerve is often in the middle of the field and is very sensitive to even mild retraction.[16] **[Q7: K]**

The results of surgery are about the same for all procedures. The biggest variable is etiology. When the etiology is an auto accident related injury, the 1-year success rate is 75–80%; when the etiology is repetitive stress at work or a work injury, the success rate is 15% lower.[15,16,19] **[Q8: B** (for auto accident etiology), **C** (for work related and repetitive stress etiology)]**

References

1. Sanders RJ, Jackson CGR, Banchero N, Pearce WH. Scalene muscle abnormalities in traumatic thoracic outlet syndrome. *Am J Surg*. 1990;159:231-236.
2. Gergoudis R, Barnes RW. Thoracic outlet arterial compression: prevalence in normal persons. *Angiology*. 1980;31:538-541.
3. Sanders RJ, Haug CE. *Thoracic Outlet Syndrome: A Common Sequela of Neck Injuries*. Philadelphia: Lippincott; 1991:71-84.
4. Sanders RJ, Hammond SL. Diagnosis of thoracic outlet syndrome. *J Vasc Surg*. 2007;46: 601-604.
5. Upton ARM, McComas AJ. The double crush in nerve-entrapment syndromes. *Lancet*. 1973;2:359-362.
6. Sanders RJ. Pectoralis minor syndrome. In: Eskandari MK, Morasch MD, Pearce WH, Yao JST, eds. *Vascular Surgery: Therapeutic Strategies*. Shelton: People's Medical Publishing House; 2009:149-160.
7. Sanders RJ, Rao NM. The forgotten pectoralis minor syndrome. 100 operations for pectoralis minor syndrome alone or accompanied by neurogenic thoracic outlet syndrome. Ann Vasc Surg 2010; 24:701-708.
8. Gilliatt RW, Willison RG, Dietz V, Williams IR. Peripheral nerve conduction in patients with a cervical rib and band. *Ann Neurol*. 1978;4:124-129.
9. Green RM, McNamara MS, Ouriel K. Long-term follow-up after thoracic outlet decompression: an analysis of factors determining outcome. *J Vasc Surg*. 1991;14:739-746.
10. Novak CB, Collins ED, Mackinnon SE. Outcome following conservative management of thoracic outlet syndrome. *J Hand Surg*. 1995;20A:542-548.
11. Roos DB. The place for scalenectomy and first rib resection in thoracic outlet syndrome. *Surgery*. 1982;92:1077-1085.
12. Sanders RJ, Pearce WH. The treatment of thoracic outlet syndrome: a comparison of different operations. *J Vasc Surg*. 1989;10:626-634.
13. Sanders RJ, Cooper MA, Hammond SL, Weinstein ES. Neurogenic thoracic outlet syndrome. In: Rutherford RB, ed. *Vascular Surgery*. 5th ed. Philadelphia: Saunders; 1999:1184-1200.
14. Cheng SWK, Reilly LM, Nelken NA, et al. Neurogenic thoracic outlet decompression: rationale for sparing the first rib. *Cardiovasc Surg*. 1995;3:617-623.
15. Thomas GI. Diagnosis and treatment of thoracic outlet syndrome. *Perspect Vasc Surg*. 1995;8:1-28.

16. Sanders RJ, Hammond SL. Complications and results of surgical treatment for thoracic outlet syndrome. *Chest Surg Clin N Am.* 1999;9:803-820.

17. Razi DM, Wassel HD. Traffic accident induced thoracic outlet syndrome: decompression without rib resection, correction of associated recurrent thoracic aneurysm. *Int Surg.* 1993;78:25-27.

18. Gockel M, Vastamaki M, Alaranta H. Long-term results of primary scalenotomy in the treatment of thoracic outlet syndrome. *J Hand Surg.* 1994;19B:229-233.

19. Ellison DW, Wood VE. Trauma-related thoracic outlet syndrome. *J Hand Surg.* 1994;19B: 424-426.

Acute Axillary/Subclavian Vein Thrombosis

37

Torbjørn Dahl, Jarlis Wesche, and Hans O. Myhre

A 34-year-old male motor mechanic was admitted with a 3-day history of severe swelling of the right arm. He had been undertaking physical activity, including weightlifting, training for about 1.5 h four times a week. There was no history of trauma. The patient felt discomfort, but no severe pain in the arm. The superficial veins were distended. The color of the hand and forearm was slightly cyanotic. The pulses in the radial and ulnar arteries were palpable. No bruits could be heard along the brachial, supraclavicular or axillary arteries. The rest of the examination was without remarks. The patient did not use any medication.

Question 1

What further diagnostic investigations would you prefer in this patient?

A. Pletysmography
B. Venography
C. Duplex scanning
D. Magnetic resonance phlebography
E. Computed tomography (CT) scanning
F. X-ray of the chest and thoracic outlet
G. Venous pressure measurements

Venography revealed a thrombosis of the axillary/subclavian veins (Fig. 37.1). The brachiocophalic vein was patent. There were no signs of skeletal deformities.

T. Dahl (✉)
Department of Surgery, St. Olavs Hospital, University Hospital of Trondheim, Trondheim, Norway

G. Geroulakos and B. Sumpio (eds.), *Vascular Surgery*,
DOI: 10.1007/978-1-84996-356-5_37, © Springer-Verlag London Limited 2011

Fig. 37.1 DSA venogram showing occlusion of the right subclavian vein, but contrast passage to the superior caval vein via jugular/supra clavicular collateral veins (note it's relation to the thoracic outlet)

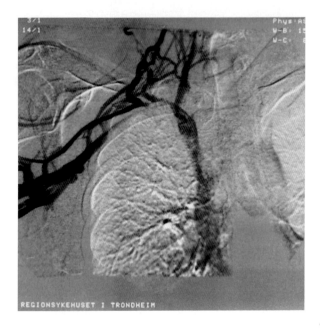

REGIONSYKEHUSET I TRONDHEIM

Question 2

Which of the following conditions could lead to axillary/subclavian vein thrombosis?

A. Venous-access catheters
B. Callus from fractured clavicle or rib
C. Local tumor/malignancy
D. Radiotherapy
E. Trauma to the vein caused by repeated strenuous exercise

Question 3

Which therapy would you recommend in the acute (2–3 days) phase?

A. Resection of the first rib
B. Balloon angioplasty of the subclavian vein
C. Stenting of the subclavian vein
D. Thrombolysis
E. Systemic Heparin
F. Thrombectomy

Question 4

Following thrombolytic therapy for axillary/subclavian vein thrombosis, what percentage of complete lysis can you expect provided the patient is treated within 3 days after start of symptoms?

A. 10%
B. 25%
C. 40%
D. 60%
E. 80%

Question 5

A control venography revealed a stenosis of the axillary/subclavian vein at the thoracic outlet. There was no residual thrombotic material. At 3 months' follow-up the patient still had pain and discomfort in the arm when going back to his job as a motor mechanic. Which of the following alternatives of treatment would you recommend at this stage?

A. Repeated attempt of thrombolytic therapy
B. Balloon angioplasty and stenting of the subclavian artery
C. Continued oral anticoagulation therapy
D. Relief of the thoracic outlet by resection of the first rib including venolysis
E. Direct reconstruction of the vein

37.1
Commentary

In patients with acute axillary/subclavian vein thrombosis, it is important to separate so-called primary from secondary thrombosis. Primary thrombosis is also known as Paget–Schroetter's syndrome, which is induced by strenuous activity of the arm or venous compression at the thoracic outlet predisposing for thrombosis formation.[1–4] The term "effort thrombosis" is also used for this condition. Men are affected more often than women, and the incidence is higher in the veins of the dominant arm. Secondary axillary/subclavian vein thrombosis could be caused by venous-access catheters, pacemaker wires, malignancies, radiotherapy or compression from local tumor formation. Secondary thrombosis is also seen as a complication of thrombophilia and in patients with dialysis fistulas.[5] [Q2: A, B, C, D, E] The preferred therapy may be different in the two groups, and in general a more conservative attitude is justified in patients with secondary thrombosis. These patients often have a limited life expectancy due to serious comobidities, such as cardiac disease or malignancy, which would also represent a contraindication to thrombolytic therapy. In addition, there is often less need for extensive activity of the upper extremities in this group of patients. There is usually a rich venous collateral network, and therefore phlegmasia coerulea dolens of the arm is extremely rare. It may occasionally be connected with hypercoagulability or malignancies.

Complications following axillary/subclavian vein thrombosis are swelling, pain and discomfort in the arm prohibiting work or daily-life activities. Furthermore, it has been reported that up to ten per cent of the patients with axillary/subclavian vein thrombosis develop pulmonary emboli and that it is more common than usually appreciated.[5,6]

In patients with primary axillary/subclavian vein thrombosis, duplex scanning can be performed as a supplement to the clinical examination.[6] However, duplex scanning is operator dependent. If the examination is negative, then venography has to be performed anyway. Three-dimensional gadolinium-enhanced magnetic resonance phlebography technique has been applied successfully.[7] However, venography, preferably by contrast injection via the basilic vein, is still the gold standard in these cases. The guide-wire could be advanced into the thrombus to investigate if it is soft enough for lysis. A chest X-ray including the thoracic outlet to investigate the possibility of bony deformation is also indicated. [Q1: B, C, F]

D-dimer levels are usually elevated in patients with thrombus. The patient should also be evaluated thoroughly for thrombophilia and blood tests should include a blood count, tests for decreased levels of anti-thrombin (III), protein C and protein S deficiencies, activated protein C (APC) resistance, antiphospholipid antibodies (lupus anticoagulans) and anticardiolipin antibodies. Contraceptive drugs can cause axillary subclavian vein thrombosis due to a decrease in the anti-thrombin levels.

As soon as the diagnosis has been established, systemic heparinisation is administered.[8] This should be followed by local thrombolysis using recombinant tissue plasminogen activator (rt-PA) unless there are contraindications.[9–14] [Q3: D, E] At introduction of the guidewire, the resistance will indicate the age of the thrombosis and the possibility of obtaining lysis of the thrombotic occlusion. The catheter for application of the thrombolytic agent should be placed within the thrombosis. Usually, a dose of 5 mg rt-PA is given as a bolus, followed by infusion of 0.01 mg/kg body weight/h for 24–72 h.

Although the most favorable results are obtained in patients with less than 1 week's duration of symptoms,[10] an attempt at thrombolysis could be justified even if the symptoms have lasted for 1 month. [Q4: E]

After thrombolysis, a repeat venography is performed to evaluate whether any intrinsic or extrinsic obstructions of the blood flow are present. Often a defect is located close to the costoclavicular ligament. Together with hypertrophic anterior scalene and subclavius muscles, this ligament could cause external compression of the vein. Intrinsic venous stenosis is thought to be due to repetitive trauma damaging venous valves or the endothelium, or producing thickening of the vein wall or intraluminal synechiae, predisposing to thrombosis.

After thrombolysis the patient should be on oral anticoagulation for 1–3 months, depending on the preferred time for thoracic outlet decompression. Some centers proceed with more radical surgery soon after thrombolysis.[11,15,16] By allowing a 3 month period of oral anticoagulation,the clinical status could be reevaluated. If the patient is asymptomatic at follow-up, we do not recommend further treatment.[13]

If the patient is symptomatic and there is a residual stenosis of the subclavian vein caused by either internal or external pathological structures, then the stenosis should not be treated by balloon angioplasty or stenting primarily.[11–13,15,17] Whenever these treatment modalities are applied before relief of the thoracic outlet, recurrence of the symptoms will inevitably occur. Furthermore, fracture of the stents has been described because of the "scissors effect" caused by the narrow thoracic outlet.[18] Decompression of the thoracic outlet is obtained by resection of the first rib, including the distal part of the anterior and middle scalene muscles and fibrous structures adhering to the first rib. Venolysis is also a part of the procedure. [Q5: D]

The surgical approach for relieving the thoracic outlet is controversial: However, most surgeons prefer a transaxillary approach. In cases where reconstruction of the vein is indicated a paraclavicular approach can be used.[3,5,11,15,16,19,20] After thoracic outlet surgery, a venous obstruction can be treated with balloon angioplasty preferably without stenting. Finally, in rare cases, direct reconstruction by endovenectomy and patch angioplasty may be indicated for relief of intravenous obstructions.[3]

Fig. 37.2 Algorithm for treatment options in acute axillary/subclavian vein thrombosis

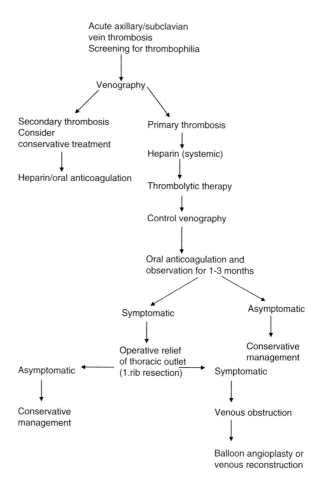

In summary the most effective sequence to restore venous patency and reduce rethrombosis seems thus to include local thrombolytic therapy, 1–3 months of oral anticoagulation, and then transaxillary first-rib resection with venolysis in patients who have significant symptoms at this stage. Thereafter, occasionally percutaneous transluminal angioplasty (PTA) or venous reconstruction may be indicated.[21,22] Following such a staged multidisciplinary treatment (Fig. 37.2) the disability rate following acute axillary/subclavian thrombosis has been significantly reduced.[19]

References

1. Hughes ESR. Venous obstruction in the upper extremity (Paget-Schroetter's syndrome). A review of 320 cases. *Int Abstr Surg*. 1949;88:89-128.
2. McCleery RS, Kesterson JE, Kirtley JA, Love RB. Subclavius and anterior scalene muscle compression as a cause of intermittent obstructin of the subclavian vein. *Ann Surg*. 1951;133:588-602.

3. Haug CE, Sanders RJ. Endovascular management of aortic transection in a multiinjured patient. Venous TOS. In: Sauders RJ, ed. *Thoracic Outlet Syndrome. A Common Sequela of Neck Injuries*, vol. 15. Philadelphia: JB Lippicott; 1991:233-236. ISBN 0-397-51097-7.

4. Daskalakis E, Bouhoutsos J. Subclavian and axilliary vein compression of musculoskeletal origin. *Br J Surg*. 1980;67:573-576.

5. Hicken GJ, Ameli M. Management of subclavian-axillary vein thrombosis: a review. *Can J Surg*. 1998;41:13-24.

6. Kerr TM, Lutter KS, Moeller DM, et al. Upper extremity venous thrombosis diagnosed by duplex scanning. *Am J Surg*. 1990;160:202-206.

7. Thornton MJ, Ryan R, Varghese JC, Farrell MA, Lucey B, Lee MJ. A three-dimensional gadolinium-enhanced MR venography technique for imaging central veins. *AJR*. 1999;173: 999-1003.

8. Gloviczki P, Kazmier FJ, Hollier LH. Axillary-subclavian venous occlusion: the morbidity of a nonlethal disease. *J Vasc Surg*. 1986;4:333-337.

9. Becker GJ, Holden RW, Rabe FE, et al. Local thrombolytic therapy for subclavian and axillary vein thrombosis. *Radiology*. 1983;149:419-423.

10. Beygui RE, Olcott C, Dalman RL. Subclavian vein thrombosis: outcome analysis based on etiology and modality of treatment. *Ann Vasc Surg*. 1997;11:247-255.

11. Lee MC, Grassi CJ, Belkin M, Mannick JA, Whittemore AD, Donaldson MC. Early operative intervention after thrombolytic therapy for primary subclavian vein thrombosis: An effective treatment approach. *J Vasc Surg*. 1998;27:1101-1108.

12. Lindblad B, Tengborn L, Bergqvist D. Deep vein thrombosis of the axillary-subclavian veins: epidemiologic data, effects of different types of treatment and late sequele. *Eur J Vasc Surg*. 1988;2:161-165.

13. Lee WA, Hill BB, Harris EJ Jr, Semba CP, Olcott C. Surgical intervention is not required for all patients with subclavian vein thrombosis. *J Vasc Surg*. 2000;32:57-67.

14. Büller HR, Agnelli G, Hull RD, Hyers TM, Prins MH, Raskob GE. Antithrombotic therapy for venous thromboembolic disease. The seventh ACCP conference on antithrombotic and thrombolytic therapy. *Chest*. 2004;126:401S-428S.

15. Azakie A, McElhinney DB, Thompson RW, Raven RB, Messina LM, Stoney RJ. Surgical management of subclavian-vein effort thormbosis as a result of thoracic outlet compression. *J Vasc Surg*. 1998;28:777-786.

16. Urschel HC Jr, Razzuk MA. Paget-Schroetter syndrome: what is the best management? *Ann Thorac Surg*. 2000;69:1663-1669.

17. Glanz S, Gordon DH, Lipkowitz GS, Butt KM, Hong J, Sclafani SJA. Axillary and subclavian vein stenosis: percutaneous angioplasty. *Radiology*. 1988;168:371-373.

18. Bjarnason H, Hunter DW, Crain MR, Ferral DW, Mitz-Miller SE, Wegryn SA. Collapse of a Palmaz stent in the subclavian vein. *Am J Radiol*. 1993;160:1123-1124.

19. Machleder HI. Evaluation of a new treatment strategy for Paget–Schroetter syndrome: spontaneous thrombosis of the axilliary-subclavian vein. *J Vasc Surg*. 1993;17:305-317.

20. Kreienberg PB, Chang BB, Darling RC III, et al. Long-term results in patients treated with thrombolysis, thoracic inlet decrompression, and subclavian vein stenting for Paget–Schroetter syndrome. *J Vasc Surg*. 2001;33:S100-S105.

21. Melby SJ, Vedantham S, Narra VR, et al. Comprehensive surgical management of the competitive athlete with effort thrombosis of the subclavian vein (Paget–Schroetter syndrome). *J Vasc Surg*. 2008;47:809-821.

22. Doyle A, Wolford HY, Davies MG, et al. Management of effort thrombosis of the subclavian vein: today's treatment. *Ann Vasc Surg*. 2007;21:723-729.

Ariane L. Herrick

A 38-year-old female patient presented to the rheumatology clinic with a 3-week history of a painful fingertip ulcer. The pain was so severe that it was keeping her awake at night. For 20 years (since her teens) her hands had been turning white then purple in the cold weather, going red (with tingling) when rewarming. Her feet also felt cold. Her family doctor had told her that this was Raynaud's phenomenon, which was very common. However, each winter her symptoms seemed to be worsening, and even a slight temperature change would bring on an attack. The previous winter she had had some finger ulcers which had, however, been less painful than the current one and which had healed spontaneously. Also of concern to her was that for 6 months the skin of her fingers had felt tight, and she had recently been experiencing some difficulty swallowing, with heartburn. There was no past medical history of note. She had smoked five cigarettes a day for 2 years. There was no history of chemical exposure nor of use of vibratory equipment.

Question 1

Which symptoms suggest that this is *not* primary (idiopathic) Raynaud's phenomenon?

A. Onset of Raynaud's phenomenon age 18 years
B. The feet were affected as well as the hands
C. Development of digital ulcers
D. The skin of the fingers felt tight
E. She was a smoker

On examination she had a healing ulcer at the tip of the left middle finger (Fig. 38.1). The fingertip was extremely tender. She had mild skin thickening of the fingers (sclerodactyly) but elsewhere the skin was normal. She had digital pitting of the right index and middle fingers. There were no other abnormal findings.

A.L. Herrick
Rheumatic Diseases Centre, University of Manchester, Manchester Academic Health Science Centre, Salford Royal NHS Foundation Trust, Salford M6, 8HD, UK.

G. Geroulakos and B. Sumpio (eds.), *Vascular Surgery*,
DOI: 10.1007/978-1-84996-356-5_38, © Springer-Verlag London Limited 2011

Fig. 38.1 Fingertip ulcer in a patient with systemic sclerosis

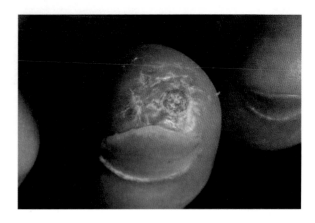

Question 2

What investigations would you perform?

A. Full blood count and erythrocyte sedimentation rate (ESR)
B. Angiography
C. Testing for antinuclear antibody (ANA)
D. Testing for anticentromere antibody
E. Nailfold capillaroscopy

Full blood count and ESR were normal. On immunological testing she was strongly ANA positive (titre 1/1,000) and she was anticentromere antibody positive. Chest X-ray showed no cervical rib. Hand X-rays were normal. Nailfold microscopy was abnormal, showing widened, dilated loops with areas of avascularity (Fig. 38.2).

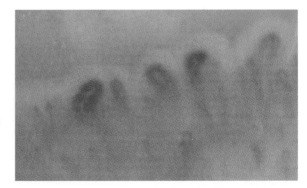

Fig. 38.2 Typical appearances on nailfold microscopy in systemic sclerosis – several capillary loops are dilated, with areas of avascularity

Question 3

What is the diagnosis?

A. It would be better to put. Limited cutaneous systemic sclerosis (previously often termed CREST [calcinosis, Raynaud's, oesophageal dysmotility, sclerodactyly, telangiectases]).
B. Hyperviscosity state, for example secondary to malignancy
C. Extrinsic vascular compression
D. Atherosclerosis
E. Buerger's disease

Question 4

Which of the following are true of systemic sclerosis (also termed "scleroderma"):

A. Digital pitting is a characteristic feature.
B. Males are more commonly affected than females.
C. The two subtypes – limited cutaneous and diffuse cutaneous – are separated on the basis of the extent of the skin involvement.
D. Raynaud's phenomenon often precedes the diagnosis of limited cutaneous systemic sclerosis by many years.
E. Anticentromere antibody is a risk factor for severe digital ischaemia requiring amputation.

The diagnosis of limited cutaneous systemic sclerosis was explained to the patient. She was told that her Raynaud's phenomenon and her upper gastrointestinal symptoms were most likely related, and that some checks of her cardiorespiratory function would be arranged on a routine basis.

Question 5

How would you have treated her Raynaud's phenomenon had you seen her 6 months previously, when there was no digital ulceration?

A. Avoidance of cold exposure.
B. Low dose prednisolone.
C. Stop smoking.
D. Nifedipine (sustained release).
E. Biofeedback.

The patient was prescribed nifedipine (sustained release) and a course of flucloxacillin. When reviewed one week later, the fingertip had deteriorated and some of the tissue had become necrotic, with surrounding erythema.

Question 6

What would you do now?

A. Admit to hospital for intravenous prostanoid therapy.
B. Intravenous antibiotics.
C. Debridement of the ulcer.
D. Cervical sympathectomy.
E. Anticoagulation.

The patient was admitted for intravenous antibiotic therapy, intravenous prostanoid infusions, and a surgical opinion. The fingertip was debrided. The patient was discharged home 6 days later, with instructions to dress warmly, avoid cold exposure, and to seek medical advice early should any further ulcers develop.

38.1
Commentary

Raynaud's phenomenon – episodic digital ischaemia usually in response to cold exposure or stress – can be either *primary* (idiopathic) or *secondary* to a number of different diseases/conditions, including connective tissue disease (most characteristically systemic sclerosis), external vascular compression (as with a cervical rib), vibration exposure, hyperviscosity, drug treatment (for example beta-blockers, ergotamine) and occupational chemical exposure. The terminology is confusing: primary Raynaud's phenomenon was previously termed "Raynaud's disease", and secondary Raynaud's phenomenon "Raynaud's syndrome". However, "primary Raynaud's phenomenon" and "secondary Raynaud's phenomenon" are now the preferred terms.[1]

The pathophysiology of Raynaud's phenomenon (either primary or secondary) is poorly understood. Raynaud's phenomenon can occur because of abnormalities in vascular structure, vascular function, or the blood itself.[2] These are interdependent and may occur together, as in systemic sclerosis when structural vascular problems inevitably impair vascular function, and platelet and white blood cell activation, together with impaired fibrinolysis, are also thought to contribute to pathophysiology. It is generally accepted that primary Raynaud's phenomenon is mainly vasospastic and does not progress to irreversible tissue damage. In contrast, Raynaud's phenomenon secondary to connective tissue disease such as systemic sclerosis is associated with structural vascular abnormality, and patients often develop ulceration, scarring, and even gangrene necessitating amputation.

The vascular surgeon is likely to encounter patients with Raynaud's phenomenon for two main reasons:

1. Diagnosis. Why does this patient have episodic digital ischaemia?
2. Treatment of a critically ischaemic digit, or of severe Raynaud's phenomenon unresponsive to medical therapy.

The onset of primary Raynaud's phenomenon is most commonly in the teens or twenties: onset in later years should always raise the suspicion of an underlying cause. Women are more commonly affected. For Raynaud's phenomenon to be primary, there should be no clinical features of underlying connective tissue disease or other disease/disorder (including absence of digital pitting or sclerodactyly), there should be no digital ulceration or gangrene, the ESR should be normal, testing for ANA negative (titre <1/100) and the nail-fold capillaries should be normal.[1] **[Q1: C, D]** In the absence of any worrying features in the history and examination, the usual investigation screen therefore comprises a full blood count and ESR, testing for ANA, nailfold capillaroscopy and, if there is any question of a cervical rib, a chest or thoracic outlet X-ray. Anaemia and/or a high ESR may indicate an underlying connective tissue disease or other illness. However, a normal haemoglobin level and ESR (as in our patient) do not exclude a diagnosis of systemic sclerosis, in which the vascular abnormalities are primarily non-inflammatory.[3] In primary Raynaud's phenomenon, the nailfold capillaries should be fairly regular "hair-pin" loops as opposed to the abnormal dilated loops, with areas of loop drop-out, that are characteristic of systemic sclerosis.[4]

Other investigations are indicated by the history and examination. For example, if there is sclerodactyly (scleroderma of the fingers) and/or digital pitting (Fig. 38.3), which are both characteristic of systemic sclerosis, then anticentromere antibodies and antibodies to topoisomerase (anti-Scl-70 antibodies) should be looked for. These antibodies are highly specific for systemic sclerosis.[5] If there is any question of a proximal vascular obstruction (absent peripheral pulses) then angiography should be considered, but in the majority of patients with systemic sclerosis and digital ischaemia this is not necessary. **[Q2: A, C, D, E]**

Systemic sclerosis, similarly to primary Raynaud's phenomenon, is more common in women than in men. There are two main subtypes of systemic sclerosis – limited and diffuse cutaneous – defined on the basis of the extent of the skin involvement. In patients with limited cutaneous disease (previously termed CREST), only the skin of the extremities and face is thickened, whereas in those with diffuse cutaneous disease there is proximal skin thickening, involving proximal limbs and/or trunk.[6] The patient described has clinical features typical of limited cutaneous disease: Raynaud's phenomenon preceding the

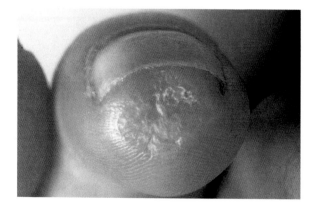

Fig. 38.3 Digital pitting in a patient with systemic sclerosis

diagnosis of systemic sclerosis by a number of years, sclerodactyly, digital pitting, and upper gastrointestinal problems. **[Q3: A]** Patients with limited cutaneous disease typically have more severe digital vascular disease than patients with diffuse cutaneous disease, and anticentromere antibody is predictive of severe digital ischaemia.[7] **[Q4: A, C, D, E]**

Treatment of Raynaud's phenomenon is initially conservative – keeping warm, avoiding cold exposure, and refraining from smoking (smoking is a risk factor for severity of digital ischaemia in patients with systemic sclerosis[8]). If these measures do not suffice, then a vasodilator is prescribed, usually a calcium channel blocker.[9,10] There is no role for steroid therapy in most patients with systemic sclerosis (and steroids are relatively contraindicated in patients with diffuse cutaneous disease). Biofeedback has gained considerable attention but was not found to be effective in a randomised trial of primary Raynaud's phenomenon.[11] **[Q5: A, C, D]** If a patient has very severe digital ischaemia, with or without digital ulceration, then the patient should be admitted for intravenous prostanoids[12] and, if there is any question of infection, then intravenous antibiotics are also indicated.

The vascular surgeon is likely to be called to see a patient with severe Raynaud's (often in the context of systemic sclerosis) because of either non-healing ulceration or because of very severe (sometimes critical) ischaemia. The reduced blood supply impairs ulcer healing. Debridement often aids healing. However, a proportion of patients come to amputation. Some patients have calcinosis at the site of the ulceration, and so this may be a complicating factor (Fig. 38.4). Severe ischaemia often coexists with ulceration. Cervical sympathectomy is no longer advocated for upper limb Raynaud's phenomenon. Recently digital sympathectomy has attracted interest for the treatment of severe digital ischaemia in patients with systemic sclerosis.[10,13] Digital sympathectomy is unlikely to be indicated at this stage in our patient, unless things do not settle with intravenous prostanoids, antibiotics and debridement. At present there is no evidence base for anticoagulation in patients with systemic sclerosis and digital ischaemia and/or ulceration although the possibility of an underlying coagulopathy, for example antiphospholipid syndrome, should always considered in patients presenting with digital ischaemia. **[Q6: A, B, C]**

Finally, although the vascular abnormalities in systemic sclerosis are predominantly microvascular, an increased prevalence of large vessel disease in patients with systemic sclerosis has recently been reported.[14] Thus the possibility of a proximal obstruction should always be considered in patients with systemic sclerosis presenting with an ischaemic digit.

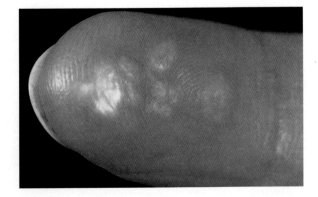

Fig. 38.4 Digital pulp calcinosis in a patient with systemic sclerosis – there is a risk that this deposit will ulcerate

References

1. LeRoy EC, Medsger TA. Raynaud's phenomenon: a proposal for classification. *Clin Exp Rheumatol.* 1992;10:485-488.
2. Herrick AL. Pathogenesis of Raynaud's phenomenon. *Rheumatology.* 2005; 44: 587-596.
3. Campbell PM, LeRoy EC. Pathogenesis of systemic sclerosis: a vascular hypothesis. *Semin Arthritis Rheum.* 1975;4:351-368.
4. Maricq HR, LeRoy EC. Patterns of finger capillary abnormalities in connective tissue disease by "wide-field" microscopy. *Arthritis Rheum.* 1973;16:619-628.
5. Harvey GR, McHugh NJ. Serologic abnormalities in systemic sclerosis. *Curr Op Rheumatol.* 1999;11:495-502.
6. LeRoy EC, Black C, Fleischmajer R, et al. Scleroderma (systemic sclerosis): classification, subsets and pathogenesis. *J Rheumatol.* 1988;15:202-205.
7. Wigley FM, Wise RA, Miller R, Needleman BW, Spence RJ. Anticentromere antibody as a predictor of digital ischemic loss in patients with systemic sclerosis. *Arthritis Rheum.* 1992;35:688-693.
8. Harrison BJ, Silman AJ, Hider SL, Herrick AL. Cigarette smoking: a significant risk factor for digital vascular diseases in patients with systemic sclerosis. *Arthritis Rheum.* 2002;46:3312-3316.
9. Thompson AE, Shea B, Welch V, Fenlon D, Pope JE. Calcium-channel blockers for Raynaud's phenomenon in systemic sclerosis. *Arthritis Rheum.* 2001;44:1841-1847.
10. Herrick AL. Treatment of Raynaud's phenomenon – update, new insights and developments. *Curr Rheumatol Rep.* 2003;5:168-174.
11. Raynaud's Treatment Study Investigators: Comparison of sustained-release nifedipine and temperature biofeedback for treatment of primary Raynaud phenomenon. Results from a randomized clinical trial with 1-year follow-up. *Arch Intern Med.* 2000;160:1101–1108.
12. Wigley FM, Wise RA, Seibold JR, et al. Intravenous iloprost infusion in patients with Raynaud phenomenon secondary to systemic sclerosis. A multicenter, placebo-controlled, double-blind study. *Ann Intern Med.* 1994;120:199-206.
13. Tomaino MM, Goitz RJ, Medsger TA. Surgery for ischemic pain and Raynaud's phenomenon in scleroderma: a description of treatment protocol and evaluation of results. *Microsurgery.* 2001;21:75-79.
14. Ho M, Veale D, Eastmond C, Nuki G, Belch J. Macrovascular disease and systemic sclerosis. *Ann Rheum Dis.* 2000;59:39-43.

Part VIII

Prevention and Management of Complications of Arterial Surgery

Christopher P. Gibbons

A 66-year-old man, an ex-smoker with hypertension and hypercholesterolaemia, had undergone a Dacron bifurcated aortic graft and bilateral ureteric stents for an inflammatory aortic aneurysm with ureteric obstruction at another hospital 4 years previously. The left limb of the graft had been anastomosed to the common femoral artery and the right limb to the common iliac bifurcation. Postoperatively he had suffered a mild groin wound infection, which had healed with antibiotics. At follow-up he complained of left calf and thigh claudication. On examination, he appeared generally well with a midline abdominal scar and a left vertical groin scar. He had good right femoral pulse but an absent left femoral pulse.

Question 1

What should be the first investigation?

A. Intra-arterial digital subtraction angiography (DSA).
B. Duplex ultrasound scan of the aortic graft.
C. ^{99}Technetium-labelled leucocyte scan.
D. CT angiography of the graft.
E. Erythrocyte sedimentation rate (ESR).

A duplex scan showed an occluded left limb of the aortic graft with patent common femoral arteries. There was no evidence of any stenosis of the left common femoral artery but a perigraft fluid collection was noted around the intra-abdominal portion of the graft.

C.P. Gibbons
Department of Vascular Surgery, Morriston Hospital, Swansea, UK

G. Geroulakos and B. Sumpio (eds.), *Vascular Surgery*,
DOI: 10.1007/978-1-84996-356-5_39, © Springer-Verlag London Limited 2011

Question 2

What further investigations should be performed?

A. CT scan of the graft.
B. Digital subtraction angiography.
C. ⁹⁹Technetium-labelled leucocyte scan.
D. Erythrocyte sedimentation rate.
E. Aspiration of the collection.

A CT scan confirmed the presence of fluid and gas around the intra-abdominal portion of the graft and the occlusion of the left limb, indicating graft infection (Fig. 39.1). Digital subtraction angiography (Fig. 39.2) confirmed the occluded left limb of the aortic graft and showed a stenosis at the origin of the right graft limb, presumably as a result of external compression. Aspiration of the perigraft collection would have allowed preoperative bacterial culture but was considered to be too difficult to perform safely.

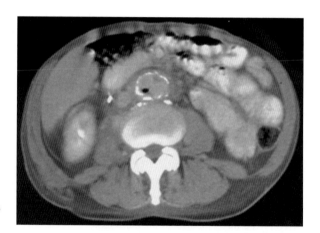

Fig. 39.1 CT scan of aortic graft showing fluid and a gas bubble around the graft

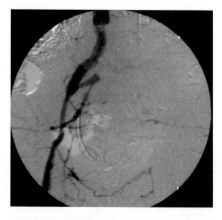

Fig. 39.2 Intra-arterial digital subtraction angiography (DSA) of the aortoiliac region

Question 3

Having confirmed the presence of infection what is the best option for management?

A. Prolonged antibiotic therapy.
B. Drainage of the perigraft pus under anaesthesia.
C. Insertion of gentamicin beads.
D. Excision of the graft.
E. Excision of the graft with in situ replacement with an antibiotic bonded graft.
F. Graft excision and extra-anatomical prosthetic bypass.
G. Graft replacement with autologous vein.
H. Graft replacement with an aortic allograft.

In situ replacement with autologous vein was chosen because of the reduced risk of persistent infection.

Question 4

Which autologous veins may be used for aortoiliac or aortofemoral graft replacement?

A. Long saphenous vein.
B. Cephalic vein.
C. Femoropopliteal vein.
D. Iliac vein.

Femoropopliteal vein was used as it is ideally suited to supra-inguinal graft replacement as it is relatively thick-walled, is of adequate diameter and has sufficient length.

Question 5

What further preoperative investigations should be performed?

A. Plain abdominal X-ray.
B. Bone scan.
C. MRI scan of the abdomen.
D. Duplex scan of the femoral veins.
E. Repeat abdominal ultrasound scan.

A duplex scan of the femoral veins confirmed that they were patent and of adequate calibre. The patient was operated on electively on the next available operating list.

Question 6

What other preoperative preparations should be undertaken?

A. Routine full blood count.
B. Urea and electrolyte estimation.

C. Chest X-ray and electrocardiogram (ECG).
D. Compression stockings.
E. Subcutaneous heparin.
F. Combination antibiotic therapy.

Routine blood investigations, chest X-ray and ECG were all performed, and in view of the magnitude of the procedure, echocardiogram and lung function tests were also ordered. They were all satisfactory. Because the bacteriology of the infection was not known pre-operatively in this patient, intravenous combination antibacterial therapy with teicoplanin, ciprofloxacin, co-amoxiclav and metronidazole was given immediately before surgery.

Question 7

How should the operation be performed?

A. Laparotomy, excision of the aortic graft, harvesting of the femoral veins and graft replacement.
B. Harvesting of femoral veins followed by laparotomy, excision of the infected graft and replacement with femoral vein.
C. Laparotomy and exposure of the infected graft, then femoral vein harvest followed by graft replacement.

The anaesthetised patient was catheterised, prepared and draped so that the abdomen and both legs were exposed. First, both superficial femoral veins were simultaneously dissected out by two operative teams and the branches divided between clips from the profunda femo-ris vein to the knee joint. The femoral veins were left in situ whilst the abdomen was opened, exposing the graft and obtaining control of the proximal infrarenal aorta and the right com-mon iliac bifurcation. The graft was encased in fibrous tissue, making dissection difficult and hazardous. The underlying prosthesis showed poor tissue incorporation and there was a loca-lised abscess between the graft and the duodenum, which was evacuated and cultured. The left groin was exposed, obtaining control of the common femoral artery, its branches and the profunda femoris artery. After systemic heparinisation, the vessels were clamped and the infected graft excised and sent for culture. The graft bed was washed repeatedly with povi-done iodine and hydrogen peroxide. One femoral vein was excised, reversed and inserted end-to-end from the infrarenal aorta to the right common iliac artery bifurcation using 4/0 polypropylene sutures. Size discrepancy at the aortic anastomosis was overcome by "fish-mouthing" the end of the vein to prevent the angulation associated with spatulation (Fig. 39.3). The other femoral vein was reversed and anastomosed end to side to the intra-abdominal part of the vein graft and to the left common femoral artery (Fig. 39.4). Both veins were led through a fresh tunnel and surrounded by greater omentum to avoid contact with the bed of the infected graft. The arterial anastomoses were covered by gentamicin-impregnated colla-gen foam and the wounds were closed with suction drainage. Antibiotic prophylaxis and low molecular weight heparin were continued postoperatively. Despite the copious pus around the graft, no organisms were grown in the laboratory. Combination antibiotic therapy was stopped after 7 days but co-amoxiclav was continued empirically for a further 5 weeks.

Fig. 39.3 "Fishmouthing" the
femoral vein to equalise
diameter with the aorta

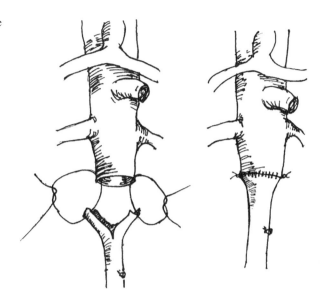

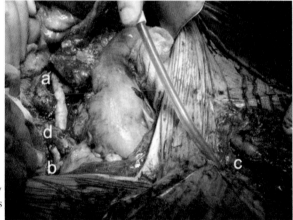

Fig. 39.4 Femoral vein reconstruction from the infrarenal
aorta (**a**) to the right iliac (**b**)
and left common femoral artery
(**c**). The right ureter (**d**) overlies
the right limb of the graft

Question 8

If the patient had presented with an exposed prosthetic graft in the groin how would this
have altered management?

A. Prolonged antibiotic therapy.
B. Use of vacuum dressings.
C. Simple coverage with a muscle flap without graft replacement.
D. Addition of a muscle flap to graft replacement with autologous vein.

Fig. 39.5 Rectus femoris muscle flap to cover a femoral anastomosis. (**a**) After mobilisation of the rectus femoris muscle (the femoral anastomosis is obscured by a sheet of gentamicin-impregnated collagen foam). (**b**) The muscle now overlies the anastomosis

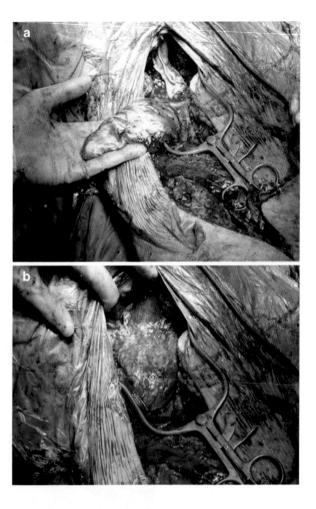

Exposed grafts present a difficult problem for achieving skin closure and the addition of a local muscle flap in the groin to graft replacement with autologous (femoropopliteal) vein is the most certain method of cure. The author´s preference is a rectus femoris flap for this (Fig. 39.5).

Question 9

What complications might occur following this operation?

A. Anastomotic haemorrhage.
B. Graft rupture.
C. Femoral deep vein thrombosis (DVT).
D. Limb swelling.
E. Seroma in the thigh.
F. Intestinal obstruction.
G. Wound infection.

The patient had the most common complication of this operation, which was a large seroma in the left thigh and a smaller one in the right thigh despite prolonged suction drainage. These were aspirated repeatedly and resolved after 3 weeks, although in other cases reoperation and reinsertion of a drain may be required. Intestinal obstruction is no more common following this operation than other abdominal procedures.

The patient otherwise made a good recovery and was discharged from hospital at 14 days. The graft and pus swabs were sterile so most of the antibiotics were stopped at 1 week but the co-amoxiclav was continued for 6 weeks on empirical grounds.

Question 10

What routine follow-up investigations should be performed?

A. Abdominal CT scan.
B. Abdominal ultrasound.
C. Graft duplex scans.
D. Abdominal X-ray.
E. Erythrocyte sedimentation rate.

Routine 3-monthly duplex scans were performed over 1 year for vein graft surveillance. The patient remains well without further intervention at 5 years.

39.1
Commentary

Aortic graft infection is thankfully rare, occurring in 1–5% of reconstructions,[1] but is one of the most feared complications in vascular surgery because of its high mortality and morbidity.[2] In a UK multicentre audit of 55 graft infections 31% died, 33% underwent amputation and only 45% left hospital alive without amputation.[3] If left untreated there is a high risk of graft occlusion and anastomotic haemorrhage, which may lead to aortoenteric fistula. Prompt curative treatment is therefore wise in patients sufficiently fit to withstand major surgery.

Graft infection may present at any time from a few days to many years after surgery. It can follow a wound infection, particularly in the groin where wound breakdown may result in exposure of the graft, or it may present later with a perigraft fluid collection or sinus at the femoral anastomosis. Infection of wholly intra-abdominal grafts may present with backache and fever but more often remain undetected until anastomotic haemorrhage or graft thrombosis occurs. Duplex ultrasound scanning or CT angiography is wise in all cases of graft thrombosis not only to confirm the occlusion but also to demonstrate any perigraft fluid which would indicate graft infection. **[Q1: B, D]**

The most common causative organism is *Staphylococcus aureus* in most series and such infections tend to present in the early postoperative period. Methicillin-resistant strains (MRSA) are said to be particularly virulent and have been associated with a high mortality in some series.[3–5] *Staphylococcus epidermidis* infections tend to be less virulent and often present many years later. They produce a slime or biofilm around the graft or occasionally thin pus. Isolation of *Staph. epidermidis* is more difficult and may require agitation of the extirpated graft with ultrasound to release it for culture. Other infections are caused by coliforms, *Salmonella, Serratia, Pseudomonas*, enterococci, streptococci or *Bacteroides*.[6] Gram-negative organisms may be more likely to present with anastomotic haemorrhage.[7] In many cases no causative organism can be isolated despite obvious infection. Possible causes of this are previous antibiotic administration or failure to isolate *Staphylococcus epidermidis*.

A preoperative diagnosis of graft infection is usually secured by ultrasound followed by CT or MRI. Aspiration of the perigraft fluid may secure a bacteriological diagnosis prior to surgery, although in many cases the responsible organism cannot be isolated. Fluid is often present in the aneurysmal sac after aortic aneurysm replacement and can be seen in smaller quantities around an aorto-bifemoral prosthesis performed for occlusive disease on ultrasound or CT for a few weeks after surgery. However, persistence of fluid around an aortic prosthesis for more than 3–6 months after surgery is highly suggestive of infection. Similarly, perigraft gas may be present for up to 10 days after surgery but indicates infection beyond this time.[9, 10]

If a groin abscess develops in relation to an aorto-bifemoral graft, aspiration under aseptic conditions in the clinic will confirm the presence of graft infection and may provide preoperative bacteriology. Perigraft fluid or gas may be absent in low-grade chronic infection or if a sinus in one or other groin allows the pus to escape. Exploration of a sinus under anaesthesia will demonstrate a connection with the infected graft and gently passing a bougie alongside the graft will determine whether or not the infection is confined to the anastomosis. If there is no sinus or perigraft fluid, a [99]technetium-labelled leucocyte scan may demonstrate increased activity over an infected graft.[11] However, this investigation has poor sensitivity and specificity and is only useful for chronic graft infection as increased leucocyte adherence is demonstrated by most prostheses for up to 6 months after insertion. The ultimate diagnosis of graft infection is made at operation by the lack of tissue incorporation into knitted Dacron or polytetrafluoroethylene (PTFE) prostheses and the presence of perigraft pus from which organisms may be cultured. Preoperative angiography is helpful for operative planning by delineating the vascular anatomy but adds no useful information about the presence of graft infection. [Q2: A, B]

There are multiple treatment options: Antibiotic therapy may buy time, but is rarely curative because the graft acts as a foreign body rendering the responsible organisms inaccessible to antibiotics. There have been occasional reports of successful treatment by drainage of the abscess around the graft followed by irrigation with antibiotic or iodine solutions[12–14] or implantation of gentamicin-impregnated beads or foam but these are anecdotal.[15, 16] Simple excision of an aortic graft is unwise unless it has already occluded without critical ischaemia as subsequent limb loss or severe lower body ischaemia is likely. Excision of the infected graft with debridement and replacement with a rifampicin-bonded or silver-impregnated graft has been advocated[17–20] but most would reserve this for chronic low-grade infections because of the risk of reinfection of the new graft. Despite their in vitro effectiveness[21] encouraging individual series, there is no convincing clinical evidence that either rifampicin-bonding or silver-impregnated Dacron grafts are less susceptible to reinfection after replacement of infected grafts.

Moreover, randomised clinical studies have failed to show that either rifampicin-bonding or silver impregnation prevents primary infection in vascular grafts, although these studies were somewhat underpowered.[22, 23]

An alternative approach, which avoids direct reimplantation of prosthetic material, is in situ replacement with fresh or cryopreserved aortic allografts. The reported results have been variable but in all series there have been instances of early or late graft disruption or aneurysm formation particularly with fresh allografts and when used for aorto-enteric fistula.[24-29]

Until the last 5 years, the mainstay of treatment has been excision of the graft with extra-anatomical reconstruction. For infected aortoiliac grafts reconstruction can be performed with an axillo-bifemoral or bilateral axillofemoral grafts. However, in those patients with infected aorto-bifemoral grafts, the lower anastomosis must be performed at the level of the superficial femoral or popliteal artery to avoid placing the new graft in an infected field. Good results can be obtained with this approach but there remains a 10–15% risk of graft reinfection.[2, 30-32] If this option is used, the extra-anatomic bypass should be performed before graft excision to reduce the risk of irreversible limb ischaemia and amputation.[2]

More recently, Claggett[33, 34] and Nevelsteen [35, 36] independently advocated aortic replacement with femoropopliteal veins for infected grafts. Femoropopliteal veins are much wider and thicker-walled than long saphenous or arm veins and have adequate length, making them ideal for aortoiliac reconstruction. Iliac veins are too short and their excision would result in severe limb swelling. Results were excellent with reduced mortality, limb loss and reinfection rates. Subsequently other authors have confirmed the effectiveness of this approach in eliminating reinfection, with mortality and amputation rates similar to or lower than reports using other techniques.[37, 38] This is now recognised as the procedure of choice in most situations. The procedure is demanding and may take several hours to perform but can be made easier by the use of two or more operative teams working together. Femoral veins may be harvested even after the removal of the long saphenous vein but it is generally advised that the profunda femoris vein should be left intact and that the popliteal vein should not be removed below the knee joint.[39, 40] Fears of venous morbidity from femoral vein harvest have not been borne out in practice although Valentine reported an 18% incidence of prophylactic or therapeutic fasciotomy for compartment syndrome.[41] However, neither Nevelsteen[42] nor the present author has found this necessary. Femoral vein harvest should be the initial step in the operation to avoid prolonged abdominal exposure or aortic clamping. Partial graft replacement is best avoided, as the remaining graft usually requires later replacement.[43] [Q3: E, F, G, H] [Q4: C] [Q7: B] If femoropopliteal aortic reconstruction is planned, it is wise to perform a preoperative venous duplex scan of the legs to confirm that the femoral veins are patent and of adequate calibre (1 cm). [Q5: D]

Whichever technique is used, the importance of adequate debridement, antiseptic washouts and drainage cannot be overstressed. Combination antibiotic cover (beginning immediately preoperatively) to cover any cultured organism and the common pathogens is essential to eliminate infection and prevent catastrophic haemorrhage from anastomotic breakdown. Routine preoperative investigations such as full blood count, urea and electrolyte estimation, chest X-ray and ECG are indicated. Compression stockings are used by some surgeons after femoropopliteal vein harvest to limit ankle swelling but cannot be used intraoperatively. Subcutaneous heparin is used postoperatively but not preoperatively as systemic heparinisation is used routinely on aortic clamping. **[Q6: A, B, C, F]**

In cases where a prosthetic graft has been exposed in the groin or the tissues overlying a femoral anastomosis are deficient, a local muscle flap is wise to protect the new femoral anastomosis. **[Q8: D]** A sartorius rotation flap may be used provided the graft does not extend in front of the inguinal ligament as in femoral-femoral or axillofemoral grafts.[44,45] Gracilis and rectus abdominis flaps or omental pedicles have also been described.[46-51] A rectus femoris flap is very quick and easy to prepare and will cover any femoral anastomosis with ease.[38] In occasional localised low-grade graft infections with exposure of the prosthesis in the groin, a simple muscle flap may be successful without excision of the graft but there is a high rate of recurrent infection.

Despite the magnitude of the procedure, graft replacement with femoral vein gives excellent results with reported mortalities in the region of 10%, amputation rates of 10% and no reinfection. Possible complications include anastomotic haemorrhage, iliac venous thrombosis, limb swelling, seroma, intestinal obstruction and wound infection. Limb swelling usually occurs but is rarely excessive and is easily controlled by elevation provided the profunda femoris vein is preserved and the popliteal vein is not harvested below the knee. Since the deep veins have been excised, lower limb DVT is unlikely. Wound and graft infection or anastomotic haemorrhage is similarly infrequent provided adequate antibiotic cover is used. **[Q9: A, D, E, F, G]**

Routine duplex surveillance of the aortofemoral vein grafts is wise as late graft stenosis due to intimal hyperplasia is common.[38] **[Q10: C]**

References

1. Seeger JM. Management of patients with prosthetic graft infection. *Am Surg.* 2000;66: 166-167.
2. Yeager RA, Porter JM. Arterial and prosthetic graft infection. *Ann Vasc Surg.* 1992;5: 485-491.
3. Naylor AR, Hayes PD, Darke S on behalf of the Joint Vascular Research Group. A prospective audit of complex wound and graft infections in Great Britain and Ireland: the emergence of MRSA. *Eur J Vasc Endovasc Surg.* 2001;21:289–294.
4. Nasim A, Thompson MM, Naylor AR, et al. The impact of MRSA on vascular surgery. *Eur J Vasc Endovasc Surg.* 2001;22:211-214.
5. Murphy GJ, Pararajasingam R, Nasim A, et al. Methicillin-resistant *Staphylococcus aureus* infection in vascular surgical patients. *Ann R Coll Surg Engl.* 2001;83:158-163.
6. Selan L, Pasariello C. Microbiological diagnosis of aortofemoral graft infections. *Eur J Vasc Endovasc Surg.* 1997;14(Suppl A):10-12.
7. Hicks RJC, Greenhalgh RM. The pathogenesis of vascular graft infection. *Eur J Vasc Endovasc Surg.* 1997;14(Suppl A):5-9.
8. Calligaro KD, Veith FJ, Schwartz ML, et al. Are Gram-negative bacteria a contraindication to selective preservation of infected prosthetic arterial grafts?. *J Vasc Surg.* 1992;136:337-345.
9. Orton DF, LeVeen RF, Saigh JA, et al. Aortic prosthetic graft infections: radiologic manifestations and implications for management. *RadioGraphics.* 2000;20:977-993.

10. Spartera C, Morettini G, Petrassi C, et al. Role of magnetic resonance imaging in the evaluation of aortic graft healing, perigraft fluid collection, and graft infection. *Eur J Vasc Surg.* 1990;4:69-73.
11. Liberatore M, Iurilli AP, Ponzo F, et al. Aortofemoral graft infection: the usefulness of [99mTc]-HMPAO-labelled leucocyte scan. *Eur J Vasc Endovasc Surg.* 1997;14(Suppl A):27-29.
12. Almgren B, Eriksson I. Local antibiotic irrigation in the treatment of arterial graft infections. *Acta Chir Scand.* 1981;147:33-36.
13. Morris GE, Friend PJ, Vassallo DJ, et al. Antibiotic irrigation and conservative surgery for major aortic graft infection. *Vasc Surg.* 1994;20:88-95.
14. Voboril R, Weberova J, Kralove H. Successful treatment of infected vascular prosthetic grafts in the groin using conservative therapy with povidone-iodine solution. *Ann Vasc Surg.* 2004;18:372-375.
15. Nielsen OM, Noer HH, Jorgensen LG, Lorentzen JE. Gentamicin beads in the treatment of localised vascular graft infection – long term results in 17 cases. *Eur J Vasc Surg.* 1991;5:283-285.
16. Holdsworth J. Treatment of infective and potentially infective complications of vascular bypass grafting using gentamicin with collagen sponge. *Ann R Coll Surg Engl.* 1999;81:166-170.
17. Bandyk DF, Novotney ML, Johnson BL, et al. Use of rifampicin-soaked gelatin-sealed polyester grafts for in situ treatment of primary aortic and vascular prosthetic infections. *J Surg Res.* 2001;95:44-49.
18. Naylor AR. Aortic prosthetic infection. *Br J Surg.* 1999;86:435–436. Hayes PD, Nasim A, London NJM, et al. In situ replacement of infected aortic grafts with rifampicin-bonded prostheses: The Leicester experience (1992–1998). *J Vasc Surg.* 1999;30:92–98.
19. Zegelman M, Gunther G. Infected grafts require excision and extra-anatomic reconstruction. Against the motion. In: Greenhalgh RM, ed. *The evidence for vascular and endovascular reconstruction.* London: WB Saunders; 2002:252-258.
20. Batt M, Magne JL, Alric P, et al. In situ revascularization with silver-coated polyester grafts to treat aortic infection: early and midterm results. *J Vasc Surg.* 2003;38:983-989.
21. Hardman S, Cope A, Swann A, et al. An in vitro model to compare the antimicrobial activity of silver-coated versus rifampicin-soaked vascular grafts. *Ann Vasc Surg.* 2004;18:308-313.
22. Sardelic F, Ao PY, Taylor DA, Fletcher JP. Prophylaxis against *Staphylococcus epidermidis* vascular graft infection with rifampicin-soaked, gelatin-sealed Dacron. *Cardiovasc Surg.* 1996;4:389-392.
23. Earnshaw JJ, Whitman B, Heather BP, on behalf of the Joint Vascular Research Group. Two-year results of a randomized controlled trial of rifampicin-bonded extra-anatomic Dacron grafts. *Br J Surg.* 2000;87:758–759
24. Vogt PR, Brunner-LaRocca HP, Lachat M, et al. Technical details with the use of cryopreserved arterial allografts for aortic infection: influence on early and midterm mortality. *J Vasc Surg.* 2002;35:80-86.
25. Verhelst R, Lacroix V, Vraux H, et al. Use of cryopreserved arterial homografts for management of infected prosthetic grafts: A multicentre study. *Ann Vasc Surg.* 2000;14:602-607.
26. Noel AA, Gloviczki P, Cherry KJ Jr. United States Cryopreserved Aortic Allograft Registry. Abdominal aortic reconstruction in infected fields: early results of the United States cryopreserved aortic allograft registry. *J Vasc Surg.* 2002;35:847-852.
27. Teebken OE, Pichlmaier MA, Brand S, et al. Cryopreserved arterial allografts for in situ reconstruction of infected arterial vessels. *Eur J Vasc Endovasc Surg.* 2004;27:597-602.
28. Gabriel M, Pukacki F, Dzieciuchowicz L, et al. Cryopreserved arterial allografts in the treatment of prosthetic graft infections. *Eur J Vasc Endovasc Surg.* 2004;27:590-596.
29. Kieffer E, Gomes D, Chiche L, et al. Allograft replacement for infrarenal aortic graft infection: early and late results in 179 patients. *J Vasc Surg.* 2004;39:1009-1017.

30. Quinones-Baldrich WJ, Hernandez JJ, Moore WS. Long-term results following surgical management of aortic graft infection. *Arch Surg.* 1991;126:507-511.
31. Yeager RA, Taylor LM Jr, Moneta GL, et al. Improved results with conventional management of infrarenal aortic infection. *J Vasc Surg.* 1999;30:76-83.
32. Seeger JM, Pretus HA, Welborn MB, et al. Long-term outcome after treatment of aortic graft infection with staged extra-anatomic bypass grafting and aortic graft removal. *Surgery.* 2000;32:451-459.
33. Clagett GP, Valentine RJ, Hagino RT. Autogenous aortoiliac/femoral reconstruction from superficial femoral-popliteal veins: feasibility and durability. *J Vasc Surg.* 1997;25:255-270.
34. Gordon LL, Hagino RT, Jackson MR, et al. Complex aortofemoral prosthetic infections: the role of autogenous superficial femoropopliteal vein reconstruction. *Arch Surg.* 1999;134:615-621.
35. Nevelsteen A, Lacroix H, Suy R. Autogenous reconstruction with lower extremity deep veins: an alternative treatment of prosthetic infection after reconstructive surgery for aortoiliac disease. *J Vasc Surg.* 1995;22:129-134.
36. Daenens K, Fourneau I. Nevelsteen a ten-year experience in autogenous reconstruction with the femoral vein in the treatment of aortofemoral prosthetic infection. *Eur J Vasc Endovasc Surg.* 2003;25:240-245.
37. Brown PM, Kim VB, Lalikos JF, et al. Autologous superficial femoral vein for aortic reconstruction in infected fields. *Ann Vasc Surg.* 1999;13:32-36.
38. Gibbons CP, Ferguson CJ, Fligelstone LJ, Edwards K. Experience with femoro-popliteal veins as a conduit for vascular reconstruction in infected fields. *Eur J Vasc Endovasc Surg.* 2003;25:424-431.
39. Coburn M, Ashworth C, Francis W, et al. Venous stasis complications of the use of the superficial femoral and popliteal veins for lower extremity bypass. *J Vasc Surg.* 1993;17:1005-1009.
40. Wells JK, Hagino RT, Bargmann KM, et al. Venous morbidity after superficial femoral-popliteal vein harvest. *J Vasc Surg.* 1999;29:282-291.
41. Modrall JG, Sadjadi J, Ali AT, et al. Deep vein harvest: predicting need for fasciotomy. *J Vasc Surg.* 2004;39:387-394.
42. Nevelsteen A, Baeyens I, Daenens K, et al. Regarding "Deep vein harvest: predicting need for fasciotomy". *J Vasc Surg.* 2004;40:403.
43. Becquemin JP, Qvarfordt P, Kron J, et al. Aortic graft infection: is there a place for partial graft removal? *Eur J Vasc Endovasc Surg.* 1997;14(Suppl A):53-58.
44. Sladen JG, Thompson RP, Brosseuk DT, Kalman PG, Petrasek PF, Martin RD. Sartorius myoplasty in the treatment of exposed arterial grafts. *Cardiovasc Surg.* 1993;1:113-117.
45. Galland RB. Sartorius transposition in the management of synthetic graft infection. *Eur J Vasc Endovasc Surg.* 2002;23:175–177. Gomes MN, Spear SL. Pedicled muscle flaps in the management of infected aortofemoral grafts. *Cardiovasc Surg.* 1994;2:70–77.
46. Thomas WO, Parry SW, Powell RW, et al. Management of exposed inguinofemoral arterial conduits by skeletal muscular rotational flaps. *Am Surg.* 1994;60:872-880.
47. Meland NB, Arnold PG, Pairolero PC, Lovich SF. Muscle-flap coverage for infected peripheral vascular prostheses. *Plast Reconstr Surg.* 1994;93:1005-1011.
48. Calligaro KD, Veith FJ, Sales CM, et al. Comparison of muscle flaps and delayed secondary intention wound healing for infected lower extremity arterial grafts. *Ann Vasc Surg.* 1994;8:31-7.
49. Illig KA, Alkon JE, Smith A, Rhodes JM, et al. Rotational muscle flap closure for acute groin wound infections following vascular surgery. *Ann Vasc Surg.* 2004;18:661-668.
50. Colwell AS, Donaldson MC, Belkin M, Orgill DP. Management of early groin vascular bypass graft infections with sartorius and rectus femoris flaps. *Ann Plast Surg.* 2004;52:49-53.
51. Morasch MD, Sam AD 2nd, Kibbe MR, et al. Early results with use of gracilis muscle flap coverage of infected groin wounds after vascular surgery. *J Vasc Surg.* 2004;39:1277-1283.

Aortoenteric Fistulas

40

David Bergqvist

A 63-year-old smoking woman presented with severe intermittent claudication for a couple of years. Her walking distance had gradually decreased to around 50–100 m. She had previously been healthy and very active. At investigation, she had no femoral pulses and a bilateral ankle brachial index of 0.6. Further evaluation with angiography showed an aortic occlusion at the level of the renal arteries, and she was reconstructed with an aorto-bi-iliac polyester graft (16 × 8 mm) after local proximal aortic endarterectomy. The proximal anastomosis was made end to end, and the iliac end to side. Polypropylene sutures were used. The operation was somewhat technically difficult, with the proximal anastomosis having to be redone; the duration of surgery was 3.5 h with a blood loss of around 800 ml. The immediate postoperative course was uneventful. After 3 years, the patient had distal septic microembolization in the left leg with an abscess around the left distal graft limb. This was extirpated, the wound was drained and a femoral–femoral cross-over graft was inserted. She was put on antibiotics for 6 months.

Five years after the aortic operation, she had melaena and a decrease in hemoglobin.

Question 1

What is the time interval between aortic surgery and the presentation of an aortoenteric fistula?

A. It usually occurs in the first 48 h following aortic surgery.
B. It typically presents within the first month following the operation.
C. It may only occur in the first 5 years following the placement of the aortic synthetic graft.
D. It may present at any time during the lifetime of the patient after the placement of the synthetic aortic graft.

The patient was investigated at her primary health care centre with gastroscopy and colon enema, with negative results. After 2 months, she again had melaena; after further melaena

D. Bergqvist
Department of Surgery, Uppsala University Hospital, Uppsala, Sweden

G. Geroulakos and B. Sumpio (eds.), *Vascular Surgery*,
DOI: 10.1007/978-1-84996-356-5_40, © Springer-Verlag London Limited 2011

3 months later, she was referred to the hospital. On this occasion, she also had slight back pain and low-grade fewer.

Question 2

What is meant by herald bleeding?

A. A bleeding where the etiology cannot be determined
B. Small bleeding(s) before a large one from a major artery
C. A "warning" bleeding before a fatal one
D. A small haematemesis before a maelena

A gastroscopy showed a very distal duodenal "ulcer" with a green colored (bile stained) graft in the bottom (Fig. 40.1). A computed tomography (CT) scan showed fluid around the proximal part of the graft, with some gas bubbles.

Question 3

How will you rule out the presence of an aortoenteric fistula?

A. Gastroscopy
B. Computerized tomography
C. Magnetic resonance imaging
D. Barium enema or barium swallow and follow-through
E. None of the above

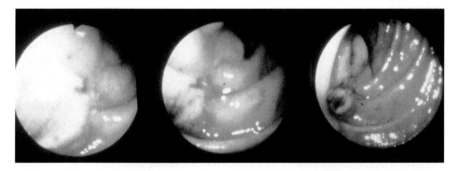

Fig. 40.1 Gastroduodenoscopy showing the dacron graft in the bottom of an ulceration, the graft being bile stained

Question 4

Which part of the bowel is involved in an aortoenteric fistula?

A. Duodenum
B. Jejunum
C. Ileum
D. Appendix
E. Any of the above could be involved

Following a diagnosis of a secondary aortoenteric fistula, and with the patient being circulatory stable, an axillo-bifemoral polyester graft was inserted. During the same period of anesthesia, the old aortic graft was extirpated. A duodenorraphy was made, and the aortic stump, which was about 2 cm below the renal arteries, was sutured and covered with omental tissue.

Question 5

Which treatment options are not to be recommended?

A. Stent grafting the anastomosis
B. Wait and see if the patient starts bleeding again
C. Extirpation of the aortic graft and then an axillofemoral reconstruction
D. Axillofemoral reconstruction and then extirpation of the aortic graft
E. In situ reconstruction with a new graft

The patient recovered and she left hospital after 12 days. After 10 months, she had melaena again and was admitted to hospital. Based on her previous history, a CT-scan was ordered, but suddenly she developed abdominal and back pain and a large gastrointestinal bleeding, both haematemesis and melaena, and went into chock. She died before any treatment could be given. Autopsy showed a blow out of the aortic stump with a fistula to the duodenum and also bleeding into the retroperitoneal space.

40.1
Commentary

The term "aortoenteric fistula" means a communication between aorta and some part of the gastrointestinal tract. It is rarely primary; most often, it is seen secondary to reconstructive vascular surgery, that is, secondary aortoenteric fistula. In the majority of cases it is seen after aortic graft insertion. It has also been reported after stent-grafting[1] and also after simple aortic suture.[2] The majority of fistulas (about 75%) involve the duodenum, but any part of the gastrointestinal tract may be involved. [**Q4: E**] A few patients have more than one fistula. In exceptional cases it can occur after other abdominal operations or radiation treatment. It is an emergent situation and should always be suspected in patients with an aortic reconstruction presenting with a gastrointestinal bleeding. It can occur at any time postoperatively, which means that the patient with an aortic graft is at risk developing a fistula for their entire lifetime. Thus, the true incidence of this condition cannot be established until all patients in a risk population have died. The longest interval reported is more than 20 years. Often there is a delay of several years. [**Q1: D**] During a period of 21 years in Sweden, there are indications that the incidence has decreased to around 0.5% after abdominal aortic operations.[3]

Two factors have been considered of major etiological importance: mechanical stress from the pulsating graft, which is in continuous contact with the intestine, and the presence of a low-grade infection. In patients with an aortoenteric fistula, there is often a history of complicated and troublesome primary graft operation or infectious problems in the postoperative course. The three most common findings at surgery are suture line contact with the bowel, pseudoaneurysn rupturing into the intestine, and graft body erosion of the intestine. To avoid the complications, atraumatic surgical technique is important, avoiding bowel trauma and large hematomas. The surgeon should try to cover the graft to avoid direct contact between the graft and the bowel.

The main symptom is gastrointestinal hemorrhage, which can range from mild melaena with anemia to a profuse, immediately fatal haematemesis. Often, this large bleeding is preceded by small "herald" bleedings, which are an important warning symptom. [**Q2: C**] About half of the patients also have septic symptoms of varying severity. In some patients, septic symptoms dominate, and the bleeding may even be occult.

There is often a long delay between onset of symptoms and final diagnosis. In some patients with a large initial bleeding, the diagnosis is established at autopsy. The cardinal importance of a high degree of clinical suspicion for obtaining a correct diagnosis must be emphasized. Unfortunately, there is no specific diagnostic test. At gastroduodenoscopy, it is important to scrutinize the whole duodenum down to the ligament of Treitz. Observation of a bile-stained graft is obviously pathognomonic. Endoscopy is also important to reveal other sources of bleeding. CT, MR and angiography may be helpful in showing pseudoaneurysm or fluid outside the graft, sometimes with gas in it. Conventional radiological methods for gastrointestinal examination are rarely helpful. One great problem is that the absence of abnormalities does not exclude the diagnosis. Exploratory laparotomy is indicated in patients with massive bleeding or where diagnostic efforts have been negative and the patient is still bleeding. [**Q3: E**]

The management is difficult. Total removal of all old graft material and revascularization seems to give the best results.[4] Just closing the fistula locally always leads to recurrence and the mortality is close to 100% and cannot be recommended.[5] It seems optimal to start with an extra-anatomical revascularization of the extremities and thereafter removal of the graft. Some authors recommend a delay of a few days between the two procedures[6]; this is possible when the hemorrhage is under control. In emergency situations, an abdominal exploration with closure of the fistula and graft removal is vital, but this may lead to a delayed revascularization with profound limb ischemia. When the graft is removed, the

Table 40.1 Treatment options for the invasive management of aortoenteric fistula

1. Extra-anatomic bypass with resection of the infected prosthesis
   - Staged
   - Simultaneous
2. Resection with in situ reconstruction
   - Antibiotic (rifampicin)-soaked graft with omental wrap
   - Homograft
   - Autologous vein
   - PTFE
3. Endovascular repair
   - As a bridging procedure
   - As a definitive solution

problem is how to deal with the aortic stump, which must be closed, preferably with double sutures. This may, however, not be possible if the distance to the renal arteries is too short. The stump is preferably covered with some vascularized tissue, and most frequently an omental pedicle has been used. Some authors advocate removal of the graft and an in situ reconstruction with expanded polytetrafluoroethylene (ePTFE) graft or an antibiotic-bonded polyester graft (often with rifampicin)[7,8] or in situ autologous vein.[2,9] Table 40.1 summarizes the treatment options for the invasive management of aortoenteric fistula. **[Q5: B]** Recently a new therapeutic option has become available and that is endovascular repair. This is especially attractive as a bridging procedure bringing a hemodynamically unstable patient into a stage where graft removal and reconstruction can be made in a controlled way.[10] In very fragile patients endovascular treatment may also be the only and final solution of a serious problem.

The prognosis is poor, with a high postoperative mortality, often several complications should the patient survive, and a risk for aortic stump blow out, which very few patients survive. Results have improved over recent years, but aortoenteric fistula still is a very serious and challenging complication.[10] The 5-year survival rate is between 50% and 60%.[3,7,10]

References

1. Bergqvist D, Bjorck M, Nyman R. Secondary aortoenteric fistula after endovascular aortic interventions: a systematic literature review. *J Vasc Interv Radiol.* 2008;19:163-165.
2. Moore RD, Tittley JG. Laparoscopic aortic injury leading to delayed aortoenteric fistula: an alternative technique for repair. *Ann Vasc Surg.* 1999;13:586-588.
3. Bergqvist D, Bjorkman H, Bolin T, et al. Secondary aortoenteric fistulae – changes from 1973 to 1993. *Eur J Vasc Endovasc Surg.* 1996;11:425-428.
4. Nagy SW, Marshall JB. Aortoenteric fistulas. Recognizing a potentially catastrophic cause ofV gastrointestinal bleeding. *Postgrad Med.* 1993;93:211-212, 215–216, 219–222.
5. Muller BT, Abbara S, Hennes N, Sandmann W. Diagnosis and therapy of second aortoenteric fistulas: results of 16 patients. *Chirurg.* 1999;70:415-421.
6. Geroulakos G, Lumley JS, Wright JG. Factors influencing the long-term results of abdominal aortic aneurysm repair. *Eur J Vasc Endovasc Surg.* 1997;13:3-8.

7. Hayes PD, Nasim A, London NJ, et al. In situ replacement of infected aortic grafts with rifampicin-bonded prostheses: the leicester experience (1992 to 1998). *J Vasc Surg.* 1999;30:92-98.

8. Young RM, Cherry KJ Jr, Davis PM, et al. The results of in situ prosthetic replacement for infected aortic grafts. *Am J Surg.* 1999;178:136-140.

9. Franke S, Voit R. The superficial femoral vein as arterial substitute in infections of the aortoiliac region. *Ann Vasc Surg.* 1997;11:406-412.

10. Bergqvist D, Bjorck M. Secondary arterioenteric fistulation – a systematic literature analysis. *Eur J Vasc Endovasc Surg.* 2009;37:31-42.

Part IX

Vascular Access

The Optimal Conduit for Hemodialysis Access

Frank T. Padberg and Robert W. Zickler

A 42-year-old type 1 diabetic of normal weight has recently progressed to chronic renal disease. Insulin-dependent diabetes mellitus (DM) has been managed by the same primary care physician for the preceding 12 years; glucose control has never been a problem in this cooperative and well-educated individual. The renal failure was initially managed with appropriate adjustments to diet and medications; the presumptive diagnosis is diabetic nephropathy. Recent laboratory tests demonstrate a creatinine of 4.1, a blood urea nitrogen of 94, a potassium of 4.8, mild proteinuria, and a creatinine clearance of 20 mL/min.

Question 1

At this juncture the physician's most appropriate course of action is:

A. Refer the individual to a surgeon for hemoaccess.
B. Refer the individual to a nephrologist to refine diagnosis and initiate specialty care. It is not time to initiate dialysis.
C. Refer the individual to a nephrologist who will refine diagnosis, and determine if there is a reversible cause for the renal insufficiency.
D. Refer the individual to a nephrologist who will evaluate the etiology of the renal insufficiency and determine if there is a reversible cause. If not, a surgeon skilled in the construction of durable hemoaccess should be consulted.
E. Refer the individual to a nephrologist to commence dialysis with a central venous catheter.

F.T. Padberg (✉)
Division of Vascular Surgery, Department of Surgery, New Jersey Medical School, University of Medicine and Dentistry of New Jersey, Newark, NJ, USA

G. Geroulakos and B. Sumpio (eds.), *Vascular Surgery*,
DOI: 10.1007/978-1-84996-356-5_41, © Springer-Verlag London Limited 2011

Question 2

A nephrology work-up finds no reversible cause and the patient's immune status precludes any further consideration of transplantation. The patient is referred for construction of a hemoaccess. The most appropriate action is to perform a clinical vascular examination with specific attention to:

A. The pedal pulses and examination of the foot; extensive arterial occlusive disease is common in diabetic patients and infection would complicate any hemoaccess procedure.
B. The radial pulses and superficial venous anatomy. Book the operating room and proceed to construct an access in the upper extremity, guided by your clinical examination.
C. The radial pulses and superficial venous anatomy supplemented by a duplex ultrasound (DU) study. Book the operating room and proceed to construct an access in the upper extremity guided by these findings.
D. Immediate hemoaccess placement. Simultaneous placement of an arteriovenous fistula (AVF) and a central venous catheter.

Question 3

Preoperative DU examination should include all *except* one of the following:

A. Both upper extremities.
B. Size and location of the arteries.
C. Location of the brachial bifurcation.
D. Assessment of the axillary and subclavian veins.
E. At least one lower extremity.
F. Size and location of the superficial veins.
G. Evaluation of the superficial veins for evidence of prior scarring.

The patient is right hand dominant. Non-invasive examination demonstrated the findings given in the caption to Fig. 41.1.

Right: Cephalic (diameter 3.3 mm) and basilic (diameter 3.5 mm) veins course through both the forearm and upper arm to their junctions with the axillary and brachial veins respectively; however, both superficial forearm veins demonstrate post-thrombotic changes in the forearm. The brachial artery (diameter 4.2 mm) bifurcates into a radial (diameter 2.8 mm) and ulnar (diameter 2.7 mm) artery 3 cm below the antecubital crease; the palmar arches are intact. The deep venous structures are normal from the forearm veins through visualization of the axillary and subclavian veins.

Left: The basilic vein is post-thrombotic and thickened in the forearm; it has a normal 3.5-mm diameter lumen just below the elbow continuing into its junction with the brachial vein at mid-humerus. The cephalic vein (diameter 3.5 mm) has a normal luminal surface, extends to the wrist, is superficial, communicates with the proximal basilic at the

Fig. 41.1 Duplex ultrasound: The patient is right hand dominant. Non-invasive examination demonstrated the following findings. Top diagram: left arm bottom diagram: right arm red=arterial antomy blue=superficial veins Dotted blue=diseased vein as described in text

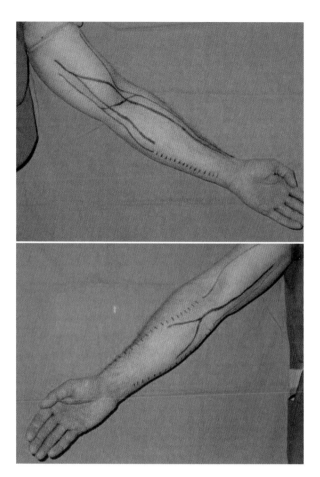

antecubital junction, and remains patent into its junction with the axillary vein. The brachial artery (diameter 4.2 mm) bifurcates into a radial (diameter 2.8 mm) and ulnar (diameter 2.7 mm) artery at mid-humerus; the palmar arches are intact. The deep venous structures are normal from the forearm veins through visualization of the axillary and subclavian veins.

Question 4

Which procedure would be the *best* option for this individual?

A. Left brachial to basilic transposition AVF in the arm.
B. Right radial to basilic transposition AVF in the forearm.
C. Left brachial to median antecubital vein forearm loop graft (PTFE).
D. Left internal jugular (IJ) tunneled, cuffed dual lumen hemodialysis catheter.
E. Left radial to cephalic AVF.

Question 5

Which of the following *best* describes when this new hemoaccess is considered mature enough to begin puncture for hemodialysis?

A. The wound is securely healed, the sutures have been removed, and there is a palpable thrill.
B. The wound is securely healed, the sutures have been removed, and there is a palpable thrill. At 2 weeks, a duplex examination demonstrates unobstructed flow, but the walls of the conduit appear to be relatively thin.
C. The wound is securely healed, the sutures have been removed, and there is a palpable thrill. At 8 weeks, a duplex examination demonstrated that there was unobstructed flow and the walls of the conduit have thickened measurably.
D. The wound is securely healed, the sutures have been removed, and there is a palpable thrill. At 6 weeks, a duplex examination demonstrates an equal volume of flow through both the fistula vein and a large branch vein at the site of the thrill.
E. Two weeks.

Your initial hemoaccess has functioned well for 6.4 years, but the hemodialysis staff has noted increasing difficulty obtaining adequate flows for the external machine circuit; arterial pressures were low at 70 mm Hg and venous pressures elevated to 350 mm Hg. You are asked to consider revision or a new hemoaccess.

A new duplex examination demonstrates progressive stenosis of the distal radial artery, and multiple sites of localized thrombosis extending into the upper arm cephalic vein. You determine that there is no role for angioplasty of the lengthy arterial stenosis or the multiple venous lesions. With the exception of the appropriate postoperative changes, the remainder of the examination is unchanged from that described in Fig. 41.1.

Question 6

Which is the *best* option to maintain hemodialysis?

A. Right radial to basilic transposition AVF in the forearm.
B. Right forearm loop graft (PTFE).
C. Left forearm loop graft (PTFE).
D. Left radial (antecubital) to basilic transposition AVF in the arm.
E. Left IJ tunneled, cuffed dual lumen hemodialysis catheter.

A new hemoaccess is constructed and an excellent thrill achieved. During initial maturation, hemodialysis is continued via the original left arm hemoaccess. Fortunately, the original left hemoaccess provides sufficient flow for adequate interval hemodialysis, but 6 weeks later has spontaneously thrombosed. Dialysis using the new hemoaccess is successful and the hemoaccess functions well for thrice weekly puncture.

Two years later you are again contacted to evaluate this individual. One year previously, an uneventful coronary bypass was performed. Subsequently, following an episode of syncope, and tachyarrhythmia, a permanent defibrillator was installed on the left anterior chest wall 2 months ago (Fig. 41.2).

Fig. 41.2 The chest X-ray
was taken at the time of the
referral for arm edema

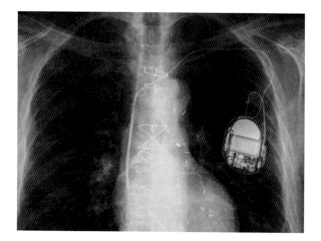

The patient is complaining of an obviously swollen left arm.

Question 7

What is wrong?

A. The patient's heart failure has worsened from a combination of a fixed heart rate and the increased output demanded for the hemoaccess.
B. Edema is a result of lymphatic disturbance from defibrillator implantation.
C. The patient is hypercoagulable and has thrombosis of the superior vena cava (SVC).
D. Unilateral swelling results from continuously increasing flow in the hemoaccess and enlargement of the arterial anastomosis.
E. The transvenous electrodes have induced a stenosis or obstruction of the left subclavian vein.

Question 8

The *best* treatment for this condition is?

A. Begin strong diuresis to counter the right heart failure.
B. Place the arm in a sling and elevate it to reduce the existing edema from the operation. The patient is reassured that edema following pacemaker insertion of these devices is usually self-limited and will soon resolve.
C. The defibrillator is removed and replaced in the right subclavian vein.
D. A fistulagram/venogram is performed. This will determine the etiology of the edema and may offer an opportunity for interventional therapy.
E. A hypercoagulable work-up is obtained.

All of the interventions aimed at reducing the left arm edema are unsuccessful, and the patient is discharged home. After multiple attempts, the dialysis staff reluctantly admit they are no longer able to reliably cannulate the left arm AVF. You are again asked to consider revision or a new hemoaccess.

A new DU is obtained. The appropriate postoperative findings are noted; otherwise, the relevant arm anatomy is unchanged from the initial survey as shown in Fig. 41.1.

Question 9

The optimal hemoaccess for this individual now is:

A. Right forearm loop graft (PTFE). Ligation of left hemoaccess.
B. Left IJ tunneled, cuffed dual lumen hemodialysis catheter. Ligation of left hemoaccess.
C. Right IJ tunneled, cuffed dual lumen hemodialysis catheter. Ligation of left hemoaccess.
D. Left femoral to femoral loop graft (PTFE). Ligation of left hemoaccess.
E. Left femoral tunneled, cuffed dual lumen hemodialysis catheter.
F. Right brachial-cephalic transposition.

The left arm symptoms resolve, and the new access functions well for 2.6 additional years. However, dilation begins to appear in two sites most commonly used for the tri-weekly puncture for hemodialysis. Duplex examination of the larger discerns the presence of a large pseudoaneurysm with a 0.6-mm neck communicating with the lumen of hemoaccess. The individual reports several recent episodes of prolonged difficulty achieving hemostasis after removal of the access needles. During duplex interrogation, a thrombotic plug is dislodged. Pulsatile bleeding ensues, which is controlled with 30–45 min of direct compression.

Question 10

The best treatment option at this time is:

A. Ligation of the hemoaccess.
B. Revision by primary closure of the pseudoaneurysm.
C. Revision with placement of an interposition, prosthetic segment.
D. Removal of the hemoaccess.
E. Continued, but close, observation of the patient with treatment initiated if the bleeding recurs.

After loss of the above hemoaccess, a new autogenous AVF was available for construction in the right arm, which remained functional until the patient's demise 3 years later.

41.1
Commentary

Question 1

The first order of business is to determine whether the individual has a reversible condition such as obstructive uropathy, drug-induced acute tubular necrosis, or another nephrotoxic condition. Commencement of hemoaccess would be unnecessary at this time since the individual has minimal symptoms; however, the degree of renal insufficiency is sufficient to predict that it will likely be required within several months to a year. Since some access procedures require several months before they are usable, an experienced surgical specialist should be contacted to construct the hemoaccess, if the nephrologist confirms that the individual has chronic progressive renal insufficiency.[1] **[Q1: D]**

Urgent or immediate hemodialysis is not indicated and because of the associated morbidity, catheter placement is contraindicated in the absence of acute renal failure. Likewise, it is inappropriate to refer directly to the surgical specialist without determining the cause of the renal insufficiency, whether it is reversible, and whether the individual should be placed on the eligibility list for transplantation. Simply referring the individual to the nephrologist is not wrong, but the best option includes the diagnostic evaluation, management of treatable etiologies, and consideration for hemoaccess assuming that commencement of hemodialysis is imminent within several months to a year. It is clear that early nephrology consultation is of benefit, from the perspective of directing appropriate therapy.[2-5] Likewise, early consideration of hemoaccess options facilitates preservation of vascular assets and reduces the incidence of catheter placement and the subsequent morbidities.

Question 2

The complete clinical vascular examination is an important adjunct to surgical planning and may direct the surgeon to either upper extremity; clearly the non-dominant upper extremity is preferred, unless a preferred access option is only available in the dominant extremity. While reliance on the clinical examination alone may be accurate in many cases, experience currently suggests that valuable information is contributed by the non-invasive ultrasound survey.[6-9]

While reliable DU examinations may not be available in all practice situations, it does provide the "best" option by decreasing the likelihood of unsuccessful operations while increasing the options for autologous conduit. Additional information from the duplex examination may reveal proximal vein occlusion, visible superficial veins which are postphlebitic, arterial abnormalities (location of the brachial bifurcation, occlusive disease, inadequate palmar arch collateralization, large branch veins, and relative size of the arteries and veins).

An added reason for preoperative DU survey is that the diabetic population is the group most likely to harbor asymptomatic upper extremity arterial occlusive disease. It is unknown whether this is the reason, but functional patency of hemoaccess is usually reduced in the diabetic population.[8,10,11] In obese patients the lack of visible superficial veins may be countered by duplex examination; the depth of the veins precludes clinical identification and may mask prior thromboses. The depth of an otherwise acceptable vein is an important consideration and may mandate transposition to a more superficial site. Failure to identify superficial upper extremity veins on clinical examination is not an acceptable rationale for commencing access at a lower extremity site; even if no superficial veins are available, a prosthetic graft can usually be constructed between the artery and one of the deep veins in the upper extremity.

As before, there is still no indication for immediate dialysis, so that placement of a catheter at the time of the permanent access is not indicated in this clinical scenario. [Q2: C]

Question 3

The list includes all of the usual information needed for proper operative planning. The goal is to construct the most durable hemoaccess from autogenous tissue. When acceptable options exist only in the dominant upper extremity, it is selected; thus, both arms should be studied.

Adequate arterial inflow is essential for the fistula or graft to function properly. Failure was universal with an arterial diameter <1.6 mm in one study.[9] A more commonly accepted criterion is >2.0 mm diameter. Although upper extremity atherosclerotic occlusive disease is uncommon in the arm, diabetics are the group most likely to have diseased arteries, and thus it should be considered for this patient. While all vascular laboratories may not subscribe to this position, no palpable pulses were described in the core scenario such that some reassurance is needed regarding adequate arterial flow.

A key function of the preoperative duplex examination is to determine the acceptability of the superficial vein network of the forearm and arm. In addition to location and diameter, identification of large branches, occluded segments, scarring, other post-thrombotic changes, and depth of vein below the skin are all critical to success. Failure was also universal when preoperative DU identified stenotic vein segments.[9] Identification of acceptable veins may increase substantially.[6] Vein diameters of less than 2.5–3 mm are generally considered unacceptable, but since there is little data to support this recommendation, the practice guidelines did not incorporate a recommendation for a minimum venous diameter.[7] Complete evaluation of superficial upper extremity veins should include the forearm basilic vein.[6,12] Transposition of the basilic vein is usually necessary whether in the forearm or upper arm, and any vein that is too deep (greater than 0.5–1.0 cm) may need to be transposed before anastomosis.

Central vein stenoses or occlusions are usually due to prior central vein catheterizations, but the surgeon should also be wary of transvenous wires from implanted pacemakers or defibrillators.[1,13,14] Forty percent of patients with known subclavian vein catheterization had moderate to severe subclavian vein stenoses that were clinically silent.[15]

In the absence of an autogenous option, the surgeon should still be informed regarding the best location for the first graft. The anatomic variant of a high brachial bifurcation occurs in ~10% of individuals. This anatomic variant may preclude placement of a prosthetic graft at a given site, but should have little adverse effect on an autogenous AVF.

Routine evaluation of the lower extremity is unnecessary, but may be considered when upper extremity sites have been completely exhausted. **[Q3: E]**

Question 4

This is a complex issue and the correct answer **[Q4: E]** is derived from a combination of experience and the recommendations of the United States Kidney Dialysis Outcomes Quality Initiative (K-DOQI). The best answer is a combination of the "best" choices summarized from the principles of all autogenous, most distal, non-dominant extremity. Thus, since almost all options are really open for this individual, the non-dominant, radiocephalic AVF is the best first choice; a potential collateral benefit is communication with (and arterialization of) the proximal basilic vein. Recognition of problems causing failure to mature are the major impediment to wider utilization of this modality.[1,8–10,16] Failure to mature a forearm AVF may occur in 34–53%, and may be less attractive in the elderly, the diabetic, and female patients.[8,9]

The proximal options of brachial and cephalic anastomoses and transpositions have experienced a higher incidence of arterial steal and ignore the basic principle of progression from distal to proximal.[1] The forearm loop graft was equated with the proximal brachial transposition by K-DOQI, but current initiatives more emphatically encourage autogenous fistula.[5,16]

Catheter access is to be avoided if at all possible, and is clearly not indicated in this situation; multiple autogenous options are available and commencement of dialysis is not emergent.[4,5,13,14]

A *left* radiocephalic AVF serves the dual purpose of increasing lifetime site options, and allows the distal AVF to develop more proximal veins for subsequent autogenous hemoaccess options. A forearm vein transposition is available, but because the distal forearm vein is post-thrombotic, the proximal vein would combine with transposition of an upper arm vein as well.[12,17]

Question 5

Although this is a common clinical question, informed decisions are difficult since there is a paucity of concrete data. There is little data to support any course of action, and the correct answer is based upon opinion.[1] **[Q5: C]** Clearly a healed wound, a palpable thrill, and unobstructed flow are essential. Two weeks is generally considered early for an AVF, and the minimum recommended interval is 6–8 weeks. For prosthetic grafts, 2–3 weeks is usually satisfactory, as long as the edema has resolved sufficiently to identify the outline of the graft. Since the functional patency is so low, a prosthetic AV graft should not be inserted until dialysis is imminent.[1]

A period of 6–8 weeks is an arbitrary interval often used in practice and supported by K-DOQI. However, if at all possible, a longer interval is preferable, since a matured access is more likely to provide durable function.

A large branch vein within 5 cm of the arteriovenous anastomosis can prevent maturation, by diversion and diffusion of fistula flow and should be ligated.[9]

Thickening of the wall is one of the few indicators of arterialization in the conduit walls
and would therefore be desirable, but there is no data to support this course of action, or to
guide the obvious question of how thick? In reality, the progression of the individual's
renal disease will likely be the best guide. If early referral can be achieved, urgent commencement of dialysis becomes a moot question and the hemoaccess is ready for use when
the time arrives.[1]

Question 6

The best option again emphasizes the principles of most distal site, autogenous if possible,
and in this instance the recruitment of additional vein collaterals from the long-standing
prior left radiocephalic AVF.[17,18] **[Q6: D]** The initial DU examination specifically noted the
communication from the cephalic feeding the basilic system; the proximal forearm basilic
has a good size and does not exhibit post-thrombotic changes from this point into its termination in the brachial veins. Thus, the transposition of the proximal basilic vein, which
may already be arterialized, is the preferred choice.[17,18] The arterial inflow for this may be
the proximal forearm radial artery if the vein length is satisfactory; if not the high bifurcation would still make the inflow from the radial the best choice. Even though the diameter
of the artery would be less than the usual brachial diameter, this should not present a problem for construction of an autogenous fistula.

The brachial arterial variant would compromise the inflow to a left forearm loop prosthetic graft and even a brachial to axillary prosthetic graft in the arm.

The right forearm loop graft would be an acceptable alternative, except that there are
good autogenous alternatives bilaterally. It moves the access to the dominant upper
extremity and fails to take advantage of the previously arterialized proximal venous
channels.

Any right forearm transposition is inappropriate because both veins have evidence of
prior thrombosis.

Central catheter access is to be avoided if at all possible. Multiple autogenous options
are available and dialysis can be maintained in the interval with the existing, but poorly
functioning left radiocephalic AVF. By mobilizing a proximal basilic vein segment that has
already been exposed to arterialized fistula flow, the time for maturation may be reduced.[1]
The arm will need to be observed for possible arterial steal, in which case the failing AVF
may need to be sacrificed and a hemoaccess catheter inserted until the new left radiobasilic
transposition has matured satisfactorily.[13]

Questions 7 and 8

The presence of subclavian vein electrodes in the subclavian vein is the inciting factor for
subclavian vein thrombosis or stenosis whether for pacing or defibrillation. **[Q7: E]**

Symptoms from acute subclavian vein thrombosis are often expressed for only a short time in patients without an AVF. Edema will be severely and continuously exacerbated from the additional limb blood flow of the AVF.[13,14] Often the edema becomes chronic, and precludes accurate puncture of an ipsilateral access. Untreated venous hypertension from this combination may produce the typical symptoms of venous stasis: edema, hyperpigmentation and even ulceration. Therefore any treatment must include ligation of the access.

Although lymphatic disruption from an infraclavicular pocket incision is possible, this would be so rare as to be remarkable. The electrodes are usually inserted indirectly and do not require surgical exposure of the vein; this reduces the likelihood of injury to the lymphatic channels in the axillary-subclavian vascular sheath. Localized swelling in the pocket would be a more likely complication than arm swelling.

There is no evidence for hypercoagulability. Since the electrodes pass through the SVC, obstruction there is theoretically possible. However, the absence of contralateral upper extremity edema or a swollen head fails to suggest SVC thrombosis. Replacing the device on the right complicates the issue immeasurably. In addition to incurring a real risk of SVC obstruction, it also places the remaining (right) upper extremity at risk for problems with subsequent hemoaccess.

The combination of a high flow AVF with probable subclavian vein obstruction suggests a rather poor prognosis for the left arm radiobasilic AVF. Thus, investigation of the etiology with a fistulagram and venogram is appropriate. **[Q8: D]** A DU should also be obtained, but since central vein visualization is poor it is inadequate to confirm the suspected diagnosis. Although unlikely, it is entirely possible that the device has nothing to do with the venous obstruction and that the outflow vein of the AVF may be stenotic from an intimal hyperplastic response in a different anatomic location more amenable to a salvage procedure. If this is a subclavian thrombosis, it may be a good opportunity to consider thrombolysis. However, even if the vein could be reopened, a subclavian vein angioplasty and/or stent has not proven a durable solution in this anatomic site.[13] Finally, thrombolysis carries a small but real risk of intracranial hemorrhage, which would be less acceptable without a real benefit. Removal of the electrodes would be complicated and risky. Unfortunately, if the obstruction is not well collateralized, the left arm should be excluded from future access options.[1,13,14,18]

Question 9

The best choice is the right forearm loop prosthetic graft. **[Q9: A]** Either an IJ or femoral catheter site has significant clinical negatives, and fails to offer a durable solution in the face of numerous better options.

The right brachial to cephalic is probably a better option, but as presented in the question, ligation of the contralateral symptomatic radiobasilic AVF is not accomplished. As presented in the question, ligation of the contralateral symptomatic radiobasilic AVF is not accomplished. More importantly, the two proximal transposition options remain available for construction of subsequent hemoaccess.

Ligation of the left radiobasilic AVF is essential to control the venous obstructive symptoms. While a jugular vein turn-down would offer preservation of the left radiobasilic

AVF, there is not likely to be sufficient length to reach a non-thrombosed segment of axillary vein. A prosthetic extension to the jugular is another alternative. Adequate central outflow from the jugular would need to be assured by venography before further consideration of either option.[14,19]

Question 10

Although there is very little data to provide a clear answer to this clinical problem, the best choice and DOQI recommendation is prosthetic interposition. **[Q10: C]** It preserves a functioning access in someone who has already lost the use of the contralateral upper extremity to venous outflow obstruction.[1,20,21]

Ligation solves the bleeding problem but sacrifices the access. Removal may subsequently be required, but is not essential at this juncture. Revision with primary closure of the aneurysm is unattractive since the tissues and graft material are friable and usually destroyed by the repetitive puncture. Close observation is doomed to fail with a real risk of bleeding and hemorrhage.

Although prosthetic interposition is the appropriate choice, this option is not without complications. Our own experience identified an increased incidence of infection, and good material to anastomose may require bypass of lengthy segments.[22] Recent introduction of the covered stent is an attractive, but expensive and unproven option. Percutaneous access, control of the neck of the pseudoaneurysm, and retention of hemoaccess function are currently offset by limited clinical data, and high expense.[13,23]

Comment

The initial use of distal sites, and judicious consumption of the available autogenous assets facilitated construction of several different hemoaccess sites during this patient's 14-year odyssey with hemodialysis. Problems such as these are common and require forethought and ingenuity for successful cumulative function and minimization of major complications.

References

1. NKF-K/DOQI Clinical Practice Guidelines for Vascular Access: Update 2000. *Am J Kidney Dis*. 2001;37:S137–81.
2. Stack AG. Impact of timing of nephrology referral and pre-ESRD care on mortality risk among new ESRD patients in the United States. *Am J Kidney Dis*. 2003;41:310-318.
3. Khan IH. Co-morbidity: the major challenge for survival and quality of life in end stage renal disease. *Nephrol Dial Transplant*. 1998;13:S176-79.
4. Powe NR. Early referral in chronic kidney disease: an enormous opportunity for prevention. *Am J Kidney Dis*. 2003;41:505-507.
5. Pisoni RL, Young EW, Dykstra DM, et al. Vascular access use in Europe and the United States: results from the DOPPS. *Kidney Int*. 2002;61:305-316.

6. Silva MB, Hobson RW, Pappas PJ, et al. A strategy for increasing use of autogenous hemodialysis access procedures: impact of preoperative noninvasive evaluation. *J Vasc Surg*. 1998;27:302-308.

7. Sidawy AN. The Society for Vascular Surgery: Clinical Practice Guidelines for surgical placement and maintenence of arteriovenous hemodialysis access. *J Vasc Surg* 2008;48:S2-255.

8. Miller PE, Tolwani A, Luscy CP, et al. Predictors of adequacy of arteriovenous fistulas in hemodialysis patients. *Kidney Int*. 1999;56:275-280.

9. Wong V, Ward R, Taylor J, Selvakumar S, How TV, Bakran A. Factors associated with early failure of arteriovenous fistulae for haemodialysis access. *Eur J Vasc Endovasc Surg*. 1996;12:207-213.

10. Hodges TC, Fillinger MF, Zwolek RM, Walsh DB, Bech F, Cronenwett JL. Longitudinal comparison of dialysis access methods: risk factors for failure. *J Vasc Surg*. 1997;26:1009-1019.

11. Kalman PG, Pope M, Bhola C, Richardson R, Sniderman KW. A practical approach to vascular access for hemodialysis and predictors of success. *J Vasc Surg*. 1999;30:727-733.

12. Choi HM, Lal BK, Cerveira JJ, Padberg FT, Hobson RW, Pappas PJ. Durability and cumulative functional patency of transposed and non-transposed arterio-venous fistula. *J Vasc Surg*. 2003;38(6):1206-1212.

13. Cerveira JJ, Padberg FT, Pappas PJ, Lal BK. Prevention and management of complications from hemoaccess. In: Pearce W, Yao J, Matsumura J, eds. *Trends in Vascular Surgery*. Chicago, IL: Greenwood Academic; 2004.

14. Currier CBJ, Widder S, Ali A, Kuusisto E, Sidawy A. Surgical management of subclavian and axillary vein thrombosis in patients with a functioning arteriovenous fistula. *Surgery*. 1986;100:25-28.

15. Surratt RS, Picus D, Hicks ME, Darcy MD, Kleinhoffer M, Jendrisak M. The importance of preoperative evaluation of the subclavian vein in dialysis access planning. *AJR Am J Roentgenol*. 1991;156:623-625.

16. Huber TS, Carter JW, Carter RL, Seeger JM. Patency of autogenous and polytetrafluoroethylene upper extremity arteriovenous hemodialysis accesses: a systematic review. *J Vasc Surg*. 2003;38:1005-1011.

17. Silva M, Hobson RW, Simonian GT, Haser PB, Jamil Z, Padberg FT, et al. Successful autogenous hemodialysis access placement after prosthetic failure: the impact of non-invasive assessment. Poster presentation at SVS/AAVS 2000, Toronto, CA.

18. Haser PB, Padberg FT Jr. Complex solutions for hemoaccess. In: Matsumura J, Pearce W, and Yao JST, eds. *Trends in Vascular Surgery*, 2003;Ch 33.

19. Puskas JD, Gertler JP. Internal jugular to axillary vein bypass for subclavian vein thrombosis in the setting of brachial arteriovenous fistula. *J Vasc Surg*. 1994;19:939-42.

20. Raju S. PTFE grafts for hemodialysis access. Techniques for insertion and management of complications. *Ann Surg*. 1987;206:666-673.

21. Ryan SV, Calligaro KD, Sharff J, Dougherty MJ. Management of infected prosthetic dialysis arteriovenous grafts. *J Vasc Surg*. 2004;39:7378.

22. Padberg FT, Lee BC, Curl GR. Hemoaccess site infection. *Surg Gynecol Obstet*. 1992;174:103-108.

23. Lin PH, Johnson CK, Pullium JK, et al. Transluminal stent graft repair with Wallgraft endoprosthesis in a porcine arteriovenous graft pseudoaneurysm model. *J Vasc Surg*. 2003;37:175-181.

Acute Ischemia of the Upper Extremity Following Graft Arteriovenous Fistula

42

Miltos K. Lazarides and Vasilios D. Tzilalis

A 65-year-old woman with end-stage renal disease and insulin-dependent diabetes was admitted for access construction in order to start haemodialysis. There was a lack of suitable veins to construct an arteriovenous (AV) fistula, and the patient underwent placement of a 6-mm polytetrafluoroethylene (PTFE) AV bridge graft between the brachial artery and the axillary vein in the left arm.

Question 1

Which of the following is the order of preference for placement of a permanent angioaccess in new patients requiring chronic haemodialysis?

A. (1) A brachio-cephalic AV fistula. (2) A wrist radial-cephalic AV fistula. (3) An AV PTFE bridge graft or a transposed brachial-basilic AV fistula. (4) A cuffed, tunnelled central venous catheter

B. (1) A wrist radial-cephalic AV fistula. (2) A brachio-cephalic AV fistula. (3) An AV PTFE bridge graft or a transposed brachial-basilic AV fistula

C. (1) A wrist radial-cephalic AV fistula. (2) A transposed brachial-basilic AV fistula. (3) A brachio-cephalic AV fistula. (4) An AV PTFE bridge graft

Question 2

Which of the following statements represent advantages of the autologous AV fistulas over AV grafts?

A. Excellent long-term patency once established

B. Lower complication rate

M.K. Lazarides (✉)
Department of Vascular Surgery, Demokritos University Hospital, Alexandroupolis, Greece

G. Geroulakos and B. Sumpio (eds.), *Vascular Surgery*,
DOI: 10.1007/978-1-84996-356-5_42, © Springer-Verlag London Limited 2011

C. Short lag time from construction to maturation
D. Easy to correct surgically when thrombosed

Immediately after surgery, the patient complained of numbness of the left hand with slight pain of the fingers. On examination the left radial pulse, which had existed previously, was absent, and the fingers were cold and cyanotic. Evaluation of the patient in the vascular laboratory with forearm Doppler pressure measurement revealed an index of 0.3. Interestingly the left forearm segmental pressure index was normalized after manual compression of the graft, while the left radial pulse reappeared with this maneuver. The evaluation confirmed an obvious hemodynamic "steal." The patient's condition deteriorated within a few hours; she developed severe, acute, painful weakness of the hand, wrist-drop, and minimal ability to flex the wrist.

Question 3

Which of the following statements regarding the incidence of steal after proximal access construction is correct?

A. The incidence of asymptomatic steal after proximal access construction, detected in the vascular laboratory, is rare.
B. Clinically obvious mild ischaemia after the construction of a proximal AV fistula occurs in about 10% of cases.
C. Severe ischaemia necessitating surgical correction complicates 2–4% of patients following a proximal AV fistula.

Question 4

Which of the following are indications for surgical correction of steal after proximal access construction?

A. Absence of ipsilateral preoperative existed radial pulse
B. Severe symptoms (rest pain, paralysis, wrist-drop)
C. Abnormal forearm segmental pressure index measurement
D. Abnormal ipsilateral nerve conduction studies
E. Reversal of flow in the distal artery in colour-flow duplex imaging

Urgent surgical correction was performed. Under local anaesthesia, a small segment of saphenous vein was harvested. The brachial artery was ligated just distal to the take-off of the graft. A vein bypass was constructed from the brachial artery 4–5 cm proximally to the inflow of the graft to a point distal to ligation (Fig. 42.1). Complete relief of symptoms occurred immediately postoperatively. The recovery of the patient was uneventful. She was discharged home on the third postoperative day with a palpable left radial pulse and a patent AV graft.

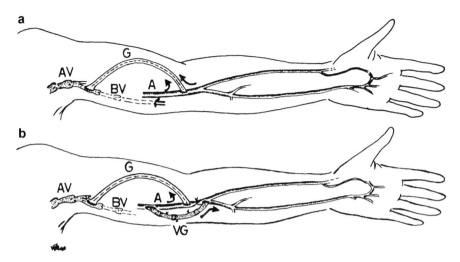

Fig. 42.1 (a) The operation before the creation of the corrective procedure. (b) The corrective procedure with ligation of the artery just distal to the AV graft take-off and the venous bypass from a point proximal to the inflow to a point just distal to ligation (DRIL procedure). A, brachial artery; AV, axillary vein; BV, basilic vein; G, arteriovenous PTFE graft; VG, vein graft

Question 5

Which of the following are acceptable corrective options for limb-threatening steal following proximal access construction?

A. Percutaneous transluminal angioplasty
B. Flow reduction procedures (banding, plication or tapering of the AV fistula)
C. AV fistula closure
D. The DRIL (distal revascularization interval ligation) procedure

---

42.1
Commentary

Construction of an AV fistula provides a sufficiently superficial arterialized vein that can be punctured with ease while its flow is high enough to permit efficient dialysis. Post-dialysis compression of a matured thick-wall arterialized vein in order to stop bleeding can be obtained readily and reliably.

The classic first-choice site for an AV fistula construction is between the radial artery and the cephalic vein at the wrist, as introduced by Brescia et al.[1] in 1966. If the cephalic vein at the wrist or forearm is not usable, then the next alternative is to move to the ante-cubital fossa. The AV fistula can be constructed at this site between the median cubital vein and the brachial artery. The superficial cephalic vein provides enough length of vein suitable for haemodialysis venipunctures. Alternatively, if the cephalic vein is not usable, then the brachial artery can be anastomosed to the basilic vein of the upper arm. However, the latter is situated under the deep fascia in the arm, and mobilisation and transposition to a subcutaneous new position is always necessary. When an autologous AV fistula either at the wrist or the elbow cannot be created, then an AV graft using synthetic material bridging an artery and a vein in the upper extremity (either forearm or arm) is the next choice. Grafts may be placed in straight, looped or curved configurations. AV grafts and fistulas are created in the lower extremity only rarely, as they are prone to infection at this site.

The order of preference for placement of AV fistulas in patients requiring chronic hae-modialysis according to dialysis outcomes quality initiative (DOQI) guidelines established by the United States Kidney Foundation is[2]:

1. A wrist radial-cephalic AV fistula.
2. An elbow (brachial-cephalic) AV fistula.

If it is not possible to establish either of these types of fistula, then access may be estab-lished using:

3. An AV graft of synthetic material (PTFE grafts are preferred over other synthetic material).
4. A transposed brachial-basilic vein fistula.

Cuffed, tunnelled central venous catheters should be discouraged as permanent vascular access. [Q1: B]

Recognising the superiority of the autologous AV fistulas over grafts, DOQI guidelines recommend an aggressive strategy increasing the number of native fistulas. DOQI guide-lines suggest that autologous AV fistulas should be constructed in at least 50% of all new patients electing to receive haemodialysis as their initial form of renal replacement ther-apy.[2] Bridge AV grafts should be reserved for those patients whose vein anatomy does not permit the construction of an autologous AV fistula.[3,4] Autologous fistulas, especially distal ones at the wrist, present a lower complication rate compared with other access options.[5] A vein must be matured before use for vascular access. The time required for maturation of an autologous fistula varies among patients. It is not correct to use a fistula within the first month after its construction. Premature cannulation may result in a higher incidence of haematoma formation, with associated compression of the still soft-wall vein, leading to thrombosis. Allowing the AV fistula to mature for 3–4 months may be ideal.[2]

In contrast, PTFE AV grafts need a shorter maturation time and can be used approxi-mately 14 days after placement. Within this period, an attempt to cannulate the still oedem-atous arm may lead to graft laceration from inaccurate needle insertion. An AV graft may be considered matured when swelling of the subcutaneous tunnel has reduced to the point that its course is easily palpable. Additionally, after the first 2 weeks, fibrous tissue forma-tion round the graft is able to seal the holes caused by each needle puncture. PTFE grafts are easily thrombectomised, with a reported unassisted patency following thrombectomy at 6 months close to 50%.[6] In contrast, autologous fistulas when thrombosed are difficult to salvage.[2] [Q2: A, B]

The reversal of flow after creation of an AV fistula in the distal artery beyond the fistula and before the point of entry of collateral vessels has been characterised as steal. This is caused by a pronounced pressure drop in the distal artery, while pressure increases with increasing distance away from the fistula as a consequence of inflow from arterial collaterals.[7] Steal occurs in more than 90% of proximal AV fistulas – when the arterial anastomosis is at the brachial artery – but in most patients, the collateral vasculature is adequate to maintain distal flow, and severe ischaemia does not develop in the hand.[8,9] Clinically obvious mild ischaemia from steal occurs in about 10% of patients. The presentation is coldness and numbness of the hand, and the symptoms resolve spontaneously within 1 month.[8] The term "steal" is used inappropriately for this condition in many reports because it means reversal of flow and not any of its potential ischaemic sequelae. A wide spectrum of symptoms and signs may occur, however, such as paraesthesias and sensory loss, weakened or absent distal pulse, muscle weakness and wrist-drop, rest pain usually getting worse during dialysis, muscle atrophy and – if left untreated – digital gangrene. The reported rate of steal-induced severe ischaemia necessitating immediate surgical treatment is 2.7–4.3%.[8,9] In contrast to proximal AV fistulas, the incidence of symptomatic steal following distal radiocephalic AV fistulas is rare, at a rate of 0.25%.[10] **[Q3: B, C]**

Clinical signs and symptoms of steal syndrome do not differ from those of leg ischaemia. Therefore it can be classified according to Fontaine´s classification: stage I, reduced wrist-brachial pressure index, coldness of the hand or no symptoms; stage II, intermitted pain during haemodialysis; stage III, continuous ischaemic rest pain; and stage IV, ulceration and necrosis. Stages I and II should be closely observed and treated conservatively (e.g., wearing gloves).[11]

In most reports, the indication for surgical correction of steal is based on clinical grounds only.[8,9] Low segmental pressure, as measured by Doppler, distal to the fistula is not an indication per se for surgical correction of steal. Additionally, absence of a radial pulse is a common finding in approximately one-third of patients following proximal access creation.[9] A corrective surgical procedure is indicated when proven haemodynamic steal causes severe stage III and/or stage IV ischaemic symptoms early after access construction (rest pain, paralysis, cyanosis of digits, wrist-drop). Mild ischaemic symptoms that persist beyond 1 month from access creation should be observed closely. When these "mild" symptoms are present for a long time, there is always a threat of irreversible neurological impairment, termed "ischaemic monomelic neuropathy." This is a serious and disabling complication causing sensorimotor dysfunction without tissue necrosis.[12] Abnormal deteriorated nerve conduction studies in the presence of even mild ischaemia are an indication for surgical correction of steal.[9] **[Q4: B, D]**

Several catheter-based and surgical techniques have been used to correct steal-induced ischaemia. Arterial stenoses proximal to the AV fistula are eligible for percutaneous transluminal angioplasty and may augment blood flow to the periphery with relief of symptoms. However, such proximal inflow stenoses contribute to steal syndrome in only 20% of patients who have distal extremity ischaemia.[13] In the vast majority of cases (80%) steal is caused by discordant vascular resistance and a poorly formed arterial collateral network. A variety of surgical techniques have been applied to correct limb-threatening steal including fistula closure with simple ligation, various flow reduction techniques (banding, placation or tapering) and the DRIL (distal revascularization interval ligation) procedure introduced by Schanzer et al.[14] Ligation provides immediate improvement but requires creation of a new access. Banding–plication techniques improve distal perfusion, but it is difficult to determine the required amount of stenosis to eliminate steal while allowing a flow sufficient to sustain patency of the graft. Flow reduction procedures are attractive options in high-flow AV fistulas (>1,500 mL/min).[15] In patients with normal flow through their AV fistulas often concomitant arteriosclerotic disease causes insufficient collateral perfusion. In these cases the DRIL procedure is the treatment of choice. With the DRIL a ligature (placed distal to the take-off of the graft) eliminates the reversal of flow, while the bypass (from a point proximal to the inflow to a point just distal to ligation) re-establishes flow to the limb (Fig. 42.1). Recent reports support the efficacy of this technique.[16,17] **[Q5: A, B, C, D]**

References

1. Brescia MJ, Cimino JE, Appel K, Hurwich BJ. Chronic hemodialysis using venipuncture and a superficially created arteriovenous fistula. *N Engl J Med.* 1966;275:1089-1092.
2. NKF-DOQI. Clinical practice guidelines for vascular access: update 2000. *Am J Kidney Dis.* 2001;30(Suppl 1):S137-S181.
3. Marx AB, Landerman J, Harder FH. Vascular access for hemodialysis. *Curr Probl Surg.* 1990;27:1-48.
4. Windus DW. Permanent vascular access: a nephrologist's view. *Am J Kidney Dis.* 1993;21:457-471.
5. Feldman H, Kobrin S, Wasserstein A. Hemodialysis vascular access morbidity. *J Am Soc Nephrol.* 1996;7:523-535.
6. Marston WA, Criado E, Jaque PF, Mauro MA, Burnham SJ, Keagy BA. Prospective randomized comparison of surgical versus endovascular management of thrombosed dialysis access grafts. *J Vasc Surg.* 1997;26:373-381.
7. Gordon IL. Physiology of the arteriovenous fistula. In: Wilson SE, ed. *Vascular access, principles and practice.* 3rd ed. St. Louis: Mosby; 1996:29-41.
8. Schanzer H, Scladany M, Haimov M. Treatment of angioaccess-induced ischemia by revascularization. *J Vasc Surg.* 1992;16:861-866.
9. Lazarides MK, Staramos DN, Panagopoulos GN, Tzilalis VD, Eleftheriou GJ, Dayantas JN. Indications for surgical treatment of angioaccess-induced arterial steal. *J Am Coll Surg.* 1998;187:422-426.
10. Wilson SE. Complications of vascular access procedures. In: Wilson SE, ed. *Vascular Access, Principles And Practice.* 3rd ed. St. Louis: Mosby; 1996:212-224.
11. Bakran A, Mickley V, Passlick-Deetjen J. *Management of the Renal Patient, Clinical Algorithms of Vascular Access for Haemodialysis.* Lengerich: Pabst Science; 2003:90.
12. Hye RJ, Wolf YG. Ischemic monomelic neuropathy: an under-recognized complication of hemodialysis access. *Ann Vasc Surg.* 1994;8:578-582.
13. Wixon CL, Mills JL. Hemodynamic basis for the diagnosis and treatment of angioaccess-induced steal syndrome. *Adv Vasc Surg.* 2000;8:147-159.
14. Schanzer H, Schwartz M, Harrington E, Haimov M. Treatment of ischemia due to steal by arteriovenous fistula with distal artery ligation and revascularization. *J Vasc Surg.* 1988;7:770-773.
15. Tordoir JH, Dammers R, van der Sande FM. Upper extremity ischemia and hemodialysis vascular access. *Eur J Vasc Endovasc Surg.* 2004;27:1-5.

16. Knox RC, Berman SS, Hughes JD, Gentile AT, Mills JL. Distal revascularization-interval ligation: a durable and effective treatment for ischemic steal syndrome after hemodialysis access. *J Vasc Surg*. 2002;36:250-255.
17. Lazarides MK, Staramos DN, Kopadis G, Maltezos C, Tzilalis VD, Georgiadis GS. Onset of arterial steal following proximal angioaccess: immediate and delayed types. *Nephrol Dial Transplant*. 2003;18:2387-2390.

Part X

Amputations

Amputations in an Ischemic Limb

43

Kenneth R. Ziegler and Bauer Sumpio

A 70 year old white male hospitalized for pneumonia is discovered to have a Stage IV heel ulcer on his left foot by the nursing staff. The patient describes no pain at the site of the ulcer, and has no previous history of sores on his lower extremities. He denies a history of diabetes, but states that he has been having progressive difficulty lately in walking distances due to cramps in his calves bilaterally. His past medical history is significant for hypertension and stable angina, for which he takes nitrates and a beta-blocker. His only previous surgery was a right inguinal herniorrhaphy 30 years ago. He admits to a 50 pack-year tobacco history, and still smokes.

The ulcer appears to have a dark base on examination, with mild malodorous discharge. His heart rate is 84 bpm, blood pressure is 140/70 mmHg, and he is afebrile on examination. He is alert, awake, and normally conversant, but states that his prolonged bedrest has reduced his normal willingness to get out of bed and ambulate.

Question 1

The most common cause of major lower extremity amputation in the United States is:

A. Trauma
B. Complications secondary to diabetes mellitus
C. Neoplasm
D. Acute limb ischemia
E. Vascular bypass graft failure

Physical examination reveals that the femoral and popliteal pulses are palpable bilaterally, but the pedal pulses are absent. Doppler exam reveals a faintly monophasic dorsalis pedis (DP) signal and absent posterior tibital (PT) signal on the left foot, while biphasic signals are present at the DP and PT on the right. Bedside pressure exams reveal an ankle-brachial index of 0.2 on the left, 0.5 on the right.

B. Sumpio (✉)
Department of Surgery, School of Medicine, Yale University, New Haven, CT, USA

G. Geroulakos and B. Sumpio (eds.), *Vascular Surgery*,
DOI: 10.1007/978-1-84996-356-5_43, © Springer-Verlag London Limited 2011

Fig. 43.1 (**a**) Left heel ulcer after uncapping of eschar and debridement of nonviable tissues. Note the pink base of the ulcer with backbleeding from the wound bed. (**b**) Plain film of the left foot. The radiolucency of the left heel reflects the ulcerated tissue; no appreciable osteomyelitis is evident.

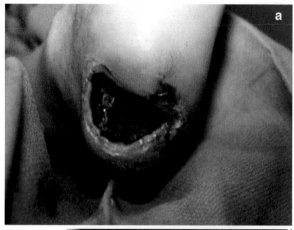

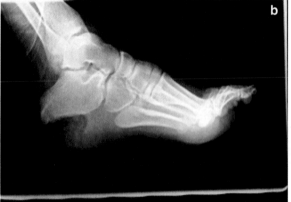

The eschar on the ulcer is uncapped, and the remainder of the wound is debrided (Fig. 43.1). Tissue samples and swabs are sent for bacterial culture and sensitivity assays. A CT angiogram is ordered for the patient.

Question 2

In anticipating the results of the angiogram, what is true about primary and secondary amputation in the treatment of chronic limb ischemia?

A. Primary amputation is the most common form of initial therapy in the treatment of chronic limb ischemia.

B. Overwhelming infection is the most common cause of secondary amputation.

C. Early graft occlusion always results in a secondary amputation within the first year after arterial reconstruction.

D. Primary amputation is indicated when extensive gangrene has compromised the foot to such a degree that it cannot be salvaged.

E. All of the above.

F. None of the above.

Question 3

If the results of the angiogram preclude vascular reconstruction and the wound remains non-healing, which of the following would be the single best non-invasive method to determine the level of appropriate amputation?

A. Pulse volume recordings/segmental systolic blood pressure measurements.
B. Transcutaneous oxygen pressure measurements.
C. Skin fluorescein uptake/radiotracer injection.
D. Skin thermography.
E. Clinical assessment of popliteal pulses, skin temperature, dependent rubor.
F. There is no test that can reliably predict primary healing by itself.

While awaiting angiography, the Vascular Surgery resident is alerted to a sudden deterioration in the patient's condition. The patient has become febrile, hypotensive, and tachycardic. He is awake, but delirious. Examination of the left foot reveals frank purulence from the wound, expressible with manual pressure on the dorsal forefoot. The Achilles tendon appears grossly infected with extensive loss of structural integrity. There is no crepitance on palpation.

Question 4

Which of the following is the most appropriate initial intervention at this time?

A. IV antibiotics and medical management alone
B. IV antibiotics, below-the-knee amputation (BKA) with flap (non-staged)
C. IV antibiotics, ankle disarticulation in expectation of a staged BKA or above-the-knee amputation (AKA)
D. IV antibiotics, immediate above-the-knee amputation
E. IV antibiotics, debridement, and vascular reconstruction

The patient is started on broad spectrum IV antibiotics and is taken urgently to the operating room for an ankle disarticulation under general anesthesia. He is extubated post-operatively after an initial stay in the ICU for resuscitation and recovers from sepsis adequately on the surgery ward. The amputated stump appears to be draining adequately without signs of expanding cellulitis. One week later, he returns to the operating room for his staged amputation.

Question 5

Which of the following is true regarding the relative advantages and disadvantages of a below-the-knee amputation as compared to an above-the-knee amputation in elderly patients?

A. Most patients who undergo unilateral AKA do not achieve independent ambulation.
B. Patients who undergo BKA experience a 10–40% increase in energy expenditure above their normal baseline when ambulating.

C. Proximal amputations are associated with a higher probability of primary healing.

D. The rehabilitative advantages of BKA over AKA are negligible in patients who are unable to ambulate due to their comorbid conditions.

E. All of the above.

Question 6

Which of the following factors and complications are NOT associated with below-knee stump failure necessitating revision and/or a more proximal amputation?

A. Intrinsic wound infection/sepsis

B. Trauma to the residual limb

C. Wound edge necrosis/ischemia

D. Stump ulceration

E. Early ambulation and weight-bearing on the stump

Question 7

Advantages of a customizable removable immediate postoperative prosthesic after BKA include which of the following?

A. Rigid support to control or prevent joint flexion contracture

B. Accelerated wound healing and stump maturation

C. Minimizing postsurgical edema and pain

D. Decreasing inactivity by assisting in early ambulation

E. Decreased need for postoperative follow-up

F. Protection from trauma

The patient recovers well on the vascular ward post-operatively. His wounds appear to be healing well without signs of infection (Fig. 43.2a); his pain is well-managed on oral narcotics, but he states that he has reduced sensation on the skin over his residual limb. He begins physical therapy in the hospital, but has initial resistance to getting out of bed due to deconditioning. Though he makes significant progress toward walking while in the hospital, he is discharged to a short-term rehabilitation facility after consultation with the physical and occupational therapy team (Fig. 43.2b).

Question 8

Which of the following statements regarding the post-operative care of amputation patients is false?

A. For optimal patient recovery, a combination of good amputation level selection and early ambulation rehabilitation is necessary.

B. The patient is best treated by a multidisciplinary team that includes the vascular surgeon, a prosthetist, physical therapy, and mental health professionals as warranted.

Fig. 43.2 The patient at his post-discharge clinic follow-up appointment. (**a**) The well-healed left BKA stump without complications. (**b**) The patient demonstrating independent ambulation with his BK prosthesis

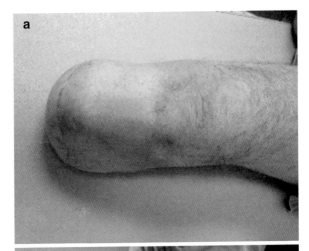

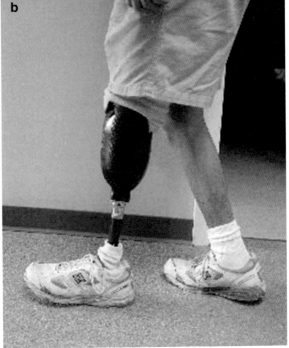

C. The 5 year life expectancy of diabetic patients is less than 50% after major lower extremity amputation.

D. Patient education and contralateral foot care are key for continued patient well-being.

E. Elderly patients commonly ambulate after bilateral above-knee amputations.

43.1
Commentary

The performance of major lower extremity amputations is an important field of expertise for the vascular surgeon. Unfortunately, the necessity of amputation has come to carry a negative connotation of "failure" of our reconstructive therapies in relationship to the treatment of chronic extremity ischemia. Instead, as physicians and surgeons, the need to perform an amputation when indicated should be viewed as an opportunity to maximize a patient's potential functional recovery, post-operative quality of life, and independence.[1,2]

In the 2007 update to the Trans-Atlantic Inter-Society Consensus Document on Management of Peripheral Artery Disease (TASC II), the reported aggregate incidence of major lower extremity amputations from large population or nation-wide data is 120–500 per million people per year, with a ratio near 1:1 between above-knee (AKA) and below-knee (BKA) amputations. Continuing debate occurs as to the impact of increasing numbers of revascularization procedures on amputation rates in patients with chronic limb ischemia (CLI). Recent data from Sweden, Denmark and Finland demonstrate a significant decrease in amputations for CLI with the increased availability and use of both endovascular interventions and surgical revascularization and data from the UK demonstrates a plateau in major amputation that may reflect increasingly successful limb salvage.[3] At the time of the TASC II study, older US studies had shown no positive impact of revascularization procedures on amputation rates. However, more recent studies of Medicare B claims between 1996 and 2006 have shown trends in congruence with the European studies, namely a marked decrease in total lower extremity amputations with increasing numbers of vascular interventions.[4]

The leading causes of amputation vary widely between countries, influenced heavily by their socioeconomic and political situation. Countries with a recent or ongoing history of conflict may experience trauma as the most common cause of major amputation, whereas vascular and metabolic disease tends to dominate in the sedentary populations of developed countries. As a single disease entity, diabetes mellitus and its attendant complications are the leading cause of non-traumatic lower extremity amputation in the United States.[5] [Q1: B] Globally, diabetes mellitus is associated with an estimated 25–90% of all amputations.[6] A 2002 analysis of discharged patients from United States hospitals showed that the underlying pathology leading to amputations were dominated by far by vascular diseases including diabetic complications (82.0%), followed by trauma (16.4%), with amputations for neoplasm (0.9%) and congenital causes (0.8%) trailing behind.[7]

Generally, the indications for lower extremity amputation in the setting of vascular disease include overwhelming infection of the foot that threatens patient life, rest pain in claudicants that cannot be controlled, and situations in which extensive necrosis has destroyed the foot. However, the advent of modern vascular surgical reconstruction strategies and improvements in endovascular techniques have markedly reduced the role of primary amputation, defined as the performance of amputation prior to revascularization attempts, in the treatment of peripheral vascular disease. Vascular reconstruction remains the mainstay of chronic limb ischemia therapy; on initial presentation of CLI, 50% of patients are initially treated with a revascularization procedure, 25% with primary amputation, and

25% undergo medical management.[3] Currently, the indications for primary amputation in the setting of vascular disease are limited to those situations where arterial reconstruction is contraindicated. This includes patients in whom the burden of peripheral vascular disease does not allow for bypass grafting (i.e., "no target for bypass"), those who have gangrene to such an extent that it would not permit the salvage of a useful extremity even if vascular reconstruction is successful, and those who have prohibitive comorbid states such as advanced CHF. [Q2: D] Patients with chronic limb ischemia who are nonambulatory pose a dilemma. Due to their preoperative condition, and often possessing flexion contractures due to their ischemic disease or pain, vascular reconstruction usually produces a limb that is neither stable nor useful; primary amputation may be appropriate for this population.[3]

Despite the focal role of arterial reconstruction in the treatment of chronic limb ischemia, the surgeon must be sensitive to the possibility of futility in repeated treatment and the need for secondary amputation in achieving the best clinical outcome. The indications for secondary amputation include early graft occlusion with fruitless attempts to attain a patent reconstruction, exhaustion of interventional possibilities in restoring flow, or the event in which the limb continues to deteriorate despite the presence of a patent reconstruction.[3,8] Indeed, the most common causes of secondary amputation are unreconstructable vascular disease (60%) and persistent infection of the lower extremity despite aggressive vascular reconstruction.[3] In a review of 2,306 lower extremity bypass procedures by the Vascular Study Group of Northern New England, 8% of the cases were found to require secondary amputation within 1 year post-intervention; 17% of these amputations were performed in the setting of a patent graft. While graft occlusion was not found to be a definitive amputation requiring event, 42% of those with early graft occlusion eventually had a major lower extremity amputation. Independent risk factors associated with amputation in this population included nonambulatory status preoperatively, dialysis dependence, diabetes mellitus, a tarsal target for the bypass graft, and preoperative housing in a nursing home.[9]

Given the societal, economic, and personal impact of an amputation to a patient, amputees report that they are willing to undergo multiple, repeated, and potentially painful interventions in an attempt at limb salvage rather than undergoing an early amputation.[10] The increasing use of endovascular techniques to treat peripheral vascular lesions has shown a potential to avoid amputation for these patients. As cited above, the decade between 1996 and 2006 saw a significant decrease in the rate of amputation. This same period also witnessed a substantial growth in Medicare B claims for endovascular intervention. It is estimated that, in conjunction with bypass surgery, this period coincided with a doubling in the total number of vascular procedures performed.[4] Likewise, endovascular specific techniques such as subintimal angioplasty could potentially salvage limbs that would otherwise have undergone primary amputation.[11]

Appropriate selection of the level of amputation is critical to the formation of an amputation stump that can be well healed and allow for functional rehabilitation. For the vascular surgeon, a badly chosen distal level can lead to the feared complication of a "creeping amputation," whereas an overly proximal cut would greatly hamper rehabilitation possibilities for the patient. However, no single noninvasive clinical test has been demonstrated to reliably predict primary healing in the ischemic amputee, particularly when dealing with below-knee amputations. [Q3: F] Objective evaluation of skin blood flow at the desired level of amputation is the best means to anticipate primary healing. Clinical assessment includes a pulse exam, looking for palpable pulses above the level of the proposed amputation, the presence or absence of dependent rubor, venous filling, skin temperature as assessed by the palm of the hand, and signs of infection at the site of incision.[12] Segmental Doppler systolic blood pressure measurements have been used for decades, but its use is hampered in distal amputation measurement by the calcification of arteries, and data defining a lower limit of systolic blood pressures at the popliteal artery for successful healing have been inconsistent, ranging from below 50 mmHg to as high as 70 mmHg. Skin injections of radiotracer dyes have been studied since the 1980s, but are highly subject to operator variability in injection level and factors affecting blood flow such as cardiac function, body temperature, and ambient temperature that proved difficult in providing standardization. In the case of fluorescein injection, cardiac arrest has been described following injection. There is little work to support the independent use of skin thermography alone in determining incision level.[13]

Much literature has been produced to support the use of transcutaneous oxygen pressure measurements ($TcPO_2$) in determining amputation level. This method utilizes a heated Clark electrode to overcome the limitations of skin injection dyes in a test that is both simple and inexpensive to perform. Early experiments found high correlations of $TcPO_2$ with ischemic rest pain, intermittent claudication, and tissue loss compared to normal controls. Like the blood pressure tests, attempts to establish a lower limit threshold to predict primary healing has varied widely, from a $TcPO_2$ 25 to 40 mmHg. Nonetheless, this method may have the highest potential for reaching significance as an adjunctive test in clinical practice, as higher $TcPO_2$ levels are consistently associated with improved rates of primary healing, and the method can be adapted to be used preoperative, intraoperatively, and postoperatively for continued evaluation.[13,14]

Given the absence of a "gold standard" method, the surgeon is best served using his or her clinical judgment, with the optional conjunction of tests the surgeon feels comfortable with to augment that judgment.

In a patient with extensive gangrene or active infection, the surgeon must follow basic surgical principles regarding control of a contaminated field. The patient with evidence of tissue loss in conjunction with peripheral vascular insufficiency is particularly vulnerable to infection in ischemic areas, and can have profound difficulty clearing disease in these locations as well. Control of infection and restoration of perfusion when limb salvage is realistic is essential.

The patient described above demonstrates ongoing septic shock; while he was initially hospitalized for pneumonia, the frank purulence from his wound and evidence of deep space infection of his foot suggest that his left lower extremity is the infectious focus. Beginning broad spectrum antibiotics is a prudent initial step in his treatment. However, given his known vascular compromise in his affected foot, it is unreasonable to expect medical management alone would be adequate to treat his infection and sepsis. The wound was previously debrided for necrotic tissue to a clean base; at this stage, the deep space infection of the foot suggests that simple debridement would not be sufficient. While the initial goal for this patient was limb salvage, loss of the Achilles tendon to disease in conjunction with the extensive infection of the foot makes the possibility of a functional foot unlikely despite revascularization. High importance should be placed on avoidance of wound infection, a complication with disastrous consequences for the patient. The most efficacious surgical intervention in this situation is an ankle disarticulation or guillotine amputation at the level of the malleoli in order to clear diseased tissue, reduce final amputation wound infection, and improve overall outcomes. [**Q4: C**] This incision should be no higher than a few centimeters proximal to the malleoli despite more proximal cellulitis, without flaps to allow for adequate drainage while treatment is continued with dressing changes and antibiotics. Completion amputation should be delayed until 1 week after the disarticulation to allow for sepsis clearance.[8]

When planning an amputation level, the surgeon must weigh competing surgical factors favoring wound healing with the desires of the patient and rehabilitation team for a highly conservative amputation. The advantages of a BKA, in comparison to an AKA, are most noticeable when considering the postoperative recovery and rehabilitation of the patient. Though factors such as presurgical fitness, mental status, and age weigh into the potential of a patient to ambulate after amputation, the presence of a preserved knee joint greatly favors positive outcomes. Amputees who have undergone a BKA achieve post-surgical bipedal amputation rates up to 80%, as opposed to 38–50% patient who have had an AKA. Similarly, while all amputees experience increased energy expenditure when compared to a non-amputated control during ambulation, BKA patients only face a 10–40% increase, as opposed to a greater than 60% increase after an AKA.[15] These findings are summarized in Table 43.1.

The primary disadvantage of a BKA when compared to an AKA in the setting of peripheral vascular disease is the decreased potential for primary healing. It is often quoted in surgical dogma that, with clinical determination of amputation level, a BKA has an 80% rate of uninterrupted primary healing, while an AKA chosen under the same guidelines has a rate of primary healing of at least 90%.[16,17] More recent data from the TASC II study confirms an overall rate of 75% of BKA stump healing: a primary healing rate of 60% is found among patients after a BKA, with an additional 15% of patients achieving secondary healing while preserving their BKA residual limb. Additionally, 15% of BKA patients require conversion to AKA in the early postoperative period, while an estimated 10% succumb to perioperative death.[3]

In light of the post-surgical well-being of the patient, the data clearly supports the preservation of a functional knee joint whenever feasible. However, there are many patients in

Table 43.1 Energy expenditure and ambulation rates as a function of amputation level. Adapted from Tang et al., JACS 2008.

Amputation level	Post-recovery ambulation rate (%)	Energy expenditure above non-amputated patient (%)
Hip disarticulation	0–10 (vascular patients)	82
Above-the-knee amputation	38–50	63
Knee disarticulation	31 (prosthesis fitting rate)	71.5
Below-the-knee amputation		
Long stump		10
Short stump	80	40
Syme amputation	n/a	43

whom essential medical conditions leave an initial AKA as the best clinical option. In patients who have had chronic ischemic damage, the surgeon may find ischemia in areas precluding a BKA, or discover irreversible tissue injury during the open amputation, signified by noncontractile gray muscle or severe knee flexion contracture or rigidity; BKA in these patients may be futile, result in a nonfunctional knee joint that may not heal and would require further surgery. Another group in which AKA may be more clinically appropriate include patients who fail to walk or would not be expected to ambulate post-operative due to underlying comorbities; examples of these patients include the elderly afflicted with severe dementia, those debilitated by the sequelae of severe or multiple cerebral vascular accidents, and people who are experiencing end-stage pulmonary or cardiac dysfunction.[17,18] Due to their bedridden status, severe knee contracture would inevitably result, predisposing to the formation of pressure ulcers on the residual limb that would necessitate revision to an AKA.[17] [Q5: E]

The patient described in the case scenario, though reporting symptoms consistent with claudication, still possesses a reasonable expectation of ambulation due to his pre-hospitalized functional status. A BKA would be an appropriate choice for his completion amputation.

Healing is a particularly complex concern for vascular and diabetic amputees, as the underlying medical comorbidities and the issues of local tissue ischemia that resulted in the pathology necessitating surgery will heavily weigh on the success of recuperation. Wound infection is the most serious complication that frequently requires an above-knee revision of the residual limb; infection greatly reduces rehabilitation potential, increases hospitalization length, and can be life-threatening. Intrinsic infection from tissues used to create the stump are more common than new extrinsic infections in this patient population.[8] Antibiotic regimens should be tailored to preoperative cultures and sensitivities from infected wound beds as the clinical timecourse allows. A statistical regression of a small UK population of BKA failures yielded an increased odds ratio of 14 toward AKA revision over noninfected residual limbs; similarly, postoperative limb trauma was shown to contribute significantly to a need for revision or AKA.[19] Wound edge necrosis in isolation does not necessarily require an AKA, its presence signifies local ischemia that may hamper adequate wound healing. The presence of necrosis and ulcerations on the stump also predispose to infection and concurrent sepsis.[8,19] While a poor-fitting prosthetic or dressing can contribute to pressure ulcer formation on the residual limb, early ambulation and weight-bearing are highly encouraged and associated with increased success rates of post-surgical rehabilitation. [Q6: E]

In carefully selected populations, conversion to an AKA and its consequent distractions from the patient's quality of life can be avoided by a revision of the BKA. Recent initial studies suggest that these patients generally have failure secondary to a history of minor trauma to the stump while possessing a palpable popliteal pulse, as opposed to a failure due to inadequate tissue perfusion. 86% of these patients were able to ambulate postoperatively, while 0% of their matched AKA controls achieved that goal.[20]

While the gold standard for dressing of a post-below-the-knee amputation has long been a bulky, rigid dressing, evolving technologies in the field of prosthetics has created an expanding role for the use of immediate postoperative prosthesis (IPOP). Modern use of IPOP is first cited in the early 1960s and 1970s with variable healing rates; Moore cites a primary healing rate of 62–75% with a 100% rehabilitation rate in amputees who were ambulatory prior to surgery.[21] These early designs were non-removable cylindrical casts that had to be cut for wound observation and recreated for additional use thereafter. Currently, IPOP is not the standard of treatment; concerns cited may stem from this legacy, as they include unfamiliarity with the technique, the need for frequent wound monitoring, and fear of placing a hard cast on a vascularly compromised limb. The purpose and results attributed to IPOP use include controlling or preventing knee flexion contracture, minimizing postsurgical edema and pain, providing psychological benefit of early ambulation, reducing phantom pain and the effects of inactivity through controlled weight bearing and ambulation, and protecting the residual limb from trauma. [Q7: A, C, D, F] In addition, IPOP use is also associated with assistance (but not acceleration) in wound healing and residual limb maturation. Experience through the last decade with the removable IPOP has demonstrated not only the ability for frequent wound examination for the surgeon, but benefit to the physical therapist in allowing for strengthening and range of motion exercises, and to the prosthetist in allowing for adjustments for residual limb volume loss and assisting in limb shaping.[15,22] Bulky rigid or semirigid dressings also possess many of the same advantages in the avoidance of wound complications and preventing the development of flexion contracture at the knee. Advocates of these dressings cite concerns about inhibiting the patient's movement in bed during the initial hours of recovery.[8] However, the unique advantage of the IPOP is the speedy path to rehabilitation and ambulation in the capable patient.

Healing from surgery is only the first hurdle for the amputee; recovery and rehabilitation is the focus of surgical therapy in these patients. In order to maximize the patient's chances for independent ambulation, adequate surgical recovery with appropriate amputation level selection must be combined with early ambulation. This can be maximized in BKA patients with the use of an IPOP. However, if the surgical team chooses to utilize rigid bulky dressings, rehabilitation for the patient should begin on the first postoperative day by getting the patient out of bed and encouraging weight bearing on the intact contralateral leg; by postoperative day 4 or 5, most patients will be ready for pylon and foot fitting and travel to physical therapy for more intense rehabilitation. Though amputees experience the dangers of atelectasis and pulmonary embolism associated with prolonged bedrest common to surgical patients, muscle atrophy in the upper body and remaining lower extremity can profoundly complicate mobility and must be avoided with an aggressive rehabilitative routine.[8] Ultimately, the ability to achieve independent survival is directly related to patient survival. In a series of 2,616 Veterans Administration patients who underwent major lower extremity amputation, those who achieved even marginal independence had a 6 month survival rate of at least 91%; patients who remained totally dependent on assistance had only a 73.5% 6 month survival rate. Unfortunately, 36% of all patients in this population were never able to recuperate beyond total dependence on assistance. Those that were able to achieve higher levels of independence tended to be younger, have undergone fewer procedures, and carried less comorbidities.[23]

Despite the most ambitious of rehabilitation protocols, about 80% of BKA patients and less than 50% of AKA patients achieve ambulation (Table 43.1).[15] These results drop dramatically when amputation is bilateral; it is uncommon for bilateral amputees to regain ambulation after surgery, regardless of their age. Even in young, otherwise healthy patients, it is rare for bilateral amputees to achieve normal gait. [Q8: E][8]

On follow-up after hospital discharge and rehabilitation, patients tend to report relatively high scores on subjective quality-of-life (QoL) measures. A 2008 study confirmed that predictors of decreased QoL scores include symptoms of depression, decreased mobility with prosthetics, number of prosthetic problems, increasing number of comorbidities, and less social support and daily social activity. Among these factors, depression was found to have the single largest impact on reported QoL.[24] Further study on depression in amputees found a rate of 17–20% at 1–3 years after surgery, compared to a 23% rate prior to admission and 2% at discharge. The post-surgical depression was found to be associated with baseline depression at admission and significant comorbidities, but not with length of hospital stay, wearing of the prosthetic, or dysvascular disease as the cause of amputation.[25] The therapy team can make the greatest impact on the quality of life of amputees by ensuring adequate mental health resources are available to the patient.

Regrettably, the morbidity and mortality profile of patients who have undergone major limb amputation is poor. Aggregate data from the TASC II study demonstrated that at 2 years after BKA, only 40% of patients were found to be fully mobile. Another 15% had undergone conversion to AKA, 15% required a contralateral amputation, and 30% were dead.[3] A series of 954 amputation from Beth Israel Deaconess found a median survival after AKA of 20 months, and 52 months after BKA; the presence of diabetes mellitus as a comorbidity showed a significant difference of survival at 60 months on the Kaplan-Meier curve of 30%, as opposed to 60% in non-diabetics.[26] Data from the Netherlands showed a 62% survival after amputation at 1 year, which dropped to 50% at 2 years and 29% at 5 years.[27] In a VA patient retrospective, a 7 year survival rate of 39% was noted; major causes of death in amputees were found to include congestive heart failure, myocardial infarction, respiratory failure, disseminated cancer, overwhelming sepsis, stroke, and renal failure.[28] Additional factors contributing to early mortality post-amputation in a West Virginia case series included advanced age, low albumin levels, undergoing an AKA, and the lack of previous cardiac intervention.[29] A rate of BKA to AKA conversion of 12–17% was reiterated in the two series from the Veterans Administration and the Netherlands.[27,28] Mortality within the first decade after amputation is significant; the etiology of death usually is the result of underlying medical issues that contributed to the need for amputation.

With the proper attention of a vascular surgeon and a multidisciplinary team, an amputation does not have to signify the failure of treatment. Rather, it should be seen as the first step toward functional recovery and regaining a quality of life comparable to the patient's pre-pathologic state. In many cases, amputation surgery may be preferable to extended distal bypass or multiple revisions of a below-knee bypass if the support infrastructure is available post-operatively. Continuing advances in prosthetic technology have the potential to improve patient outcomes in terms of energy expenditures, recovery of ambulatory ability, and gait improvement. It is incumbent on the vascular surgeon to remain actively engaged in the post-operative care of the amputee.

References

1. Sumpio BE. Foot ulcers. *N Engl J Med.* 2000;343(11):787-793.
2. Sumpio BE, Paszkowiak J, Aruny JA, Blume PA. Lower Extremity Ulceration. In: Creager M, Loscalzo J, Dzau V, eds. *Vascular Medicine.* 3rd ed. W.B. Saunders. Philadelphia; Chap. 62, 2005:880-893.

3. Norgren L, Hiatt WR, Dormandy JA, Nehler MR, Harris KA, Fowkes FGR. Inter-society consensus for the management of peripheral arterial disease (TASC II). *J Vasc Surg*. January 2007;45(1):S5A-S67A.

4. Goodney PP, Beck AW, Nagle J, Welch HG, Zwolak RM. National trends in lower extremity bypass surgery, endovascular interventions, and major amputations. *J Vasc Surg*. July 2009;50(1):54-60.

5. U.S. Department of Health and Human Services. Healthy People 2010: Understanding and Improving Health. Vol 1. Washington DC, U.S. Department of Health and Human Services, Government Printing Office, January 2000:5–22.

6. Global Lower Extremity Amputation Study Group. Epidemiology of lower extremity amputation in centres in Europe, North America and East Asia. *Br J Surg*. 2000;87:328-337.

7. Dillingham TR, Pezzin LE, MacKenzie EJ. Limb amputation and limb deficiency: epidemiology and recent trends in the United States. *South Med J*. 2002;95(8):875-883.

8. Jacobs LA, Durance PW. Below-the-knee amputation. In: Ernst CB, Stanley JC, eds. *Current Therapy in Vascular Surgery*. 4th ed. 2001:674-677.

9. Goodney PP, Nolan BW, Schanzer A, Eldrup-Jorgensen J, Bertges DJ, Stanley AC, Stone DH, Walsh DB, Powell RJ, Likosky DS, Cronenwett JL (Vascular Study Group of Northern New England). Factors Associated with Amputation or Graft Occlusion One Year after Lower Extremity Bypass in Northern New England. Ann Vasc Surg. September 2009, epub.

10. Reed AB, Delvecchio C, Giglia JS. Major lower extremity amputation after multiple revascularizations: was it worth it? *Ann Vasc Surg*. 2008;22(3):335-340.

11. Met R, Koelemay MJ, Bipat S, Legemate DA, van Lienden KP, Reekers JA. Always contact a vascular interventional specialist before amputating a patient with critical limb ischemia. Cardiovasc Intervent Radiol. August 2009. epub.

12. Collins KA, Sumpio BE. Vascular assessment. Blume P, ed. *Clinics in Podiatric Medicine and Surgery*. Vol. 17, No. 2. Chap. 1, 2000:171–192.

13. Provan JL. Noninvasive methods of determining amputation levels. In: Ernst CB, Stanley JC, eds. *Current Therapy in Vascular Surgery*. 4th ed. 2001:669-672.

14. Poredos P, Rakovec S, Guzic-Salobir B. Determination of amputation level in ischaemic limbs using tcPO2 measurement. *Vasa*. 2005;34(2):108-112.

15. Tang PCY, Ravji K, Key JJ, Mahler DB, Blume PA, Sumpio B. Let them walk! current prosthesis options for leg and foot amputees. *J Am Coll Surg*. March 2008;206(3):548-560.

16. Lim RC Jr, Blaisdell FW, Hall AD, Moore WS, Thomas AN. Below-knee amputation for ischemic gangrene. *Surg Gynecol Obstet*. 1967;125(3):493-501.

17. Endean ED. Above-the-knee amputation and hip disarticulation. In: Ernst CB, Stanley JC, eds. *Current Therapy in Vascular Surgery*. 4th ed. 2001:677-680.

18. Taylor SM, Kalbaugh CA, Cass AL, et al. "Successful outcome" after below-knee amputation: an objective definition and influence of clinical variables. *Am Surg*. July 2008;74(7): 607-612.

19. Yip VSK, Teo NB, Johnstone R, et al. An analysis of risk factors associated with failure of below knee amputations. *World J Surg*. 2006;30:1081-1087.

20. Stasik CN, Berceli SA, Nelson PR, Lee WA, Ozaki CK. Functional outcome after redo below-knee amputation. *World J Surg*. 2008;32:1823-1826.

21. Moore WS. Below-knee amputation. In: Moore WS, Malone JM, eds. *Lower Extremity Amputation*. Philadelphia: WB Saunders; 1989:118-131.

22. Walsh TL. Custom removable immediate postoperative prosthesis. *J Prosthet Orthot*. 2003;15(4):158-161.

23. Stineman MG, Kurichi JE, Kwong PL, et al. Survival analysis in amputees based on physical independence grade achievement. *Arch Surg*. June 2009;144(6):543-551.

24. Asano M, Rushton P, Miller WC, Deathe BA. Predictor of quality of life among individuals who have a lower limb amputation. *Prosthet Orthot Int*. June 2008;32(3):231-243.

25. Singh R, Ripley D, Pentland B, et al. Depression and anxiety symptoms after lower limb amputation: the rise and fall. *Clin Rehabil*. 2009;23:281-286.

26. Subramaniam B, Pomposelli F, Talmor D, Park KW. Perioperative and long-term morbidity and mortality after above-knee and below-knee amputations in diabetics and nondiabetics. *Anesth Analg.* 2005;100:1241-1247.
27. Ploeg AJ, Lardenoye JW, Vrancken Peeters MPFM, Beslau PJ. Contemporary series of morbidity and mortality after lower limb amputation. *Eur J Vasc Endovasc Surg.* June 2005;29: 633-637.
28. Cruz CP, Eidt JF, Capps C, Kirtley L, Moursi MM. Major lower extremity amputations at a Veterans affair hospital. *Am J Surg.* 2003;186:449-454.
29. Stone PA, Flaherty SK, Aburahma AF, et al. Factors affecting perioperative mortality and wound-related complications following major lower extremity amputations. *Ann Vasc Surg.* March 2006;20(2):209-216.

Part XI

Vascular Malformations

Congenital Vascular Malformation

44

Byung-Boong Lee

A 10-year-old girl presented with a history of recurrent painful swelling of the left knee with mild ecchymosis. The latest episode of tender swelling of soft tissue along the left knee was preceded by a direct blow to the area during a ball game. In addition, she has had an abnormally grown left lower limb with scattered multiple soft tissue masses throughout the limb since birth.

- Physical examination revealed diffuse swelling of the entire left limb, which was longer and larger than the opposite limb and more pronounced along the foot and lower leg. The swollen limb had slightly increased firmness on palpation throughout its entire length except for the soft tissue mass areas.
- Multiple soft tissue masses were easily compressible and scattered from the dorsum of foot to the upper thigh; their diameters varied between 2 and 8 cm.
- Similar lesions were also noticed at the left perineum, left labia, left lower abdomen, and left flank. Diffuse swelling along the medial side of left foot collapsed spontaneously when the foot was elevated.
- Further evaluation of the skeletal system revealed the left lower extremity to be 5.0 cm longer – 3.0 cm longer in the tibia and 2.0 cm longer in the femur – in total length than the right lower extremity, accompanied by pelvic tilt and compensatory scoliosis of the lower spine.
- However, the patient had minimal limitation of her daily activities except for moderate limping.
- Family history and past history were unremarkable except for a vague history of cellulitis along the affected limb.

B.-B. Lee
Department of Vascular Surgery, Georgetown University
School of Medicine, Washington, DC, USA

G. Geroulakos and B. Sumpio (eds.), *Vascular Surgery*,
DOI: 10.1007/978-1-84996-356-5_44, © Springer-Verlag London Limited 2011

Question 1

What is the most fundamental problem on which clinician should focus in order to establish the proper diagnosis and treatment of this condition?

A. Scoliosis with pelvic tilt
B. Abnormal long-bone growth with length discrepancy
C. Abnormal swelling of lower limb with scattered soft tissue tumors
D. Mechanical problem of knee joint with symptoms

Question 2

What is the most basic laboratory test required to verify the nature of the problem?

A. Lumbosacral spine assessment
B. Radiologic assessment of bone length discrepancy
C. Duplex ultrasonography for the hemodynamic assessment
D. Locomotive test including gait evaluation

Question 3

Which of the following non-invasive studies could be most useful in the clinical diagnosis of the disease complex in our patient?

A. Volumetric assessment of limb size
B. Special radiologic study of epiphyseal plate of abnormally long bone
C. Magnetic resonance imaging (MRI) study of soft tissue masses
D. Transarterial lung perfusion scintigraphy
E. Bone scan

Question 4

Which of the following non-invasive tests is not appropriate to assist in the differential diagnosis for the extremity lesions in our patient?

A. Whole-body blood-pool scintigraphy (WBBPS)
B. Computed tomography (CT) scan
C. Radionuclide lymphoscintigraphy
D. Transarterial lung perfusion scintigraphy (TLPS)
E. Lymphangiography (lymphography)

44.1
Clinical Evaluation

This patient underwent a thorough investigation of the nature and extent of the congenital vascular malformation (CVM) involved.

A combination of various non- to minimally-invasive studies were performed to confirm the clinical impression of venolymphatic malformation (VLM): duplex ultrasonography, whole-body blood-pool scintigraphy (WBBPS), magnetic resonance image (MRI) study, transarterial lung perfusion scintigraphy (TLPS), and/or radionuclide lymphoscintigraphy.

The primary hemodynamic impact and the secondary musculoskeletal impact of the venous malformation (VM) were assessed as the main CVM lesion in addition to the extent/degree of each component of the VM, truncular (T) and extratruncular (ET) form, involved in the extremity.

A thorough skeletal evaluation of the long-bone growth discrepancy of the lower extremity and the degree of pelvic tilt with its compensatory scoliosis was also made with conventional bone X-rays.

The TLPS assessment was performed substituting arteriographic investigation of the lower extremity for the possible hidden micro-arteriovenous malformation (AVM) lesion, which was marginally indicated due to an unusually increased venous flow by the isolated VM lesion alone on the duplex scan under the normally developed and functioning deep vein system.

An ascending phlebography was also performed together with the percutaneous direct-puncture phlebography as a therapeutic guide; mandatory confirmation of the presence of a normal deep vein system of the lower extremity was made before starting the treatment to the infiltrating ET-form lesion of the VM.

The final diagnosis confirmed extensive involvement of the VM as an infiltrating type of the ET form causing serious clinical impact directly to the venous system hemodynamically as well as to the skeletal system to induce abnormal long-bone growth of the left lower extremity. A moderate degree of venectasia as a T form of VM along the left femoral-popliteal vein segment was also found, by WBBPS, MRI and duplex scan, and subsequently confirmed by separate ascending phlebography.

A venectasia of the femoral vein was assessed to have a limited clinical significance at this stage in comparison to the ET-form lesions of the VM.

The lymphatic malformation (LM) component which is mixed with the ET form of VM, was confirmed as the ET form, giving minimum and limited clinical impact so that a conservative management/observation was instituted for this LM component.

Therefore, the ET-form lesions of VM along the knee region were selected for active treatment as a priority; this was followed by the ankle and foot lesions.

The primary indication to initiate the treatment immediately was that these lesions were potentially limb-threatening (e.g., hemarthrosis) due to their proximity to the joints with increased vulnerability to repeated trauma, especially as a cause of her knee symptoms.

The treatment was further indicated to arrest/slow down their impact on abnormal long-bone growth.

Multiple infiltrating ET lesions of the VM along the knee region, which is surgically not amenable, were selected for ethanol sclerotherapy as independent therapy. Multisession ethanol sclerotherapy was given using the absolute ethanol in the range of 80 to 100% concentration in calculated dosage – not exceeding 1.0 mg/kg of body weight as maximum dose per session – by direct puncture technique under general anesthesia. Close cardiopulmonary monitoring during the procedure was ensured to control and/or prevent transient pulmonary hypertension by the unavoidable spillage of ethanol into the systemic circulation from the lesion during treatment.

The symptomatic lesions along the knee with recurrent painful swelling following minor injuries were controlled well without complication/morbidity and substantially reduced the risk of intra-articular bleeding and subsequent hemarthrosis. Subsequently, the ET-form VM lesions at the foot and ankle underwent surgical excision following preoperative multisession ethanol and N-butyl cyanoacrylic glue embolosclerotherapy with much reduced perioperative morbidity to improve foot function.

Following successful control of multiple VM lesions along the knee, ankle, and foot with priority as a potentially limb-threatening condition, other VM lesions, scattered throughout the lower extremity, were also treated with absolute ethanol to assist further attempts to arrest the abnormal long-bone growth of the lower extremity. The abnormal long-bone growth is attributed to these VM lesions scattered within the muscular structure of the lower extremity in the extensive infiltrating type of ET, with significant impact on the venous circulation along the epiphyseal plate.

In addition to the multisession embolosclerotherapy as independent and/or adjunct perioperative therapy to the VM lesions, the conservative supportive measures to improve and/or maintain overall venous function have been supplemented with the use of a graded compression above-knee stocking to prevent chronic venous insufficiency.

The final decision for the T-form lesion was left femoral-popliteal venectasia, but it was decided to defer treatment until urgent treatment of the ET form of the VM was finished, but to keep it under close observation. It might eventually require treatment (e.g., venorrhaphy, venous bypass) to prevent development of venous thromboembolism when significant venous flow/volume reduction should occur following successful control of the ET form of VM lesions. The hemodynamic consequences of the treatment of such extensive ET-form lesions directly affect total venous blood volume through the deep vein system.

The LM component in this patient was treated only with complex decongestive therapy (CDT) in order to prevent full development of lymphedema. The infiltrating ET form of LM detected together with the ET form of VM has been shown to put extra burden on the marginally normal lymph-conducting system on lymphoscinti-graphic evaluation. Therefore, continuous surveillance for aggressive preventive measurement of local to systemic cellulitis along this ET form of LM lesions is mandated.

This patient will continue to be managed by the multidisciplinary team of the CVM Clinic at regular intervals for her entire lifetime, through periodical follow-up assessment of the treatment results and the natural course of the untreated lesions.

Question 5

What is the first priority in the management of this patient?

A. Correction of scoliosis
B. Correction of bone length discrepancy
C. Control of abnormal hemodynamic status of lower extremity by vascular lesions

D. Correction of gait with physical therapy and shoe adjustment
E. Biopsy of the soft tissue mass

Question 6

Which of the following is not an indication for the treatment of venous malformation?

A. Lesion located near to the limb threatening region
B. Life threatening lesion
C. Symptomatic lesion
D. Lesion with complication
E. All the lesions regardless of their condition

Question 7

What is the International Society for the Study of Vascular Anomaly (ISSVA) recommended and most popular strategy with respect to limb length discrepancy?

A. Immediate surgical intervention to the epiphyseal plate to arrest further abnormal growth of the affected bone
B. Conservative treatment of limb length discrepancy only with physical therapy and shoe adjustment
C. Hemodynamic control of venous malformation as a priority whenever possible
D. Corrective surgery of bone for length discrepancy with the unaffected limb as a priority
E. None of the above

Question 8

What is the current trend of therapeutic strategy for venous malformation lesions in the lower extremity?

A. Surgical excision of the vascular lesions and related procedure only
B. Transarterial embolotherapy only
C. Transvenous sclerotherapy only
D. Multidisciplinary approach with surgical therapy and embolosclerotherapy
E. Percutaneous direct puncture sclerotherapy only

Question 9

What is the general consensus on invasive investigations (e.g., arteriography; phlebography) for venous malformation?

A. There is no indication for invasive investigation for the diagnosis and treatment of venous malformation.
B. Invasive investigations are indicated in every suspected case of venous malformation for the confirmation of the diagnosis.

C. Invasive investigation can be reserved for the therapeutic regimen as a road map and/ or occasional differential diagnosis.
D. Invasive investigation should be used only for the follow-up assessment.
E. None of the above.

Question 10

What is the most important precondition for the treatment of venous malformation in the lower extremity?

A. History of deep vein thrombosis
B. Combined lymphatic malformation
C. Vascular-bone syndrome: length discrepancy of the long bone
D. Existence of deep vein system
E. Skin lesion with ulcer and necrosis

Question 11

What has to be included in the differential diagnosis of venous malformation?

A. Lymphatic malformation
B. AV shunting malformation
C. Infantile hemangioma
D. Capillary malformation
E. All of the above

44.2
Commentary

Congenital vascular malformation (CVM) is regarded as one of the most difficult diagnostic and therapeutic enigmas in the practice of medicine. Vascular surgeons often take this vascular malformation quite casually without any specific knowledge, and this cavalier approach can end in failure. Clinical presentations of the CVMs are extremely variable, ranging from an asymptomatic birthmark to a life-threatening condition. This variability in the clinical presentation has been a major challenge to even the most experienced clinicians.[1,2] Many attempts to control this ever-challenging problem, especially in the twentieth century, were led by surgeons alone, but with mostly disastrous results because of poorly planned and over-aggressive surgical treatment carried out on the basis of limited knowledge.[3,4] Recently, a multidisciplinary approach was introduced with a new concept based on Hamburg classification.[5,6] The Hamburg classification gives excellent clinical applicability with minimum confusion because the new terminology itself provides substantial information on the anatomico-pathophysiological status of vascular malformation; it has become the most fundamental rationale for the advanced concept of vascular malformation[7-9] (Table 44.1). It classifies complex groups of various vascular malformations based on the predominant type: VM, LM, AVM, and combined form which is mostly hemolymphatic malformation (HLM). The VM is the most common type of CVM together with LM and they often combine together to make the clinical condition quite complicated.

When this HLM consists of only two components, that is, VM and LM, it is grouped separately as VLM which is almost equivalent to Klippel–Trenaunay syndrome, where our patient belongs.

The new Hamburg classification provides critical information relating to recurrence based on precise information of embryonal stage when the developmental arrest has occurred.[9,10]

Table 44.1 Hamburg classification of congenital vascular malformation: 1988 consensus with modification

Species	Anatomical form
Predominantly: Arterial defects	Truncular forms: Aplasia or obstruction Dilatation Extratruncular forms: Infiltrating Limited
Predominantly: Venous defects	Truncular forms: Aplasia or obstruction Dilatation Extratruncular forms: Infiltrating Limited
Predominantly: Arteriovenous (AV) shunting defects	Truncular forms: Deep AV fistula Superficial AV fistula Extratruncular forms Infiltrating Limited
Combined: Vascular defects	Truncular forms: Arterial and venous Hemolymphatic Extratruncular forms Infiltrating hemolymphatic Limited hemolymphatic
Predominantly: Lymphatic defects	Truncular forms: Aplasia or obstruction Dilatation Extratruncular forms: Infiltrating Limited

When this developmental arrest occurs in an early stage of embryonal life, it remains with mesenchymal cell characteristics so it is grouped as ET form; when it occurs in the later stage of embryogenesis, it is grouped as T form with lack of mesenchymal cell characteristics, which is extremely crucial for the clinical management.

This patient presented with the most common clinical manifestation of CVM, with various findings related to the venous malformation (VM) as primary lesion as well as its secondary phenomena since birth (Fig. 44.1). Among many clinical findings, this patient presented with multiple, scattered, soft tissue mass lesions along the lower extremity, extending from the toe to flank, which provide the necessary clues to initiate proper investigation of VM as the etiology of this condition.[11,12] **[Q1: C]**

Relatively firm diffuse swelling of the entire left lower extremity, in addition to the abnormal long-bone growth with length discrepancy, may give further clues to the investigation on the combined nature of VM and LM as the cause of the vascular-bone syndrome.[13,14]

The VM in particular has a significant incidence of secondary abnormal long-bone growth with subsequent bone length discrepancy. In addition, it is also known to have a relatively high incidence of combined LM, which is still called Klippel–Trenaunay syndrome.[15,16]

Of the many clinical clues this patient presented with that suggested VM among various CVMs, immediate collapse of the bulging soft lesion along the foot upon elevation was the most important.

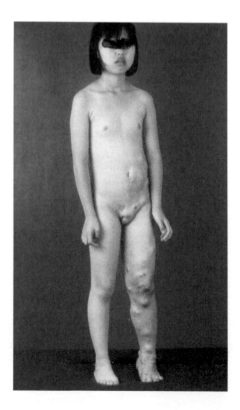

Fig. 44.1 Clinical appearance of the patient, with extensive VM lesions scattered along the left lower extremity from toe to thigh, with extension to the perineum, labia, lower abdomen and flank, left

Therefore, hemodynamic assessment of the lower extremity along the scattered soft tissue tumors has to be the starting point for the work-up of proper diagnosis and treatment of this disease complex; duplex ultrasonographic study provides most of the essential hemodynamic information and an excellent guideline for further management (Fig. 44.2). [Q2: C]

Further study to assess scoliosis with pelvic tilt and/or abnormal long-bone growth with length discrepancy may be carried out once primary diagnosis of the vascular malformation has been made. In this case report, the patient presented recurrent episodes of tender swelling of the left knee following minor trauma. This was probably due to the bleeding/leaking from the VM lesion near to the knee joint to the surrounding soft tissue. A detailed evaluation of the knee joint itself can be deferred until the basic evaluation of VM, presented as soft tissue swelling along the knee joint, is completed with MRI, WBBPS, and

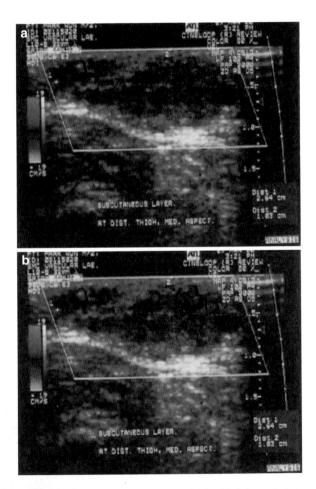

Fig. 44.2 (**a**) Sonographic identification of the communicating/draining vein between VM lesion and deep vein system. (**b**) Sonographic assessment of the VM lesion located superficially in the lower extremity

duplex ultrasonography.[17,18] This approach will delineate the accurate relationship of this VM lesion to the periarticular structure including the joint space, and the potential risk of inducing hemarthrosis by repeated bleeding following trauma.

Radiological assessment of lumbosacral spine together with long-bone length discrepancy should be made *after* hemodynamic assessment to identify the extent of VM, starting with duplex scan as the most basic laboratory test.[19]

Although duplex ultrasonographic study can provide most of the crucial first-line hemodynamic information about vascular malformation, MRI of T1 and T2 images is the most valuable non-invasive study for clinical diagnosis, and has become the new gold standard for the diagnosis, especially for the VM[17] (Fig. 44.3). **[Q3: C]**

MRI study of the soft tissue along the entire left lower extremity extending from toe to the torso can confirm the clinical diagnosis of VM already made preliminarily by ultrasonographic study. MRI can provide precise delineation of the anatomical relationship of the malformation lesion with its surrounding tissues like muscle, tendon, nerve, vessels, and bone from the foot to the retroperitoneal, pelvic, and gluteal regions. In addition to the duplex scan and MRI study in this patient, various non-invasive tests are needed for further differential diagnosis.

Lymphoscintigraphic study based on radioisotope-tagged sulfur colloid is indicated to assess lymphatic function and the lymph-conducting system in general and rule out chronic lymphedema due to the T form of LM.[20,21]

The extremity involved was felt to be firmer than usual for a VM-affected leg, with general diffuse swelling throughout the entire length of the lower limb; this finding suggested primary lymphedema combined with venous stasis so that further evaluation of the lymphatic function is indicated with radionuclide lymphoscintigraphy. The lymphatic function assessment of this patient with lymphoscintigraphy has shown the marginal status of the lymphatic system and its vulnerability to further insult by the ET form of LM.

WBBPS based on radioisotope-tagged red blood cell pooling is also indicated as one of three basic tests for the diagnosis of VM. This relatively new investigation is very sensitive in detecting abnormal blood pooling throughout the body (Fig. 44.4). It can be used not only as a practical test to assess treatment results but also as a screening test for hidden vascular malformation. It also has a unique role in the differentiation between venous and lymphatic malformation.[22,23]

CT scanning also has practical value in providing information on the relationship of vascular malformation to its surrounding skeletal and soft tissue of the lower extremity.

Transarterial lung perfusion scintigraphy (TLPS) can provide crucial information on possible involvement of a micro-, if not, macro-AVM lesion to the VM (Fig. 44.5).

AVM involvement is a critical condition for the management strategy of VM; the VLM in particular is seldom combined with the AVM, especially in micro-AVM, which can be overlooked by conventional arteriography alone. Positive confirmation of no existence of micro-AVM is extremely important before the initiation of the treatment to the symptomatic VM lesions, especially when it is combined with LM.

The TLPS can therefore provide necessary guidance for the further invasive study of arteriography.[24,25]

However, classical lymphangiography (or lymphography) using oil-based contrast material is *no longer* performed for the screening lymphatic function because of the potential risk of further damaging the lymphatic vessel with the procedure. **[Q4: E]**

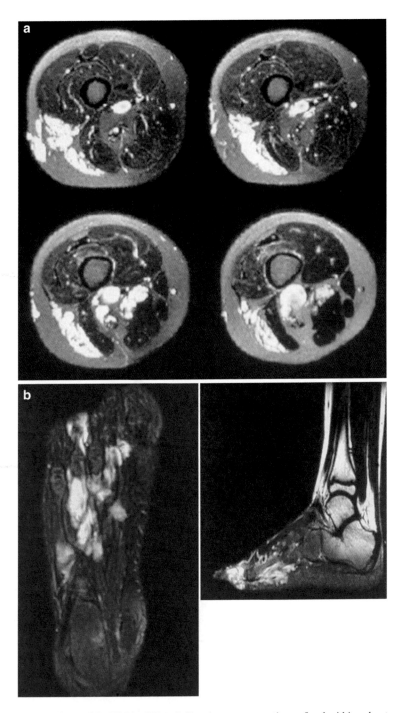

Fig. 44.3 (**a**) ET form of the VM in diffuse infiltrating status mostly confined within subcutaneous soft tissue, and T form of lesion along the deep vein system as femoral-popliteal venectasia. (**b**) ET form of the VM lesion, infiltrating into foot muscle structure as well as sole soft tissue

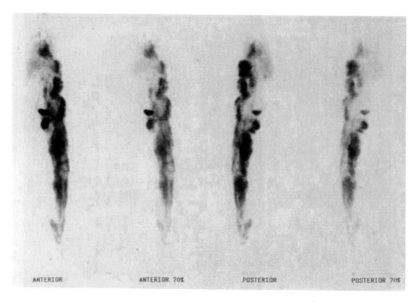

Fig. 44.4 Extensive abnormal blood pooling by the ET lesions and T lesion of the VM, diffusely involving entire lower extremity

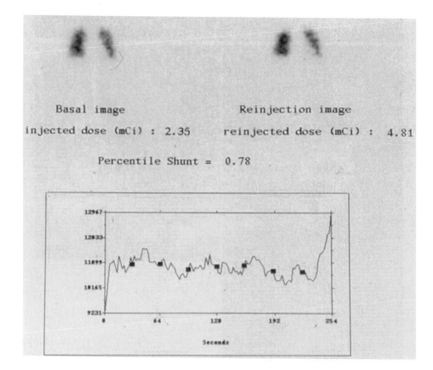

Fig. 44.5 TLPS investigation of arteriovenous (AV) shunting status in lower extremity to assess potential risk of the AVM lesion involved to the VM lesion. Normal TLPS finding with no evidence of micro-AV shunting can rule out AVM without further investigation by arteriography

Once the final diagnosis of a combination of VM and LM has been made, then the next decision should be whether treatment is indicated. In view of the abnormal long-bone growth involvement to this vascular malformation, immediate treatment of this particular VM is generally preferred.

Treatment priority should be given to the primary etiology, i.e., vascular malformation. Therefore, the control of abnormal hemodynamic status of the lower extremity secondary to the VM should have priority.[26,27] **[Q5: C]**

All the other clinical problems secondary to this primary lesion, including scoliosis with pelvic tilt, abnormal long-bone growth with bone length discrepancy, and abnormal gait, can be deferred while treatment is aimed at the VM itself.[5,6,26] Not all the VM lesions are indicated or feasible for treatment. In general, VM lesions located near limb-threatening regions (e.g., proximity to the joint space) or potentially life/critical function-threatening regions (e.g., proximity to the airway), symptomatic lesions, and/or lesions with complications are generally considered for treatment.[5,11] **[Q6: E]**

There is significant controversy over how to manage limb-length discrepancy as the secondary phenomenon of the VM in the lower extremity. Surgical intervention directly to the epiphyseal plate to arrest further abnormal growth of the affected long bone has brought mixed results, with further controversy on its long-term value.[13,14] Therefore, general the consensus on this issue of vascular-bone syndrome accepted by most ISSV A members these days is to endorse a new strategy to control the hemodyamic abnormality of VM *first*, since hemodynamic impact/stimulation by the VM lesions to the intraosseous tissue along the epiphyseal plates is known to be the cause of abnormal long-bone growth.[14,26] The strategy based on conservative treatment only with physical therapy and shoe adjustment until the long-bone growth is completed is also not acceptable due to increasing morbidity in gait and spine, as well as the unpredictable outcome of late correction. Meanwhile, too aggressive an approach with early correction of long-bone discrepancy has also been abandoned due to significant difficulty in achieving good long-term results. **[Q7: C]**

The traditional surgical approach of removing the entire lesion is still theoretically acceptable if the lesion is located in a surgically accessible area and localized enough to be completely removable with limited or no morbidity. However, this condition is generally very rare and for most VM lesions there will be significant morbidity with a surgical approach aimed at complete removal of the lesion.

Therefore, a multidisciplinary approach that combines traditional surgical therapy with newly introduced embolosclerotherapy utilizing various embolscleroagents is the treatment strategy of choice.[5,6,8] This can substantially reduce overall treatment-related morbidity with good long-term therapy results.[11,12]

A lesion located along the surgically inaccessible area and/or with prohibitively high surgical morbidity is generally treated with sclerotherapy alone. The current trend in the management of VM of the lower extremity involves a multidisciplinary approach combining surgical therapy, sclerotherapy, and/or embolotherapy, whenever feasible.[5,27] **[Q8: D]**

Most of the diagnosis of VM in the lower extremity in particular can be made efficiently on the basis of non-invasive studies. However, classical invasive studies, including arteriography and phlebography, are still considered to be the gold standard for the management of all vascular malformations, but they are generally reserved for use as a road map for the final therapeutic regimen (Fig. 44.6). These invasive imaging techniques are also used to rule out hidden micro-AVM combined with the VM, especially when TLPS findings indicate a high possibility of a micro-AV shunting condition.[6,8,25] **[Q9: C]**

Numerous embolosceroagents have been tested for the treatment of VM; most recently, absolute ethanol has been accepted as the scleroagent of choice not only for VM but also for AVM, with excellent long-term outcome with no recurrence when treated properly.[11,12,25,28–30] However, this has significant side effects, resulting in various acute and/or chronic complications/morbidity, such as deep vein thrombosis, pulmonary embolism, nerve palsy, and various degrees of skin to soft tissue damage from bullae to full thickness necrosis. Therefore, the selection of ethanol as the scleroagent to treat VM has to be based on the risk involved of recurrence, acute morbidity during the therapy, and long-term sequelae of the treatment.[6] In order to treat VM of the lower extremity safely, careful hemodynamic assessment of the deep vein system is also mandatory, including confirmation of the existence of a normal deep vein system. This is crucial before treatment of the T-form lesion of VM, the marginal (lateral embryonic) vein in particular. Once the deep vein system is properly documented, proper treatment of VM can be initiated. **[Q10: D]** However, all the other issues raised in Question 10, including history of deep vein thrombosis, combined LM, and history of skin damage during previous sclerotherapy, will also require careful assessment to improve overall safety of the planned treatment.

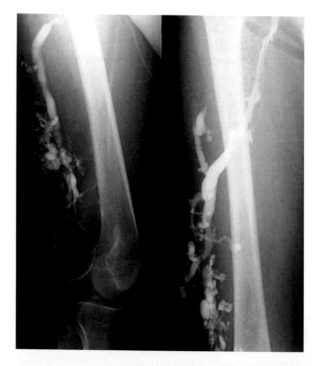

Fig. 44.6 Percutaneous direct puncture phlebographic findings of the ET-form lesions of VM in the thigh; it may become a road map for the subsequent endovascular management with embolo/sclerotherapy

Differential diagnosis with other forms, T or ET forms, as well as other kinds of vascular malformation, VM. LM, VLM, or AVM, is mandatory, in view of their different behavior with different clinical impact. This is particularly important for the ET form of various vascular malformations whose behavior is totally unpredictable. The ET form retains the original evolutional ability of mesenchymal cells, in contrast to the T form, so that it can grow when the condition/stimulation should meet (e.g., trauma, surgery, pregnancy, hormone therapy).[10] Regarding the VM of the lower extremity, precise differential diagnosis of other conditions such as LM or AVM is extremely important, because the treatment strategy is substantially different.[6,27] Besides, initial differential diagnosis for VM, like any vascular malformation, should start from the infantile (neonatal) hemangioma which also belongs to the vascular anomaly together with the vascular malformation. Hemangioma is a true vascular tumor and not a vascular malformation, possessing distinctively different pathophysiology, anatomico-histology, and clinical behavior.[1,31] **[Q11: E]** The clinical significance of capillary malformation is not understood properly yet, but it should be included in the evaluation of any vascular malformation although the modified Hamburg classification did not include it in the classification of various CVMs, due to the lack of clinical significance for the vascular surgeon.[32]

References

1. Mulliken JB. Cutaneous vascular anomalies. *Semin Vasc Surg*. 1993;6:204-218.
2. Rutherford RB. Congenital vascular malformations: diagnostic evaluation. *Semin Vasc Surg*. 1993;6:225-232.
3. Malan E. *Vascular malformations (angiodysplasias)*. Milan: Carlo Erba Foundation; 1974:17.
4. Szilagyi DE, Smith RF, Elliott JP, Hageman JH. Congenital arteriovenous anomalies of the limbs. *Arch Surg*. 1976;111:423-429.
5. Lee BB, Bergan JJ. Advanced management of congenital vascular malformations: a multidisciplinary approach. *J Cardiovasc Surg*. 2002;10(6):523-533.
6. Lee BB. Critical issues on the management of congenital vascular malformation. *Ann Vasc Surg*. 2004;18(3):380-392.
7. Belov ST. Anatomopathological classification of congenital vascular defects. *Semin Vasc Surg*. 1993;6:219-224.
8. Lee BB. Advanced management of congenital vascular malformation (CVM). *Int Angiol*. 2002;21(3):209-213.
9. St B. Classification of congenital vascular defects. *Int Angiol*. 1990;9:141-146.
10. Bastide G, Lefebvre D. Anatomy and organogenesis and vascular malformations. In: Belov DT, Loose DA, Weber J, eds. *Vascular Malformations*. Reinbek: Einhorn-Presse Verlag; 1989:20-22.
11. Lee BB, Kim DI, Huh S, et al. New experiences with absolute ethanol sclerotherapy in the management of a complex form of congenital venous malformation. *J Vasc Surg*. 2001;33: 764-772.
12. Lee BB, Do YS, Byun HS, Choo IW, Kim DI, Huh SH. Advanced management of venous malformation with ethanol sclerotherapy: mid-term results. *J Vasc Surg*. 2003;37(3):533-538.
13. Mattassi R. Differential diagnosis in congenital vascular-bone syndromes. *Semin Vasc Surg*. 1993;6:233-244.

14. St B. Correction of lower limbs length discrepancy in congenital vascular-bone disease by vascular surgery performed during childhood. *Semin Vasc Surg.* 1993;6:245-251.

15. Lee BB. Klippel–Trenaunay syndrome and pregnancy. *Int Angiol.* 2003;22(3):328.

16. Servelle M. Klippel and Trenaunay's syndrome. *Ann Surg.* 1985;201:365-373.

17. Lee BB, Choe YH, Ahn JM, et al. The new role of MRI (magnetic resonance imaging) in the contemporary diagnosis of venous malformation: can it replace angiography? *J Am Coll Surg.* 2004;198(4):549-558.

18. Lee BB. Current concept of venous malformation (VM). *Phlebolymphology.* 2003;43:197-203.

19. Lee BB, Mattassi R, Choe YH, et al. Critical role of duplex ultrasonography for the advanced management of venous malformation (VM). *Phlebology.* 2005;20:28-37.

20. Lee BB, Seo JM, Hwang JH, et al. Current concepts in lymphatic malformation (LM). *J Vasc Endovasc Surg.* 2005;39(1):67-81.

21. Lee BB, Kim DI, Whang JH, Lee KW. Contemporary management of chronic lymphedema – personal experiences. *Lymphology.* 2002;35(Suppl):450-455.

22. Lee BB, Mattassi R, Kim BT, Kim DI, Ahn JM, Choi JY. Contemporary diagnosis and management of venous and AV shunting malformation by whole body blood pool scintigraphy (WBBPS). *Int Angiol.* 2004; 23(4):355-367.

23. Lee BB, Kim BT, Choi JY, Cazaubon M. Prise en charge des malformations vasculaires congénitales (MVC) en 2003: rôle de la scintigraphy corps entier dans las surveillance évolutive. *Angeiologie.* 2003;55(3):17-26.

24. Lee BB, Mattassi R, Kim BT, Park JM. Advanced management of arteriovenous shunting malformation with transarterial lung perfusion scintigraphy (TLPS) for follow up assessment. *Int Angiol.* 2005;24(2):173-184.

25. Lee BB, Do YS, Yakes W, et al. Management of arterial-venous shunting malformations (AVM) by surgery and embolosclerotherapy. A multidisciplinary approach. *J Vasc Surg.* 2004;39(3):590-600.

26. Lee BB, Kim HH, Mattassi R, Yakes W, Loose D, Tasnadi G. A new approach to the congenital vascular malformation with new concept – Seoul Consensus. *Int J Angiol.* 2004;12:248-251.

27. Lee BB, Beaujean M, Cazaubon M. Nouvelles strategies dans la prise en charge des malformations vasculaires congenitales (MVC): un aperc[,]u de l'experience clinique coreenne. *Angeiologie.* 2004;56(2):11-25.

28. Yakes WF, Pevsner PH, Reed MD, Donohu HJ, Ghaed N. Serial embolizations of an extremity arteriovenous malformation with alcohol via direct percutaneous puncture. *AJR.* 1986;146:1038-1040.

29. Yakes WF, Haas DK, Parker SH, et al. Symptomatic vascular malformations: ethanol embolotherapy. *Radiology.* 1989;170:1059-1066.

30. Yakes WF, Parker SH, Gibson MD, Haas DK, Pevsner PH, Carter TE. Alcohol embolotherapy of vascular malformations. *Semin Intervent Radiol.* 1989;6:146-161.

31. Mulliken JB, Young AE, eds. *Vascular birthmarks: hemangiomas and malformations.* Philadelphia: W.B. Saunders; 1988.

32. Van Der Stricht J. Classification of vascular malformations. In: Belov ST, Loose DA, Weber J, eds. *Vascular Malformations.* Reinbek: Einhorn-Presse Verlag; 1989:23.

Klippel-Trenaunay Syndrome

45

Magdiel Trinidad-Hernandez and Peter Gloviczki

A 38-year-old woman with the diagnosis of Klippel-Trenaunay Syndrome (KTS) presents with severe pain over venous malformations on the left thigh and severe hyperhidrosis of the left leg and foot. She has a history of pulmonary embolism at age 17. Otherwise, she is healthy and compliant with the use of compression garments. The diagnosis of KTS was made soon after birth because of the port wine stains, slightly larger and longer leg and lateral varicose veins of her left leg. Physical examination shows a port wine nevus on the left buttock with varicose veins and soft tissue hypertrophy along the anterolateral aspect of the left leg and thigh. These areas are tender to palpation and leg elevation eases their appearance. Hyperhidrosis behind the knee and dorsum of the foot and in the interdigital spaces is obvious. Limb length discrepancy is 1 cm. The remainder of the exam is unremarkable.

Question 1

Which of the following is not a characteristic finding in patients with KTS?

A. High-flow arteriovenous shunting
B. Long bone hypertrophy
C. Lateral varicosity
D. Port wine nevus

No bruits or thrills were detected during the physical examination. If arteriovenous shunting is suspected further studies should be performed to characterize the anomaly. These include segmental limb pressures and ankle-brachial indices.

P. Gloviczki (✉)
Division of Vascular and Endovascular Surgery,
Gonda Vascular Center, Mayo Clinic, Rochester, MN, USA

G. Geroulakos and B. Sumpio (eds.), *Vascular Surgery*,
DOI: 10.1007/978-1-84996-356-5_45, © Springer-Verlag London Limited 2011

Question 2

The patient's pain is affecting her quality of life and she seeks surgical treatment. What conditions should be present prior to offering any type of surgical procedure?

A. Duplex ultrasound showing valvular incompetence and absence of DVT
B. Patent deep venous system
C. Sufficient collateral circulation
D. Outflow plethysmography without evidence of venous obstruction

The patient underwent a complete venous duplex ultrasound with valvular competence evaluation and magnetic resonance venography (MRV) (Fig. 45.1a and b). The deep venous system was found to be patent. Only mild left popliteal vein incompetence was encountered. The MRV confirms a patent and normal deep venous system. A large lateral vein perforates the fascia and gives rise to multiple varicosities in the lower thigh.

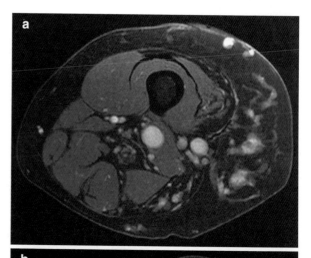

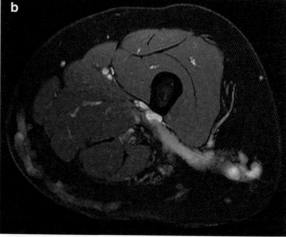

Fig. 45.1 (**a**) Magnetic resonance venography of the left thigh demonstrates low flow venous malformation of the lateral left thigh. There is a dilated lateral superficial vein and a dilated profunda femoris vein visible. Soft tissue hypertrophy are present in the lateral portion of the thigh. (**b**) A large lateral perforator vein is connected to multiple congenital varicose veins in the distal thigh

Question 3

What treatment options are suitable for this patient?

A. Vein stripping and phlebectomy
B. Endovenous closure
C. Sclerotherapy
D. Lumbar sympathectomy

The patient underwent lumbar sympathectomy, a temporary IVC filter placement, and ambulatory phlebectomy with ligation of the perforating embryonic vein and avulsion and excision of varicose veins and venous malformations of the left leg. There was no long lateral vein for treatment with endovenous closure. The operation was uneventful. The hyperhidrosis resolved and the limb swelling and pain improved. She continues to wear compression garments.

A 13-year-old boy with KTS presents for follow-up. He was first evaluated at 6 years of age when the diagnosis was made. Since then, he has been managed conservatively with elastic compression stockings. He has a prominent lateral vein with varicose veins of the right lateral leg and thigh. There are venular blebs in the lateral leg that occasionally bleed. There is a 1.5 cm limb discrepancy. He has never had cellulitis nor has he suffered thromboembolism. Otherwise, he is healthy. The patient is seeking surgical treatment for his varicose veins.

Question 4

What are the indications for treatment in patients with KTS?

A. Bleeding
B. Refractory venous ulcers
C. Soft tissue infection
D. Acute thromboembolism

Although the patient has not developed venous ulcers, infection or thromboembolism he has suffered from mild bleeding episodes and has significant pain. He is a candidate for varicose vein surgery.

Question 5

What tests should be performed to evaluate this patient prior to surgical intervention?

A. Outflow plethysmography and exercise plethysmography (calf muscle pump function) with and without thigh tourniquets
B. MRV

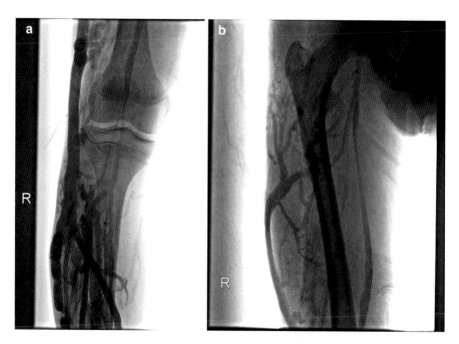

Fig. 45.2 (a) Ascending venogram demonstrates large lateral embryonic vein connected to multiple incompetent perforating veins in the right leg. The popliteal vein appears to be hypoplastic.(b) The lateral embryonic vein drains into the deep femoral vein

C. Ascending venogram
D. Duplex scanning

Ascending venogram demonstrates a large and distended lateral embryonic vein arising from multiple perforators in the leg and draining into the deep femoral vein (Fig. 45.2a and b). The paired popliteal veins are hypoplastic.

Question 6

What are the expected findings in outflow plethysmography?

A. The application of a tourniquet will decrease venous outflow.
B. The application of a tourniquet will have minimal effect on venous outflow.
C. Tourniquet use will not be helpful for the evaluation of this patient.

Outflow plethysmography demonstrated moderate right side venous obstruction in this patient. However, when a tourniquet was applied to the thigh and below the knee the venous outflow became severely obstructed (Fig. 45.3). This is strong evidence that the superficial veins are the primary route of venous drainage in the right limb.

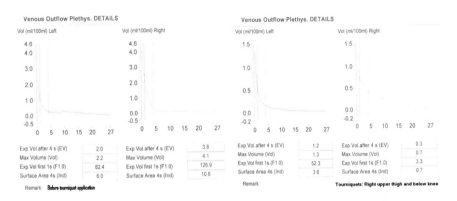

Fig. 45.3 Venous outflow plethysmography shows mild obstruction in the right limb. After tourniquet application there is a severe decrease in outflow

Question 7

What are the expected findings on exercise plethysmography?

A. Normal calf ejection fraction in the left limb
B. Reduced calf ejection fraction in the right limb
C. Both
D. Neither

Exercise plethysmography demonstrated a normal left calf ejection fraction. The right calf ejection fraction is severely reduced. The patient was encouraged to continue wearing elastic compression stockings. He will be evaluated again in 1 year. This may be enough time for the deep venous system to develop.

45.1
Commentary

Clinical Presentation

The triad of capillary malformation with port wine nevus, long bone hypertrophy, and lateral varicosity characterizes KTS (Fig. 45.4).[1][2] These lesions are frequently of lateral distribution and rarely cross the midline. Typically, one lower extremity is involved, but bilateral presentation or upper extremity involvement is possible. Occasionally, capillary or venous malformations can cause bleeding and cellulitis in patients with poor skin coverage. The same can occur through defects in the mucosa. Pelvic involvement with venous malformation may present with rectal bleeding or hematuria.[3] The hallmark of venous malformations in KTS is persistence of embryonic veins. The lateral marginal vein of Servelle has been the most typical finding.[4] Another persistent embryonic vein is

Fig. 45.4 Characteristic triad
of KTS: port wine stains,
lateral varicose veins, and
slightly longer extremity

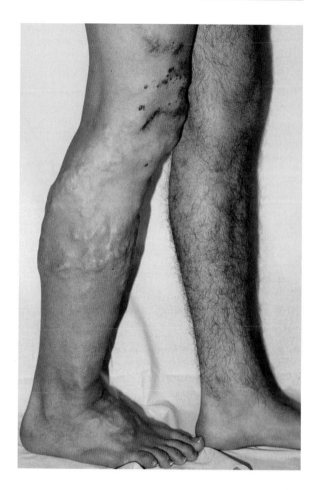

the sciatic vein.[5] The deep venous system may be anomalous. It may be hypoplastic, atretic, or much less frequent, non-existent. The deep venous valves may be hypoplastic or absent. [**Q1: A**]

Evaluation

Diagnostic tests in KTS should focus on the evaluation of the type, extent, and severity of the malformation. The absence of a clinically significant arteriovenous shunt should be confirmed. A thorough physical examination is complemented by color duplex of the venous system. This test can detect anomalies such as atresia, hypoplasia, and aneurysms of the deep veins. In addition, duplex can confirm patency and incompetence of deep, superficial, and perforator veins.

Plain X-rays of the long bones (scanogram) are helpful to measure length of bones. Magnetic resonance imaging can differentiate between muscle, bone, fat, and vascular tissue. Contrast venography can be performed through multiple injections in the limb. A tourniquet can be used to force contrast into the deep system to visualize it. Venography is frequently the only test that can help estimate the degree of deep venous occlusion and the presence of sufficient collateral circulation to permit excision or ablation of large incompetent superficial embryonic veins.[6] **[Q5: A, B, C, D]**

Strain gauge or air plethysmography has been utilized to compare the limbs of patients with KTS and normal controls. The limbs of patients with KTS are characterized by complex reflux patterns, severe valvular incompetence, calf muscle pump impairment, and venous hypertension.[7] **[Q6: A] [Q7: C]**

Treatment

Absolute indications for treatment in KTS include hemorrhage, infections, acute thromboembolism or refractory venous ulcers. Relative indications include pain, functional impairment, swelling due to chronic venous insufficiency, limb asymmetry or major cosmetic reasons. **[Q4: A, B, C, D]**

The management is mostly conservative. The mainstay has been compression therapy in the form of elastic garments, non-elastic bandages, and intermittent pneumatic compression. For venous swelling and chronic lymphedema physical therapy using massage treatment and physical decongestive therapy has been used with good success. The psychological impact caused by a visible deformity of KTS should not be underestimated. Participation of patients and families in support groups is strongly encouraged.[8]

Intervention is reserved for selectively symptomatic patients with KTS. A careful evaluation must precede any intervention. The extent of malformations and patency of the deep system must be assessed. High ligation of the incompetent marginal vein, invagination stripping of long superficial veins and ambulatory phlebectomy through stab wounds are the most commonly used techniques, although endovenous thermal ablation is gaining popularity and can be used in patients who do not have the lateral vein immediately under the skin. Tumescent anesthesia can be used to carefully separate the distance between the skin and the treated vein. **[Q2: A, B, C, D]**

Lumbar sympathectomy is helpful for occasional severe hyperhidrosis in these patients. The placement of a temporary IVC filter is indicated in patients with a history of pulmonary thromboembolism.

The use of subfascial endoscopic perforator surgery in patients with large incompetent perforating veins and venous ulcers has been useful and some patients benefit from deep venous reconstructions. Limb exsanguination with Esmarque bandage and tourniquet use help to reduce intraoperative blood loss during varicose vein avulsion or SEPS.[9]

Endovenous therapies have included sclerotherapy and embolotherapy with alcohol, sodium tetradecyl sulfate, and polidocanol. Serial sclerotherapy with alcohol has excellent results in 75–90% of patients with low-flow malformations according to Burrows.[10] However, caution should be used in malformations close to peripheral nerves. Foam sclerotherapy with Polidocanol or Sodium Tetradecyl sulfate is being used with success with increasing frequency.[11, 12] **[Q3: A, B, C, D]**

References

1. Baskerville PA, Ackroyd JS, Lea Thomas M, Browse NL. The Klippel-Trenaunay syndrome: clinical, radiological and haemodynamic features and management. *Br J Surg.* 1985;72(3): 232-236.
2. Jacob AG, Driscoll DJ, Shaughnessy WJ, Stanson AW, Clay RP, Gloviczki P. Klippel-Trenaunay syndrome: spectrum and management. *Mayo Clin Proc.* 1998;73(1):28-36.
3. Servelle M, Bastin R, Loygue J, et al. Hematuria and rectal bleeding in the child with Klippel and Trenaunay syndrome. *Ann Surg.* 1976;183(4):418-428.
4. Servelle M. Klippel and Trenaunay's syndrome. 768 operated cases. *Ann Surg.* 1985;201(3):365-373.
5. Cherry KJ, Gloviczki P, Stanson AW. Persistent sciatic vein: diagnosis and treatment of a rare condition. *J Vasc Surg.* 1996;23(3):490-497.
6. Gloviczki P, Driscoll J. Klippel-Trenaunay syndrome: current management. *Phlebology.* 2007;22(6):291-298.
7. Delis KT, Gloviczki P, Wennberg PW, Rooke TW, Driscoll DJ. Hemodynamic impairment, venous segmental disease, and clinical severity scoring in limbs with Klippel-Trenaunay syndrome. *J Vasc Surg.* 2007;45(3):561-567.
8. http://www.k-t.org/index/html
9. Noel AA, Gloviczki P, Cherry KJ, Rooke TW, Stanson AW, Driscoll DJ. Surgical treatment of venous malformations in Klippel-Trenaunay syndrome. *J Vasc Surg.* 2000;32:840-847.
10. Burrows PE, Mason KP. Percutaneous treatment of low flow vascular malformations. *J Vasc Interv Radiol.* 2004;15:431-445.
11. Cabrera J, Cabrera J Jr, Garcia-Olmedo MA, Redondo P. Treatment of venous malformations with sclerosant in microfoam form. *Arch Dermatol.* 2003;139(11):1409-1416.
12. Bergan J, Cheng V. Foam sclerotherapy of venous malformations. *Phlebology.* 2007;22(6): 299-302.

Part XII

Management of Venous Disorders

Deep Venous Thrombosis

46

Fahad S. Alasfar, Dwayne Badgett, and Anthony J. Comerota

A 67-year-old male had a history of a right calf deep venous thrombosis (DVT) following a flight from California to New York. He was treated on that occasion with anticoagulation with unfractionated heparin then Coumadin for 3 months. Recently, he was diagnosed with sigmoid cancer. He is now on postoperative day 3 from exploratory laparotomy, sigmoid colectomy and extensive lysis of adhesions. Although he was haemodynamically stable, he required a transfusion of three units of blood. DVT prophylaxis for the perioperative period included graded knee-high compressive stockings and intermittent pneumatic compression (IPC).

Question 1

What are the risk factors that predispose to DVT?

Question 2

What is the clinical presentation of a patient with anti-thrombin III (ATIII) deficiency?

Question 3

Regarding antiphospholipid antibody (APA) syndrome, which of the following is not correct?

A. Procainamide has been associated with the development of APA syndrome.
B. Thrombotic complications associated with APA syndrome are limited to the venous system.
C. Long-term anticoagulation has been recommended in managing APA syndrome, maintaining the international normalized ratio (INR) at 3 or higher.
D. Recurrent venous and arterial thrombosis is a major feature of the APA syndrome.

A.J. Comerota (✉)
Department of Surgery, Temple University Hospital, Philadelphia, PA, USA

G. Geroulakos and B. Sumpio (eds.), *Vascular Surgery*,
DOI: 10.1007/978-1-84996-356-5_46, © Springer-Verlag London Limited 2011

Question 4

Regarding Factor V Leiden gene mutation, which of the following is/are correct?

A. Factor V Leiden mutation is an important risk factor for pulmonary embolism and DVT during pregnancy or use of oral contraceptives.
B. Factor V Leiden mutation is associated with an increased risk of myocardial infarction and angina.
C. Hyperhomocystinaemia increases the risk of Factor V Leiden carriers having any Venous Thromboembolic Episodes (VTE) from 2% to 10%.
D. A single-point mutation in the gene coding for coagulation Factor V results in the formation of a Factor V molecule that is not inactivated properly by activated protein C (APC).

Question 5

Which of the following statements are true concerning prophylaxis for DVT?

A. There are many prospective randomised studies supporting the efficacy of graded compression stockings in preventing DVT in patients with malignancy.
B. IPC is as effective as low-dose unfractionated heparin (LDUH) in reducing the risk of DVT.
C. LDUH and low-molecular-weight heparin (LMWH) are most effective in preventing DVT.
D. Dextran is an excellent alternative to LDUH in preventing DVT.

On the fifth postoperative day, the patient began complaining of mild left calf pain and swelling. On physical examination, his lower extremities were warm with normal pulses. The left calf was mildly swollen with slight tenderness. A venous duplex of the lower extremity revealed thrombosis of the left popliteal, posterior tibial and peroneal veins.

Question 6

Which of the following statements regarding perioperative DVT is/are correct?

A. In general surgery, the overall incidence of DVT as assessed by labelled fibrinogen uptake (FUT) is 25%.
B. In surgical patients with malignant disease, the incidence of postoperative DVT is 60%.
C. The incidence of postoperative DVT after total hip replacement is 45–55%.
D. Major trauma patients have a low risk for DVT.
E. Patients undergoing elective neurosurgical procedures have a 20–25% incidence of DVT documented by radioisotopic scanning.

The patient was started on a therapeutic regimen of LMWH (enoxaparin) 1 mg/kg every 12 h and a daily dose of Coumadin. The patient's baseline coagulation profile was normal and his platelet count was 190,000.On day 3 of anticoagulation, his INR was 2.2 and his platelet count dropped to 67,000.

Question 7

Regarding heparin-induced thrombocytopoenia (HIT), which of the following is/are correct?

A. It is caused by IgM antibodies that recognise the complex of heparin and platelet factor 4.
B. The peak incidence occurs 4–14 days after initiation of heparin.
C. It occurs more commonly with unfractionated heparin than with LMWH.
D. It can be treated by reducing the dose of LMWH.
E. Argatroban and hirudin are acceptable agents used for the treatment of HIT.

LMWH was discontinued and the patient started on Argatroban. On the tenth postoperative day, the patient started complaining of left flank pain and his haemoglobin level dropped to 6 g/dL. A computed tomography (CT) scan of his abdomen revealed a 6 × 7-cm retroperitoneal haematoma. Because of the haematoma, anticoagulation was discontinued and an inferior vena cava (IVC) filter inserted.

Question 8

Which of the following are acceptable indications for an IVC filter?

A. Complication or contraindication to anticoagulation in a patient diagnosed with a pulmonary embolism
B. Recurrent thromboembolism despite therapeutic anticoagulation
C. Acute iliofemoral DVT
D. Recurrent pulmonary embolism with pulmonary hypertension

Question 9

Regarding thrombolysis for acute DVT, which of the following is/are correct?

A. Studies show no difference in lysis capability between anticoagulation and lytic therapy.
B. Randomised studies support lytic therapy for all lower-extremity DVT.
C. Patients with iliofemoral DVT treated with catheter-directed thrombolysis have a better quality of life than patients treated with anticoagulation alone.
D. Lytic agents are more effective when delivered by catheter-directed intrathrom-bus infusion rather than systemic intravenous infusion.

46.1
Commentary

The natural history of DVT has been described well in the literature. Complications of venous thromboembolism continue to be a major cause of death and morbidity each year. In the USA, there are approximately 50,000–200,000 deaths each year secondary to pulmonary embolism. Fifty-two percent of patients with DVT develop pulmonary embolism,[1] most of which occur from the proximal venous segments of the lower extremities.

Patients with proximal DVT had a pulmonary embolism incidence of 66%, whereas tibial thrombi had a 33% incidence.[1] Multiple studies have shown a 50% reduction in fatal pulmonary embolism when prophylaxis with LDUH is used.[2] Moreover, natural history studies have shown that the long-term morbidity of post-thrombotic syndrome (PTS) is significant following DVT. PTS has been reported in 33–79% of patients following proximal DVT and 2–29% of patients with calf DVT. Masuda et al.[3] reported valve reflux in 30% of individuals with calf DVT followed for 3 years. Furthermore, they reported that 23% of patients with calf DVT have ongoing pain and swelling of the affected extremity.

Thus, proper prophylaxis, early diagnosis and appropriate therapy are of paramount importance in preventing the short- and long-term complications of DVT.

An understanding of the risk factors for DVT is helpful for appropriate DVT prophylaxis. These risk factors include prior DVT/pulmonary embolism, prolonged immobilisation or paralysis, malignancy, major surgery (especially abdominal, hip and lower-extremity surgery), age over 40 years, and severe heart disease. There are also hypercoagulable states that predispose to thrombosis. Haematological abnormalities include protein C and protein S deficiency, Factor V mutation, disorders of plasminogen activation and antiphospholipid antibodies.

Lupus anticoagulant and HIT are also associated with DVT. Proteins C and S are part of the naturally occurring balance of coagulation that prevents thrombosis by inactivating Factors Va and VIIIa. Deficiency of these factors leads to an increased risk of thrombosis. Proteins C and S, like Factors II, VII, IX and X, depend on vitamin K. Because of the shorter half-life of protein C, a transient hypercoagulable state can be induced early in the course of treating patients with a warfarin compound due to the acute reduction in protein C level. A search for an underlying hypercoagulable disorder should be undertaken in patients with recurrent DVT or unexplained arterial or graft occlusion.

Chronic warfarin therapy may reduce the level of proteins C and S by 30–50%; therefore, these levels should be measured after the patient has discontinued warfarin. Indefinite oral anticoagulation is indicated in patients with confirmed deficiency. **[Q1]**

ATIII is an important naturally occurring anticoagulant that inhibits the enzymatic activation of thrombin and other naturally occurring clotting factors. The heterozygous form of ATIII deficiency is asymptomatic and may affect 1 in 2,000 people. A chronic deficiency of ATIII can occur with protein loss in nephrotic syndrome, liver disease, sepsis and Disseminated Intravascular Coagulation (DIC). When complications occur, heparin followed by Coumadin is the treatment of choice. **[Q2]**

APA is a heterogeneous group of circulating autoantibodies directed primarily against negatively charged phospholipid compounds. These antibodies interfere with the thromboplastin reaction against the activated platelet. Recurrent venous and arterial thrombosis is a major feature of APA syndrome. Thrombosis associated with APA syndrome has occurred in diverse anatomic locations, causing a wide spectrum of clinical manifestations. DVT and pulmonary embolism are common complications of APA.[4] Similarly, arterial thrombosis involving carotid,[5] hepatic, splenic, mesenteric and retinal arteries causing infarction has occurred. APA syndrome should be suspected in young patients with stroke or arterial occlusion.

APA syndrome has been associated with multiple medications. However, procainamide has been implicated more commonly than other drugs.[6]

The diagnosis should be suspected based on the clinical presentation or the unexplained prolonged PTT. Diagnostic tests for APA syndrome include serology testing for APA and clotting assays. The primary treatment remains anticoagulation, maintaining an INR at or above 3.0.[7,8] [Q3: B]

Protein C is one of the key regulatory proteins for coagulation cascade. APC cleaves and inactivates Factors Va and VIIIa. A single-point mutation in the gene coding for Factor V results in the formation of a Factor V molecule that is not inactivated properly by APC.[9] Factor V Leiden mutation is an important risk factor for pulmonary embolism and DVT, especially during pregnancy or oral contraceptive use.[10]

Hyperhomocystinaemia increases the relative risk of a Factor V leiden carrier having any VTE.[11] There is no increased risk of myocardial infarction or angina in patients with Factor V Leiden mutation.[12] [Q4: A, C, D]

Among the available methods of DVT prophylaxis, LDUH and LMWH are the most effective in reducing DVT as assessed by FUT.[13] LDUH was the first anti-thrombotic agent evaluated in early randomised studies. LDUH, dextran, IPC and graded elastic stockings also significantly reduce the incidence of postoperative DVT.[13]

LDUH given subcutaneously (5,000 U) every 8 or 12 h started preoperatively and continued postoperatively for 7 days has been shown to decrease the incidence of DVT from 25% to 8%.[14] Moreover, these studies have shown a 50% reduction of fatal pulmonary embolism when patients are treated with LDUH. LMWH and LDUH have been shown to be equally effective in preventing DVT in general surgery patients.[14]

Advantages of LMWH include improved bioavailability, once-daily dosing, and a lower incidence of HIT.[15]

IPC is an attractive method of DVT prophylaxis since there are no observed complications. This device provides intermittent compression lasting 10 s/min with insufflation pressures of 35–40 mmHg. In a trial comparing IPC with LDUH, both agents were effective in reducing lower-extremity DVT in high-risk patients.[16]

Graded compression stockings decrease the risk of DVT, but data are limited regarding the effect on the prevention of DVT and pulmonary embolism. There are no randomised trials on the use of these stockings alone in high-risk patients, although current recommendations suggest the use of more effective methods. Fifteen to 20% of patients will not receive benefit from elastic stockings because of their leg shape or size. Dextran has not been shown to be as effective as either LMWH or LDUH in preventing DVT; however, it may reduce the incidence of pulmonary embolism. Disadvantages of dextran include its high price, risk of anaphylaxis, potential for volume overload, and need for intravenous access. It is also contraindicated in patients with impaired renal and cardiac function. [Q5: B, C]

The incidence of DVT in general surgery patients has been well established. Overall, the incidence of DVT was 25% in general surgery patients not receiving prophylaxis. In patients with other risk factors, i.e., malignancy, the risk of DVT is 29%. Overall, the risk of pulmonary embolism is 1.6% while the risk of fatal pulmonary embolism is 0.8%.[13]

Patients undergoing major orthopaedic surgery of the lower extremity are at high risk of postoperative DVT, despite improved techniques and early mobilisation. The incidence of postoperative DVT after total hip replacement is 45–57%, with the risk of proximal DVT being 23–36%.[17] The incidence of pulmonary embolism in this group is 6–30% and that of fatal pulmonary embolism is 3–6%. Because many pulmonary embolisms are asymptomatic, and because of the high incidence of DVT in the postoperative period, proper prophylaxis is mandatory.[18]

DVT and pulmonary embolism are considered common complications after major trauma. A recent study using a venographic endpoint demonstrated that major trauma patients (injury severity score >9) have an exceptionally high risk of venous thromboembolism (58%). This study also revealed that there is a greater than 50% incidence of DVT in the major trauma subset.[19]

Pulmonary embolism is the most frequent reason for death following spinal cord injury. Clinically recognised DVT and pulmonary embolism occur in only 15% and 5% of cases, respectively.[20] However, the incidence of DVT in patients with acute spinal cord injury by venography has been reported to be between 18% and 100%, with an average of 40%. The incidence of fatal pulmonary embolism is 4.6%, with the greatest risk occurring in the first 2–3 months after spinal-cord injury.[21] **[Q6: A, C, E]**

Approximately 2–5% of patients exposed to heparin will develop HIT. This is caused by IgG antibodies that recognise complexes of heparin and platelet factor 4, leading to platelet activation via platelet Fc gamma IIa receptors. Formation of a procoagulant, platelet-derived microparticles generates thrombin and makes patients especially vulnerable to venous thromboembolism.[22,23]

When examined directly, the clot appears white due to the concentration of fibrin and platelets. HIT should be suspected if a patient develops DVT or pulmonary embolism while receiving heparin, especially if the platelet count drops below 35%. HIT usually develops between the 4th and 14th days after initiation of heparin, although a rapid fall in platelet count can occur in response to heparin if the patient has had recent heparin exposure.

HIT occurs much more commonly with unfractionated heparin than with LMWH.[15] Upon recognition of HIT, heparin should be discontinued; however, appropriate anticoagulation should be continued to avoid a thrombotic complication, which has been observed in up to 50% of patients within 30 days of the diagnosis of HIT.[15]

Current treatment options include lepirudin,[24] argatroban and danaparoid. Lepirudin is recombinant hirudin (r-hirudin) and is approved for the treatment of patients with HIT. It is a potent direct thrombin inhibitor and is given in a bolus dose of 0.4 mg/kg/min followed by an infusion of 0.2 mg/kg/h, but the dosage should be adjusted in patient with renal dysfunction. Argatroban is a synthetic peptide that binds to and inhibits thrombin. It is given in doses of 0.5–4 μg/kg/min and has the advantage of normal excretion (hepatic) in patients with impaired renal function. Danaparoid is a mixture of heparan sulphate and dermatan sulphate, which inhibits thrombin generation indirectly via inhibition of Factor

Xa, with some direct anti-thrombin activity as well. The disadvantage of danaparoid includes a 10–20% in vitro cross-reactivity with HIT antibodies and long half-life. **[Q7: B, C, E]**

IVC filters are intended to prevent pulmonary emboli following filter insertion. Anticoagulation should be continued whenever possible to prevent further thrombosis.[25,26] The primary indication for the insertion of an IVC filter is the occurrence of a complication of or contraindication for anticoagulation therapy. Less frequent indications for the insertion of an IVC filter are recurrent thromboembolism despite adequate anticoagulation therapy and chronic recurrent pulmonary embolism with pulmonary hypertension.

Finally, IVC filters have been used for pulmonary embolism prophylaxis in patients with proximal DVT who are at high risk for bleeding and selected trauma patients (pelvic fracture) who are at high risk for VTE and cannot be managed with effective prophylaxis. **[Q8: A, B, D]**

Restoring patency by eliminating the thrombus in the deep venous system is the ideal goal of therapy for acute DVT. Many reports have shown that lysis can be achieved and patency restored with thrombolysis, and that long-term sequelae occur less often with successful treatment.[27] Systemic thrombolytic therapy for lower-extremity DVT is associated with a 40–60% success rate. While recanalisation is better than standard anticoagulation, the increased risk of bleeding complications has reduced enthusiasm for thrombolysis.

It has been shown that patients with iliofemoral DVT treated with catheter-directed thrombolysis have better functioning and wellbeing than patients treated with anticoagulation alone.[28] Currently, it is recommended that lytic agents be delivered via catheter-directed technique into the thrombus. Thrombolytic therapy is recommended for patients with iliofemoral DVT and selected patients with infrainguinal DVT who are severely symptomatic due to multilevel thrombosis. **[Q9: C, D]**

References

1. Kistner RL, Ball JJ, Nordyke RA, Freeman GC. Incidence of pulmonary embolism in the course of thrombophlebitis. *Am J Surg*. 1972;124:169-176.
2. Collins R, Scrimgeour A, Yusuf S, Peto R. Reduction in fatal pulmonary embolism and venous thrombosis by perioperative administration of subcutaneous heparin: overview of results of randomized trials in general, orthopaedic, and urologic surgery. *N Engl J Med*. 1988;318: 1162-1173.
3. Masuda EM, Kessler DM, Kistner RL, Eklof B, Sato DT. The natural history of calf vein thrombosis: lysis of thrombi and development of reflux. *J Vasc Surg*. 1998;28:67-74.
4. Lechner K, Pabinger-Fasching I. Lupus anticoagulant and thrombosis: a study of 25 cases and review of the literature. *Haemostasis*. 1985;15:254-262.
5. Baker WH, Potthoff WP, Biller J, McCoyd K. Carotid artery thrombosis associated with lupus anticoagulant. *Surgery*. 1985;98:612-615.
6. Li GC, Greenberg CS, Currie MS. Procainamide-induced lupus anticoagulant and thrombosis. *South Med J*. 1988;81:262-264.
7. Asherson RA, Chan JK, Harris EN, Gharavi AE, Hughes GR. Anticardiolipin antibody, recurrent thrombosis, and warfarin withdrawal. *Ann Rheum Dis*. 1985;44:823-825.

8. Khamashta MA, Cuadrado MJ, Mujic F, Taub NA, Hunt BJ, Hughes GR. The management of thrombosis in the antiphospholipid-antibody syndrome. *N Engl J Med*. 1995;332:993-997.
9. Bertina RM, Koeleman BPC, Koster T, et al. Mutation in blood coagulation factor V associated with resistance to activated protein C. *Nature*. 1994;369:64-67.
10. Hirsh DR, Mikkola KM, Marks PW, et al. PE and DVT during pregnancy or oral contraceptive use: prevalence of factor V Leiden. *Am Heart J*. 1996;131:1145-1148.
11. Ridker PM, Glynn RJ, Miletich JP, Goldhaber SZ, Stampfer MJ, Hennekens CH. Age-specific incidence rates of venous thromboembolism among heterozygous carriers of factor V mutation. *Ann Intern Med*. 1997;126:528-531.
12. Cushman M, Rosendaal FR, Psaty BM. Factor V Leiden is not a risk factor for arterial vascular disease in the elderly: result from the cardiovascular health study. *Thromb Haemost*. 1998;79:912-915.
13. Geerts WH, Heit JA, Clagett GP, et al. Prevention of venous thromboembolism. *Chest*. 2001;119:132S-175S.
14. Clagett GP, Reisch JS. Prevention of venous thromboembolism in general surgical patients. Results of meta-analysis. *Ann Surg*. 1988;208:227-240.
15. Warkentin TE, Levine MN, Hirsh J, et al. Heparin-induced thrombocytopenia in patients treated with low-molecular-weight heparin or unfractionated heparin. *N Engl J Med*. 1995;332:1330-1335.
16. Nicolaides AN, Miles C, Hoare M, Jury P, Helmis E, Venniker R. Intermittent sequential pneumatic compression of the legs and thromboembolism-deterrent stockings in the prevention of postoperative deep venous thrombosis. *Surgery*. 1983;94:21-25.
17. Hoek JA, Nurmohamed MT, Hamelynck KJ, et al. Prevention of deep vein thrombosis following total hip replacement by low molecular weight heparinoid. *Thromb Haemost*. 1992;67:28-32.
18. Turpie AG, Levine MN, Hirsh J, et al. A randomized controlled trial of low-molecular-weight heparin (enoxaparin) to prevent deep-vein thrombosis in patients undergoing elective hip surgery. *N Engl J Med*. 1986;315:925-929.
19. Geerts WH, Code KI, Jay RM, Chen E, Szalai JP. A prospective study of venous thromboembolism after major trauma. *N Engl J Med*. 1994;331:1601-1606.
20. Waring WP, Karunas RS. Acute spinal cord injuries and the incidence of clinically occurring thromboembolic disease. *Paraplegia*. 1991;29:8-16.
21. Myllynen P, Kammonen M, Rokkanen P, Bostman O, Lalla M, Laasonen E. Deep venous thrombosis and pulmonary embolism in patients with acute spinal cord injury: a comparison with nonparalysed patients immobilized due to spinal fractures. *J Trauma*. 1985;25:541-543.
22. Warkentin TE. Heparin-induced thrombocytopenia: a ten-year retrospective. *Ann Rev Med*. 1999;50:129.
23. Magnani HN. Heparin induced thrombocytopenia (HIT): an overview of 230 patients treated with Orgaran (Org 10172). *Thromb Haemost*. 1993;70:554.
24. Greinacher A, Janssens U, Berg G, et al. Lepirudin (recombinant hirudin) for parenteral anticoagulation in patients with heparin-induced thrombocytopenia. *Circulation*. 1999;100:587-593.
25. Decousus H, Leizorovicz A, Parent F, et al. A clinical trial of vena caval filters in the prevention of pulmonary embolism in patients with proximal deep-vein thrombosis. *N Engl J Med*. 1998;338:409-415.
26. Becker DM, Philbrick JT, Selby JB. Inferior vena cava filters: indications, safety, effectiveness. *Arch Intern Med*. 1992;152:1985-1994.
27. Duckert F, Muller G, Nyman D, et al. Treatment of deep vein thrombosis with streptokinase. *BMJ*. 1975;1:479-481.
28. Comerota AJ, Throm RC, Mathias SD, Haughton S, Mewissen M. Catheter-directed thrombolysis for iliofemoral deep venous thrombosis improves health-related quality of life. *J Vasc Surg*. 2000;32:130-137.

Endoluminal Ablation of Varicose Veins

47

Cassius Iyad N. Ochoa Chaar and Jeffrey Indes

A 48-year-old male was referred by his primary care physician (PCP) for evaluation of varicose veins (VV) in his right leg. The patient noted the varicosities in his twenties. Initially, he was not concerned with the cosmetic appearance and decided not to seek medical attention. The VV became progressively more prominent. He started to complain of right leg pain and fatigue associated with mild edema 6 months prior to referral. The pain increased during the day and was unbearable in the evening after work. The patient works as a barber and needs to stand most of the day. His past medical history is significant for a motor vehicle accident 10 years ago. He only takes NSAIDs occasionally to relieve his leg pain. The patient finally decided to seek medical attention. His primary care physician prescribed him compression stockings that he used for 3 months with minimal improvement.

Question 1

At this point, what other information would you like to obtain?

A. What where the circumstances of the motor vehicle accident?
B. Does the patient have family history of VV?
C. Was the diagnosis of deep vein thrombosis (DVT) entertained by the PCP and was there any duplex ultrasound (DU) performed?
D. Was the patient compliant with the compression stocking, and did he wear the appropriate stocking?

The patient recalled the car accident. He was a front seat passenger and the car was hit on his side at a moderate speed. He remembers receiving a CT scan. The doctors told him his only injury was a rib fracture on the right side. He did not require hospitalization and was ambulating the same day. The patient has two sisters with VV that were first noticed during

C.I.N.O. Chaar (✉)
General Surgery Department, Yale New Haven Hospital, New Haven, CT, USA

G. Geroulakos and B. Sumpio (eds.), *Vascular Surgery*,
DOI: 10.1007/978-1-84996-356-5_47, © Springer-Verlag London Limited 2011

491

pregnancy but did not require surgical intervention. He denies receiving an ultrasound recently. He shows you the compression stockings which were fitted by the same company you routinely refer your patients to. He tells you:

I wear those socks as soon as I wake up in the morning and take them off before sleeping.

Question 2

Which statement(s) is/are true regarding VV?
A. VV are extremely common and are present in 90% of the population.
B. Risk factors are age, female sex hormones, and hereditary.
C. Most patients present because of leg pain.
D. Venous ulcers typically occur over the metatarsal heads and other weight baring spots in the foot.

Question 3

Which of the following statement(s) is/are true regarding compression stockings?

A. Stockings decrease venous reflux and leg swelling but increase veno-muscular efficiency.
B. Prescription of stockings is classified according to the pressure level required – Class 1 stockings exert the least sub-bandage pressure (14–21 mmHg).
C. The classification of compression stockings is internationally standardized.
D. The application of compression stockings is safe and has no reported complications.
E. The treatment of VV with compression stockings as first line modality is supported by level 1 evidence.

You examine the patient and you notice significant dilatation along the antero-medial aspect of the right thigh and leg as shown in Fig. 47.1. There is no ulceration or pigmenta-tion. The left leg is normal.

Question 4

How would you like to proceed with the evaluation? What information would you like to obtain?

A. Hand held Doppler can help to assess reflux.
B. DU will provide most of the information needed.
C. Rule out the presence of a DVT.
D. Assess saphenofemoral junction (SFJ) and sapheno-popliteal junction (SPJ) for reflux.
E. Look for incompetent perforators.

You obtain a DU that does not show evidence of DVT. There is reflux only at the SFJ without the presence of incompetent perforators.

Fig. 47.1 Patient's right leg with VV upon presentation

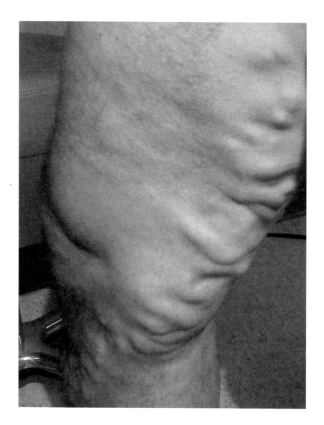

Question 5

What treatment options can you offer to the patient?

A. High Ligation and Stripping
B. Endovenous laser therapy (EVLT)
C. Endovenous radiofrequency ablation (RFA)

Initially the patient asks you to explain to him what would be the most conservative treatment modality. He has a conservative mentality and does not want to "try anything new."

Question 6

The True statement(s) about high ligation and stripping is (are):

A. High ligation without stripping predisposes patient to recurrence.
B. High ligation and stripping of the small saphenous vein (SSV) is associated with a higher rate of complications as compared with high ligation alone.

C. High ligation and stripping is no longer the gold standard of treatment of VV after the introduction of endoluminal therapy.
D. The improvement in quality of life with VV surgery is comparable to the improvement that patients with billiary colic get after laparoscopic cholecystectomy.

After explaining what an open procedure entails, you explain to the patient the different endoluminal options. He finds endoluminal treatment appealing and elects to proceed with EVLT. After obtaining informed consent, the patient's right leg is prepped and draped sterile. The patient is initially positioned in reverse Trendelenburg and venous access is obtained in the greater saphenous vein (GSV) just below the knee with a 4F micropuncture set. The micropuncture sheath is replaced with the long 5F sheath and the laser fiber is exposed and positioned at 2.0 cm below the SFJ and 1.55 cm below the superficial epigastric vein (SEV) under ultrasound guidance (Fig. 47.2).

The patient is then positioned in Trendelenburg and 500cc of tumescent anesthesia are administered around the GSV. The power is set at 14J and the treatment starts while simultaneously pulling back on the sheath and the laser probe at 1 cm every 5 s. You examine the vein with DU and find it devoid of flow with evidence of thrombosis of the entire treatment length. The absence of extension of thrombosis into the superficial femoral vein through the SFJ is confirmed. There is no evidence of DVT with good flow observed within the common femoral vein. In addition, the very proximal GSV and SEV have evidence of flow proximal to the ablated segment. An ACE wrap is applied to the right lower extremity for two days. The patient is recommended to continue using compression stockings for one month.

Question 7

Which statement(s) is/are true about tumescent anesthesia?

A. It is a unique type of anesthesia used only with EVLT.
B. It is administered around the vein and helps prevent conduction of heat to surrounding tissue.

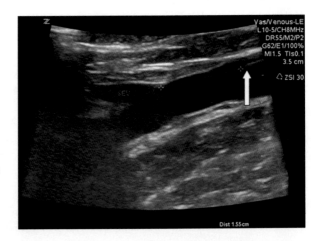

Fig. 47.2 DU showing the tip of the probe in the GSV (*arrow*) positioned at 1.55 cm distal to the Superficial Epigastric Vein (SEV)

C. It increases the efficacy of treatment by compressing the vein and causing vasospasm.

D. It is associated with a small increase in nerve injury because of the increase in tissue pressure.

Question 8

Which of the following is/are characteristic of EVLT?

A. EVLT is more effective than high ligation and stripping for treatment of VV.

B. The ideal position of the catheter tip should be right at the SFJ to accomplish complete thrombosis of the dilated GSV and prevent recurrence.

C. here is no significant difference in the effectiveness of the different laser wavelengths (810, 980, 1,320, and 1,470 nm) used.

D. DVT can occur from extension of thrombosis into the deep system. Most clots resolve within 3 months and do not lead to pulmonary embolization (PE).

Question 9

The statement(s) that is/are correct about RFA is (are):

A. RFA relies on direct contact of the catheter with vessel wall.

B. Most studies on RFA were performed using the VNUS Closure device with a continuous catheter pullback technique.

C. Body Mass Index (BMI) and catheter pullback rate are predictors of failure of RFA.

D. The RFA probe typically heats the vein wall to a temperature of 250°C for successful obliteration.

The patient presents for follow up one week after the procedure. DU shows obliteration of the GSV and a competent proximal GSV (Fig. 47.3). There is no evidence of DVT. The large dilated vessels did not show however complete resolution externally. He returns 3 months later asking for removal of the residual varices. You proceed with stab avulsions in the operating room resulting in complete resolution of the VV.

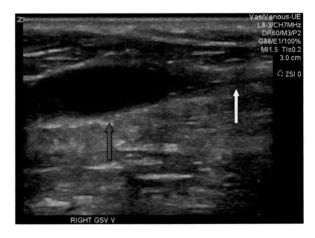

Fig. 47.3 DU showing complete obliteration of the treated segment (*white arrow*). The proximal GSV is patent (*red arrow*) and there is no extension of the thrombosis into the deep system

47.1
Commentary

VV are visible dilatation involving predominantly the two major superficial veins of the lower extremities: the GSV and the SSV. It is a common disease in adults affecting 15% of men and 25% of women.[1] [**Q 2-A: F**] Incidence increases with age and with positive family history. The ratio of progesterone to estrogen seems to affect venous insufficiency. Most women have increase in symptoms during pregnancy. [**Q 2-B: T**] Patient with varicose veins seek treatment mostly for cosmetic reasons. [**Q 2-C: F**] Some patients present with pain especially at the end of the day after standing for long periods of time and causing excess engorgement of their varicosities. They may also complain of leg cramping and a sensation of heaviness. Lower extremity swelling is sometimes associated with VV. Overlying skin changes may occur and consist of brown discoloration, lipodermatosclerosis, or frank ulceration. Venous ulcers are typically located over the malleoli while arterial ulcers arise on the toes and the metatarsal heads. [**Q 2-D: F**]

Compression stocking is the first line treatment for VV despite the lack of level 1 evidence as recently reviewed by Palfreyman and Michaels.[2] [**Q 3-E: F**] Stocking increase veno-muscular efficiency, and reduce venous reflux and leg edema. [**Q 3-A: T**] The classification of stockings is based on the level of compression applied. Class 1 has the lowest sub-bandage pressure between 14 and 21 mmHg. [**Q 3-B: T**] The classification is not standardized and varies between different countries. [**Q 3-C: F**] In the United States, Class 1, 2, and 3 stockings exert 15–20, 20–30, and 30–40 mmHg respectively. There is no consensus whether thigh or knee length is better. The class prescribed depends on the size and shape of the leg as well as the level of activity of the patient. Poorly fitted stockings can cause tissue necrosis and potentially amputation especially in patients with arterial insufficiency. [**Q 3-D: F**] It is safer to measure an ABI on elderly patients before prescribing stockings.[2]

Surgical treatment of VV underwent a dramatic evolution with the introduction of endoluminal therapy. The traditional procedure is ligation and stripping of the involved vein that has been practiced for over 100 years.[3] Newer technology using laser or radiofrequency ablation can achieve the same goal using often a single small incision. The short-term effectiveness of endoluminal therapy seems to be comparable to open ligation and stripping. However, long term results and safety profile are still under investigation.

Current surgical options include high ligation and stripping of the refluxing vein, as well as ablation with RFA or EVLT. [**Q 6-C: F**] High ligation alone is not sufficient and predisposes patients to recurrence as shown by the group from Gloucestershire. [**Q 6-A: T**] They followed 100 patients that underwent high ligation with and without routine stripping of the GSV. Patients undergoing high ligation only had significantly higher rates of recurrence at 5 years[4] and 11 years.[5] O'Hare et al. examined surgical treatment of SSV varicosities in 234 legs in 219 patients. Patients that had stripping in addition to SPJ ligation had significantly lower incidence of SPJ reflux at 1 year (13%) as compared to patients who had isolated SPJ ligation (32%). The complication rate was comparable between the two groups.[6] [**Q 6-B: F**] High ligation and stripping is very effective for the treatment of VV. The improvement in quality of life is remarkable and comparable to the improvement in quality of life of patients with billiary colic who undergo laparoscopic cholecystectomy.[7] [**Q 6-D: T**]

Tumescent anesthesia is the injection of a solution of local anesthetic around the VV to be treated with an endoluminal modality. [**Q7-A: F**] The injection is done under DU guidance to avoid inadvertent injection into the vein or injury to adjacent nerves or arteries. Large volume of fluid should be used especially with the SSV to separate it from the sural nerve. The injection facilitates the dissection of the vein from the surrounding soft tissue. It also protects neighboring structures and overlying skin from thermal injury by acting as a heat sink. [**Q7-B: T**; **7-D: F**] In addition to providing prolonged analgesia lasting to the postoperative period, tumescence compresses the vein and causes it to spasm making the delivery of thermal energy more effective.[8] [**Q7-C: T**]

EVLT relies on the introduction of a catheter into the dilated vein under DU guidance. The tip of the catheter is a laser fiber placed 1.5–2.0 cm distal to the junction of the superficial vein with the deep venous system. [**Q8-B: F**] After confirmation of the location of the tip, energy is delivered to denature collagen in the vessel wall and denude the endothelium. Eventually, the vessel contracts and gets obliterated by fibrosis. The optimal wavelength of the laser used is a subject of ongoing research. Kabnick compared the wavelength of 810 nm and 980 nm in 51 patients. His results showed less pain using the 980 nm wavelength.[9] More recent reports have looked at a higher wavelength (1,470 nm) that is preferentially absorbed by water as opposed to hemoglobin. It may better target the vessel wall and allow closure of the veins with less total energy delivered and consequently less pain and ecchymosis.[10] [**Q8-C: F**]

Rasmussen et al. conducted a randomized trial comparing EVLT of GSV with high ligation and stripping. Both procedures were performed in an office setting with tumescent anesthesia. The success rates and the complication rates for the two procedures were comparable. The only difference was that patients undergoing high ligation and stripping had increased postoperative pain and bruising.[11] Darwood et al. showed similar results in 118 patients. EVLT with SFJ ligation and stripping had comparable efficacy in abolishing reflux and had comparable safety profile. [**Q8-A: F**] Patients returned to normal activity and resumed work earlier after EVLT. The authors did not do a cost analysis but postulated that earlier return to normal activity (5 days earlier) and work (13 days earlier) might confer a socioeconomic advantage to EVLT.[12]

Endovenous techniques for treatment of VV can be complicated by DVT and occasionally PE. Thus, most specialists recommend follow up DU within a week of the procedure. The imaging can document success of the procedure and detect the presence of DVT resulting from clot extension into the deep system. To avoid this complication, most vascular surgeons leave the proximal 1.5–2.0 cm of the GSV untreated. The incidence of DVT is less than 1% in most series with occasional PEs.[13] [**Q8-D: T**] The use of perioperative DVT prophylaxis with heparin products may help decrease the incidence of thrombosis.

The application of RFA is analogous to EVLT. A catheter is introduced in the dilated veins with an electrode extending from the tip. A generator delivers the radiofrequency energy necessary to keep the vein wall heated to 85–120°C. [**Q9-D: F**] The catheter contains a feedback mechanism that evaluates vein wall impedance and adjusts the energy delivered to keep the temperature at a set target. Heat causes contraction of the vessel wall and complete obliteration. [**Q9-A: T**] Emptying the vein from blood by putting the patient in Trendelenburg and compression are crucial since the effectiveness of the treatment relies on the contact with the vein wall. The first catheter used for RFA is the VNUS closure system (VNUS Medical Technologies Inc., San Jose, CA, USA). It requires a continuous pullback technique and it is the catheter used in most published papers. [**Q9-B: T**] In 2006, VNUS introduced the ClosureFast segmental ablation catheter. The new catheter allows RFA of a 7 cm segment of superficial vein in 20 s without continuous pull-back. The advantage is a faster and more consistent ablation.[14] Merchant et al. reported the largest series of patients undergoing RFA. They followed 1,006 patients (1,222 limbs) up to 5 years and reported occlusion rate of 87.2% at the end of the follow up period. Linear regression showed that BMI and speed of catheter pullback were predictors of failure.[15] [**Q9-C: T**]

References

1. Callam MJ. Epidemiology of varicose veins. *Br J Surg*. 1994;81(2):167-173.
2. Palfreyman SJ, Michaels JA. A systematic review of compression hosiery for uncomplicated varicose veins. *Phlebology*. 2009;24(Suppl 1):13-33.
3. Perkins JM. Standard varicose vein surgery. *Phlebology*. 2009;24(Suppl 1):34-41.
4. Dwerryhouse S, Davies B, Harradine K, Earnshaw JJ. Stripping the long saphenous vein reduces the rate of reoperation for recurrent varicose veins: five-year results of a randomized trial. *J Vasc Surg*. 1999;29(4):589-592.
5. Winterborn RJ, Foy C, Earnshaw JJ. Causes of varicose vein recurrence: late results of a randomized controlled trial of stripping the long saphenous vein. *J Vasc Surg*. 2004;40(4):634-639.
6. O'Hare JL, Vandenbroeck CP, Whitman B, et al. A prospective evaluation of the outcome after small saphenous varicose vein surgery with one-year follow-up. *J Vasc Surg*. 2008;48(3):669-673. discussion 674.
7. Sam RC, Darvall KA, Adam DJ, Silverman SH, Bradbury AW. A comparison of the changes in generic quality of life after superficial venous surgery with those after laparoscopic cholecystectomy. *J Vasc Surg*. 2006;44(3):606-610.
8. Bhayani R, Lippitz J. Varicose veins. *Dis Mon*. 2009;55(4):212-222.
9. Kabnick LS. Outcome of different endovenous laser wavelengths for great saphenous vein ablation. *J Vasc Surg*. 2006;43(1):88-93.
10. Almeida J, Mackay E, Javier J, Mauriello J, Raines J. Saphenous laser ablation at 1470 nm targets the vein wall, not blood. *Vasc Endovascular Surg*. 2009;43(5):467-472.
11. Rasmussen LH, Bjoern L, Lawaetz M, Blemings A, Lawaetz B, Eklof B. Randomized trial comparing endovenous laser ablation of the great saphenous vein with high ligation and stripping in patients with varicose veins: Short-term results. *J Vasc Surg*. 2007;46(2):308-315.
12. Darwood RJ, Theivacumar N, Dellagrammaticas D, Mavor AI, Gough MJ. Randomized clinical trial comparing endovenous laser ablation with surgery for the treatment of primary great saphenous varicose veins. *Br J Surg*. 2008;95(3):294-301.
13. Mozes G, Kalra M, Carmo M, Swenson L, Gloviczki P. Extension of saphenous thrombus into the femoral vein: A potential complication of new endovenous ablation techniques. *J Vasc Surg*. 2005;41(1):130-135.
14. Gohel MS, Davies AH. Radiofrequency ablation for uncomplicated varicose veins. *Phlebology*. 2009;24(Suppl 1):42-49.
15. Merchant RF, Pichot O, Closure Study Group. Long-term outcomes of endovenous radiofrequency obliteration of saphenous reflux as a treatment for superficial venous insufficiency. *J Vasc Surg*. 2005;42(3):502-509. discussion 509.

Ultrasound Guided Foam Sclerotherapy for the Management of Recurrent Varicose Veins

Christopher R. Lattimer and George Geroulakos

A 67-year old man presented with left leg discomfort and gaiter itch which interfered with his retirement lifestyle. His symptoms were worse after prolonged standing and towards the end of the day. Below knee graduated compression stockings (GCS) provided him with some relief. He suffered with poliomyelitis at 12 years old which caused leg muscle wasting. Seven years previously he had his left great saphenous vein (GSV) stripped with multiple avulsions with removal of all varicosities. This alleviated similar symptoms but resulted in persistent ankle edema.

Question 1

Which of the following are recurrent varicose veins?

A. Varicose veins emptying into a neovascularisation following crossectomy.
B. Residual veins after incomplete phlebectomy.
C. Remaining varicosities after endovenous laser ablation.
D. Remaining varicosities after foam sclerotherapy.
E. Primary short saphenous varicosities after a GSV strip.

The patient had already undergone surgical treatment for his varicose veins in the same leg so he has recurrences.

Question 2

Which investigation is the most useful in the management of recurrent varicose veins and why?

A. CT Venography
B. Venous Duplex
C. Air plethysmography
D. Contrast venography

C.R. Lattimer (✉)
Department of Vascular Surgery, Ealing Hospital NHS Trust, Middlesex, UK

G. Geroulakos and B. Sumpio (eds.), *Vascular Surgery*,
DOI: 10.1007/978-1-84996-356-5_48, © Springer-Verlag London Limited 2011

A venous Duplex scan demonstrated a large varicosity 5 mm in diameter in the calf which was fed by an incompetent medial calf perforator. There was no communication with the below knee GSV remnant which was patent, only 1 mm in diameter and without reflux. All deep veins were patent and all without reflux.

Question 3

The treatment aims can best be described as:

A. Prophylaxis against venous ulceration
B. Normalisation of calf muscle pump function
C. Improvement on quality of life
D. Improvement of cosmetic appearance
E. Removal of all duplex abnormalities

The patient was told that he had recurrent varicose veins and that his symptoms were typical. Treating them was therefore likely to improve matters. He was warned that he may require further injections to completely eradicate his varicose veins, and a DVT and PE risk of less than 1%. Varying degrees of phlebitis with pain, hyperpigmentation and induration were likely and reflected the treatment process.

Question 4

Why is foam better than liquid sclerotherapy?

A. Through a transmural chemical injury to the vein wall.
B. It causes thrombosis of the injected vein.
C. It displaces venous blood.
D. Through improved surface contact.
E. Foam is compressible, liquids are not.

Question 5

What is the recommended maximum amount of foam that can be injected in a single treatment session?

A. 10 ml.
B. 12 ml.
C. 16 ml.
D. 24 ml.
E. The volume depends on the size of the varicose reservoir on ultrasound.

The patient was scanned by ultrasound whilst standing to confirm the extent of superficial venous reflux and determine a suitable site for cannulation. A medial calf perforator was identified and marked with a pen (Fig. 48.1). The patient was placed supine and a distal part

Fig. 48.1 The varicosity distends as foam is injected up to the site of a perforator (marked)

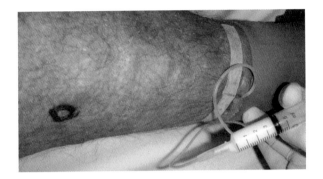

Fig. 48.2 The treated varicosity is isolated between a partially applied stocking and direct digital pressure on the perforator

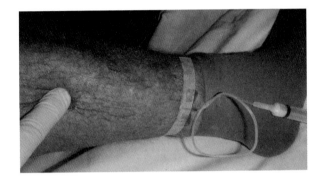

of the varicosity was cannulated with a 21 gauge butterfly needle and secured with tape. A high thigh GCS was partially applied over the foot and ankle and the leg was elevated to empty the veins. The leg was then injected with foam under ultrasound guidance. After 5 ml, syringe resistance increased and further injections were stopped. Digital pressure was applied over the perforator for 2 min and the patient remained resting for a further 10 min (Fig. 48.2). The rest of the stocking was applied and the waist attachment was secured.

Question 6

Which of the following methods may improve the efficacy of foam?

A. Multiple small dose injections.
B. Type of gas used.
C. Leg elevation.
D. Gas/liquid ratio.
E. Elastic graded compression bandaging.

Foam was prepared in 6 ml aliquots by agitating 1.2 ml of 1% liquid sodium tetradecylsulphate (STD Pharmaceuticals™) with 4.8 ml of air in separate syringes connected by a partially opened three way stopcock. The syringes were alternately depressed in rapid succession for several cycles immediately prior to injection.

Question 7

Suggest a possible cause for ankle swelling after long saphenous stripping and why this complication may be avoided by using foam for recurrences?

The ankle swelling could have been related to a DVT following the last operation but there was no evidence of this on the venous Duplex examination.

Question 8

Place the following complications and side effects of foam in ascending order of incidence?

A. Headache
B. Deep vein thrombosis
C. Induration and skin discolouration/hyperpigmentation
D. Pulmonary embolism
E. Visual disturbance

There were no side effects at the time of injection. At a 3 week follow up there was induration and mild hyperpigmentation along the course of the destroyed varicosity but no tenderness or concerns from the patient. His symptoms had all resolved and the ankle edema had disappeared. This may have been related to the GCS. A routine venous Duplex scan demonstrated complete obliteration. The femoral, popliteal and deep calf veins were all patent.

48.1
Commentary

Ultrasound guided foam sclerotherapy (UGFS) has become an effective and safe treatment option for symptomatic recurrent varicose veins. A single sclerotherapy session is adequate in over half of patients. Over an 18 month period with repeated sessions, 87% of legs may achieve immediate elimination of all varicosities. Potential complications such as deep vein thrombosis or systemic side-effects are rare. The superficial nature of recurrences however predispose to thrombophlebitis in 8.2% of patients without proximal reflux and up to 33% of those patients with reflux.[1]

Recurrent varicose veins following open surgery range from 20% to 80% between 5 and 20 years.[2] A formal definition of recurrence is imprecise. The international consensus meeting defined recurrent varicose veins after surgery (REVAS) as the presence of varicose veins in a lower limb previously treated surgically for varices with or without adjuvant therapies. This definition is clinical and includes "true recurrences," residual veins and varicose veins as a consequence of disease progression.[2] [Q1: A, B, C, E] Foam sclerotherapy is now both a primary therapy as well as an adjuvant treatment and it is not clear if it should be considered as an operation. Furthermore, several treatment sessions are often required to complete a treatment period which makes this definition grey between individual treatment sessions.

Venous duplex imaging should be considered mandatory in the investigation of recurrent varicose veins. It provides anatomy and quantifies reflux in varicosities and individual superficial and deep veins following a manual calf compression and release manoeuvre. It is also an essential tool in the classification of surgical recurrences.[3,4] **[Q2: B]** CT Venography is rarely necessary but may be helpful in the diagnosis of unilateral limb swelling such as occult pelvic vein thrombosis or May Thurner Syndrome.[5] Air plethysmography is a non-invasive investigation in the assessment of calf muscle pump function and global venous reflux. A rapid venous filling index (>2.5 ml/s) or large venous reservoir may help in the assessment in patients with complex symptoms and concomitant pathologies.[6] A diminished ejection fraction would suggest weakness of the calf muscle. Contrast venography is the most invasive of all the tests and useful for the assessment of the deep venous system in patients with malformations such as Klippel-Trenaunay syndrome[7] or deep venous obstruction prior to stent insertion.

The aim of any individual treatment should be to improve the quality of life during the everyday activities of a patient. The treatment of recurrent varicose veins is no exception. **[Q3: C]** Both generic and venous disease specific assessments are complimentary and advocated as a reporting standard.[8] Patient satisfaction depends on the success of treating the presenting complaint in parallel with the patients expectations and the potential side-effects or complications of any proposed treatment. The Aberdeen Questionnaire has been validated as a measurement of disease specific health outcome in patients with varicose veins and is scored from 0 to 100.[9]

The mechanism of action of foam is through a chemical injury to the vein endothelium resulting in a chemical phlebitis. The injury is endothelial but the inflammation is transmural. External compression with a GCS is required to prevent luminal thrombosis and subsequent thrombothlebitis. Foam is far more effective that liquids because of the increased surface area provided by the micro bubbles which make contact with the venous endothelium. Foam also has the property of displacing any remaining blood within its path as it is being injected. Furthermore, the compressible nature of foam hampers its progression within the circulation. **[Q4: C, D, E]**

Current European safety recommendations limit foam administration to 10 ml.[10] **[Q5: A]**This is 2 ml less than the recommended maximum in 2004.[11] Despite this advice, serious complications can still occur after an injection of only 10 ml as illustrated in a 52 year old woman with a patent foramen ovale who suffered a TIA for 30 min.[12] When the volume of injected foam becomes excessive, strokes are possible.[13]

Foam is prepared using the three way tap technique described by Tessari.[14] A vigorous movement is required over a partially occluded tap to ensure maximal agitation of liquid and gas. The foam should be used immediately before the micro bubbles have a chance of uniting and enlarging. The sclerosant is usually polidocanol or sodium tetradecylsulphate which are both detergents and come in concentrations from 1% to 3%. With larger caliber and relatively straight veins a catheter is advised to facilitate foam delivery because there is a diminished risk of intra-arterial injection and extravasation.[15] There is evidence that the physiological gas carbon dioxide is safer than air with a reduction in overall side-effects from 39% to 11%.[16] [**Q6: B**] Multiple small-dose injections have been shown to reduce the passage of sclerosant foam into the deep veins using ultrasound inspection immediately post sclerotherapy.[17] [**Q6: A**]The optimum ratio of gas to liquid is 4:1 although a large range of ratios are reported. [**Q6: D**] Leg elevation is advised prior to injection to empty the venous reservoir and reduce the amount of blood contact which can de-activate foam.[18] [**Q6: C**] A high thigh GCS applied for 2–3 weeks has been shown to be more effective and cheaper than compression bandaging with a reduction in thrombophebitis.[19] [**Q6: E**] Our protocol is to apply this stocking at the time of sclerotherapy and instruct the patient to wear this continuously for 2 weeks, but only during the day on the third week.

Ankle swelling is part of the staging and severity in venous disease and is therefore most likely to be related to venous insufficiency.[20,21] Oedema after surgical treatment however raises the possibility of a DVT or lymphatic compromise. Conventional varicose vein surgery has been shown to cause lymphatic damage.[22] It is likely that this may contribute to ankle swelling and lymphedema in predisposed patients. Foam sclerotherapy has not been shown to cause lymphatic disruption and subsequent lymphedema. Its use in recurrent disease will prevent this complication by removing the need for redo groin surgery. [**Q7**]

The incidence of complications and side effects are as follows: headache (4.2%), deep vein thrombosis (under 1%), induration/pigmentation (17.8%), pulmonary embolism (under 1%) and visual disturbance (1.4%).[23] [**Q8**] The incidence of a patent foramen ovale is 27%[24] which may explain the presence of left sided heart micro bubbles after foam treatment in several patients.[25] Their clinical significance and correlation with transient neurological complications however remains unclear.

References

1. Kakkos SK, Bountouroglou DG, Azzam M, Kalodiki E, Daskalopoulos M, Geroulakos G. Effectiveness and safety of ultrasound-guided foam sclerotherapy for recurrent varicose veins: immediate results. *J Endovasc Ther*. 2006;13:357-364.
2. Perrin MR, Guex JJ, Ruckley CV, et al. Recurrent varices after surgery (REVAS), a consensus document. *Cardiovasc Surg*. 2000;8(4):233-245.
3. Fischer R, Linde N, Duff C, Jeanneret C, Chandler JG, Seeber P. Late recurrent saphenofemoral junction reflux after ligation and stripping of the greater saphenous vein. *J Vasc Surg*. 2001;34:236-240.
4. Winterborn RJ, Foy C, Earnshaw JJ. Causes of varicose vein recurrence: Late results of a randomized controlled trial of stripping the long saphenous vein. *J Vasc Surg*. 2004;40: 634-639.
5. Lamont JP, Pearl GJ, Patetsios P, et al. Prospective evaluation of endoluminal venous stents in the treatment of the May-Thurner syndrome. *Ann Vasc Surg*. 2002;16:61-64.
6. Christopoulos DC, Nicolaides AN, Szendro G. Venous reflux: quantitation and correlation with the clinical severity of chronic venous disease. *Br J Surg*. 1988;75:352.
7. Gloviczki P, Driscoll DJ. Klippel-Trenaunay syndrome: current management. *Phlebology*. 2007;22:291-298.
8. Kundu S, Lurie F, Millward SF, et al. Recommended reporting standards for endovenous ablation for the treatment of venous insufficiency: Joint Statement of the American Venous Forum and the Society of Interventional Radiology. *J Vasc Surg*. 2007;46:582-589.

9. Smith JJ, Garratt AM, Guest M, Greenhalgh RM, Davies AH. Evaluating and improving health-related quality of life in patients with varicose veins. *J Vasc Surg*. 1999;30:710-719.
10. Breu FX, Guggenbichler S, Wollmann JC. Second European consensus meeting on foam sclerotherapy 2006, Tegernsee, Germany. *Vasa*. 2008;37(71):1-29.
11. Breu FX, Guggenbichler S. European consensus meeting on foam sclerotherapy, April, 4–6, 2003, Tegernsee, Germany. *Dermatol Surg*. 2004;30(5):709-717.
12. Gillet JL, Guedes JM, Guex JJ, et al. Side-effects and complications of foam sclerotherapy of the great and small saphenous veins: a controlled multicentre prospective study including 1025 patients. *Phlebology*. 2009;24:131-138.
13. Morrison N, Cavezza A, Bergan J, Partsch H. Regarding 'Stroke after varicose vein foam injection sclerotherapy'. *J Vasc Surg*. 2006;44:224-225.
14. Tessari L, Cavezzi A, Frullini A. Preliminary experience with a new sclerosing foam in the treatment of varicose veins. *Dermatol Surg*. 2001;27:58-60.
15. Parsi K. Catheter-directed sclerotherapy. *Phlebology*. 2009;24:98-107.
16. Morrison N, Neuhardt DL, Rogers CR, et al. Comparisons of side effects using air and carbon dioxide foam for endovenous chemical ablation. *J Vasc Surg*. 2008;47:830-836.
17. Yamaki T, Nozaki M, Sakurai H, Takeuchi M, Soejima K, Kono T. Multiple small-dose injections can reduce the passage of sclerosant foam into deep veins during foam sclerotherapy for varicose veins. *Eur J Vasc Endovasc Surg*. 2009;37(3):343-348.
18. Parsi K, Exner T, Connor DE, Ma DDF, Joseph JE. In vitro effects of detergent sclerosants on coagulation, platelets and microparticles. *Eur J Vasc Endovasc Surg*. 2007;34:731-740.
19. Scurr JH, Coleridge-Smith P, Cutting P. Varicose veins: optimum compression following sclerotherapy. *Ann Royal Coll Surg Eng*. 1985;67:109-111.
20. Eklof B, Rutherford RB, Bergan JJ, et al. Revision of the CEAP classification for chronic venous disorders: consensus statement. *J Vasc Surg*. 2004;40:1248-1252.
21. Kakkos SK, Rivera MA, Matsagas MI, et al. Validation of the new venous severity scoring system in varicose vein surgery. *J Vasc Surg*. 2004;39:696-697.
22. Van Bellen B, Gross WS, Verta MJ Jr, Yao JS, Bergan J. Lymphatic disruption in varicose vein surgery. *Surgery*. 1977;82(2):257-259.
23. Jia X, Mowatt G, Burr JM, Cassar K, Cook J, Fraser C. Systematic review of foam sclerotherapy for varicose veins. *Br J Surg*. 2007;94:925-936.
24. Hagen PT, Scholz DG, Edwards WD. Incidence and size of patent foramen ovale during the first 10 decades of life: an autopsy study of 965 normal hearts. *Mayo Clin Proc*. 1984;59:17-20.
25. Hansen K, Morrison N, Neuhardt DL, Salles-Cunha SX. Transthoracic echocardiogram and transcranial Doppler detection of emboli after foam sclerotherapy of leg veins. *J Vasc Ultrasound*. 2007;31(4):213-216.

Venous Ulcers Associated with Deep Venous Insufficiency

49

Seshadri Raju

A 46-year-old female schoolteacher and non-smoker presented with an ulcer on the medial side of the ankle. The ulcer had persisted for the past year despite compressive dressings at a hospital wound care center. Ulcers in the same general area had occurred intermittently in the past but had healed with local wound care and dressings. The ulcer was very painful, particularly with dependency of the leg (7/10 over a visual analogue scale) and frequently at night. The patient had made a habit of elevating her legs during the day whenever feasible, and to sleep with her legs elevated on a pillow at night. She had been using a nonsteroidal anti-inflammatory drug once or twice a day at work for pain relief, but lately a narcotic prescribed by her physician was required for sleep at night. Even so, on some nights, she had to "walk off" the pain for 20–30 min before she could fall asleep.

Past medical history: She had been hospitalized on two occasions during the past year for cellulitis of the leg, which required intravenous antibiotics. Her saphenous vein was stripped 15 years ago when the ulcer initially appeared. This resulted in healing of the ulcer but it recurred 2 years later. During adolescence, she sustained a closed tibial fracture of the same extremity during a ski accident and was in a plaster cast and crutches for several weeks. Family history: No one in the family had varicose veins or deep venous thrombosis.

Examination: The patient was found to be healthy except for the affected extremity, which had a large 5 Ð 10-cm indolent ulcer on the medial aspect of the lower third of the leg. The ulcer bed had clean granulation tissue with serous drainage. The ulcer was surrounded by a broader area of hyperpigmentation in the "gaiter" area. No obvious varicosities or "blow outs" were noted. Good pedal pulses were present.

S. Raju
Department of Surgery, University of Mississippi Medical Center, Flowood, MS, USA

G. Geroulakos and B. Sumpio (eds.), *Vascular Surgery*,
DOI: 10.1007/978-1-84996-356-5_49, © Springer-Verlag London Limited 2011

Question 1

Which of the following is *least* likely in this patient?

A. "Primary" deep vein valve reflux
B. Post-thrombotic syndrome
C. Popliteal artery entrapment
D. Recurrent saphenous reflux from neovascularization
E. Perforator incompetence

The patient was referred to the vascular laboratory, where a detailed duplex venous examination was performed. Extensive reflux throughout the deep venous system in the affected extremity was found. Both the femoral and popliteal valves were refluxive, with valve closure times of 7 s and 6 s, respectively. The great saphenous was confirmed absent with no evidence of tributary or collateral reflux around the short sapheno-femoral stump. Neovascularization was not detectable. No significant perforator reflux was found, and the short saphenous vein was not refluxive. The deep venous system was widely patent without evidence of prior thromboses. Air-plethysmography (APG) results were as follows: venous filling index (VFI90) 7 ml/s; venous volume (VV) 135 ml; ejection fraction (EF) 60%; residual volume fraction (RVF) 48%.

Based on the above findings and the clear failure of conservative therapy to heal the ulcer, surgical intervention was discussed with the patient. She consented to this approach. Other preoperative work-up included a hypercoagulation profile and ascending and descending venography.

Question 2

Which of the following statements is true?

A. Duplex is more specific than descending venography in assessing reflux.
B. Valve closure time (VCT) is a reliable quantitative measure of reflux.
C. Venous filling index (VFI90) with APG correlates best with ambulatory venous pressure.
D. Absence of varicosities or "blow outs" on physical examination rules out neovascularization or perforator reflux as a significant source of reflux.
E. Palpable pedal pulses rule out arterial insufficiency as the etiology in patients with painful leg ulcer.

The patient underwent internal valvuloplasty (Kistner technique) of the femoral vein valve under general anesthesia. Postoperative recovery was uneventful. DVT prophylaxis included low-molecular-weight heparin (LMWH) started preoperatively and continued until discharge, intraoperative intravenous heparin (5,000 units), and daily warfarin sodium. Pneumatic compression was started during surgery and continued postoperatively when not ambulatory. She was discharged on 5 mg warfarin with instructions to the local physician to maintain the international normalized ratio (INR) at or above 2.5 for 6 weeks, after which the dosage could be lowered for a target INR of 1.7–2.0. The patient was instructed to wear elastic stockings for at least 6 weeks on a daily basis, after which she could adjust the usage as desired.

The patient was seen on follow-up at 6 weeks, at which time the surgical incision was well healed and the ulcer had become epithelialized to 90% of the original surface area. She requested and was granted permission to go back to full-time work. When seen in follow-up at 4 months, the patient reported that the ulcer had healed completely 2 weeks after the first clinic visit and had remained healed since. She was free of pain and had abandoned regular use of her stockings. She found it necessary to use them only occasionally when she expected her day to be more strenuous than usual. Physical examination revealed good-quality skin coverage over the previous ulcer, and the limb was free of edema. Interval follow-up duplex examination showed competence of the repaired femoral valve with valve closure time of 0.4 s. Popliteal valve reflux was unchanged. Postoperative APG showed that the VFI90 had been nearly normalized at 2.3 ml/s. Other values were essentially unchanged from preoperative levels.

Question 3

Which of the following is *not* true?

A. Postoperative DVT (30 day) is relatively rare after valve reconstruction procedures for correction of "primary" valve reflux.
B. Arm swelling occurs infrequently after axillary vein harvest for valve reconstruction.
C. Valve reconstruction is contraindicated in post-thrombotic veins.
D. Saphenous vein ablation can be safely undertaken in chronic deep venous obstruction (secondary saphenous varix).
E. In combined obstruction/reflux, stent placement to correct the obstruction alone often results in healing of stasis ulceration.

49.1
Commentary

The differential diagnosis of venous ulcers includes ischemic ulcers, diabetic foot ulcers, ulcers related to vasculitis from hypertension or other causes, ulcers related to connective tissue disorders (rheumatoid arthritis, scleroderma, etc.), neuropathic ulcers, Marjolin's ulcer, and numerous other conditions that are clinically quite rare. Popliteal *vein* (not artery) entrapment is a rare cause of venous ulcers.[1] The clinical features of venous ulcers are so characteristic and obvious that a positive diagnosis can be made on the basis of clinical examination alone in all but a few cases. When doubt exists, or when combined pathologies are suspected, a punch biopsy of the skin should be performed without hesitation to clarify the situation. Relevant testing for specific connective tissue, immunological or hematological conditions may be required in some cases. Venous ulcers are differentiated quite easily from arterial (ischemic) ulcers in most instances. The former are indolent and recurring with episodes of healing and breakdown and are generally confined to the gaiter area of the leg. In contrast, the arterial ulcer is progressive without periods of remission and has a wider distribution in the leg with characteristic gangrenous or ischemic appearance devoid of granulation tissue and covered with necrotic tissue. There is seldom the surrounding hyperpigmentation or dermatitis that occurs so commonly with venous ulcers. Palpable pedal pulses virtually rule out ulcers of ischemic origin, with the notable exception of diabetic foot ulcers and less common entities in which vasculitis or small-vessel disease is often implicated (e.g., collagen disorders such as scleroderma and rheumatoid arthritis). It is usually possible, however, to narrow down the possibilities by a combination of clinical features (history, appearance and location of the ulcer), skin biopsy, and specific testing directed toward suspected non-venous pathology. Ankle/arm arterial index and toe pressure measurements may be required in some cases to clarify the issue. Because of their wide prevalence, venous ulcers can and do occur in combination with the other pathologies listed above. To establish the presence of venous ulcers in concert with other nonvenous pathology, it is necessary to confirm that significant reflux is present based on venous duplex examination and venous hemodynamic tests such as ambulatory venous pressure measurement and/or air plethysmography. In combined arterial/venous ulcers, treatment should be directed initially towards improving arterial perfusion.

However obvious the diagnosis, patients with venous ulcers should be evaluated through a detailed assessment protocol to assess severity and form a base for later outcome assessment. Use of CEAP classification[2] and venous clinical severity scoring[3] provides a standardized format to accomplish this. Quality-of-life assessment methodologies[4] in venous disease have been validated and provide a way for outcome assessment from the patient's perspective. [**Q1: C**]

Many patients with chronic venous insufficiency will not volunteer information such as relief of leg pain with leg elevation and stocking use, night leg cramps and restless legs, or their developed habit of sleeping with the leg elevated at night, unless specifically asked. Perhaps because of the chronicity of the condition, these details have become an integral part of their daily lives and may not be mentioned as complaints without direct questioning. Even potentially important information, such as previous attacks of cellulitis or "phlebitis" that occurred years or decades ago and required hospitalization and a period of anticoagulant treatment may not be forthcoming unless specifically inquired, because the patient has forgotten the episode or does not consider it relevant to their current condition. Besides solidifying the diagnosis of venous ulcer, such information may be important in narrowing down the differential diagnosis in doubtful cases or combined pathologies. For example, ischemic rest pain at night is often relieved by hanging the leg over the side of the bed at night, whereas patients with venous pain seldom resort to this practice. Pain of claudication (arterial or venous) worsens with ambulation, whereas patients with limb pain from venous reflux have often learned to "walk off" their nocturnal pain. Venous claudication is estimated to occur in about 15% of patients with chronic venous insufficiency. Climbing up stairs is particularly difficult for these patients. Pain out of proportion to clinical signs is a characteristic of deep venous pathology. Pain, nocturnal leg cramps or restless legs may be the only clinical feature(s) in some patients. Recording the level of pain preoperatively by a visual analogue scale[5] is a simple reliable tool in severity assessment. The type and frequency of analgesic use (narcotic, non-narcotic, non-steroidal) is also useful. Past and current list of medications, particularly estrogen-type hormones and anticoagulants/platelet inhibitors, are relevant parts of the history and useful information in future management.

Limb swelling is a frequent manifestation of venous disease. It is hard to quantify by examination except in very gross terms. Plethysmographic techniques including the commonly used limb circumference measurement are unreliable as swelling is quite variable during the day with the extent of orthostasis. Patients' own perception of limb swelling is strongly influenced by the degree of accompanying pain. Patients themselves may not be aware of swelling obvious to the examiner if painless; conversely, even mild swelling, when painful, may be rated as severe by the patient. For these reasons, quantification of swelling either by history or by examination is subject to considerable variance and error. Although some clinical features are described as unique to lymphedema in texts, differentiation of venous from lymphatic swellings on clinical grounds alone is generally not possible. Furthermore, the two pathologies frequently coexist. Lymphatic dysfunction appears to be secondary to venous obstruction in many cases; relief of venous obstruction can reverse the lymphatic dysfunction.[6] A thorough venous investigation is essential even when lymphoscintigraphy is abnormal.

The investigation of venous ulcers is directed toward positive establishment of venous etiology, identification of regional pathology, and assessment of hemodynamic severity. Hypercoagulability work-up provides guidance to the institution of anticoagulation, its duration and intensity. Duplex examination has replaced venography as the primary investigation for both screening and definitive assessment of chronic venous insufficiency. Overall accuracy of duplex ultrasound is superior to that of descending venography in the assessment of reflux.[7,8] Duplex examination in the erect position yields more accurate results than does examination in the sitting or recumbent position.[9] Quick inflation/deflation cuffs with pressures set for various levels provide for standardized compression maneuvers and allow measurement of valve closure times; reflux is present when these exceed threshold values for the various valve stations. Disappointingly, valve closure times do not correlate with clinical or hemodynamic severity of reflux[10] and cannot be used in a quantitative way as originally hoped. The size and location of perforators can be assessed by duplex and is superior to physical examination. Patency of venous structures can be confirmed positively and post-thrombotic changes can be identified. Despite evolving refinement, duplex remains a largely qualitative morphologic technique.

Descending venography can document reflux through valve stations. The best results are obtained when the test is performed in the near-erect position with standardized Valsalva maneuver.[11] Comparison with duplex has led to the realization that the test, though sensitive, is not very specific. Descending venography is easily combined with transfemoral ascending venogram for assessment of the iliac veins, which may not visualize adequately by pedal injections of contrast. Even transfemoral venogram is only about 50% sensitive for detection of iliac vein obstructions.[12] Intravascular ultrasound (IVUS) is the gold standard for assessment of iliac veins for stent placement.[13]

Ambulatory venous pressure is a global test of venous function. About 25% of patients with venous stasis ulceration have normal ambulatory venous pressure measurement parameters. Factors other than venous reflux, such as compliance, ejection fraction and arterial inflow, affect ambulatory venous pressure.[14] The latter factors are often abnormal in patients with chronic deep venous insufficiency. Consequently, ambulatory venous pressure often improves after valve reconstruction surgery but complete normalization is less frequent.[15] Measurement of ambulatory venous pressure via the dorsal foot vein has been believed to accurately reflect deep venous pressure changes with calf exercise. Recent data throw considerable doubt on this long-held assumption.[16]

Air-plethysmography is a non-invasive test of calf venous pump and can be used to assess surgical outcome.[17] Residual volume correlates with ambulatory venous pressure. However, venous filling index (VFI90) has been a more consistent index of reflux with normalization after corrective surgery.[18,19]

Venous endothelial injury that occurs with deep venous surgery takes about 6 weeks to heal.[20] Patients should be anticoagulated adequately during this vulnerable period. With proper management, the thromboembolic complication rate is surprisingly low.[21] Patients who have suffered from previous bouts of thromboembolism and those with known hypercoagulable abnormalities are under increased risk of recurrent thrombosis and are candidates for long-term or even permanent anticoagulation. [**Q2: A**]

Once thought a rarity, primary deep venous reflux comprises about 30–40% of all deep venous reflux in centers active in deep venous reconstruction. Differentiating "primary" deep venous reflux from secondary or post-thrombotic reflux is problematic. The presentation and clinical features may be similar. Negative history for prior DVT may be unreliable as some thromboses are silent; and others might have been overlooked, ascribing limb pain to trauma or orthopedic surgery that initiated it. Preoperative venography is a poor guide, and surgical exploration of the valve station is often the final arbiter.[22] Some patients with primary reflux develop actual distal thrombosis that can be recurrent. Correction of proximal reflux in this group of patients may alleviate these recurrent symptoms.[23] Conversely, deep venous thrombosis initiates by unknown mechanisms eventual development of reflux in adjacent and remote valve stations.[24]

Correction of primary deep venous reflux by internal valvuloplasty was first described by Kistner in 1964. Subsequently, he described an external technique as well. A variety of open and closed techniques for correction of primary and post-thrombotic deep venous reflux are currently in use.[25,26] The internal valvuloplasty technique has provided excellent results[21,23,27–29] and remains the standard. The newer techniques provide a wider choice that may be more appropriate in certain circumstances, and yield clinical results similar to the original internal technique.[21,30] Direct valvuloplasty may be feasible in some cases of post-thrombotic reflux where the valves have escaped destruction.[22,31] Axillary vein valve transfer is the standard commonly used for correction of post-thrombotic reflux. It can be used with some modifications even in trabeculated veins with surprisingly good long-term patency and clinical success.[32] Arm swelling after axillary vein harvest is rare. [**Q3: C**]

The recent introduction of vein stent technology has decreased the number of valve reconstructions in our institution. Surprisingly, stent application appears to yield excellent clinical results in a broad spectrum of symptomatic chronic venous disease patients, including those with severe associated reflux.[33] This finding portends a major paradigm shift in the treatment of chronic venous disease. In the last three centuries the diagnosis and treatment of chronic venous disease had focused on the reflux component. It appears that the prevalence and

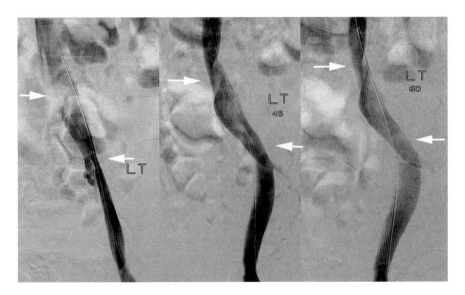

Fig. 49.1 Proximal and distal NIVL. Notice appearance and disappearance of the lesions as the projection is rotated from frontal to oblique lateral[37]

importance of obstructive component present in iliac veins had been underestimated in the past.[34] This is mainly due to deficiencies of traditional diagnostic modalities. The diagnostic sensitivity of venography even using transfemoral injection of contrast is only about 50% in frontal projections.[12,33] Higher diagnostic yield may be obtained by using biplane projections (Fig. 49.1). Specialized duplex techniques are required for examination of iliac veins[35] and are not routinely carried out in most institutions.

Post-thrombotic syndrome is now known to be due to a combination of obstruction and reflux in the majority of patients[36]; iliac obstructive lesions are commonly present. Use of intravascular ultrasound (IVUS) has shown Cockett's syndrome (alias May–Thurner syndrome, iliac vein syndrome) is surprisingly frequent in "primary" reflux as well.[37] These lesions may be extrinsic compression, intrinsic webs and membranes or often a combination. The generic term "Non-thrombotic iliac vein lesion (NIVL)" has been suggested instead for this reason.[37] They are thought to result from injury of repetitive pulsations of the proximate artery.[12] Lesions have been detected in all age groups, both sexes, both sides of the limb and in distal as well as proximal iliac vein segments. Retro inguinal lesions may also be present in some patients. Iliac vein lesions are pathogenic in about 30–40% of patients without associated reflux.[33] Absence of reflux or presence of only trivial reflux (eg. single station segmental reflux) by duplex examination in the context of symptoms should prompt investigation of the iliac vein segment.[38] Modern imaging techniques have shown such lesions to be present in over half the general population,[39] most remaining silent during lifetime. The very high incidence (>90%) of these lesions in symptomatic limbs suggests a "permissive" role[37] allowing symptom expression when additional pathology such as trauma, infection, venosclerosis or onset of reflux is superimposed. Permissive lesions are known to play a role in many disease processes such as, for example, patent foramen ovale (PFO) associated stroke.PFO in silent form is present in about 25% of the general population and becomes symptomatic when paradoxical embolus occurs.

Correction of the obstructive component with stent placement in thrombotic and non-thrombotic cases results in excellent relief of pain and swelling and improvement in quality of life measures. Long-term cumulative stent patency rate is excellent (93% in 603 limbs at 6 years in one series).[8-10] Stent occlusions are exclusive to postthrombotic limbs and very rare in primary disease.

Even totally occluded iliac veins (Fig. 49.2) and even more extensive occlusions of the inferior vena cava can be successfully recanalized and stented.[43-45] Venous stasis ulcers are

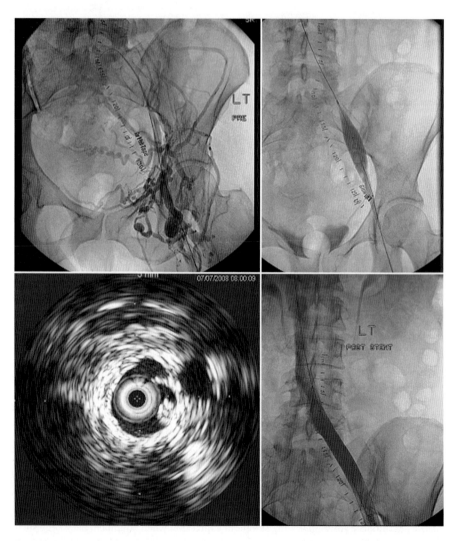

Fig. 49.2 Percutaneous recanalization of occluded iliac vein. Dilation of the recanalized channel and its IVUS appearance prior to stenting are shown.[44]

generally believed to be the result of reflux, not obstruction. Yet this relatively simple percutaneous outpatient stent technique results in healing of about 60% of venous stasis ulceration,[42] even when the associated reflux remains uncorrected. Iliac vein stent placement is currently the first choice in most highly symptomatic patients resistant to compression, whether primary or postthrombotic in origin. Stent deployment does not preclude later open surgery (reverse, often not the case) such as valve reconstruction or venous bypass if the stent were to fail. It is often combined with percutaneous laser ablation of the saphenous vein when refluxive.[46] Saphenous ablation can be carried out safely, even in the presence of chronic deep venous obstruction (secondary varix).[47]

References

1. Raju S, Neglen P. Popliteal vein entrapment: a benign venographic feature or a pathologic entity? *J Vasc Surg*. 2000;31(4):631-641.
2. Beebe HG, Bergan JJ, Bergqvist D, et al. Classification and grading of chronic venous disease in the lower limbs. A consensus statement. *Eur J Vasc Endovasc Surg*. 1996;12(4):487-491. discussion 491–2.
3. Rutherford RB, Padberg FT Jr, Comerota AJ, Kistner RL, Meissner MH, Moneta GL. Venous severity scoring: an adjunct to venous outcome assessment. *J Vasc Surg*. 2000;31(6):1307-1312.
4. Launois R, Rebpi-Marty J, Henry B. Construction and validation of a quality of life questionnaire in chronic lower limb venous insufficiency (CIVIQ). *Qual Life Res*. 1996;5:539-554.
5. Scott J, Huskisson EC. Graphic representation of pain. *Pain*. 1976;2(2):175-184.
6. Raju S, Owen S Jr, Neglen P. Reversal of abnormal lymphoscintigraphy after placement of venous stents for correction of associated venous obstruction. *J Vasc Surg*. 2001;34(5):779-784.
7. Neglen P, Raju S. A comparison between descending phlebography and duplex Doppler investigation in the evaluation of reflux in chronic venous insufficiency: a challenge to phlebography as the "gold standard". *J Vasc Surg*. 1992;16(5):687-693.
8. Masuda EM, Kistner RL. Prospective comparison of duplex scanning and descending venography in the assessment of venous insufficiency. *Am J Surg*. 1992;164(3):254-259.
9. Masuda EM, Kistner RL, Eklof B. Prospective study of duplex scanning for venous reflux: comparison of Valsalva and pneumatic cuff techniques in the reverse Trendelenburg and standing positions. *J Vasc Surg*. 1994;20(5):711-720.
10. Neglen P, Egger JF III, Raju S. Hemodynamic and clinical impact of venous reflux parameters. *J Vasc Surg*. 2004;40:303-319.
11. Morano JU, Raju S. Chronic venous insufficiency: assessment with descending venography. *Radiology*. 1990;174(2):441-444.
12. Negus D, Fletcher EW, Cockett FB, Thomas ML. Compression and band formation at the mouth of the left common iliac vein. *Br J Surg*. 1968;55(5):369-374.
13. Neglen P, Raju S. Intravascular ultrasound scan evaluation of the obstructed vein. *J Vasc Surg*. 2002;35(4):694-700.
14. Raju S, Neglén P, Carr-White PA, Fredericks RK, Devidas M. Ambulatory venous hypertension: component analysis in 373 limbs. *Vasc Surg*. 1999;33:257-267.
15. Kistner RL, Eklof B, Masuda EM. Deep venous valve reconstruction. *Cardiovasc Surg*. 1995;3:129-140.
16. Neglen P, Raju S. Ambulatory venous pressure revisited. *J Vasc Surg*. 2000;31(6):1206-1213.
17. Christopoulos D, Nicolaides AN, Galloway JM, Wilkinson A. Objective noninvasive evaluation of venous surgical results. *J Vasc Surg*. 1988;8(6):683-687.

18. Sakuda H, Nakaema M, Matsubara S, et al. Air plethysmographic assessment of external valvuloplasty in patients with valvular incompetence of the saphenous and deep veins. *J Vasc Surg*. 2002;36(5):922-927.

19. Criado E, Farber MA, Marston WA, Daniel PF, Burnham CB, Keagy BA. The role of air plethysmography in the diagnosis of chronic venous insufficiency. *J Vasc Surg*. 1998;27(4):660-670.

20. Raju S, Perry JT. The response of venous valvular endothelium to autotransplantation and in vitro preservation. *Surgery*. 1983;94(5):770-775.

21. Raju S, Fredericks RK, Neglen PN, Bass JD. Durability of venous valve reconstruction techniques for "primary" and postthrombotic reflux. *J Vasc Surg*. 1996;23(2):357-366. discussion 366-7.

22. Raju S, Fredericks RK, Hudson CA, Fountain T, Neglen PN, Devidas M. Venous valve station changes in "primary" and postthrombotic reflux: an analysis of 149 cases. *Ann Vasc Surg*. 2000;14(3):193-199.

23. Masuda EM, Kistner RL. Long-term results of venous valve reconstruction: a four- to twenty-oneyear follow-up. *J Vasc Surg*. 1994;19(3):391-403.

24. Killewich LA, Bedford GR, Beach KW, Strandness DE Jr. Spontaneous lysis of deep venous thrombi: rate and outcome. *J Vasc Surg*. 1989;9(1):89-97.

25. Raju S, Berry MA, Neglen P. Transcommissural valvuloplasty: technique and results. *J Vasc Surg*. 2000;32(5):969-976.

26. Raju S, Hardy JD. Technical options in venous valve reconstruction. *Am J Surg*. 1997;173(4): 301-307.

27. Perrin M. Reconstructive surgery for deep venous reflux: a report on 144 cases. *Cardiovasc Surg*. 2000;8(4):246-255. 2000;8:246-55.

28. Eriksson I. Reconstructive venous surgery. *Acta Chir Scand Suppl*. 1988;544:69-74.

29. Sottiurai VS. Surgical correction of recurrent venous ulcer. *J Cardiovasc Surg (Torino)*. 1991;32(1):104-109.

30. Camilli S, Guarnera G. External banding valvuloplasty of the superficial femoral vein in the treatment of primary deep valvular incompetence. *Int Angiol*. 1994;13(3):218-222.

31. Raju S, Fountain T, Neglen P, Devidas M. Axial transformation of the profunda femoris vein. *J Vasc Surg*. 1998;27(4):651-659.

32. Raju S, Neglen P, Doolittle J, Meydrech EF. Axillary vein transfer in trabeculated postthrombotic veins. *J Vasc Surg*. 1999;29(6):1050-1062. discussion 1062-4.

33. Raju S, Darcey R, Neglen P. Unexpected major role for venous stenting in deep reflux disease. *J Vasc Surg*. 2010;51:401-408.

34. Neglen P, Thrasher TL, Raju S. Venous outflow obstruction: An underestimated contributor to chronic venous disease. *J Vasc Surg*. 2003;38:879-885.

35. Labropoulos N, Borge M, Pierce K, Pappas PJ. Criteria for defining significant central vein stenosis with duplex ultrasound. *J Vasc Surg*. 2007;46:101-107.

36. Johnson BF, Manzo RA, Bergelin RO, Strandness DEJ. Relationship between changes in the deep venous system and the development of the postthrombotic syndrome after an acute episode of lower limb deep vein thrombosis: a one- to six-year follow-up. *J Vasc Surg*. 1995;21: 307-312. discussion 13.

37. Raju S, Neglen P. High prevalence of nonthrombotic iliac vein lesions in chronic venous disease: a permissive role in pathogenicity. *J Vasc Surg*. 2006;44:136-143. discussion 44.

38. Raju S, Neglen P. Clinical practice. Chronic venous insufficiency and varicose veins. *N Engl J Med*. 2009;360:2319-2327.

39. Kibbe MR, Ujiki M, Goodwin AL, Eskandari M, Yao J, Matsumura J. Iliac vein compression in an asymptomatic patient population. *J Vasc Surg*. 2004;39:937-943.

40. Hartung O, Loundou AD, Barthelemy P, Arnoux D, Boufi M, Alimi YS. Endovascular management of chronic disabling ilio-caval obstructive lesions: long-term results. *Eur J Vasc Endovasc Surg*. 2009;38:118-124.

41. Knipp BS, Ferguson E, Williams DM, et al. Factors associated with outcome after interventional treatment of symptomatic iliac vein compression syndrome. *J Vasc Surg*. 2007;46:743-749.
42. Neglen P, Hollis KC, Olivier J, Raju S. Stenting of the venous outflow in chronic venous disease: long-term stent-related outcome, clinical, and hemodynamic result. *J Vasc Surg*. 2007;46:979-990.
43. Kolbel T, Lindh M, Akesson M, Wasselius J, Gottsater A, Ivancev K. Chronic iliac vein occlusion: midterm results of endovascular recanalization. *J Endovasc Ther*. 2009;16:483-491.
44. Raju S, Neglen P. Percutaneous recanalization of total occlusions of the iliac vein. *J Vasc Surg*. 2009;50:360-368.
45. Raju S, Hollis K, Neglen P. Obstructive lesions of the inferior vena cava: clinical features and endovenous treatment. *J Vasc Surg*. 2006;44:820-827.
46. Neglen P, Hollis KC, Raju S. Combined saphenous ablation and iliac stent placement for complex severe chronic venous disease. *J Vasc Surg*. 2006;44:828-833.
47. Raju S, Easterwood L, Fountain T, Fredericks RK, Neglen PN, Devidas M. Saphenectomy in the presence of chronic venous obstruction. *Surgery*. 1998;123:637-644.

Venous Ulcers Associated with Superficial Venous Insufficiency

50

Guðmundur Daníelsson and Bo Eklöf

A 59-year-old female secretary was referred for evaluation and treatment of a non-healing painful ulcer on the medial aspect of her right lower leg. The ulcer had been recurrent almost every year for the past 9 years, often healing during the winter season. She had since early childhood been overweight (currently 87 kg, 170 cm, body mass index 30) and had difficulty in using compression stocking. She was otherwise healthy. She had two children, the first child born when she was 32 year of age and her second child 2 years later. After the birth of her second child she began to notice varicose veins on the lower leg on both sides and she often felt tiredness and heaviness in the leg in the afternoon. There was no history of deep venous thrombosis. She had been on birth control pills for 10 years and was currently on hormone replacement therapy because of severe postmenopausal symptoms. She had been treated at a local dermatological clinic for the past 2 years and was now being evaluated by a vascular surgeon. Clinical evaluation showed that she had 5×5 cm well-granulated ulceration above the right median malleolus which was surrounded by brownish leathery skin. She had slight swelling of the right leg with large varicosities below the knee. The left leg had large varicosities below the knee but no swelling or skin changes. Doppler examination revealed clear reflux in the groin that could be followed over both great saphenous veins (GSV) down the thigh. A possible minimal reflux was also noted in the popliteal fossa on the right side, although it was difficult to confirm this when the Doppler examination was repeated. Foot arteries were palpable on the dorsum of the foot on both sides.

Question 1

What should be the next step in this patient evaluation?

A. Measurement of ankle-brachial index.
B. Duplex ultrasound scanning of the venous system.
C. Plethysmography.

G. Daníelsson (✉)
Department of Vascular Surgery, The National University Hospital of Iceland,
Fossvogi, 108 Reykjavík, Iceland

G. Geroulakos and B. Sumpio (eds.), *Vascular Surgery*,
DOI: 10.1007/978-1-84996-356-5_50, © Springer-Verlag London Limited 2011

D. Ascending phlebography.

E. Biopsy of the ulcer.

Doppler measurement revealed a normal ankle/brachial index with systolic blood pressure 130 in both legs and right arm. Duplex ultrasound scanning of the venous system performed with the patient in 60° reversed-Trendelenburg position, using pneumatic cuff with automatic inflation/release on the lower leg to evaluate the reflux, showed bilateral reflux in the GSV, from the common femoral vein down to below knee, as well as two incompetent perforator veins on the medial aspect of the right calf with a diameter of 4 mm. The diameter of the GSV at the groin was 12 mm on the right side and 9 mm on the left side. The reflux time exceeded 4 s in both GSV, with peak reverse flow velocity more than 30 cm/s. Reflux less than 0.5 s was noted in the lesser saphenous vein on right side. No reflux was present in the deep veins except for minimal reflux in the common femoral vein with reflux duration of approximately 1 s on the right side. There were no signs of post-thrombotic changes.

Question 2

How should this patient be classified?

A. Leg ulcer

B. Varicose ulcer

C. C 6, S, Ep, As, p, d, Pr

D. C2, 3, 4b, 5, 6, S, Ep, As, p, d, Pr2, 3, 11, 18

The patient was classified according to the CEAP (clinical, (a)etiological, anatomical, pathophysiological) classification based on history and results of duplex ultrasound.

Question 3

Which of the following is not regarded as a risk factor for venous ulcer?

A. Diabetes

B. Essential hypertension

C. Smoking

D. Overweight

E. Resistance to activated protein C

Question 4

What would be appropriate management for the right leg in this patient?

A. Conservative treatment with below-knee compression bandage, rest and leg elevation

B. High ligation and stripping of GSV to below knee, with local extirpation of varicose veins

C. High ligation of GSV with extirpation of varicose veins

D. Obliteration of GSV using laser or radiofrequency heating with local extirpation of varicose veins

E. Sclerotherapy with or without foam

Question 5

How should the incompetent perforator veins be managed?

A. Subfascial endoscopic perforator surgery (SEPS)

B. Ligation through Linton-Cockett incisions

C. Disregard them

D. Ligation through small skin incisions

E. Duplex-guided sclerotherapy

Question 6

How should the left leg be managed?

A. Observation

B. Sclerotherapy

C. High ligation and stripping of GSV and local extirpation of varicose veins

D. Obliteration of GSV using laser or radiofrequency heating and local extirpation of varicose veins

The patient was treated with four-layer compression therapy until the operation day, which was postponed for 4 months. The ulcer and the swelling both decreased during this period; the ulcer measured 2×2 cm the day before operation. Both the right and the left leg GSV were treated with the closure method using radiofrequency derived heating, and varicose veins on the lower leg were extirpated through multiple small incisions. Intraoperative duplex ultrasound scanning revealed that both GSV were occluded with no sign of reflux and the deep veins were patent with no sign of deep venous thrombosis. No specific treatment was performed for the incompetent perforator veins. The patient was discharged the same day after uneventful postoperative recovery and was scheduled for new duplex ultrasound scanning after 2 and 7 days. The postoperative duplex ultrasound scanning was normal, with no sign of deep venous thrombosis, and the remnant of GSV was occluded. The patient continued with four-layer bandaging and went back to work on the fifth day after operation. The ulcer was healed at the last visit, which was 4 weeks later. Treatment with compression stocking during the daytime was planned for another 6 months.

50.1
Commentary

Investigation of both the arterial and the venous system is mandatory in cases of non-healing ulcer on the leg. Although Doppler examination had only revealed a clear reflux in

GSV it is worthwhile to continue with duplex ultrasound scanning as deep venous incompetence and post-thrombotic changes can otherwise be overlooked. This is especially important when reflux is noted at the back of the knee where it is difficult with certainty to differentiate between deep venous reflux in the popliteal vein and reflux in the lesser saphenous vein. Although the history (no claudication or rest pain, no diabetes) and the location of the ulcer (medial aspect of lower leg) strongly suggest a venous ulcer, sometimes an arterial component is also present that might reduce the ability of the ulcer to heal. Palpable pulse on the dorsum of the foot (dorsalis pedis) or behind the medial malleolus (posterior tibial artery), as was evident in this case, almost rules out an arterial component. Although plethysmography can estimate the overall venous function it is not mandatory as a first line of investigation. Obtaining an ascending phlebography is also not necessary as it does not add any information that duplex ultrasound scanning does not provide and it is also an invasive method with the risk of complications. Non-healing ulcer with unusual appearance should be considered for other etiology and investigated with biopsy in the early stage of evaluation. [Q1: A, B]

The old concept that the majority of venous ulcers are due to previous deep venous thrombosis[1,2] has been altered during the last 20 years when duplex ultrasound studies have shown the importance of primary reflux in all venous segments.[3-7] Superficial venous incompetence is often noted to be the sole pathology in patients presenting with non-healing venous ulcer.[8] Formerly the venous ulcer was often judged as being related to a post-thrombotic condition without any objective diagnosis. Because of the benign course of varicose veins in the majority of patients with superficial venous incompetence, the need for thorough evaluation is often neglected. Formerly used classifications of chronic venous disease used the term varicose ulcer if varicose veins were present, or post-thrombotic ulcer if they were less evident or if there was a previous history of deep venous thrombosis. The importance of classification, based on findings from duplex ultrasound scanning, has become more evident during the last decades as treatment and prognosis is largely dependent on the background history and the results of clinical investigation. CEAP (clinical, (a)etiological, anatomical, pathophysiological) classification has gained more acceptance as the "gold standard" for classifying all aspects of venous pathology such as clinical class, etiological background, anatomical distribution and pathophysiological findings (Table 50.1). There is a clear correlation between the CEAP clinical class and the venous function as measured by plethysmography (foot volumetry), indicating that the clinical classification has a realistic meaning concerning the functional evaluation of venous disease. The duration of reflux in venous segments, on the other hand, does not correlate with clinical class, but the peak reverse flow velocity is significantly higher in patients with skin changes/ulcer (C4–C6).[9] The basic part of CEAP indicates the highest clinical class (C6, active venous ulcer) and the anatomical distribution in superficial, perforator or deep system (As, p, d) with reflux (Pr). S is added behind clinical class to indicate that the patient is symptomatic. The basic classification is sufficient for most clinical doctors. [Q2: C, D] The detailed version of CEAP is used when more information is needed as in longitudinal studies comparing treatment alternatives (Table 50.2). For more detailed information regarding the disease and its effect on daily life it is possible to use a venous severity scoring system.[11] Venous severity scoring is used as a complement to the

Table 50.1 CEAP classification

Clinical classification
C0: no visible or palpable signs of venous disease
C1: telangiectases or reticular veins
C2: varicose veins
C3: edema
C4a: pigmentation and/or eczema
C4b: lipodermatosclerosis and/or atrophie blanche
C5: healed venous ulcer
C6: active venous ulcer
S: symptoms including ache, pain, tightness, skin irritation, heaviness, muscle cramps, as well as other complaints attributable to venous dysfunction
A: Asymptomatic
Etiological classification
Ec: Congenital
Ep: Primary
Es: Secondary (post-thrombotic)
En: No venous etiology identified
Anatomic classification
As: Superficial veins
Ap: Perforator veins
Ad: Deep veins
An: No venous location identified
Pathophysiological classification
Pr: Reflux
Po: Obstruction
Pr,o: Reflux and obstruction
Pn: No venous pathophysiology identifiable

CEAP classification (Fig. 50.1). Some medical conditions are clearly a risk factor for venous ulcer while others are less important. Venous ulcers are overrepresented in patients with diabetes although it is not clear if it is the venous pathology or if it is the diabetic microangiopathy that is the reason for this. Neither essential hypertension nor smoking is a proven risk factor for venous ulcer. The prevalence of varicose veins is increased in overweight individuals but the role of obesity is less clear when it comes to the risk of developing skin changes or ulcer. The apparent association between overweight and varicose veins in women suggests that it is a risk factor even in the more severe form of chronic venous disease.[12–14] In a consecutive series of 272 patients with chronic venous disease investigated with duplex ultrasound scanning, 58% of patients with healed or open ulcer (C5–C6) had body mass index >30 kg/m^2 (obese) as compared to 15% of those with varicose veins but without skin changes or ulcer.[15] [**Q3: A, B, C**] Most thrombophilic conditions are risk factors for deep venous thrombosis and venous ulceration, as is resistance to activated protein C.[16] The prevalence of thrombophilia is high in patients with

Table 50.2 Advanced CEAP

Same as basic CEAP with the addition that any of 18 named venous segments can be utilized as locators for venous pathology.
Superficial veins:
1. Telangiectases/reticular veins
2. Great saphenous vein above knee
3. Great saphenous vein below knee
4. Small saphenous vein
5. Non-saphenous veins
Deep veins:
6. Inferior vena cava
7. Common iliac vein
8. Internal iliac vein
9. External iliac vein
10. Pelvic: gonadal, broad ligament veins, other
11. Common femoral vein
12. Deep femoral vein
13. Femoral vein
14. Popliteal vein
15. Crural: anterior tibial, posterior tibial, peroneal veins (all paired)
16. Muscular: gastrocnemial, soleal veins, other
17. Perforating veins, thigh
18. Perforating veins, calf

venous ulceration despite no history or duplex ultrasound findings of deep venous thrombosis.[17]

Surgical treatment is mandatory in cases of isolated superficial incompetence as the likelihood of ulcer recurrence otherwise will remain high. Conservative treatment alone with below-knee compression had not been successful in keeping the ulcer healed, but it is important to continue with compression therapy while the ulcer is open and for some time after operation. Four-layer bandage is effective in healing venous ulcer.[18] High ligation with stripping of the GSV down to below the knee, with local extirpation of varicose veins, is the method of choice. It decreases the risk of ulcer recurrence and has a low incidence of nerve damage to the saphenous nerve. Stripping of the vein from the groin to the ankle increases the risk of damage to the saphenous nerve (5% versus 29%), although the recurrence rate is still the same.[19] Just doing high ligation without stripping the vein is less feasible as the recurrence rate is significantly higher.[20] Other promising methods for ablation of the refluxing GSV have emerged recently and might become the methods of choice in the future. As the diameter of the GSV was less than 15 mm it was possible to use the radiofrequency closure method to obliterate the vein. The main advantage of using less invasive methods is increased patient satisfaction, as the recovery time after operation has been reported to be shorter. Follow-up time up to 5 years with the radiofrequency method indicates that the method is durable. The long-term results after ablation of GSV using laser technique or foam sclerotherapy are still unknown. [**Q4: B, D**]

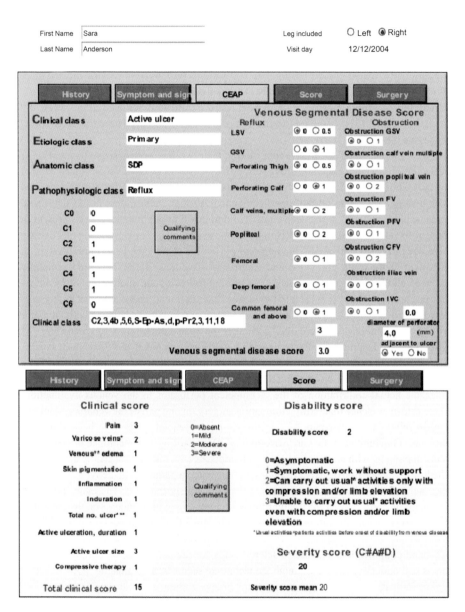

Fig. 50.1 Venous severity scoring is used as a complement to the CEAP classification

The varicose veins on the lower leg are dealt with by using multiple stab incisions and bringing them out using hooks. The cosmetic results are better and the risk of nerve damage is less. Care should be taken not to operate close to the ulcer area as healing problems and infection are more common if the incisions are made in damaged skin.

Even though the role of surgery in venous ulcer disease has been unclear,[21] a recently reported randomized controlled study comparing surgery with compression therapy, to compression therapy alone, could clearly show a significantly lower recurrence rate in the surgically treated group.[22] Altogether 500 patients with open or recently healed ulcer (6 months) were included in the study. The healing rate was similar during the study period, but 12-month ulcer recurrence rates were significantly reduced in the surgically treated group or 12%, compared to the compression-only group where the ulcer recurrence rate was 28%.

The pathophysiology behind venous ulcer is mainly reflux as opposed to obstruction or occlusion. In a study on a consecutive series of 98 legs with an open venous ulcer, 85% of the extremities had some form of superficial venous incompetence that might be treated with a simple operation on the superficial venous system. Axial reflux in the superficial (great saphenous vein) or the deep veins (femoral down to popliteal level) was present in 79% of the legs.[23] Incompetent perforator veins and their role in chronic venous disease have been debated for years.[24] Incompetent perforator veins have been implicated as an important factor in the formation and recurrence of venous ulcers. This view is mainly based on clinical reports of excellent ulcer healing following the interruption of incompetent perforators. There is substantial evidence that subfascial endoscopic perforator surgery (SEPS) is effective in interrupting perforator veins, and it can be done without major wound complications that were often seen after the open subfascial Linton procedure.[25–28] Also, the ulcer healing rate after venous procedures that included SEPS has been satisfying.[25,26] Patients undergoing surgery for incompetent perforator veins almost always have surgery simultaneously on the superficial venous system and therefore it is difficult to judge the actual contribution of the incompetent perforator to the venous dysfunction. There is also evidence that reflux-eliminating surgery on one part of the venous system can abolish reflux in another part.[29–31] Operations on superficial veins have been shown to eliminate concomitant reflux in perforators.[32] Disregarding the incompetent perforator veins in patients with superficial venous incompetence seems therefore to be appropriate. The low incidence of isolated perforator incompetence in patients with active venous ulcer does indicate that they are less important than previously thought.[8] The main indication (although not proven yet) for treating them is in patients with primary venous incompetence with recurrent ulceration despite optimal treatment of the superficial venous incompetence. The method of choice for treatment is then SEPS, mainly because of the low risk of wound complication. The use of sclerotherapy for the purpose of obliterating perforators is still under evaluation although the technique seems to be promising. [Q5: A, C]

The indication for treating varicose veins in legs without skin changes or ulcer is less clear. The decision of recommending treatment for asymptomatic legs with varicose veins has to be judged individually; often it is the patient's preference that will decide. The cosmetic results of sclerotherapy on local varicose veins are poor if the refluxing GSV is left in place. The risk of future problems with skin changes or ulcer is increased when axial reflux is present in the GSV, as was the case with this patient, and that might be a sufficient reason to recommend even surgery for the asymptomatic left leg. A simultaneous operation on both legs in an otherwise healthy person does not seem to add any risk to the operation. If a catheter-based ablation is used to obliterate the GSV it is feasible to treat both legs at the same time as one catheter can then be used to treat both legs as the catheter is expensive. [**Q6: A, C, D**]

References

1. Homans J. The etiology and treatment of varicose ulcer of the leg. *Surg Gynecol Obstet.* 1917;24:300-11.
2. Bauer G. A roentgenological and clinical study of the sequels of thrombosis. *Acta Chir Scand.* 1942;86.
3. Lees TA, Lambert D. Patterns of venous reflux in limbs with skin changes associated with chronic venous insufficiency. *Br J Surg.* 1993;80:725-8.
4. Hoare MC, Nicolaides A, Miles C. The role of primary varicose veins in venous ulceration. *Surgery.* 1983;82:450.
5. Sethia KK, Darke SG. Long saphenous incompetence as a cause of venous ulceration. *Br J Surg.* 1984;71:754-5.
6. Labropoulos N, Landon P, Jay T. The impact of duplex scanning in phlebology. *Dermatol Surg.* 2002;28:1-5.
7. Wong JK, Duncan JL, Nichols DM. Whole-leg duplex mapping for varicose veins: observations on patterns of reflux in recurrent and primary legs, with clinical correlation. *Eur J Vasc Endovasc Surg.* 2003;25:267-75.
8. Danielsson G, Eklof B, Grandinetti A, Lurie F, Kistner RL. Deep axial reflux, an important contributor to skin changes or ulcer in chronic venous disease. *J Vasc Surg.* 2003;38:1336-41.
9. Danielsson G, Norgren L, Jungbeck C, Peterson K. Global venous function correlates better than duplex derived reflux to clinical class in the evaluation of chronic venous disease. *Int Angiol.* 2003;22:177-81.
10. Eklof B, Rutherford RB, Bergan JJ, Carpentier PH, Gloviczki P, et al. Revision of the CEAP classification for chronic venous disorders. A consensus statement. *J Vasc Surg.* 2004;40: 1248-52.
11. Rutherford RB, Padberg FT Jr, Comerota AJ, Kistner RL, Meissner MH, Moneta GL. Venous severity scoring: an adjunct to venous outcome assessment. *J Vasc Surg.* 2000;31:1307-12.
12. Iannuzzi A, Panico S, Ciardullo AV, et al. Varicose veins of the lower limbs and venous capacitance in postmenopausal women: relationship with obesity. *J Vasc Surg.* 2002;36:965-8.
13. Brand F, Dannenberg A, Abbott R, Kannel W. The epidemiology of varicose veins: the Framingham study. *Am J Prev Med.* 1988;4:96-101.
14. Sadick NS. Predisposing factors of varicose and telangiectatic leg veins. *J Dermatol Surg Oncol.* 1992;18:883-6.
15. Danielsson G, Eklof B, Grandinetti A, Kistner RL. The influence of obesity on chronic venous disease. *Vasc Endovasc Surg.* 2002;36:271-6.
16. Munkvad S, Jorgensen M. Resistance to activated protein C: a common anticoagulant deficiency in patients with venous leg ulceration. *Br J Dermatol.* 1996;134:296-8.
17. Bradbury AW, MacKenzie RK, Burns P, Fegan C. Thrombophilia and chronic venous ulceration. *Eur J Vasc Endovasc Surg.* 2002;24:97-104.
18. Nelson EA, Iglesias CP, Cullum N, Torgerson DJ. Randomized clinical trial of four-layer and short-stretch compression bandages for venous leg ulcers (VenUS I). *Br J Surg.* 2004;91: 1292-9.

19. Holme K, Matzen M, Bomberg AJ, Outzen SL, Holme JB. Partial or total stripping of the great saphenous vein. 5-year recurrence frequency and 3-year frequency of neural complications after partial and total stripping of the great saphenous vein. *Ugeskr Laeger*. 1996;158:405-8.

20. Dwerryhouse S, Davies B, Harradine K, Earnshaw JJ. Stripping the long saphenous vein reduces the rate of reoperation for recurrent varicose veins: five-year results of a randomized trial. *J Vasc Surg*. 1999;29:589-92.

21. Clinical evidence, Option: Vein surgery. *BMJ*. 2001;1510.

22. Barwell JR, Davies CE, Deacon J, et al. Comparison of surgery and compression with compression alone in chronic venous ulceration (ESCHAR study): randomised controlled trial. *Lancet*. 2004;363:1854-9.

23. Danielsson G, Arfvidsson B, Eklof B, Kistner RL, Masuda EM, Sato DT. Reflux from thigh to calf, the major pathology in chronic venous ulcer disease: surgery indicated in the majority of patients. *Vasc Endovascular Surg*. 2004;363:1854-9.

24. Danielsson G, Eklof B, Kistner RL. What is the role of incompetent perforator veins in chronic venous disease? *J Phlebol*. 2001;1:67-71.

25. Nelzen O. Prospective study of safety, patient satisfaction and leg ulcer healing following saphenous and subfascial endoscopic perforator surgery. *Br J Surg*. 2000;87:86-91.

26. Gloviczki P. Subfascial endoscopic perforator vein surgery: indications and results. *Vasc Med*. 1999;4:173-80.

27. Wittens CH, Bollen EC, Kool DR, van Urk H, Mul T, van Houtte HJ. Good results of subfascial endoscopy as treatment of communicating vein insufficiency. *Ned Tijdschr Geneeskd*. 1993;137:1200-4.

28. Quiros RS, Kitainik E, Swiatlo MR, Breyter E. Cutaneous complications of the subaponeurotic surgery of the communicating venous system. *J Cardiovasc Surg*. 1967;8:206-8.

29. Walsh JC, Bergan JJ, Beeman S, Comer TP. Femoral venous reflux abolished by greater saphenous vein stripping. *Ann Vasc Surg*. 1994;8:566-70.

30. Stuart WP, Adam DJ, Allan PL, Ruckley CV, Bradbury AW. Saphenous surgery does not correct perforator incompetence in the presence of deep venous reflux. *J Vasc Surg*. 1998;28:834-8.

31. Sales CM, Bilof ML, Petrillo KA, Luka NL. Correction of lower extremity deep venous incompetence by ablation of superficial venous reflux. *Ann Vasc Surg*. 1996;10:186-9.

32. Gohel MS, Barwell JR, Wakely C, et al. The influence of superficial venous surgery and compression on incompetent calf perforators in chronic venous leg ulceration. *Eur J Vasc Endovasc Surg*. 2005;29:78-82.

Iliofemoral Venous Thrombosis

51

William P. Paaske

A 72-year-old man was admitted in the late evening because of a turgid, white, painful left leg. Over the course of 4 months, he had lost 8 kg of weight (from 82 to 74 kg); his height was 175 cm. There were general symptoms, such as tiredness, slight nausea, lack of appetite and increasing apathy. Over the last 12 h, he had been increasingly confused and aggressive. He had been bedridden for 3 weeks but had refused to see a doctor. There was no history of psychiatric disease, focal cerebrovascular events, ischaemic heart disease, hypertension, intermittent claudication, or venous insufficiency. He had been smoking about 20 cigarettes a day since he was 14 years old, and for many years he had had slight functional dyspnoea, but otherwise no pulmonary symptoms. Stools had been light yellow to grey/white for the last week. His renal function had never been examined, and it had not been noticed whether he had passed urine in the last 24 h. Diazepam was the only medication. The history was provided by his wife, who had called the ambulance. Medical records were not available.

The patient was confused, with delusions; he was intermittently agitated and possibly psychotic, but he could be calmed down. He looked chronically ill, slightly emaciated, possibly anemic and dehydrated. Temperature and blood pressure (arms) were normal. There was tachycardia with a regular rhythm. The abdomen was slightly distended, but there was neither a palpable mass nor peritoneal reactions. Digital rectal exploration was unremarkable. The right leg was normal with distal pulses.

The left leg had diffuse swelling from the groin to the toes; there was moderate pallor, and no visible varicosities when standing. There was no evidence of superficial thrombophlebitis. Minor venous collaterals were noticed in the groin and just above the inguinal ligament. During palpation over the deep femoral veins, the patient groaned and became increasingly aggressive. The consistency of the calf muscle groups was increased with tenderness but not woody. There was less floppiness of the left leg muscles compared with those of the right. Spontaneous dorsiflexion of the foot was noticed, but sensory function could not be assessed due to lack of patient cooperation.

W.P. Paaske
Department of Cardiothoracic and Vascular Surgery,
Aarhus University Hospital, Aarhus, Denmark

G. Geroulakos and B. Sumpio (eds.), *Vascular Surgery*,
DOI: 10.1007/978-1-84996-356-5_51, © Springer-Verlag London Limited 2011

The quality of the pulses in the groin and knee was good, and the pulse in the dorsal pedal artery was possibly present. Capillary filling in the pulp of the toes could not be assessed. The plantar pallor did not increase during elevation, but discrete color change was noticed at the back of the foot during post-elevation dependency.

Bladder catheterisation did not produce urine. Electrocardiogram (ECG) was normal apart from a rate of 114 bpm.

Question 1

What is the most likely diagnosis?

A. Thrombosis of the crural veins
B. Thrombosis of the femoral veins
C. Thrombosis of the iliac and femoral veins
D. Thrombosis of the superficial femoral artery
E. Thrombosis of the external iliac and superficial femoral arteries

Blood samples were taken, and the patient was admitted.

Question 2

Which investigation should be ordered and carried out at once?

A. Intravenous arteriography
B. Intra-arterial arteriography
C. Ascending phlebography
D. Color duplex sonography
E. Plethysmography

Due to an unusually large number of emergency admissions, the patient had to wait several hours before he could be examined by color duplex sonography and have his chest X-ray taken. An hour before the scheduled time for these examinations (8 h after admission), and before the results of the blood tests were available, the patient deteriorated and the pulse rose further. His temperature was now 38.9°C. He had become increasingly agitated and complained of severe pain in the left leg.

Haemorrhagic bullae developed on the back of the foot and around the medial ankle, and the skin of the rest of the foot and the distal calf showed numerous petechiae. There was increased swelling, and the color of the leg turned deeply cyanotic, even during elevation. The tips of all the toes were black. A weak pulse could be felt in the femoral artery in the groin, but distal pulses were absent. The consistency of the muscle groups of the thigh as well as the lower leg was clearly increased, and the patient suffered severe pain when femoral muscles were assessed by compression. He did not react to pain induced by pinching the skin from the knee and distally. At this point, the right leg exhibited slight but definite swelling, and the skin was beginning to become cyanotic. Pulses could still be felt in the right groin and popliteal artery, but pedal pulses had disappeared.

Question 3

What is/are the common name(s) for this clinical presentation?
A. Iliofemoral venous thrombosis
B. Iliofemoral phlebothrombosis
C. Phlegmasia alba dolens
D. Phlegmasia cerulea dolens
E. Venous gangrene

Question 4

What ideally should have been done, and what should be done at this stage at 4 a.m. on the basis of this clinical presentation and with the additional information provided above?

At this point, the results of the blood tests taken in the emergency room became available: they showed anaemia with haemoconcentration, thrombocytopenia and electrolyte derangements; S-creatinine was 410 mmol/l, and the leucocyte count was 14 times above the upper normal limit. The large amount of fluid sequestered in the gangrenous left leg may account for part of the haemo-concentration.

Question 5

Would you consider a surgical thrombectomy at this stage? If so, how would you perform it?

The situation was deemed hopeless and beyond medical therapy. The patient was given intravenous morphine to relieve the pain, and he died 13 h after admission.

50.1
Commentary

The tentative diagnosis at admission was acute left-sided iliofemoral venous thrombosis with the clinical picture of phlegmasia alba dolens. [**Q1: C**] It was highly probable – but not proven – that this bedridden patient suffered from active malignant disease with secondary venous thrombosis. His general appearance in connection with the specific signs and symptoms, including apparent lack of urine production, indicated a disaster in progression. The association of cancer and deep venous thrombosis is well established.[1] If a malignancy is definitely diagnosed, or suspected with a high degree of certainty, disseminated and/or in an advanced stage where expected residual lifespan is very short, then ultrasonically or phlebographically verified iliofemoral venous thrombosis with venous gangrene (ischaemic venous thrombosis) must be interpreted as one of the signs indicating imminent termination of life, and treatment (medical as well as operative) is generally contraindicated, including on compassionate grounds.

With unreliable, rudimentary or uncertain information, it is essential that diagnosis is established not merely as soon as possible but at once; it is not acceptable to wait several hours for the diagnostic test, color duplex sonography. [Q2: D] The patient should be taken immediately to the ultrasound examination room and, if necessary, scanned by the surgeon. [Q4]

In our case, the color duplex sonography after a phase of phlegmasia cerulea dolens progressing to manifest venous gangrene on the left side and phlegmasia cerulea dolens in development on the right, showed bilateral thrombosis of both femoral and iliac veins in addition to thrombosis of the inferior vena cava up to and above the renal veins, which explained the lack of urine production. [Q3: E]

Certain assessment algorithms have been devised for the management of this condition,[2] but the remotest suspicion of deep venous thrombosis should result either in color duplex sonography or ascending phlebography (with digital subtraction technique), or in magnetic resonance venography with gadolinium enhancement plus T1 images (bull's eye sign),[3] if available, in patients with renal impairment or allergy to angiographic contrast media. Some centers have the option of computed tomographic (CT) venography (possibly with spiral/slip-ring technique), which has the additional advantage of being able to visualise extravascular morphology. Plethysmography (strain gauge, impedance, air, etc.) must be considered obsolete for precise diagnosis; isotope uptake tests have generally been disappointing and should be avoided. Both legs, rather than only the symptomatic leg, should be examined in all patients. In patients with coexisting arterial insufficiency of the lower extremities, the diagnosis can be even more difficult, so investigations should be performed at a lower level of clinical suspicion. Where phlegmasia cerulea dolens is surmised, or where venous gangrene is apparent, then one of these examinations must be performed without delay. If pulmonary embolism is suspected, then lung scintigraphy, pulmonary angiography or magnetic resonance or CT scanning of the pulmonary arteries should be performed.

Treatment aims to prevent or decrease further thrombus formation or propagation, to reduce or stop acute (pulmonary embolism) and chronic (post-thrombotic syndrome) complications, and to reduce pain.

In principle, the thrombus can be reduced, or removed, by chemical or mechanical means. A fresh thrombus is generally less adherent than an old thrombus. The preferred treatment of iliofemoral venous thrombolysis is heparin administered for 3–4 days as a continued intravenous infusion (high-dose heparin) concomitant with oral phenprocoumon, dicoumarol or warfarin, which should be given for a further 3–6 months.[4] This regime probably has on influence on the development of chronic post-thrombotic syndrome.

Thrombolysis with streptokinase, urokinase or recombinant tissue plasminogen activator (rt-PA) can be attempted for thrombi less than about 10 days old under close monitoring with repeated color duplex sonography examinations.[5–9] Although many series have been published, the effect on pulmonary embolism is dubious, and the long-term clinical results of properly conducted studies are still poorly documented.

Interruption of the venous system between the thrombus and the heart prevents pulmonary embolism and may be considered in highly selected cases; it is performed by partial or complete occlusion of the inferior caval vein by either open surgery[10] or deployment of temporary or permanent caval filters,[11] of which several types are commercially available. The long-term outcomes of both techniques are not clear. The incidence of filter complications – early as well as late – is not negligible.

Once again, as in many other aspects in the treatment of venous disease, there are widely diverging opinions as to the place of surgical thrombectomy of iliofemoral venous thrombosis with or without construction of an arteriovenous fistula. In pregnancy or during puerperium, surgical thrombectomy should not be attempted.[12] A balanced view, based on the available literature, would be that it may be a possibility that could be considered in limb-threatening phlegmasia cerulea dolens.[13–17]

The operation is performed with the supine patient in the reversed Trendelenburg position (legs down), and under general anaesthesia with continuous positive airway pressure. The femoral veins, which may bulge with thrombus, and arteries are exposed in the groin by a longitudinal incision. After slings have been applied, a longitudinal phlebotomy is made, and a venous Fogarty catheter is advanced toward the heart. The balloon is inflated, and the catheter is withdrawn together with the thrombus. The procedure is repeated until no more thrombus is delivered. The leg is now elevated, and by manual compression (possibly followed by compressing bandage, e.g. Esmarch´s), one aims to remove the thrombus within the leg. The phlebotomy is then closed. The patient should have the leg elevated until mobilization after a few days. Thrombectomy often results in incomplete clot removal and recurrence.[18]

In certain centers, the contralateral groin vessels are also routinely exposed, a Fogarty catheter is introduced into the common femoral vein, and the tip is positioned in the upper part of the inferior caval vein. The balloon of this catheter is insufflated during the manoeuvres on the contralateral side, and it is retracted with inflated balloon after each of the Fogarty thrombectomy procedures. The aim is to retract fragments of thrombus and avoid (additional) pulmonary embolism.

Some surgeons advocate construction of an arteriovenous fistula in addition to the surgical thrombectomy. The great saphenous vein is transected as appropriate below the saphenofemoral junction, and the distal part of the proximal segment is anastomosed to an arteriotomy in the common femoral artery. The aim is to increase blood flow, thereby reducing the risk of recurrent thrombus formation, in the proximal part of the femoral vein and veins proximal to that. [**Q5**]

Although the extremity with phlegmasia cerulea dolens may look very bad indeed, a conservative approach is warranted (careful monitoring, elevation of the leg, heparin, fluid replacement). If systemic symptoms or signs occur, or if the situation deteriorates into manifest venous gangrene, then amputation must be performed without delay.

Operative treatment of chronic iliofemoral venous thrombosis and its sequelae, notably post-thrombotic syndrome, remains controversial. Reports with various reconstructions, e.g. with polytetrafluoroethylene (PTFE), remain anecdotal.[19]

Endovascular treatment options are emergent, some in combination with open surgery (hybrid procedures). Combined application of transcutaneous thrombectomy devices, balloon angioplasty, stenting etc. with thrombolysis may lead to a new level of therapeutic aggressiveness,[20] but proper scientific documentation is so far not available, and these new developments must be considered experimental.

References

1. Prandoni P, Lensing AW, Buller HR, et al. Deep-vein thrombosis and the incidence of subsequent symptomatic cancer. *N Engl J Med.* 1992;327:1128-1133.
2. Wells PS, Hirsh J, Anderson DR, et al. Accuracy of clinical assessment of deep-vein thrombosis. *Lancet.* 1995;345:1326-1330.
3. Froehlich JB, Prince MR, Greenfield LJ, Downing LJ, Shah NL, Wakefield TW. "Bull's-eye" sign on gadolinium-enhanced magnetic resonance venography determines thrombus presence and age: a preliminary study. *J Vasc Surg.* 1997;26:809-816.
4. Gallus A, Jackaman J, Tillett J, Mills W, Wycherley A. Safety and efficacy of warfarin started early after submassive venous thrombosis or pulmonary embolism. *Lancet.* 1986;2:1293-1296.
5. Semba CP, Dake MD. Catheter-directed thrombolysis for iliofemoral venous thrombosis. *Semin Vasc Surg.* 1996;9:26-33.
6. Verhaeghe R, Stockx L, Lacroix H, Vermylen J, Baert AL. Catheter-directed lysis of iliofemoral vein thrombosis with use of rt-PA. *Eur Radiol.* 1997;7:996-1001.
7. Patel NH, Plorde JJ, Meissner M. Catheter-directed thrombolysis in the treatment of phlegmasia cerulea dolens. *Ann Vasc Surg.* 1998;12:471-475.
8. Mewissen MW, Seabrook GR, Meissner MH, Cynamon J, Labropoulos N, Haughton SH. Catheter-directed thrombolysis for lower extremity deep venous thrombosis: report of a national multicenter registry. *Radiology.* 1999;211:39-49.
9. Grossman C, McPherson S. Safety and efficacy of catheter-directed thrombolysis for iliofemoral venous thrombosis. *Am J Roentgenol.* 1999;172:667-672.
10. Silver D, Sabiston DC Jr. The role of vena caval interruption in the management of pulmonary embolism. *Surgery.* 1975;77:3-10.
11. Magnant JG, Walsh DB, Juravsky LI, Cronenwett JL. Current use of inferior vena cava filters. *J Vasc Surg.* 1992;16:701-706.
12. Torngren S, Hjertberg R, Rosfors S, Bremme K, Eriksson M, Swedenborg J. The long-term outcome of proximal vein thrombosis during pregnancy is not improved by the addition of surgical thrombectomy to anticoagulant treatment. *Eur J Vasc Endovasc Surg.* 1996;12:31-36.
13. Röder OC, Lorentzen JE, Hansen HJB. Venous thrombectomy for iliofemoral thrombosis. Early and long-term results in 46 consecutive cases. *Acta Chir Scand.* 1984;150:31-34.
14. Hood DB, Weaver FA, Modrall JG, Yellin AE. Advances in the treatment of phlegmasia cerulea dolens. *Am J Surg.* 1993;166:206-210.
15. Perkins JM, Magee TR, Galland RB. Phlegmasia caerulea dolens and venous gangrene. *Br J Surg.* 1996;83:19-23.
16. Eklöf B, Kistner RL. Is there a role for thrombectomy in iliofemoral venous thrombosis? *Semin Vasc Surg.* 1996;9:34-45.
17. Plate G, Eklöf B, Norgren L, Ohlin P, Dahlström JA. Venous thrombectomy for iliofemoral vein thrombosis – 10-year results of a prospective randomised study. *Eur J Vasc Endovasc Surg.* 1997;14:367-374.
18. Patel KR, Paidas CN. Phlegmasia cerulea dolens: the role of non-operative therapy. *Cardiovasc Surg.* 1993;1:518-523.
19. Alimi YS, Dimauro P, Fabre D, Juhan C. Iliac vein reconstructions to treat acute and chronic venous occlusive disease. *J Vasc Surg.* 1997;25:673-681.
20. Hood DB, Alexander JQ. Endovascular management of iliofemoral venous occlusive disease. *Surg Clin North Am.* 2004;84:1381-1396. viii.

Iliofemoral Deep Venous Thrombosis During Pregnancy

52

Anthony J. Comerota

A 24-year-old female who was 32 weeks pregnant presented to the emergency department at 7 pm with a swollen, painful left lower extremity. Her left leg had become progressively more symptomatic during the past 48 h. During the past 24 h, she began feeling lethargic, had slight shortness of breath, and began to experience right chest discomfort with deep breathing.

Upon physical examination, her heart rate was 106/min, respiratory rate was 18/min, and blood pressure was 112/70. Her lungs were clear, and her abdomen was appropriate for her gestational age.

She had a swollen left leg from the foot to the inguinal ligament, which had a bluish hue. She had pain upon palpation of the left femoral vein. Her arterial examination was normal.

A venous duplex was ordered and scheduled to be performed in approximately 3 h.

Question 1

At this point, what would be your next course of action?

A. Obtain an immediate ventilation/perfusion lung scan.
B. Perform a venogram.
C. Start intravenous heparin at 100 mg/kg bolus followed by a continuous infusion at 15 mg/kg/h; or, an injection of subcutaneous enoxaparin at 1 mg/kg.
D. Maintain the patient at bed rest until the duplex is completed. If the duplex confirms deep vein thrombosis (DVT), begin treatment with heparin.
E. Perform an echocardiogram.

The patient had an intravenous line started and a bolus of unfractionated heparin was given, followed by a continuous infusion. Four hours later, the venous duplex examination demonstrated venous thrombosis in the posterior tibial vein, popliteal vein, femoral vein, proximal great saphenous vein, common femoral vein, and external iliac vein to the visible limit of the examination. The veins of the right lower extremity were normal. The patient asks, "What can I expect if treated with continued anticoagulation?"

A.J. Comerota
Department of Surgery, Temple University Hospital, Philadelphia PA, USA

G. Geroulakos and B. Sumpio (eds.), *Vascular Surgery*,
DOI: 10.1007/978-1-84996-356-5_52, © Springer-Verlag London Limited 2011

Question 2

You tell the patient that she has iliofemoral and infrainguinal deep vein thrombosis, and with continued anticoagulation

A. She will do much better following delivery if she remains anticoagulated for 1 year.
B. She faces a 15–40% likelihood of venous claudication at 5 years.
C. She faces a 90% likelihood of venous insufficiency and 15% likelihood of venous ulceration.
D. It is difficult to predict the natural consequences of her disease.

Question 3

This patient's father has long suffered with post-thrombotic chronic venous insufficiency, and she expresses a strong desire to avoid post-thrombotic complications.

However, she does not want to accept the risks of bleeding associated with thrombolytic therapy; therefore, she asks for your treatment recommendation. Your best recommendation to this patient would be

A. Intravenous heparin for 5 days, followed by oral anticoagulation with a warfarin compound.
B. Heparin (unfractionated or low-molecular-weight) until the delivery, followed by warfarin anticoagulation.
C. Rheolytic thrombectomy.
D. Catheter-directed thrombolysis.
E. Operative venous thrombectomy.

Because of her painful lower extremity and her concern for post-thrombotic complications, the patient requested that the thrombus be removed. She was reluctant to accept the potential bleeding complications of catheter-directed thrombolysis, and the attending radiologist was reluctant to treat with catheter-directed lysis. Therefore, venous thrombectomy was planned

Question 4

The next appropriate step is

A. Obtain a ventilation/perfusion scan or spiral CT scan of the chest to evaluate for suspected pulmonary embolism.
B. Obtain a contralateral iliocavagram prior to taking the patient to the operating room.
C. Take the patient directly to the operating room and perform the procedure in order to avoid progressive deterioration.
D. Anticoagulate overnight and proceed with operative thrombectomy the next day.

The patient was anticoagulated with intravenous heparin overnight. The next morning a contralateral iliocavagram was performed (Fig. 52.1) prior to taking the patient to the operating room. A large volume of nonocclusive thrombus was found throughout the infrarenal vena cava.

Fig. 52.1 A contralateral iliocavagram demonstrates a large volume of nonocclusive thrombus in the vena cava. Note fetal skeleton in normal position

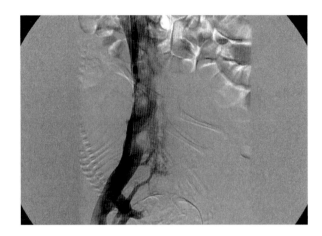

Question 5

In light of the findings on the cavagram, what is the best next step?

A. Abandon operative venous thrombectomy and anticoagulate.
B. Perform an AngioJet mechanical thrombectomy of the vena cava and iliofemoral venous system.
C. Perform a pulmonary arteriogram to confirm/exclude pulmonary embolism.
D. Obtain an echocardiogram.
E. Insert a suprarenal vena caval filter and proceed with venous thrombectomy under fluoroscopic guidance.

The patient was presumed to have had a pulmonary embolism. A echocardiogram failed to show right ventricular dysfunction, an enlarged right ventricle, tricuspid insufficiency, or elevated pulmonary artery pressures. Because of the potential risk of dislodging nonocclusive thrombus during the venous thrombectomy, a removable suprarenal vena caval filter was inserted (Fig. 52.2).

Question 6

Important considerations during thrombectomy include

A. Shield the fetus from all X-ray exposure.
B. Perform the venous thrombectomy under fluoroscopic guidance.
C. Monitor the fetus throughout the procedure.
D. Let the nonocclusive thrombus in the vena cava remain undisturbed and perform a thrombectomy of the iliofemoral venous system only.

The patient was taken to the operating room for a venous thrombectomy with fluoroscopic guidance and fetal monitoring. A cut-down was performed on the left common femoral and femoral veins, with exposure of the saphenofemoral junction. A longitudinal venotomy was

Fig. 52.2 X-ray demonstrates suprarenal vena caval filter in proper position

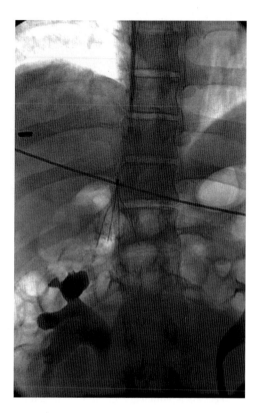

performed at the level of the saphenofemoral junction, followed by protrusion of a large amount of acute thrombus. The leg was raised and a tight rubber bandage applied with minimal extrusion of the infrainguinal thrombus. Attempts to pass a catheter from the inguinal ligament distally into the femoral vein and attempts to pass a guidewire distally were unsuccessful.

Question 7

The next appropriate step would be

A. Perform iliofemoral and caval thrombectomy with AV fistula, leaving the infrainguinal thrombus.
B. Abandon thrombectomy and anticoagulate.
C. Perform an infrainguinal venous thrombectomy aided by a cut-down on the left posterior tibial vein.

A cut-down on the posterior tibial vein was performed. Following a posterior tibial venotomy, a no. 3 Fogarty catheter was passed upwards through the thrombosed venous system, exiting the common femoral venotomy. This catheter was used to guide a no. 4 Fogarty catheter distally through the venous valves by placing both catheter tips within a 14-gauge Silastic intravenous catheter sheath after the hub was amputated. Following a mechanical balloon catheter thrombectomy, the leg was flushed using a bulb syringe with a large volume of heparin/saline solution, which flushed additional thrombus from the common femoral venotomy. After clamping the femoral vein, the deep venous system was then filled with 300 ml of a dilute recombinant tissue plasminogen solution (6 mg rt-PA in 300 ml).

The iliofemoral and vena caval thrombectomy was performed under fluoroscopic guidance, filling the balloon with contrast to ensure that the suprarenal caval filter was not dislodged. After completing the thrombectomy, an operative iliocavagram was performed to assess the adequacy of thrombectomy and to ensure unobstructed venous drainage into the vena cava. An iliac vein stenosis was observed.

Question 8

The appropriate next step is

A. Close the venotomy and anticoagulate, since a common iliac vein stenosis is frequently observed due to normal vascular anatomy.
B. Close the venotomy and perform an AV fistula.
C. Perform angioplasty and insert a self-expanding stent if recoil occurs.
D. Operatively expose the common iliac vein and perform an endovenectomy and transpose the vein above the right common iliac artery.

A balloon angioplasty catheter was placed into the lesion and an angioplasty performed. The iliac vein was dilated to 14 mm without evidence of recoil (Fig. 52.3).

Question 9

Now that patency has been restored to the infrainguinal and iliofemoral venous systems, are there any additional techniques that can be performed to reduce risk of rethrombus?

A. An AV fistula, using the end of the proximal saphenous vein sewn to the side of the superficial femoral artery.
B. The saphenous vein should not be used for AV fistula, since it represents collateral drainage from the leg in the event of recurrent thrombosis.
C. Placement of a catheter into the posterior tibial vein for anticoagulation with unfractionated heparin.
D. Elevate the legs and avoid ambulation for the next 4–5 days.
E. Therapeutic anticoagulation.

An arteriovenous fistula (AVF) using the proximal saphenous vein anastomosed to the superficial femoral artery increases flow velocity through the iliofemoral venous system, reducing the risk of rethrombosis. A thrombectomy of the proximal great saphenous vein was required in this patient, as is often the case. Since the goal of the AVF is to increase venous blood flow velocity, the size of the anastomosis is limited to 3.5–4 mm in order to avoid a steal and avoid venous hypertension. A small piece of PTFE is wrapped around the saphenous AVF and looped with a 2-cm piece of O-Prolene, which is left in the subcutaneous tissue (Fig. 52.4). This will serve as a guide should the AVF require closure.

Fig. 52.3 (**a**) A completion phlebogram following iliofemoral thrombectomy shows stenosis of the left common iliac vein. (**b**) Balloon dilation corrects the lesion without evidence of recoil, providing unobstructed venous drainage into the vena cava

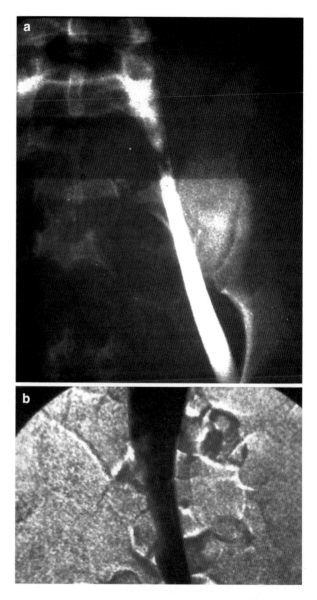

However, since the AVF is small, it is considered permanent and closure is not anticipated. To further reduce the risk of rethrombosis, a heparin infusion catheter (pediatric feeding tube) is placed into the proximal posterior tibial vein and brought out through a separate stab wound adjacent to the lower leg incision. Infusing unfractionated heparin through this catheter to achieve a therapeutic PTT ensures a high concentration of heparin in the target vein, a concentration much higher than would be achieved if the patient was treated with standard intravenous anticoagulation through an arm vein. A monofilament suture is looped around the catheter in the posterior tibial vein and brought out through

Fig. 52.4 The construction of the arteriovenous fistula (AVF) using a large side branch of the great saphenous vein sutured end-side to the superficial femoral artery. Note sleeve of PTFE wrapped around the AVF and looped with a 2-cm piece of O-monofilament suture. The purpose of this is to assist in operative closure should obliteration of the AVF become necessary

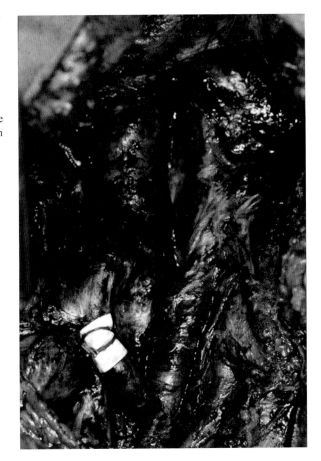

the skin and secured with a sterile button. This is used to occlude the vein after 5–6 days when the catheter is removed following full oral anticoagulation with warfarin. In the case of this pregnant patient, intravenous anticoagulation through the leg veins was maintained for 4 days, after which she was converted to subcutaneous enoxaparin at 1 mg/kg every 12 h. The catheter was removed and the patient discharged. The patient was maintained on subcutaneous enoxaparin 1 mg/kg twice a day until she delivered a healthy baby 6 weeks later.

Question 10

The patient does not wish to breastfeed her baby. What is your best recommendation for ongoing therapy?

A. Six more weeks of Lovenox.
B. Oral anticoagulation for 6–12 months.

C. Patients' risk for recurrence is determined by the amount of residual thrombus. If there is no residual thrombus on venous duplex, additional anticoagulation is unnecessary.

D. Stop anticoagulation and start aspirin.

Question 11

What is your recommendation regarding a thrombophilia evaluation?

A. It is not necessary to perform an expensive thrombophilia evaluation since this was a DVT of pregnancy.

B. Defer the thrombophilia evaluation until after the patient discontinues anticoagulation.

C. Since this patient will be on indefinite anticoagulation, a thrombophilia evaluation is not necessary.

D. Perform tests not affected by anticoagulation and complete the evaluation after anticoagulation has been discontinued.

An abbreviated thrombophilia evaluation of: lupus anticoagulant, antiphospholipid/anticardiolipin antibody, factor V Leiden, prothrombin gene mutation, and homocysteine was negative. The remainder of the thrombophilia evaluation will be completed in 1–2 years, at which time it is anticipated that the patient's Coumadin will be discontinued.

52.1
Commentary

In 2008, it was recognized by the ACCP guidelines on antithrombotic therapy for venous thromboembolism[1] that iliofemoral deep venous thrombosis represents a condition with a uniquely high incidence of post-thrombotic morbidity.[2–4]

This patient's presentation was clinically consistent with iliofemoral deep venous thrombosis associated with a pulmonary embolism. The adventitia of the femoral vein is innervated with sensory nerves; therefore, pain on palpation of the femoral vein as a result of its distension is a frequent physical finding. The femoral vein distends as a result of the associated venous hypertension and thrombosis, and there may be an associated inflammatory response.

Patients presenting during off hours to the emergency department who are at high clinical risk of a venous thromboembolic condition should be anticoagulated **[Q1: C]** until a definitive diagnosis is made.[1] A ventilation/perfusion (V/Q) lung scan is not performed in this patient because she is pregnant and the clinical probability of a pulmonary embolism is high. Likewise, a CT angiogram is not performed because of the excessive amount of radiation. The likelihood of the venous duplex demonstrating acute DVT is also high. This patient's treatment will not be altered by the V/Q scan or CTA findings. There is appropriate reluctance to expose the pregnant patient to a radioisotope or the radiation of a CTA. Standard ascending phlebography is not necessary, since the clinical presentation and venous duplex will establish the diagnosis with a high degree of accuracy.

Once anticoagulation is established, it is not necessary and actually counterproductive to maintain the patient at bed rest.[5] An echocardiogram is advisable in all patients who have the diagnosis of pulmonary embolism to evaluate its impact on right ventricular function; however, it is not necessary in this patient to perform an "off hours" echocardiogram since the patient can be adequately treated until the next business day.

This patient's thrombus extends from the posterior tibial vein to the external iliac vein, as documented on venous duplex. The natural history of these patients is one of significant post-thrombotic morbidity. **[Q2: B, C]** Akesson and colleagues[3] demonstrated that within 5 years of anticoagulation for iliofemoral deep venous thrombosis, 95% of patients had documented venous insufficiency, 15% had venous ulceration, and 15% suffered with venous claudication. Delis et al.[4] studied in greater detail a similar but larger cohort of patients with iliofemoral deep venous thrombosis and performed exercise testing. They demonstrated that 40% developed symptoms of venous claudication. While pregnancy is an induced hypercoagulable state, delivery of the present patient's child is not known to alter the natural history of the patient's acute venous thrombosis. In order to reduce the high risk of post-thrombotic sequelae, a strategy of thrombus removal should be considered. Operative venous thrombectomy **[Q3: E]** is the best recommendation in light of the fact that the patient does not wish to face any risk of bleeding with thrombolytic therapy. Rheolytic thrombectomy is in its early stages, and to date has not been shown to be effective by itself in the absence of incorporating a plasminogen activator.[6] Oral anticoagulation during pregnancy is not recommended. Although this patient is in her third trimester and warfarin embryotrophy is not a concern, the potential exaggerated coagulopathy of the fetus due to its immature liver and potential fetal bleeding complications during delivery as a result of passage through the birth canal make oral anticoagulation inadvisable. Heparin anticoagulation until delivery followed by oral anticoagulation is commonly offered to these patients; however, their post-thrombotic morbidity is high.

A decision was made to proceed with venous thrombectomy. Patients can be anticoagulated overnight and the operation performed the next business day. Venous thrombectomy does not need to be performed as an "emergency operation." **[Q4: B, D]** In all patients in whom a venous thrombectomy is performed, it is important to know the proximal extent of thrombus, particularly whether there is thrombus in the inferior vena cava. Therefore, a contralateral iliocavagram is performed prior to the iliofemoral venous thrombectomy. As mentioned earlier, it is assumed that this patient has had a pulmonary embolism and the radiation exposure of a CT scan or a V/Q scan is unnecessary, since their results are unlikely to change this patient's management. However, in the non-pregnant patient, a spiral CT scan of the head, chest, abdomen, and pelvis would be performed. The rationale for CT scanning is that approximately 50% of patients with proximal DVT will have an asymptomatic pulmonary embolism. Up to 25% of these patients will develop subsequent pulmonary symptoms.[7] When the symptoms surface during anticoagulation, the symptoms are often misinterpreted as "failure" of anticoagulation, when in reality it is the natural evolution of the patient's initially asymptomatic (undiagnosed) pulmonary embolism. The proximal extent of thrombus in the vena cava or iliac veins often can be identified, as well as screening for associated intra-abdominal, retroperitoneal, or pelvic pathology.

The patient was treated with anticoagulation overnight. Before going to the operating room a contralateral iliocavagram was performed. Information regarding the proximal extent of thrombus is particularly important, since the details of thrombus extension may alter the procedure. Nonocclusive thrombus in the vena cava is concerning because of its potential for fragmentation and embolization. This author believes that most of these patients should be protected against potential embolization during the procedure. This can be accomplished either with a suprarenal vena caval filter, as was inserted in this patient, since it was presumed that she already had suffered a symptomatic pulmonary embolism. Alternatively, suprathrombus balloon occlusion during the caval thrombectomy can be performed. This patient also underwent a preoperative echocardiogram (which was normal) to evaluate the impact of her presumed pulmonary embolism on right ventricular function. Echocardiography should be performed in all patients with pulmonary embolism, since it is a predictor of chronic thromboembolic pulmonary hypertension, and patients who have rightsided abnormalities should be considered for thrombolytic therapy or mechanical thromboembolectomy. **[Q5: D, E]**

During the operative procedure, fluoroscopy is used to guide the placement of the balloon catheter so as not to dislodge the vena caval filter. Fluoroscopy is also used to assess the success of thrombectomy and to evaluate for underlying venous lesions and their correction (Fig. 52.3). Since the fetus is well developed by the third trimester, the risk to the fetus from modest X-ray exposure is low. Fetal monitoring is routinely performed throughout the procedure. The monitoring devices must be checked so as not to interfere with appropriate imaging of the venous system during the procedure. Shielding of the fetus would obscure the iliac veins and distal vena cava. **[Q6: B, C]** Previous descriptions of iliofemoral venous thrombectomy focus only on the iliofemoral venous system. An occluded infrainguinal venous system reduces venous return through the thrombectomized iliofemoral veins, and leaves substantial thrombus burden infrainguinally with its resultant post-thrombotic sequelae. Current techniques of infrainguinal venous thrombectomy allow the procedure to be performed successfully following a cut-down on the posterior tibial vein.[8] **[Q7: C]** Therefore, contemporary venous thrombectomy should be viewed much the same as arterial thrombectomy, that is, removing as much thrombus from the venous circulation as is physically and pharmacologically possible, correcting any underlying lesion, and perform mechanical and pharmacological maneuvers to avoid recurrent thrombosis.

An iliac venous stenosis observed on completion phlebography is common. Correcting the underlying iliac vein stenosis is considered an important part of the procedure (Fig. 52.3). This is performed under fluoroscopic guidance and if recoil occurs, a self-expanding stent is used to maintain unobstructed venous drainage from the iliac venous system into the vena cava. **[Q8: C]** Direct endophlebectomy of the iliac vein lesion and transposition above the right common iliac artery is a large operation, which has been replaced by the relatively simple balloon dilation and stenting.

Following successful thrombectomy of the infrainguinal and iliofemoral venous systems and correction of any underlying iliac vein stenosis, prevention of recurrent thrombosis is paramount. There are mechanical and pharmacologic measures which, if used, minimize recurrence. These include the construction of a femoral AV fistula using the end of the transected proximal saphenous vein (or a large side branch) anastomosed to the side of the proximal superficial femoral artery (Fig. 52.4). Frequently, the proximal saphenous vein must undergo a thrombectomy to restore its patency. The saphenous vein is not a collateral pathway of venous drainage for patients with iliofemoral venous thrombosis. On occasion, it may be a collateral drainage pathway for patients with infrainguinal DVT. Since the infrainguinal venous system had patency restored, that is not an issue in this patient. The AV fistula is constructed to increase venous velocity in the iliofemoral veins; however, it should not increase venous pressure. Limiting the size of the anastomosis to approximately 4 mm usually accomplishes this goal. Pressure monitoring of the common femoral vein before and after flow is initiated through the AVF is important. If the venous pressure increases, one must suspect a proximal (iliac vein) stenosis or excessive flow through the AVF, either (or both) of which should be corrected.

An additional, effective adjunctive technique is the placement of a catheter into the posterior tibial vein, which is used to anticoagulate the patient with unfractionated heparin postoperatively. A pediatric feeding tube is inserted into the posterior tibial vein and brought out through a separate stab wound in the skin adjacent to the lower leg incision. This small catheter is used for postoperative anticoagulation with unfractionated heparin. Targeting a therapeutic PTT ensures a high concentration of heparin in the diseased vein, which should substantially reduce the risk of recurrence. In the author's experience, when these adjunctive techniques have been used, no patient has experienced rethrombosis. **[Q9: A, C, E]**. Following delivery, women can be anticoagulated with Coumadin, even if they wish to breastfeed.[9] Warfarin is not excreted in the breast milk. Among the options, oral anticoagulation for 6–12 months is the most appropriate. **[Q10: B]** While it is true that residual thrombus increases the risk of recurrent thrombosis,[10] and it appears that she has little if any residual thrombus, it would be inappropriate to treat this patient with less than a full course of anticoagulation.

Since this patient had extensive venous thrombosis and a positive family history, an underlying thrombophilia is suspected and the author would extend the duration of anticoagulation to 1 year or more. In patients on extended or indefinite anticoagulation, repeat evaluation for risk versus benefit is performed at least every 6 months. A thrombophilia evaluation is appropriate in this patient. A complete thrombophilia evaluation cannot be performed while the patient is on anticoagulation, since antithrombin III, proteins C and S, and factor VIII will be affected. However, lupus anticoagulant, antiphospholipid antibody, factor V Leiden, prothrombin gene mutation, and homocysteine levels can be obtained during anticoagulation and, if positive, may play a role in the subsequent management of this patient. **[Q11: D]**

References

1. Kearon C, Kahn SR, Agnelli G, Goldhaber SZ, Raskob G, Comerota AJ. Antithrombotic therapy for venous thromboembolic disease: ACCP evidence-based clinical practice guidelines (8th ed). *Chest*. 2008;133(6):454S-545S.
2. O'Donnell TF Jr, Browse NL, Burnand KG, Thomas ML. The socioeconomic effects of an iliofemoral venous thrombosis. *J Surg Res*. 1977;22:483-488.
3. Akesson H, Brudin L, Dahlstrom JA, Eklof B, Ohlin P, Plate G. Venous function assessed during a 5 year period after acute ilio-femoral venous thrombosis treated with anticoagulation. *Eur J Vasc Surg*. 1990;4:43-48.

4. Delis KT, Bountouroglou D, Mansfield AO. Venous claudication in iliofemoral thrombosis: long-term effects on venous hemodynamics, clinical status, and quality of life. *Ann Surg.* 2004;239:118-126.

5. Partsch H, Kaulich M, Mayer W. Immediate mobilisation in acute vein thrombosis reduces postthrombotic syndrome. *Int Angiol.* 2004;23:206-212.

6. Kasirajan K, Gray B, Ouriel K. Percutaneous AngioJet thrombectomy in the management of extensive deep venous thrombosis. *J Vasc Interv Radiol.* 2001;12:179-185.

7. Monreal M, Rey-Joly BC, Ruiz MJ, Salvador TR, Lafoz NE, Viver ME. Asymptomatic pulmonary embolism in patients with deep vein thrombosis. Is it useful to take a lung scan to rule out this condition? *J Cardiovasc Surg (Torino).* 1989;30:104-107.

8. Comerota AJ, Gale SS. Technique of contemporary iliofemoral and infrainguinal venous thrombectomy. *J Vasc Surg.* 2006;43(1):185-191.

9. Bates SM, Greer IA, Pabinger I, Sofaer S, Hirsh J. Venous thromboembolism thrombophilia, antithrombotic therapy, and pregnancy: ACCP evidence-based clinical practice guidelines (8th ed). *Chest.* 2008;133(6):844S-886S.

10. Prandoni P. Risk factors of recurrent venous thromboembolism: the role of residual vein thrombosis. *Pathophysiol Haemost Thromb.* 2003;33:351-353.

Part XIII

Lymphodema

Management of Chronic Lymphedema of the Lower Extremity

53

Byung-Boong Lee and James Laredo

A 19 year old female was brought in to the Emergency Room (ER) in a "septic shock" condition with massively swollen bilateral lower limbs (Fig. 53.1).

This patient was well known to the ER staff for many years with recurrent episodes of systemic sepsis often triggered by local cellulitis and/or erysipelas involving one of her swollen limbs. The intervals between her sepsis got shorter lately and the control of her sepsis became more difficult, to manage.

Question 1

Which of the following would you deter in your first step towards managing the situation?

1. Initiation of the differential diagnosis
2. Resuscitation
3. Blood cultures before the antibiotic administration
4. Anticoagulation
5. Thorough investigation on the cause of sepsis (Answer – 4)

The past history reveals that she was born with a swelling of the left lower leg, including her toes but did not receive any treatment. Before she reached her menarche she developed a similar swelling on her right side starting from the mid-thigh region downwards. Initially her limb swellings were relieved by nocturnal elevation but soon improvements diminished following recurrent local sepsis.

B.-B. Lee (✉)
Department of Vascular Surgery, Georgetown University School of Medicine, Washington, DC, USA

G. Geroulakos and B. Sumpio (eds.), *Vascular Surgery*,
DOI: 10.1007/978-1-84996-356-5_53, © Springer-Verlag London Limited 2011

Fig. 53.1 The clinical photo shows 19 years old female in a bed-ridden condition at the ICU after successful resuscitation from the septic shock. Massively swollen bilateral lower extremities is due to the primary lymphedema in the end stage complicated with recurrent sepsis

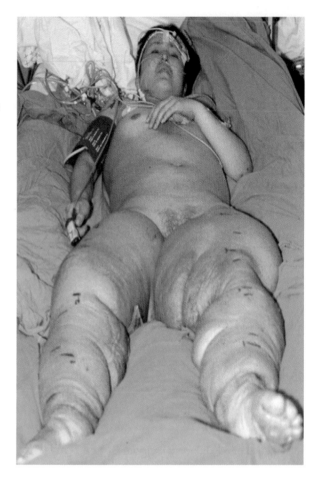

Question 2

What is the most probable cause of her bilateral lower limb swellings?

1. Chronic deep vein thrombosis
2. Congenital vascular malformation, probably of lymphatic origin
3. Early stage of cardiac failure
4. Early stage of anasarca from congenital hypothyroidism
5. Secondary chronic lymphedema, probably from filariasis infection (Answer – 2)

The patient neglected medical care until puberty, and her limb condition deteriorated steadily following repeated episodes of sepsis through the year. The pitting nature of her swelling was now replaced with a rubbery firm leg, which became massively swollen during the last few months.

Examination in the ER revealed extremely swollen bilateral limbs. There was a resolving patch of redness along the left buttock but no clear evidence of infection. A shallow decubitus ulcer (3.0 × 3.0 × 0.5 cm) was identified in right presacral region without evidence of invasive infection.

This ulcer recently developed lately when the patient became bed-ridden secondary to the debilitating swelling of her lower limbs (Fig. 53.1).

The patient was promptly resuscitated to stabilize her condition. Due to her labile vital signs however, the patient required admission to the intensive care unit for further management.

Question 3

What is the next stage of her management?

1. Parenteral antibiotic administration
2. Immediate application of compression bandages
3. Immediate application of sequential pneumatic compression therapy
4. Radical debridement of the decubitus ulcer
5. Absolute bed rest under full anticoagulation (Answer – 1)

Following the control of systemic sepsis, the management of her limb swelling remained a challenge especially since she gained over 40 kg from 55 to 99 kg following abandoned therapy.

Question 4

What is the most appropriate way to reduce her massive swelling and improve her mobility?

1. Vigorous application of high pressure compression therapy
2. Weight control regimen with strict dietary control
3. Immediate plan for the surgical excision of swollen tissue
4. Timed initiation of complex decongestive therapy
5. Angioplasty and/or stent insertion to iliac vein stenosis (Answer – 4)

Question 5

What is the most frequent and potentially serious risk involved in the management of massive edema?

1. Acute tissue gangrene
2. Acute pulmonary thromboembolism
3. Acute pulmonary edema
4. Acute limb paralysis
5. Acute deep vein thrombosis (Answer – 3)

Following successful management of her crisis, further investigations and assessments of her swollen limbs were carried out to establish a long term care plan. A home maintenance care regimen was also prescribed.

Question 6

Which of the following tests would not be needed in general for diagnosis and assessment?

1. Oil contrast lymphography/lymphangiography
2. Duplex assessment of the deep venous system
3. Volume measurements
4. Radionuclide lymphoscintigraphy
5. Magnetic Resonance Imaging study (Answer – 1)

Question 7

The aim of the investigations on the current condition include all of the following EXCEPT?

1. Clinical and laboratory staging of the edematous limb
2. Assessment of deep vein status of the lower extremity
3. Selective investigation on the iliac vein stenosis/occlusion
4. Assessment for the possibility of coexisting vascular malformation
5. Patient compliance to maintain her care (Answer – 3)

Question 8

What is the most essential and reliable part of the therapy in general?

1. Diet
2. Compression bandage
3. Exercise
4. Bed rest with leg elevation
5. Anticoagulation (Answer – 2)

Despite the rigorous home care regimen, her current limb condition continued to deteriorate. Physical therapy became increasingly difficult with very limited response. Her leg became much firmer and more frequent episodes of aborted and/or full blown cellulitis occurred through the year.

Question 9

What kind of the treatment can be instituted as a supplement to her current physical therapy?

1. Mercury bath-combined microwave therapy
2. Cross-femoral bypass surgery to relieve venous hypertension
3. Thromboembolectomy of the iliac-femoral vein

4. Reconstructive surgery to restore lymph transport
5. Excisional surgery to remove overgrown fibrosclerotic tissue (Answer – 5)

Treatment failure, despite a full year of maximum conventional care, was accepted as the indication of additional treatment by the multidisciplinary team.

Question 10

What is NOT an essential part for the treatment in such an advanced stage?

1. Encouraging patient compliance to maintain physical therapy
2. Multidisciplinary team approach to improve quality of life
3. Repeated assessments of lymphatic function with lymphography
4. Active mobilization for better social and psychological rehabilitation
5. Vigorous control and prevention of infection (Answer – 3)

53.1
Commentary

The clinical history of this young lady illustrates how primary lymphedema progresses when timely appropriate care is neglected.

Her left lower limb swelling since the birth should have been recognized as a primary lymphedema until proven otherwise. A basic assessment of her clinical appearance should not have been delayed especially after the contralateral limb went down the same path of the swelling as a 'precox' type.[1–8]

It would have ideal for basic investigations to confirm primary lymphedema when both limbs got involved. Focused management combined with active prevention of infection could then have been started at a much earlier point.

With early aggressive management, her lymphedema condition would have not reached such an advanced stage so quickly with suchlife-threatening sepsis.

If lymphedema advances to a late stage, a simple edematous condition of the soft tissue becomes a fibrosclerotic one. This will then resist conventional treatments such as manual lymphatic drainage (MLD)-based complex decongestive therapy (CDT).[9–14] hardened local tissue becomes a harbinger for infection which often advances to systemic sepsis.

Sepsis is the most serious complication as it is a potentially life-threatening. This often leads a vicious cycle with more tissue damage and subsequent vulnerability condition to recurrent sepsis/infection.[15–18]

This young lady is a typical example of advanced lymphedema (Fig. 53.1).

Neglect care without regular CDT accelerated the deterioration of her tissues provoking local sepsis and septic shock prior to her emergency admission

Prompt management of septic shock is warranted with appropriate resuscitation to stabilize her vital signs. Antibiotics should be given as soon as possible after the blood culture specimen is obtained and continued parenterally until suitable selection of culture-sensitive antibiotics. Once the patient condition is stabilized, the diagnosis of her primary condition should be initiated. For an appropriate differential diagnosis on such limb swellings, not only the local causes but also the regional and systemic causes should be included, especially if there is any doubt on currently established diagnosis.

In addition, a thorough investigation on the cause of sepsis should be repeated (e.g., fungal infection: tinea pedis). [Q1: 4]

Limb swelling since birth along the left lower leg and toes and subsequently on the right lower limb, gives ample evidence for primary lymphedema as her diagnosis. Nevertheless the causes of secondary lymphedema should also be ruled out regardless of age of onset.

Primary lymphedema represents a "truncular" type of lymphatic malformation (LM)[19–22] since the majority have associated congenital structural abnormalities of the lymphatic system (e.g., aplasia, hypoplasia, hyperplasia).

LMs are a common form of congenital vascular malformations (CVMs)[23–26] either as an independent (predominant) lesion or as a combined condition with other CVMs: venous malformations (VMs),[27–30] arterio-venous malformations (AVMs),[31–34] and/or capillary malformations (CMs).

The diagnosis and management of primary lymphedema should therefore consider such coexistence with other CVMs, including the extratruncular LM (e.g., Klippel-Trenaunay Syndrome)[35–38] (Fig. 53.2).

A basic understanding on the LM as a CVM, including its embryological background is required in order to lead appropriate investigations on primary lymphedema.

Like other CVMs, these LMs are also classified into two different groups[39–41] depending upon the embryological stage of developmental arrest: extratruncular and truncular LM's.

Extratruncular LMs are also known as "lymphangiomata" – and they are embryonic tissue remnants as a result of developmental arrest/defect occurring in the "earlier" stage of lymphangiogenesis. Mesenchymal cell characteristics are maintained with the evolutionary potential to grow when stimulated (Fig. 53.3).

In contrast truncular lesions are a result of developmental arrest/defect at the "later" stage of lymphangiogenesis and lack these critical embryonic characteristics.[42,43]

Following stabilization from septic shock, the treatment of sepsis should start with parenteral antibiotic administration while searching for the source of the infection. Compression therapy with MLD-based CDT or a pneumatic compression device is contraindicated until the sepsis is under full control. Early ambulation is recommended to control decubitus development. [Q3: 1]

Vigorous application of high pressure compression therapy should be deferred until the cardiovascular system is fully stabilized. CDT is under close observation when the overall cardiovascular condition can afford the additional loading of mobilized edema fluid. [Q4: 4]

Rapid fluid mobilization from a massively swollen limb is dangerous soon after septic shock. If the forceful evacuation of fluid from the interstitial space is too effective, massive influx into the intravascular space will accompany a high risk of acute pulmonary edema. [Q5: 3]

In order to provide an appropriate treatment strategy for long term care, a full assessment can be achieved based on a combination of basic non- to less-invasive tests[44–46]: Radionuclide lymphoscintigraphy (LSG),[47–49] Duplex ultrasonographic assessment,[50–52] Limb volume measurement,[53–55] and Magnetic Resonance Imaging (MRI) study.[56–58] Although the MRI is NOT essential for the investigation of primary lymphedema caused by the truncular LM

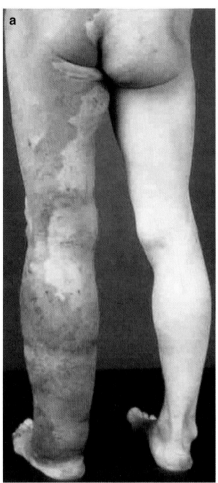
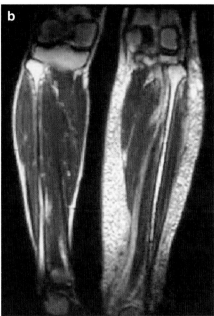

Fig. 53.2 The clinical photo (**a**) belonging to another patient shows typical appearance of Klippel-Trenaunay syndrome (KTS) involving the left lower extremity; entire left lower limb swelling is not only due to the primary lymphedema caused by the lymphatic malformation (LM) but also by coexisting venous malformation (VM) as well. MR Image (**b**) depicts typical soft tissue swelling along the lower limb as a hall mark of the chronic lymphedema. However, as the whole body blood pool scintigraphy (**c**) demonstrates, there are two VM lesions, truncular-marginal vein- as well as extratruncular VM involving to the left lower limb to accentuate the swelling. The radionuclide lymphoscintigraphy (**d**) confirms advanced lymphatic dysfunction due to the primary lymphedema, displaying extensive dermal backflow along the left lower limb due to a lack of normal clearance condition/lymphatic transportation. Therefore, whenever the "primary" lymphedema is encountered as the cause of limb swelling, possible coexisting of another congenital vascular malformations (CVMs) should be ruled out first. Because, the majority of the primary lymphedema represents the clinical manifestation of the truncular LM

Fig. 53.2 (continued)

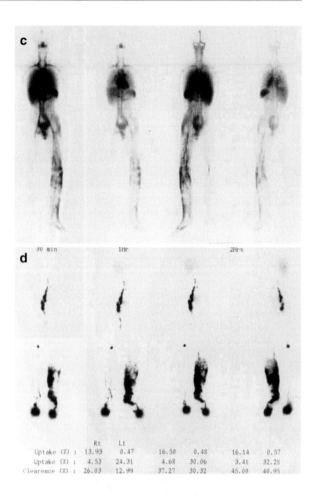

itself, the MRI may give not only additional information on the lymphedema status as well as coexisting CVMs like extratruncular VM's and/or LM's. [**Q6: 1**]

Oil contrast lymphography[59,60] is invasive and not needed for the diagnosis. Due to the risk of further damaging the lymph vessels it's use is now strictly limited as a special indication for the selection of surgical reconstruction candidates.

Such investigations to provide the critical information needed to set up a adequate home maintenance care regimen following discharge from acute care.

Accurate information on the clinical and laboratory stage of the lymphedema[46,61] is important for the selection of the right therapy. Abnormalities of the deep venous system would affect the response to therapy. Coexisting CVMs may also give a profound impact to the overall management.

Finally, an accurate evaluation on self-motivation to maintain care is absolutely essential since the life-time commitment to CDT based home maintenance therapy is totally depending on patient compliance.[18,44] [**Q7: 3**]

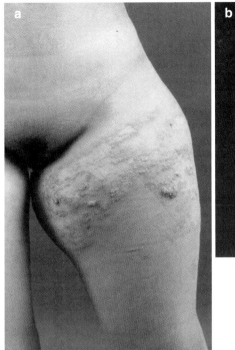
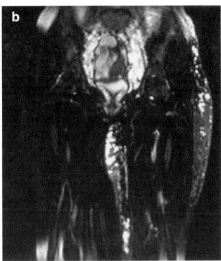

Fig. 53.3 Clinical photo (**a**) shows diffuse swelling along the upper thigh extended to the groin, which is due to the extratruncular LM, different from the truncular LM causing the primary lymphedema. This extratruncular LM, often called as "lymphangioma," is the outcome of developmental arrest/defect from the "early" stage of lymphangiogenesis. Therefore, it possesses a mesenchymal cell characteristic to grow when the condition should meet (e.g., hormone, menarche, pregnancy, trauma, surgery). As shown in MRI (**b**), this extratruncular lesion in upper thigh is extended to the pelvic cavity affecting entire pelvic soft tissue and the *left* lower limb lesion/swelling is a tip of the iceberg. The lesion is now complicated with the lymphatic leakage and sepsis

CDT[9–14] remains a main stay of contemporary treatment of chronic lymphedema although it does not cure the condition. It is the most effective means to prevent the progress of the condition. Among various components of CDT, MLD is the most essential part together with compression bandage.[62,63] MLD is a physiological means to stimulate paralyzed lymph vessels to restore peristalsis and relieve lymph stasis. Although MLD lacks theoretical evidence, it is now accepted as an effective therapy in the early stages of lymphedema (Fig. 53.4).

In contrast the sequential pneumatic compression-therapy (SIPC)[64–66] remains controversial due to risk of selective transfer of the fluid component out of the interstitial tissue leaving the protein component of the lymph behind to precipitate progressive tissue damage.

Among the many different components of CDT, compression bandage therapy remains the most effective and proven component. These recommendations are based on the grading according to scientific evidence,[67] where compression therapy belongs to 1C or 2A. 1C represents a strong recommendation based on low-quality evidence where as 2A is a weak recommendation based on high-quality evidence (Table 53.1). **[Q8: 2]**

However, when CDT-based conservative therapy fails, despite maximum care, surgical therapy is generally considered as a supplemental regimen to improve its efficacy of the CDT.[68,69]

Reconstructive surgery[70-74] is generally aimed at the early stages of the lymphedema where the paralyzed lymph vessels can be rescued before they become permanently damaged by chronic lymphatic hypertension. Methods to repair a damaged lymph transport system and restore lymphatic function include lymphatico-venous anastomosis, lymphatico-lymphatic bypass, lymphatico-lymphatic segmental interposition, and free lymph node transplantation.

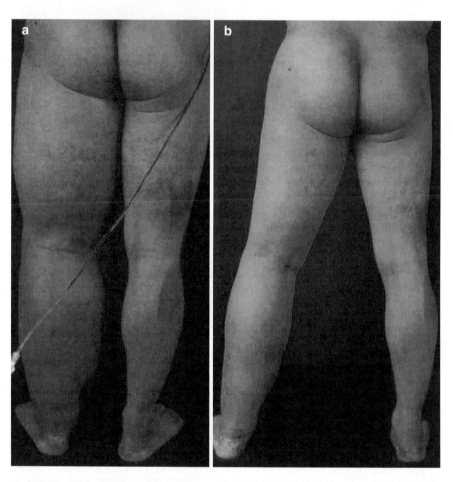

Fig. 53.4 Two clinical photos (**a** and **b**) show a clinical condition of another/different patient with primary lymphedema before (**a**) and after (**b**) the CDT instituted, showing how effective this MLD-based CDT is. As displayed by the radionuclide lymphoscintigraphy (LSG) (**c** and **d**), the pre-CDT LSG (**c**) shows extensive dermal backflow due to the lymph stasis in the soft tissue while the post-CDT LSG (**d**) demonstrates excellent response of the lymph stasis to the CDT

Fig. 53.4 (continued)

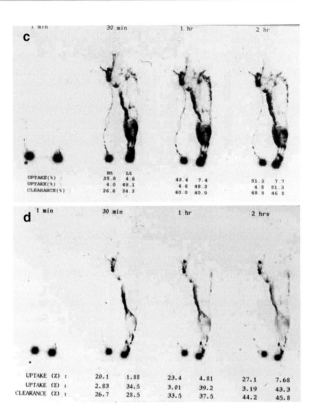

In advanced lymphedema however, there are no more salvageable lymphatic vessels remaining and therefore, it is too late for reconstructive surgery.

Since overgrown fibrosclerotic tissue is a known harbinger for t recurrent sepsis (e.g., cellulitis/erysipelas) (Fig. 53.5). Excisional surgery[18,44,75] and [76] would improve not only the efficacy of CDT but also the overall risk of sepsis thereby improving quality of life. Although surgery remains as a valid option to assist CDT, current evidence-based recommendations still classify this as 2C (Table 53.2).

Liposuction[77,78] obliterates the epifascial compartment by a selective removal of excessive adipose tissue. This procedure is not indicated for advanced lymphedema. In end stage lympedema entire tissues become fibrosclerotic with very limited fat tissue available for liposuction.

Therefore, excisional surgery remains the only viable option among the various surgical treatment modalities in end stage disease. All candidates for the excisional surgery, require mandatory postoperative CDT with a life-time. The guarantee of satisfactory outcome of the surgery should not be expected without appropriate postoperative CDT.[18,44]
[Q9: 5]

This patient met the indication for excisional surgery in order to improve the efficacy of CDT, this followed the documented failure of CDT alone despite maximum care for 2

Table 53.1 Guidelines 6.3.0 of the American venous forum on lymphedema: medical and physical therapy

No.	Guideline	Grade of recommendation (1, we recommend; 2, we suggest)	Grade of evidence (A, high quality; B, moderate quality; C, low or very low quality)
6.3.1	To reduce lymphedema we recommend multimodal complex decongestive therapy that includes manual lymphatic drainage; multilayer short-stretch bandaging; remedial exercise; skin care; and instruction in long-term management	1	B
6.3.2	To reduce lymphedema, we recommend short-stretch bandages that remain in place for longer than 22 h/day	1	B
6.3.3	To reduce lymphedema we recommend treatment daily, a minimum of 5 days per week, and continue until normal anatomy or a volumetric plateau is established	1	B
6.3.4	To reduce lymphedema we suggest compression pumps in some patients	2	C
6.3.5	For maintenance of lymphedema we recommend an appropriately fitting compression garment	1	A
6.3.6	For maintenance of lymphedema in patients with advanced (stages II or III) disease we recommend using short-stretch bandages during the night. Alternatively, compression devices may substitute for short-stretch bandages	1	B
6.3.7	For remedial exercises we recommend wearing compression garments or bandages	1	C
6.3.8	For cellulitis or lymphangitis we recommend antibiotics with superior coverage of Gram-positive cocci, particularly streptococci. Examples include cephalexin, penicillin, clindamycin, cefadroxii	1	A
6.3.9	For prophylaxis of cellulitis in patients with more than three episodes of infection we recommend antibiotics with superior coverage of Gram-positive cocci, particularly streptococci, at full strength for 1 week/month, Examples include cephalexin, penicillin, clindamycin, cefadroxil	1	C

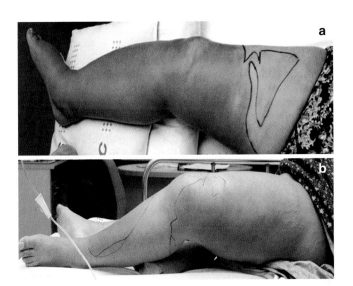

Fig. 53.5 Two clinical photos (**a** and **b**) depict extensive cellulitis involving two different sites of the limb through recurrent episodes. This condition is potentially life threatening condition to warrant immediate control to prevent systemic sepsis. Along the end stage of the lymphedema, such recurrent infections become a major challenge and would become an indirect indication for the excisional surgery to reduce the fibrosclerotic tissue as a major harbinger of the recurrent infection

Table 53.2 Guidelines 6.4.0 of the American venous forum on principles of surgical treatment of chronic lymphedema

No.	Guideline	Grade of recommendation (1, we recommend; 2, we suggest)	Grade of evidence (A, high quality; B, moderate quality; C, low or very low quality)
6.4.1	All interventions for chronic lymphedema should be preceded by at least 6 months of non-operative compression treatment	1	C
6.4.2	We suggest excisional operations or liposuction only to patients with late stage non-pitting lymphedema, who fail conservative measures	2	C
6.4.3	We suggest microsurgical lymphatic reconstructions in centers of excellence for selected patients with secondary lymphedema, if performed early in the course of the disease	2	C

years. A modified Homan-Auchincloss procedure[79,80] was implemented to remove, the entire skin and soft tissues including the muscle fascia, to facilitate lymph absorption through the deep system. An excellent surgical outcome was maintained with a postoperative CDT regimen during the follow up period of 4 years (Fig. 53.6).

A multidisciplinary team approach should always be organized to support surgical therapy. This should improve quality of life provided patient compliance is good enough for maintenance CDT.

Active mobilization for better social and psychological rehabilitation should accompany CDT in order to provide an incentive to the patient to remain on therapy.

Vigorous control and prevention of infection should always remain the ultimate goal for end stage lymphedema. [**Q10: 3**]

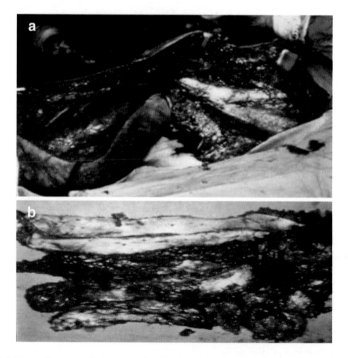

Fig. 53.6 (a) Photo illustrates the magnitude of the excisional surgery to remove entire soft tissue together with the skin, which all became sclerotic; Homan-Auchincloss technique was modified and excision was further extended to remove the muscle fascia as well to promote the absorption of the lymph by the deep lymphatic system. (**b**) Photo demonstrates the surgical specimen showing the staging excision for the optimum amount of the tissue removal. Clinical photo (**c**) shows clinical outcome of the surgery 6 months later, achieving the goal of effective mobilization from the bed and increased efficacy of the postoperative CDT. This approach delivered improved quality of life with better social/physical/ psychological adaptation

Fig. 53.6 (continued)

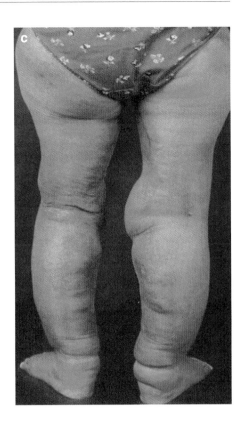

References

1. Browse NL, Stewart G. Lymphoedema: pathophysiology and classification. *J Cardiovasc Surg (Torino)*. 1985;26(2):91-106. Review.
2. Lee BB. Chronic lymphedema, no more stepchild to modern medicine! *Eur J Lymphol.* 2004;14(42):6-12.
3. Szuba A, Rockson SG. Lymphedema: classification, diagnosis and therapy. *Vasc Med.* 1998;3(2):145-156. Review.
4. Bernas MJ, Witte CL, Witte MH. The diagnosis and treatment of peripheral lymphedema. *Lymphology*. 2001;34:84-91.
5. Esterly JR. Congenital hereditary lymphedema. *J Med Genet.* 1965;2:93-98.
6. Lewis JM, Wald ER. Lymphedema praecox. *J Pediatr.* 1984;104:641-648.
7. Burnand KG, Mortimer PS. Lymphangiogenesis and genetics of lymphoedema. In: Browse N, Burnand KG, Mortimer PS, eds. *Diseases of the Lymphatics*. London: Arnold; 2003:102-109.
8. Wheeler ES, Chan V, Wassman R, Rimoin DL, Lesavoy MA. Familial lymphedema praecox: Meige disease. *Plast Reconstr Surg.* 1981;67:362-364.
9. Szolnoky G, Lakatos B, Keskeny T, Dobozy A. Advantage of combined decongestive lymphatic therapy over manual lymph drainage: a pilot study. *Lymphology.* 2002;35(Suppl):277-282.
10. Leduc O, Bourgeois P, Leduc A. Manual of lymphatic drainage: scintigraphic demonstration of its efficacy on colloidal protein reabsorption. In: Partsch, ed. *Progress in Lymphology IX. Excerpta Medica*. Amsterdam: Elsevier; 1988.

11. Foldi E, Foldi M, Weissletter H. Conservative treatment of lymphedema of the limbs. *Angiology*. 1985;36:171-180.
12. Morgan RG, Casley-Smith, Judith R, Mason MR, et al. Complex physical therapy of the lymphoedematous arm. *J Hand Surg (Brit)*. 1992;17B:437-441.
13. Leduc O, Leduc A, Bourgeois P, Belgrado JP. The physical treatment of upper limb edema. American Cancer Society Lymphedema Workshop; Supplement to Cancer; 1998:2835–2839
14. Hwang JH, Kwon JY, Lee KW, et al. Changes in lymphatic function after complex physical therapy for lymphedema. *Lymphology*. 1999;32:15-21.
15. Babb RR, Spittell JA Jr, Martin WJ, Schirger A. Prophylaxis of recurrent lymphangitis complicating lymphedema. *JAMA*. 1966;195(10):871-873.
16. Swartz MN M.D. Cellulitis. *N Engl J Med*. 2004;350:904-912.
17. Vaillant L. Erysipelas and lymphedema. *Phlebolymphology N°56*. 2007;14(3):120-124.
18. Lee BB. Current issue in management of chronic lymphedema: Personal Reflection on an Experience with 1065 Patients. *(Commentary) Lymphology*. 2005;38:28-31.
19. Lee BB, Seo JM, Hwang JH, et al. Current concepts in lymphatic malformation (LM). *J Vasc Endovascular Surg*. 2005;39(1):67-81.
20. Lee BB, Laredo J, Seo JM, Neville R. Treatment of lymphatic malformations. In: Mattassi R, Loose DA, Vaghi M eds. *Hemangiomas and Vascular Malformations,* Chap. 29. Italia: Milan, Italy: Springer; 2009:231–250.
21. Lee BB. Lymphedema-Angiodysplasia Syndrome: a Prodigal form of Lymphatic Malformation (LM). *Phlebolymphology*. 2005;47:324-332.
22. Lee BB. Lymphedema-diagnosis and treatment. In Tredbar M, Lee S, Blondeau (eds) *Lymphatic Malformation*, Chap 4. London: Springer; 2008:31–42
23. Lee BB, Bergan JJ. Advanced management of congenital vascular malformations: a multidisciplinary approach. *Cardiovasc Surg*. 2002;10(6):523-533.
24. Lee BB. Statues of new approaches to the treatment of congenital vascular malformations (CVMs) – single center experiences – (editorial review). *Eur J Vasc Endovasc Surg*. 2005;30(2):184-197.
25. Lee BB. Critical issues on the management of congenital vascular malformation. *Ann Vasc Surg*. 2004;18(3):380-392.
26. Lee BB. Changing Concept on Vascular Malformation: No longer Enigma. *Ann Vasc Dis*. 2008;1(1):11-19.
27. Lee BB. Current concept of venous malformation (VM). *Phlebolymphology*. 2003;43:197-203.
28. Lee BB, Do YS, Byun HS, Choo IW, Kim DI, Huh SH. Advanced management of venous malformation with ethanol sclerotherapy: mid-term results. *J Vasc Surg*. 2003;37(3):533-538.
29. Lee BB, Laredo J, Lee SJ, Huh SH, Joe JH, Neville R. Congenital vascular malformations: general diagnostic principles. *Special Issue, Phlebology*. 2007;22(6):253-257.
30. Lee BB, Laredo J, Kim YW, Neville R. Congenital vascular malformations: general treatment principles. *Special Issue, Phlebology*. 2007;22(6):258-263.
31. Lee BB, Do YS, Yakes W, et al. Management of arterial-venous shunting malformations (AVM) by surgery and embolosclerotherapy. A multidisciplinary approach. *J Vasc Surg*. 2004;39(3):590-600.
32. Lee BB Mastery of vascular and endovascular surgery. Zelenock GB, Huber TS, Messina LM, Lumsden AB, Moneta GL eds. Arteriovenous malformation, Chap. 76. Lippincott: Williams and Wilkins; 2006:597– 607.
33. Lee BB, Lardeo J, Neville R. Arterio-venous malformation: how much do we know? *Phlebology*. 2009;24:193-200.
34. Lee BB, Mattassi R, Kim BT, Park JM. Advanced management of arteriovenous shunting malformation with Transarterial Lung Perfusion Scintigraphy (TLPS) for follow up assessment. *Int Angiol*. 2005;24(2):173-184.

35. Klippel M, Trenaunay J. Du noevus variqueux et osteohypertrophique. *Arch Gén Méd.* 1900;3:641-672.
36. Servelle M. Klippel and Trenaunay's syndrome. *Ann Surg.* 1985;201:365-373.
37. Gloviczki P, Driscoll DJ. Klippel–Trenaunay syndrome: current management. *Phlebology.* 2007;22:291-298.
38. Gloviczki P, Stanson AW, Stickler GB, et al. Klippel-Trenaunay syndrome: the risks and benefits of vascular interventions. *Surgery.* 1991;110(3):469-479.
39. Lee BB, Laredo J, Lee TS, Huh S, Neville R. Terminology and classification of congenital vascular malformations. *Phlebology.* 2007;22(6):249-252.
40. St B. Classification of congenital vascular defects. *Int Angiol.* 1990;9:141-146.
41. St B. Anatomopathological classification of congenital vascular defects. *Semin Vasc Surg.* 1993;6:219-224.
42. Bastide G, Lefebvre D. Anatomy and organogenesis and vascular malformations. In: St B, Loose DA, Weber J, eds. *Vascular Malformations.* Reinbek: Einhorn-Presse Verlag GmbH; 1989:20-22.
43. Leu HJ. Pathoanatomy of congenital vascular malformations. In: Belov S, Loose DA, Weber J, eds. *Vascular Malformations*, vol. 16. Reinbek: Einhorn; 1989:37-46.
44. Lee BB, Kim DI, Whang JH, Lee KW. Contemporary management of chronic lymphedema – personal experiences. *Lymphology.* 2002;35(Suppl):450-455.
45. Lee BB, Mattassi R, Kim BT, Kim DI, Ahn JM, Choi JY. Contemporary diagnosis and management of venous and AV shunting malformation by whole body blood pool scintigraphy (WBBPS). *Int Angiol.* 2004;23(4):355-367.
46. Lee BB, Bergan JJ. New clinical and laboratory staging systems to improve management of chronic lymphedema. *Lymphology.* 2005;38(3):122-129.
47. Choi JY, Hwang JH, Park JM, et al. Risk assessment of dermatolymphangioadenitis by lymphoscintigraphy in patients with lower extremity lymphedema. *Kor J Nucl Med.* 1999;33(2):143-151.
48. Carena M, Campini R, Zelaschi G, Rossi G, Aprile C, Paroni G. Quantitative lymphoscintigraphy. *Eur J Nucl Med.* 1988;14:88-92.
49. Brautigam P, Foldi E, Schaiper I, Krause T, Vanscheidt W, Moser E. Analysis of lymphatic drainage in various forms of leg edema using two compartment lymphoscintigraphy. *Lymphology.* 1998;31:43-55.
50. Lee BB, Mattassi R, Choe YH, et al. Critical role of Duplex ultrasonography for the advanced management of a venous malformation (VM). *Phlebology.* 2005;20:28-37.
51. Dubois J, Patriquin HB, Garel L, et al. Soft-tissue hemangiomas in infants and children: diagnosis using Doppler sonography. *AJR Am J Roentgenol.* 1998;171(1):247-252.
52. Trop I, Dubois J, Guibaud L, et al. Soft-tissue venous malformations in pediatric and young adult patients: diagnosis with Doppler US. *Radiology.* 1999;212(3):841-845.
53. Leduc O, Klein P, Rasquin C, Demaret P. *Reliability of a volume measuring device (volumeter®) for human limbs.* Elsevier: Science B.V; 1991:617-620.
54. Thibaut G, Durand A, Schmidt Cl. The use of electronic optovolumeter to measure lymphedema limb volume. *Lymphology.* 2002;35(Suppl):261-264.
55. Stanton AW, Northfield JW, Holroyd B, Mortimer PS, Levick JR. Validation of an optoelectronic limb volumeter (Perometer). *Lymphology.* 1997;30(2):77-97.
56. Lee BB, Choe YH, Ahn JM, et al. The new role of MRI (Magnetic Resonance Imaging) in the contemporary diagnosis of venous malformation: can it replace angiography? *J Am Coll Surg.* 2004;198(4):549-558.
57. Rak KM, Yakes WF, Ray RL, et al. MR imaging of symptomatic peripheral vascular malformations. *AJR Am J Roentgenol.* 1992;159:107-112.
58. Dobson MJ, Hartley RW, Ashleigh R, Watson Y, Hawnaur JM. MR angiography and MR imaging of symptomatic vascular malformations. *Clin Radiol.* 1997;52(8):595-602.

59. Lindeman GJ, Carr P, Kenneth W, Tiver M, Allan O, Angland S. The role of bipedal lymphangiography in testicular seminoma. *Australas Radiol.* 2008;34(4):293-296.
60. Munro DD, Craig O, Fejwel M. Lymphangiography in dermatology. *Br J Dermatol.* 2006;81(9):652-660.
61. Michelini S, Failla A, Moneta G, Campisi C, Boccardo F. Clinical staging of lymphedema and therapeutical implications. *Lymphology.* 2002;35(Suppl):168.
62. Damstra RJ, Partsch H. Compression therapy in breast cancer-related lymphedema: a randomized, controlled comparative study of relation between volume and interface pressure changes. *J Vasc Surg.* 2009;49(5):1256-1263.
63. Damstra RJ, Brouwer ER, Partsch H. Controlled, Comparative study of relation between volume changes and interface pressure under short-stretch bandages in leg lymphedema patients. *Dermatol Surg.* 2008;34(6):773-779.
64. Hwang JH, Kim TU, Lee KW, Kim DI, Lee BB. Sequential intermittent pneumatic compression therapy in lymphedema. *J Korean Acad Rehab Med.* 1997;21(1):146-153.
65. Pflug JJ. Intermittent compression in the management of swollen legs in general practice. *Lancet.* 1975;215:69-76.
66. Theys S, Deltombe TH, Scavée V, Legrand C, Schoevaerdts JC. Safety of long-term usage of retrograde-intermittent pneumatic compression in lower limb lymphedema. *Lymphology.* 2002;35(Suppl):293-297.
67. Guyatt GH, Gutterman D, Baumann MH, Addrizzo-Harris D, Hylek EM, et al. Grading strength of recommendations and quality of evidence in clinical guidelines. *Chest.* 2006;129:174-181.
68. Lee BB. Lymphedema-diagnosis and treatment. Tredbar LT, Morgan CL, Lee BB, Simonian SJ, Blondeau B, eds. *Surgical Management of Lymphedema*, Chap. 6. London: Springer; 2008: 55–63.
69. Lee BB, Kim YW, Kim DI, Hwang JH, Laredo J, Neville R. Supplemental surgical treatment to end stage (stage IV –V) of chronic lymphedema. *Int Angiol.* 2008;27(5):389-395.
70. Baumeister RGH, Siuda S. Treatment of lymphedemas by microsurgical lymphatic grafting: what is proved? *Plast Reconstr Surg.* 1990;85:64-74.
71. Campisi C, Boccardo F, Zilli A, Maccio A, Gariglio A, Schenone F. Peripheral lymphedema:new advances in microsurgical treatment and long-term outcome. Microsurgery 2003;23(5):522–5. PMID: 14558015
72. Gloviczki P. Review. Principles of surgical treatment of chronic lymphoedema. *Int Angiol.* 1999;18(1):42-46.
73. Olszewski WL. The treatment of lymphedema of the extremities with microsurgical lymphovenous anastomoses. *Int Angiol.* 1988;7(4):312-321.
74. Becker C. Hidden G, Godart S et al. Free lymphatic transplant. *Eur J Lymphol* 1991;6:75-80.
75. Servelle M. Surgical treatment of lymphedema: a report on 652 cases. *Surgery.* 1987; 101(4): 485-495.
76. Kim DI, Huh S, Lee SJ, Hwang JH, Kim YI, Lee BB. Excision of subcutaneous tissue and deep muscle fascia for advanced lymphedema. *Lymphology.* 1998;31:190-194.
77. Brorson H, Svensson H. Liposuction combined with controlled compression therapy reduces arm lymphedema more effectively than controlled compression therapy alone. *Plast Reconstr Surg.* 1998;102(4):1058-1067. discussion 1068.
78. Brorson H, Svensson H, Norrgren K, Thorsson O. Liposuction reduces arm lymphedema without significantly altering the already impaired lymph transport. *Lymphology.* 1998;31:156-172.
79. Auchincloss H. New operation for elephantiasis. *Puerto Rico J Publ Health Trop Med.* 1930;6:149.
80. Homans J. The treatment of elephantiasis of the legs. *N Engl J Med.* 1936;215:1099.

Corradino Campisi and Francesco Boccardo

A 59 year old woman presented with an 8 year history of edema of the left arm. Initially, the edema appeared in the upper arm. The patient was treated with combined decongestive physiotherapy (manual and mechanical lymphatic drainage), bandaging and exercises three to four times over a 12 month period. Despite these measures, the edema later extended to the forearm and hand (Fig. 54.1). In the months preceding her admission she developed several episodes of erysipeloid lymphangitis and pain. There were no warts or wounds on the skin. Her past medical history included lumpectomy with axillary lymphadenectomy and radiotherapy for left breast cancer. There was no suggestion of local recurrence on routine follow-up.

Initially, the edema had a rhizomelic distribution. It was hard to the touch and did not pit. There were no dystrophic or dyschromic skin lesions, except for signs of acute reticular erysipeloid lymphangitic attacks caused by Gram-positive Staphylococci. A lymphangioscintigram was performed, which showed features compatible with lymphatic impairment in the left arm (Fig. 54.2). This was followed by lymphangio-magnetic resonance imaging (MRI) of the arm and hemithorax which showed no signs of loco-regional recurrence but confirmed lymph stasis, predominantly in the epifascial compartment. Dilated medial arm lymphatic collectors, interrupted at the proximal third of the arm, were also demonstrated. A Duplex of the left subclavian and axillary veins was normal. A diagnosis of chronic secondary lymphoedema was made.

Question 1

How would you classify lymphoedema?

A. Primary (congenital) and secondary (acquired)
B. Phlebo-lymphoedema and lipo-lymphoedema

C. Campisi (✉)
Department of General Surgery, University Hospital, San Martino, Genoa, Italy

G. Geroulakos and B. Sumpio (eds.), *Vascular Surgery*,
DOI: 10.1007/978-1-84996-356-5_54, © Springer-Verlag London Limited 2011

Fig. 54.1 Patient before treatment

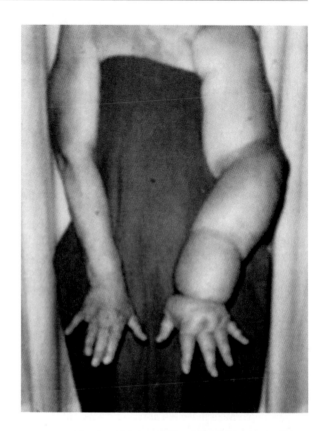

Fig. 54.2 Lymphangio-scintigram before microsurgery. Evident dermal back flow (*arrows*)

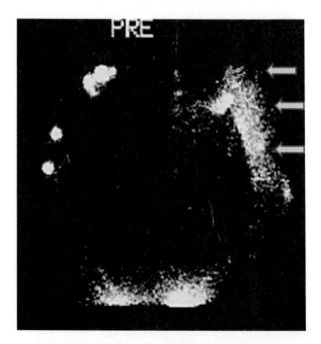

Question 2

Which of the following statements regarding the diagnosis of lymphoedema are correct?

A. Lymphangiography is currently the best diagnostic investigation for all types of lymphoedema.
B. Duplex has an important role in determining the correct treatment.
C. Lymphangioscintigraphy is the most popular non-invasive first-line investigation.
D. It is difficult to diagnose early lymphoedema.
E. Lymphangio-MRI offers precise morphological imaging on edema distribution and topography of dilated lymphatic pathways, without requiring contrast.

The patient underwent microsurgical lymphatic-venous anastomoses in the proximal third of the volar surface of the arm using 8/0 nylon sutures (Fig. 54.3).

Question 3

Which of the following statements regarding the management of lymphoedema are correct?

A. Microsurgery can reduce edema in all patients, but the best outcome is seen in patients operated on in the second and third stages.
B. Elastic graded compression garments are an important adjunct to optimize long-term results.

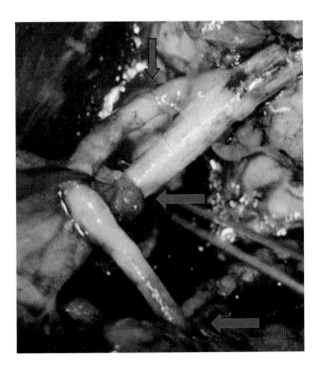

Fig. 54.3 Lymphatic-venous anastomoses seen through the operating microscope (30x). Arrows indicate anastomoses and blue dye inside the vein (direct evidence of patency)

Fig. 54.4 Long-term clinical outcome after microsurgery

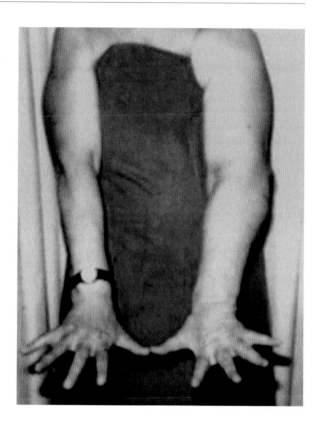

C. Surgical intervention is not indicated in the advanced stages of lymphoedema.
D. Microsurgical lymphatic-venous anastomoses are used more frequently than recon-
   structive microsurgical methods.
E. Microsurgery cannot be applied in primary lymphoedema.

The postoperative recovery was uneventful. The patient was discharged home the fifth
postoperative day. The incidence of lymphangitic attacks decreased significantly. A reduction of arm volume was seen within 3 days of the operation, and further improvements
were observed at medium and longterm follow-up, particularly between the first and the
fifth years after surgery. From the fifth year onwards, the clinical condition of the arm
stabilized (Fig. 54.4). Lymphangioscintigraphy at 10 years demonstrated that the lymphatic-venous anastomoses remained patent (Fig. 54.5).

Question 4

What are the long-term results of derivative and reconstructive microsurgery for
lymphoedema?

A. Long term results are better in the early stages.
B. Long term results are better for derivative than reconstructive microsurgery.
C. Long term results depend mainly on the surgical technique.

Fig. 54.5 Lymphangio-scintigram performed after microsurgery shows the patency of the lymphatic-venous anastomoses more than 10 years after the operation. Site of LVA (*arrow*)

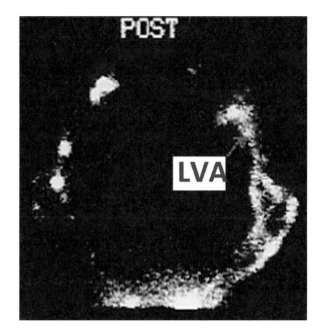

Question 5

Which of the following statements are true?

A. It is not possible to prevent secondary lymphoedema.
B. Arm Reverse Mapping (ARM) is able to identify arm lymphatics.
C. The Lymphatic Microsurgical Preventive Healing Approach (LYMPHA) offers the possibility of a primary surgical approach in the prevention of secondary lymphoedema.

54.1
Commentary

Lymphoedema is a significant worldwide problem. It can be divided into primary and secondary. Primary lymphoedemas do not have any recognizable cause (idiopathic), although triggering etiological factors can often be found. Lymphoedemas that present at birth (congenital) are included in this category. These can be hereditary-familial (Nonne-Milroy's disease), and are often associated with chromosomal abnormalities. Other primary lymphoedemas, may have an early or late onset, which can be triggered by minor trauma, infection or surgery. In females, the predisposing factors are often thought to be alterations in neurohormonal status (neuroendocrine lymphoedema).

Primary lymphoedemas can also be due lymphatic or lymph node dysplasia, hypoplasia or even hyperplasia, with increased lymph production, either together or in combinations. In most cases of hypoplasia, lymph node involvement is demonstrated and leads to the progressive secondary alteration of lymphatic vessels. This pattern is similar to that seen with secondary lymphoedemas resulting from lymphoadenectomy with or without radiotherapy.[1] Approximately 90% of all primary lymphoedemas are characterized by hypodysplastic alterations involving lymph nodes and lymphatics. This is characterized by a diminished ability to form an adequate collateral circulation in response to trauma, infection or surgery. In a further 8–10% of primary lymphoedemas, an increase in the number and size of lymphatic collectors can be demonstrated and are associated with lymphatic and lymph nodal dysplasia.[2]

Disorders in lymphogenesis often contribute to altered lymphodynamics. Increased lymph formation may result from pre-existing arterio-venous malformations, arterio-venous fistulae or angiodysplasias. In contrast, reduced or absent production of lymph can result from, agenesis, hypoplasia, or impaired permeability of lymphatics, and is very rare. Lymphodynamic disorders also include gravitational and chylous reflux pathologies. Lymph backflow (reflux) can be caused by insufficient anti-gravitational structures, normally represented by valves, the reticular myoelastic layer of the lymphatic walls, and the lymph node architecture.

The etiology of secondary lymphoedema can generally be identified in the patient's history or physical examination. This can be secondary to trauma, infection, inflammation, infestation (filarial), radiotherapy, surgery, paralysis or neoplasia. Secondary lymphoedemas often have some congenital predisposition. Arm lymphoedema secondary to breast carcinoma treatment, for example, occurs in 5–35% of patients, depending on whether axillary surgery is associated with radiotheraphy.[3] This is more likely to occur when there is no deltoid pathway.[4] The deltoid route allows the drainage of lymph from the arm directly into the supraclavicular lymph nodes. The axillary nodes are therefore bypassed because of the congenital presence of an alternative route. With preoperative lymphoscintigraphic studies, both ipsilateral and contralateral arms can be compared to enable patients with a higher risk of developing secondary lymphoedema to be identified. Based on these observations, Tosatti's classification of lymphoedemas (Fig. 54.6), proposed more than 30 years ago,[5] remains valid. [Q1:A]

The differentiation between lymphoedema and phleboedema is by a history and clinical examination, paying attention to the time and conditions of onset, location, evolution, extent and volume of the edema. Lymphoedema is hard to the touch, while venous edema is soft and pits under finger compression. This difference reflects the underlying pathophysiology: stagnant lymph in the subcutaneous connective tissue is an excellent culture medium for fibroblasts. These mature into fibrocytes and form dense fibrosclerotic tissue.

Lymphoedema typically begins proximally, whereas venous edema affects the distal part of the lower limbs with the notable exception of phlegmasia dolens, caused by acute deep thrombophlebitis of the iliofemoral veins. Unlike phleboedema, lymphoedema does not usually evolve into dystrophic and dyschromic skin lesions or ulcers. It is more likely, however, to be complicated by acute reticular erysipeloid lymphangitis, caused by Gram-positive cocci infections. Mixed types of lympho-phleboedema may also exist, with predominance of either the venous or lymphatic component. These include stage III postphlebitic syndrome and angiodysplasias with arteriovenous shunting, as seen in Mayall's syndrome.[6]

Currently, lymphangioscintigraphy and conventional oil contrast lymphography are the most suitable investigations of lymphatic and chylous edemas. Lymphangioscintigraphy is the most popular method used in screening lymphoedemas[7, 8] as it is a non-invasive way of imaging both superficial and deep lymphatic circulations. Since it is non-invasive, it can easily be repeated in patients, especially after microsurgery. A small tracer dose of [99m]technetium adsorbed in colloid spherules (colloid sulfide, rhenium, dextran) is injected. The

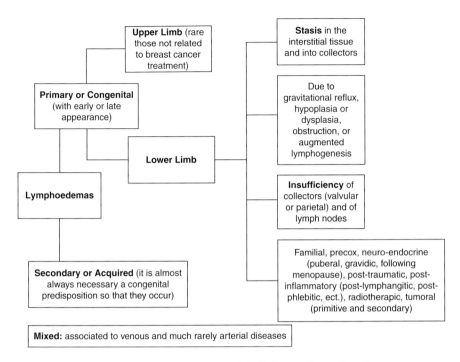

Fig. 54.6 Classification of chronic lymphoedema of the limb according to Tosatti

lymphotropic nature of these substances permits visualization of the preferential lymphatic pathways with a gamma-camera. This allows measurements of the flow rate and lymph node uptake. Tracer clearance evaluations are a useful measure of lymphodynamics especially in early lymphoedema.[9] Direct lymphangiography[10] is preferred, however, in the study of gravitational reflux and chylous edema of the lower limb and external genitalia especially if a surgical intervention is proposed.[11, 12] In this examination, ultrafluid "Lipiodol" is injected into a lymphatic collector, isolated with a microsurgical technique, on the dorsum of the both feet. This type of investigation is minimally invasive and, if performed according to well-established standards, has minimal complications. Rare adverse reactions include pulmonary micro embolism, especially in the presence of peripheral lymphovenous fistulas, or contrast allergy. Infection at the site of skin incision, acute lymphangitis and lymphorrhea may also occur. Direct lymphangiography can also be performed in children. It enables a morphological and functional study of the superficial and the deep lymphatic circulations to take place.[12]

Computer tomography (CT), ultrasonography, and lymphangio-MRI may also provide information on lymphatic and chylous dysfunction. Indirect lymphangiography[13] is performed using a dermo-hypodermic injection of a water-soluble contrast medium ("Iotasul") and is useful to clarify aetio-pathological aspects of primary lymphoedemas. Fluorescent micro-lymphography[14] can be helpful in assessing the status of the superficial dermal lymphatics, which reflects peripheral lymphatic function. The conventional Houdack-McMaster dye test with the injection of a highly lymphotropic vital stain (Patent Blue V) is used today as a rapid preliminary investigation before direct lymphangiography and microsurgery. Recent studies by Olszewski[15] and Campisi et al.[16] have developed a system to measure endolymphatic pressure and lymphatic flow rate. These parameters, together with a venous pressure assessment, help to measure the lymph-venous pressure gradient which is essential prior to microsurgical treatment. With this method, a lymphatic vessel is isolated and cannulated at the lower third of the leg's medial surface. Changes in the flow and pressure can be recorded during microsurgery, elevation and dependency, at rest and under dynamic conditions. These studies have shown that a lymphatic-venous pressure gradient is essential to achieve good medium and long term results after microsurgery. [Q2:B,C,E]

Manual lymphatic drainage has been shown to be a highly effective treatment in the conservative management of lymphoedema.[17–19] This followed by the application of bandaging and eventually graded compression stockings. The use of intermittent compression pneumatic devices is usually complementary to manual lymphatic drainage and may contribute to further reduction of the lymphoedema. Pharmacotherapy includes the use of antibiotics, particularly penicillin,[20] anti-inflammatory drugs, and benzopyrones.[21] The positive effect of benzopyrones was described by Casley-Smith et al.,[21] but their role in the treatment of lymphoedemas has yet to be clarified.

Thirty years ago, only the most severe cases of elephantiasis were treated surgically, mainly to achieve a reduction in volume. The most popular surgical methods were those proposed by Charles[22] (total resection of skin-lipid layers), Thompson[23] (drainage with scarred subfascial skin flap), and Servelle[24] (total surface lymphangectomy). They were highly destructive and invasive operations and as such they could not be recommended in less advanced or initial stages or in childhood disease.[25] More recently, microsurgical lymphatic-venous and lymph node-venous anastomoses were introduced for the management of lymphoedema resistant to conservative treatment.[26, 27] These techniques are beneficial in secondary, as well as primary lymphoedemas.[28] Early intervention is possible, even in children, where lymphatic-capsule-venous anastomoses are preferred.[29]

Lymphostatic disease may be associated with venous impairment such as varices, superficial thrombophlebitis, deep venous thrombosis and post-phlebitic sequelae. These conditions are a contraindication to traditional lymphatic-venous anastomoses. Novel reconstructive lymphatic surgery techniques however provide hope for these patients.[30] This includes segmental autotransplantation of lymphatic collectors[31] for the treatment of unilateral lymphoedema or the personally described method of interposition autologous venous grafting or lymphatic-venous-lymphatic plasty.[32]

The clinical use of microvascular lymphatic or lymph nodal flaps[33, 34] is still under evaluation. They may provide future treatment options in refractory secondary lymphoedema and for the primary lymphoedemas which cannot benefit from microsurgical techniques.

Elastic stockings are usually worn for an average period of 1–5 years after microsurgery according to the stage of the pathology at the time of operation. The stockings aim to prevent the closure of anastomoses because a rapid reduction of edema, pressure and flow is expected as a result of the improved drainage.[35] [Q3:A,B,D]

Patients are followed up at 1, 3, 6 and 12 months post surgery and then annually for 5 years. Lymphatic microsurgery results in improvement in more than 80% of cases. Better outcomes have been observed in patients undergoing prophylactic microsurgery (at stages II

Lymphoedema Staging

STAGE I
A. "Latent" lymphedema, without clinical evidence of edema, but with impaired lymph transport capacity (provable by lymphoscintigraphy) and with initial immuno-histochemical alterations of lymph nodes, lymph vessels and extracellular matrix.

B. "Initial" lymphedema, totally or partially decreasing by rest and draining position, with worsening impairment of lymph transport capacity and of immuno-histochemical alterations of lymph collectors, nodes and extracellular matrix.

STAGE II
A. "Increasing" lymphedema, with vanishing lymph transport capacity, relapsing lymphangitic attacks, fibroindurative skin changes, and **developing disability**.

B. "Column shaped" limb fibrolymphedema, with lymphostatic skin changes, suppressed lymph transport capacity and **worsening disability.**

STAGE III
A. Properly called "elephantiasis", with scleroindurative pachydermitis,papillomatous lymphostatic verrucosis, no lymph transport capacity and **life-threatening disability**.
B. "Extreme elephantiasis" with **total disability.**

Fig. 54.7 Recent clinical staging of lymphoedema, including functional disability and pathological findings

and III; see Fig. 54.7). The frequency of lymphangitic attacks also decreases. The reduction in edema volume is seen within the first three postoperative days, and a further decrease is observed between the first and fifth years after operation. From the fifth year onwards, the clinical condition of the limb tends to remain static and this effect is maintained for more than 10 years after surgery. Lymphangioscintigraphy provides evidence that the flow through the venous grafts parallels the clinical improvement.[36][**Q4:A,C**]

Early identification, diagnostic lymphangioscintigraphy[37] and prophylactic treatment of high risk patients has been suggested as a means of preventing secondary lymphoedema.[38,][39] These include patients undergoing oncological lymphadenectomies, particularly in combination with radiotherapy. Microsurgery is a reasonable option on lymphoedemas that are expected to show unrelenting progression.[40] The Arm Reverse Mapping (ARM) technique allows the precise identification of arm lymphatics and lymph nodes. Selective preservation is therefore possible but at a risk of leaving behind undetected metastatic disease. Since both arm lymphatics and breast efferents drain into the common axillary basin, its removal may interrupt the lymphatic flow from the arm. If a microsurgical lymphatic-venous anastomosis (LVA), is performed immediately after nodal excision this problem may be avoided. A LVA is a surgical technique proposed for selected patients with operable breast cancer requiring an axillary dissection. Blue dye is injected into the arm lymphatics and a simultaneous LVA is then performed between these and an axillary vein branch (Lymphatic Microsurgical Preventive Healing Approach – LY.M.P.H.A.) (Fig. 54.8).[41] [**Q5:B,C**]

Fig. 54.8 LYMPHA technique for surgical primary prevention of arm lymphedema during axillary nodal dissection

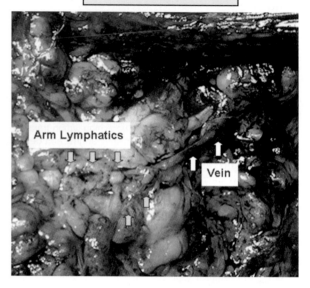

References

1. Badini A, Fulcheri E, Campisi C, Boccardo F. A new approach in histopathological diagnosis of lymphoedema: pathophysiological and therapeutic implications. *Lymphology*. 1996;29 S:190-198.
2. Papendieck CM. *Temas de Angiologia Pediatrica*. Buenos Aires: Editorial Medica Panamericana; 1992.
3. Farrar WB, Lavalle G, Kim JA. Breast cancer. In: McKenna RJ, Murphy GP, eds. *Cancer Surgery*. Philadelphia: Lippincott; 1994:209-259.
4. Witte CL. Breast cancer – an overview. *Lymphology*. 1994;27S:397-400.
5. Tosatti E. *Lymphatique profonds et lymphoedèmes chroniques des membres*. Paris: Masson; 1974.
6. Mayall JC, Mayall ACDG. Standardization of methods of treatment of Lymphoedema. Progress in Lymphology XI – Excerpta Medica 1988;517.
7. Mariani G, Campisi C, Taddei G, Boccardo F. The current role of lymphoscintigraphy in the diagnostic evaluation of patients with peripheral lymphoedema. *Lymphology*. 1998;31 S:316-319.
8. Witte C, McNeill G, Witte M et al. Whole-body lymphangioscintigraphy: making the invisible easily visible. Progress in Lymphology XII, Elsevier Science BV 1989;123.
9. Bourgeois P, Leduc O, Leduc A. Imaging techniques in the management and prevention of posttherapeutic upper limb oedemas. *Cancer*. 1998;83(12 Suppl American):2805-2813.
10. Kinmonth JB. *The Lymphatics. Surgery, Lymphography and Diseases of the Chyle and Lymph Systems*. London: Edward Arnold; 1982.
11. Bruna J. Indication for lymphography in the era of new imaging methods. *Lymphology*. 1994;27 S:319-320.
12. Campisi C, Boccardo F, Zilli A, Borrelli V. Chylous reflux pathologies: diagnosis and microsurgical treatment. *Int Angiol*. 1999;18:10-13.
13. Partsch H. Indirect lymphography in different kinds of leg oedema. In: Lymphology: advances in Europe. Genova, Ecig; 1989:95–9.

14. Bollinger A, Jager K, Sgier F, Seglias J. Fluorescence microlymphography. *Circulation*. 1981;64:195-200.
15. Olszewski W. Lymph and tissue pressures in patients with lymphoedema during massage and walking with elastic support. *Lymphology*. 1994;27 S:512-516.
16. Campisi C, Olszewski W, Boccardo F. Il gradiente pressorio linfo-venoso in microchirurgia linfatica. Minerva Angiologica; 1994;19.
17. Vodder E. *La Méthode Vodder – Le Drainage Lymphatique Manuel*. Bagsvaer: Institute for Lymphdrainage; 1969.
18. Földi M. The therapy of lymphoedema. *EJLRP*. 1993–1994;14:43-49.
19. Leduc A. Le drainage lymphatique. Théorie et pratique. Masson, 1980.
20. Olszewski WL. Recurrent bacterial dermatolymphangioadenitis (DLA) is responsible for progression of lymphoedema. *Lymphology*. 1996;29S:331.
21. Casley-Smith JR, Casley-Smith RJ. *High-Protein Oedemas and the Benzo-Pyrones*. Sydney: Lippincott; 1986.
22. Charles RH. A system of treatment. In: Latham A, English TC, eds. *lymphoedema* London: Churchill,1912.
23. Thompson N. The surgical treatment of chronic lymphoedema of the extremities. *Surg Clin North Am*. 1967;47:2.
24. Servelle M. *Pathologie Vasculaire*. Paris: Masson; 1975.
25. O'Brien B. Microlymphatic-venous and resectional surgery in obstructive lymphoedemas. *World J Surg*. 1979;3:3.
26. Degni M. New techniques of lymphatic-venous anastomosis for the treatment of lymphoedema. *Cardiovas Riv Bras*. 1974;10:175.
27. Campisi C. Rational approach in the management of lymphoedema. *Lymphology*. 1991;24:48-53.
28. Campisi C, Davini D, Bellini C, et al. Lymphatic microsurgery for the treatment of lymphedema. *Microsurgery*. 2006;26(1):65-69.
29. Campisi C. Lymphatic microsurgery: a potent weapon in the war on lymphoedema. *Lymphology*. 1995;28:110-112.
30. Campisi C, Boccardo F. Frontiers in lymphatic microsurgery. *Microsurgery*. 1998;18:462-471.
31. Baumeister RGH. Clinical results of autogenous lymphatic grafts in the treatment of lymphoedemas. In: Partsch H, ed. *Progress in Lymphology XI*. Elsevier: Science BV; 1988:419-420.
32. Campisi C. Use of autologous interposition vein graft in management of lymphoedema. *Lymphology*. 1991;24:71-76.
33. Becker C, Hidden G, Godart S, Maurage H, Pecking A. Free lymphatic transplant. *EJLRP*. 1991;2:75-77.
34. Trévidic P, Marzelle J, Cormier JM. Apport de la microchirurgie au traitement des lymphoedèmes. Editions Techniques -Encycl. Méd. Chir. (Paris-France), Techniques chirurgicales – Chirurgie Vasculaire, 1994;F.a. 43–225, 3.
35. Campisi C. Lymphoedema: modern diagnostic and therapeutic aspects. *Int Angiol*. 1999;18: 14-24.
36. Campisi C, Boccardo F. Role of microsurgery in the management of lymphoedema. *Int Angiol*. 1999;18:47-51.
37. Pecking AP et al. Upper limb lymphedema's frequency in patients treated by conservative therapy in breast cancer. *Lymphology*. 1996;29S:293-296.
38. Campisi C, Davini D, Bellini C, et al. Is there a role for microsurgery in the prevention of arm lymphedema secondary to breast cancer treatment? *Microsurgery*. 2006;26(1):70-72.
39. Pissas A. Prevention of secondary lymphoedema. Proceedings of the International Congress of Phlebology, Corfù, Greece, 113, September 4–8, 1996.
40. Casley-Smith JR. Alterations of untreated lymphedema and its grades over time. *Lymphology*. 1995;28:174-185.
41. Boccardo F, Casabona F, De Cian F, et al. Lymphedema microsurgical preventive healing approach: a new technique for primary prevention of arm lymphedema after mastectomy. *Ann Surg Oncol*. 2009;16:703-708.

Index